The New Public Health
and STD/HIV Prevention

Sevgi O. Aral • Kevin A. Fenton
Judith A. Lipshutz
Editors

The New Public Health and STD/HIV Prevention

Personal, Public and Health Systems Approaches

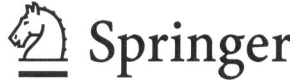 Springer

Editors
Sevgi O. Aral
Division of STD Prevention, NCHHSTP
Centers for Disease Control
 and Prevention
Atlanta, GA, USA

Kevin A. Fenton
National Center for HIV/AIDS
Viral Hepatitis, STD and TB Prevention
Centers for Disease Control
 and Prevention
Atlanta, GA, USA

Judith A. Lipshutz
Office for State, Tribal, Local
 and Territorial Support
Centers for Disease Control
 and Prevention
Atlanta, GA, USA

The findings and conclusions in this book are those of the authors and do not necessarily represent the views of the Centers for Disease Control and Prevention.

ISBN 978-1-4614-4525-8   ISBN 978-1-4614-4526-5 (eBook)
DOI 10.1007/978-1-4614-4526-5
Springer New York Heidelberg Dordrecht London

Library of Congress Control Number: 2012950330

Printed on acid-free paper

Springer is part of Springer Science+Business Media (www.springer.com)

Foreword

Public health, public health research, and STI/HIV prevention science are all at crossroads. "Expansion," "Advancement," "Repositioning," and "Paradigm shift" have become frequent expressions associated with prevention science and public health. As it became increasingly clear that prevention of HIV infection and many other sexually transmitted infections (STIs) remained beyond reach, even in the presence of efficacious interventions, attention has shifted to the importance of dissemination and implementation of effective interventions. Differences between efficacy in clinical trials, effectiveness in the real world, and large impact at the population level have become increasingly evident. Contextual understanding of STD/HIV epidemiology now includes understanding of social and structural determinants; sexual and social networks; and geographic, demographic, and subpopulation concentrations. Effective preventive interventions must focus on issues of targeting, coverage, and scale-up. Current economic realities highlight the importance of cost-effective resource allocation and maximization of return-on-investment in public health. Public health leaders and practitioners are considering how STI/HIV prevention fits into a system that creates a positive and sustainable dynamic between public health and health care institutions and trains individual providers to appreciate and incorporate population health.

The editors have brought together a team of international experts to present the evolution of promising new approaches in *"The New Public Health and STD/HIV Prevention: Personal, Public and Health Systems Approaches."* The concise and thoughtful "Introduction" provides an excellent summary of the new directions in the field. The section on social determinants and other influences on STI/HIV represent emerging paradigms in public health (e.g., sexual networks, concentration, and geographic and temporal dispersion of STI/HIV).

Critical factors in approaches to prevention are also addressed, including scaling up, targeting, and coverage, and distribution of prevention resources and its impact on sexual health. The book further highlights prevention approaches for population groups, as well as specific programs taking decidedly systemic, multicomponent approaches. The critical reviews of specific prevention programs in different developed countries provide interesting historical accounts of focused prevention efforts.

This book will be of great interest and value to experts in STI/HIV prevention and beginning students in health sciences alike, whether their background is in medicine, public health, the social sciences, or systems science.

Seattle, WA, USA   King K. Holmes, MD, PhD
                                                          William H. Foege Chair,
                                        Department of Global Health Professor,
                                              Departments of Global Health,
                                    Medicine, Microbiology, and Epidemiology
                                                  University of Washington

About the Editors

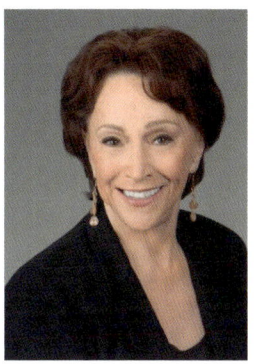

Sevgi O. Aral, MA, MS, PhD, has been the Associate Director for Science in the Division of STD Prevention, Centers for Disease Control since 1993. She holds professorial appointments at the University Of Washington in Seattle; University of Manitoba in Winnipeg and Emory University in Atlanta. Dr. Aral has authored more than 230 scientific articles and edited 16 journal issues and 2 books. Dr. Aral has served on many national and international work groups, boards and committees; and has consulted for the World Health Organization, The European Union and the World Bank. She has received the ASTDA Achievement Award and the Thomas Parran Award. Over the years, her research interests have included social and behavioral aspects of sexually transmitted disease epidemiology and prevention; including gender, age and race effects; mixing patterns; sexual and social networks; contextual factors; social determinants and most recently, program science. Dr. Aral came to the Centers for Disease Control in 1978 from Middle East Technical University in Ankara, Turkey where she was the chair of the Department of Social Sciences.

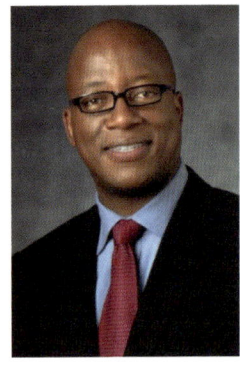 **Kevin A. Fenton, MD, PhD, FFPH,** is the Director of the National Center for HIV/AIDS, Viral Hepatitis, STD, and TB Prevention (NCHHSTP), Centers for Disease Control and Prevention (CDC), a position he has held since November 2005. Previously, he was chief of CDC's National Syphilis Elimination Effort and has worked in research, epidemiology, and the prevention of HIV and other STDs since 1995. Before coming to CDC, he was the Director of the HIV and STI Department at the United Kingdom's Health Protection Agency. At CDC, Dr. Fenton has led a number of critical efforts to address the U.S. HIV epidemic, including the release of revised HIV screening recommendations to make HIV testing a routine part of medical care for all Americans, and the implementation of a new surveillance system to provide more precise estimates of new HIV infections in the United States. Under Dr. Fenton's leadership, CDC has also expanded its efforts to engage, mobilize, and partner with at-risk communities to address health disparities, and CDC launched *Act Against AIDS,* the first national HIV/AIDS public health communications campaign in 20 years. He has authored or co-authored more than 200 peer-reviewed scientific articles and policy reports.

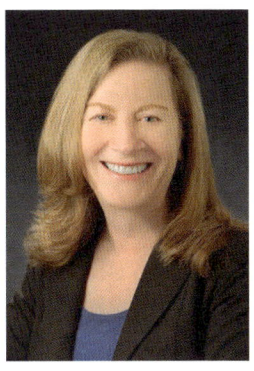**Judith A. Lipshutz, MPH**, is Deputy Associate Director for Policy in the Office for State, Tribal, Local and Territorial Support at the Centers for Disease Control and Prevention (CDC) where she has worked since June 2010. Her work focuses on policy issues related to public health systems infrastructure strengthening. Prior to this position, she worked in the Division of STD Prevention (DSTDP) in CDC's National Center for HIV/AIDS, Hepatitis, STD and TB Prevention for 17 years. Between 1996 and 2010, she coordinated both scientific and programmatic aspects of the National STD Prevention Conference, the premier domestic STD prevention meeting in the U.S. As part of the Office of the Associate Director for Science, she authored or edited a number of publications, including peer-reviewed journal articles and books. For 7 years in DSTDP, she served as the chief of the Communications and External Relations Office during which time she coordinated CDC's National STD Prevention Partnership. Prior to coming to CDC, she spent over 11 years as the Project Director for AIDS Initiatives and the Venereal Disease Action Coalition at United Community Services in Detroit, where she initiated and oversaw the city's largest AIDS case management system. Earlier, she coordinated adolescent health services at Su Clinica Familiar, a migrant health center in south Texas. Ms. Lipshutz received her B.A. from Mt. Holyoke College in 1975 and her M.P.H. from the University of Michigan in 1980.

Contents

Contributors

Adaora A. Adimora, MD, MPH Division of Infectious Diseases, University of North Carolina, School of Medicine, Chapel Hill, NC, USA

Sevgi O. Aral Division of STD Prevention, Centers for Disease Control and Prevention, Atlanta, GA, USA

Andrew Ball HIV Department, World Health Organization, Geneva, Switzerland

Robert C. Bollinger Center for Clinical Global Health Education, School of Medicine, Johns Hopkins University, Baltimore, MD, USA

Ailsa R. Butler Department Infectious Disease Epidemiology, School of Public Health, Imperial College London, London, UK

Harrell W. Chesson Division of STD Prevention, Centers for Disease Control and Prevention, Atlanta, GA, USA

Hazel D. Dean National Center for HIV/AIDS, Viral Hepatitis, STD, and TB Prevention, Centers for Disease Control and Prevention, Atlanta, GA, USA

Susan J. DeLisle Health Consultant, Atlanta, GA, USA

Kevin A. Fenton National Center for HIV/AIDS, Viral Hepatitis, STD and TB Prevention, Centers for Disease Control and Prevention, Atlanta, GA, USA

J. Dennis Fortenberry Section of Adolescent Medicine, Department of Pediatrics, Indiana University School of Medicine, Indianapolis, IN, USA

Mark S. Friedman Department of Behavioral and Community Health Sciences, University of Pittsburgh Graduate School of Public Health, Pittsburgh, PA, USA

William M. Geisler Division of Infectious Diseases, University of Alabama, Birmingham, AL, USA

Thomas E. Guadamuz Department of Behavioral and Community Health Sciences, University of Pittsburgh Graduate School of Public Health, Pittsburgh, PA, USA

Timothy B. Hallett Department Infectious Disease Epidemiology, Imperial College London, School of Public Health, London, UK

Susan Hariri Division of STD Prevention, Centers for Disease Control and Prevention, Atlanta, GA, USA

Devon J. Hensel Section of Adolescent Medicine, Department of Pediatrics, Indiana University School of Medicine, Indianapolis, IN, USA

Amy L. Herrick Department of Behavioral and Community Health Sciences, University of Pittsburgh Graduate School of Public Health, Pittsburgh, PA, USA

David R. Holtgrave Bloomberg School of Public Health, Johns Hopkins University, Baltimore, MD, USA

Edward W. Hook III Division of Infectious Diseases, University of Alabama at Birmingham and Jefferson County Department of Health, Birmingham, AL, USA

Ann M. Jolly, PhD Infectious Disease Emergency Preparedness Branch, Centre for Communicable Disease and Infection Control, Public Health Agency of Canada, Ottawa, ON, Canada

Peter R. Kerndt Sexually Transmitted Disease Program, Los Angeles County Department of Public Health, Los Angeles, CA, USA

Susan Kippax Social Policy Research Centre, University of New South Wales, Sydney, NSW, Australia

Sin How Lim Centre of Excellence for Research in AIDS (CERiA), Faculty of Medicine, University of Malaya, Kuala Lumpur, Malaysia

Judith A. Lipshutz Office for State, Tribal, Local and Territorial Support, Centers for Disease Control and Prevention, Atlanta, GA, USA

Nicola Low Division of Clinical Epidemiology and Biostatistics, Institute of Social and Preventive Medicine, University of Bern, Bern, Switzerland

Lauri E. Markowitz Division of STD Prevention, Centers for Disease Control and Prevention, Atlanta, GA, USA

Jeanne M. Marrazzo Division of Allergy and Infectious Diseases, Department of Medicine, University of Washington and Harborview Medical Center, Seattle, WA, USA

Michael P. Marshal Department of Psychiatry, University of Pittsburgh School of Medicine, Pittsburgh, PA, USA

Mary McFarlane Division of STD Prevention, Centers for Disease Control and Prevention, Atlanta, GA, USA

Adrian Mindel University of Sydney, Camperdown, NSW, Australia

Sasha Mital Division of Global HIVAIDS, Centers for Disease Control and Prevention, Atlanta, GA, USA

Ranell L. Myles National Center for HIV/AIDS, Viral Hepatitis, STD, and TB Prevention, Centers for Disease Control and Prevention, Atlanta, GA, USA

Richard Needle Office of the Global AIDS Coordinator, Washington, DC, USA

David H. Peters Bloomberg School of Public Health, Johns Hopkins University, Baltimore, MD, USA

Steven D. Pinkerton Center for AIDS Intervention Research (CAIR), Department of Psychiatry and Behavioral Medicine, Medical College of Wisconsin, Milwaukee, WI, USA

Cornelis A. Rietmeijer Department of Community and Behavioral Health, Colorado School of Public Health, Denver, CO, USA

Victor J. Schoenbach Department of Epidemiology, University of North Carolina Gillings School of Global Public Health, Chapel Hill, NC, USA

Gita Sinha Center for Clinical Global Health Education, School of Medicine, Johns Hopkins University, Baltimore, MD, USA

Ron Stall Department of Behavioral and Community Health Sciences, University of Pittsburgh Graduate School of Public Health, Pittsburgh, PA, USA

Judith M. Stephenson Institute for Women's Health, University College London, Medical School Building, London, UK

Ronald Valdiserri Office of HIV/AIDS and Infectious Disease Policy, U.S. Department of Health and Human Services, Washington, DC, USA

Jo A. Valentine Division of STD Prevention, Centers for Disease Control and Prevention, Atlanta, GA, USA

Chongyi Wei Department of Behavioral and Community Health Sciences, University of Pittsburgh Graduate School of Public Health, Pittsburgh, PA, USA

Peter J. White Department of Infectious Disease Epidemiology, MRC Centre for Outbreak Analysis & Modelling, Imperial College London, School of Public Health, London, UK

Dan Wohlfeiler Office of Policy and Communications, STD Control Branch, California Department of Public Health, Richmond, CA, USA

John L. Wylie, PhD Cadham Provincial Laboratory, Winnipeg, MB, Canada

Introduction

Sevgi O. Aral, Kevin A. Fenton,
and Judith A. Lipshutz

Sexually Transmitted Infections (STI), including HIV, remain among the most prevalent and costly health conditions facing western industrialized countries. In the United States alone, more than 19 million STIs are believed to occur each year, costing approximately $17 billion in diagnosis, treatment, and care costs [1, 2]. In Europe there are more than two million people living with HIV, and in 2010, 27,116 newly diagnosed HIV infections were reported across the European Union and the European Economic Area (EU/EEA) [3]. As with the US, the STI epidemics are remarkably distinct in individual countries. While some conditions such as chlamydia and the viral STIs are highly prevalent and demonstrate patterns consistent with generalized epidemics, STIs overall continue to disproportionly affect certain key populations, in particular men who have sex with men (MSM), persons originating from countries with generalized HIV epidemics and people who inject drugs. In many industrialized settings, governments continue to struggle with bringing these epidemics under control as they face stable or increasing STI/HIV rates among MSM, high prevalence of undiagnosed infection among young people, and poor coverage of treatment, care, and vaccination services for at-risk populations.

Recent advances in prevention, treatment, and care options for these conditions combined with improved political awareness and support provide opportunities for hope. Advances in biomedical prevention approaches for HIV, including the use of highly active antiretroviral treatment that both improves the clinical outcomes for people living with HIV and reduces onward transmission of HIV infection, have drawn attention to the importance of balancing individual and population approaches to health as part of STI/HIV prevention efforts. In contrast, many challenges now faced by programs directly reflect the difficulties in public health funding, design, and implementation of effective prevention and clinical interventions. Chief among these are the funding challenges imposed by the global economic downturn; reforming of health and public health systems towards greater accountability, quality, and impact; changing public expectations for individual, family, and community health; and changing perceptions of the role of government, private, and community sectors in the delivery of health and healthcare. While

S.O. Aral, MA, MS, PhD (✉)
Division of STD Prevention, Centers for Disease Control and Prevention, 1600 Clifton Rd., NE, MS E-02, Atlanta, GA 30333, USA
e-mail: saral@cdc.gov

K.A. Fenton, MD, PhD, FFPH
NCHHSTP, Centers for Disease Control and Prevention, 1600 Clifton Rd., NE, MS E-07, Atlanta, GA 30333, USA
e-mail: KFenton@cdc.gov

J.A. Lipshutz, MPH
OSTLTS, Centers for Disease Control and Prevention, 4770 Buford Hwy, MS E-70, Atlanta, GA 30341, USA
e-mail: JLipshutz@cdc.gov

S.O. Aral, K.A. Fenton, and J.A. Lipshutz (eds.), *The New Public Health and STD/HIV Prevention: Personal, Public and Health Systems Approaches*, DOI 10.1007/978-1-4614-4526-5_1,
© Springer Science+Business Media New York 2013

these changes promise a new approach to public health, they also threaten to fundamentally change the way health systems, and therefore STI/HIV prevention, treatment, and care efforts, are delivered in the twenty-first century.

The understanding that STI epidemics are determined by the dynamic interplay between the individual, the infectious agent, the environment, and prevention and care interventions is now well established. Indeed, much of the historical response to STI/HIV epidemics have traditionally been led by partnerships between the clinical and public health sectors. It is therefore critical that our efforts to enhance the impact and effectiveness of STI/HIV prevention occur within the context of understanding and leveraging developments in public health systems and policy. Traditionally, public health's unique contribution to STI control has included ensurance of robust clinical, behavioral, and laboratory surveillance; social marketing, health communication, and public education; policy formulation, implementation, and evaluation; partner notification; multisectoral collaboration; quality assurance and improvement; and research. As we move into the second decade of the twenty-first century, understanding how these traditional roles of public health are evolving and what might lie ahead will be important strategies for those interested in STI/HIV prevention.

The New Public Health in Historical Context

The definition, scope, challenges, and opportunities in public health change and evolve continuously—hence the repeated use of the term "The New Public Health" in the literature. Half a century ago, in an article dated September 1959, the late Milton Terris stated: "The changing character of public health is evident to anyone who wishes to see. This change implies consequences, however, and these are too often overlooked" [4]. Terris argued that the importance of epidemiologic research in the noninfectious diseases was not understood; most research funds went to laboratory and clinical studies; training in

biostatistics and epidemiology was inadequately funded; and only two state health departments— California and New York—had developed strong programs of research into the epidemiology of cancer, heart disease, and other noninfectious diseases. The challenges facing public health in the United States at the end of the 1950s included the present and potential shortages of physicians, dentists, nurses, and other health personnel. State health departments were encouraged to provide leadership to help meet these educational and training needs. At the same time Terris noted, "The responsibilities of public health today are much greater than ever before" [4]. Between 1950 and 1959, the real expenditures of local health departments failed to keep pace with the increase in population [5]. "Thus, at a time when under budgeted and understaffed state and local health departments face new and greater demands for their services, federal support for public health services is being curtailed rather than expanded" [4]. This description could easily fit public health in 2012.

Three and a half decades later (1995), a discussion paper by the World Health Organization[6] used the specific term, "The New Public Health" in the global context, and suggested that it was not so much a concept as it was a philosophy which endeavored to broaden the older understanding of public health so that, for example, it included the health of the individual in addition to the health of populations, and sought to address contemporary health issues concerned with equitable access to health services, the environment, political governance, and social and economic development. The new public health philosophy sought to put health in the development framework to ensure that health is protected through enactment of public policy, and included interest in identifying implementable strategies to solve the issues of the time,[6] again, a call for change that could have been formulated in 2012.

Reminiscent of the often observed generalization, the more things change the more they stay the same. Robert Wood Johnson's 2010 issue brief entitled, "Preventing Chronic Disease: The New Public Health" [7] focused on the need for policy change at the community level to change people's lifestyles. The authors point to the recent global economic recession and the chronic disease epidemic in the United States that necessitate difficult decisions regarding the allocation of limited public health dollars. Their analysis supports proven community prevention programs in that they help to modify lifestyles that improve health, and policy interventions that constitute a powerful tool toward the success of such prevention programs.

The definition and scope of public health evolve continuously as a consequence of changing challenges including: shifting demographics, epidemiology, and the political, social, and economic environment; and changing opportunities in the form of biological, social and management science, and tools and technologies. Such change has important implications for public health in general and the control and prevention of specific diseases and conditions in particular.

Preventing Sexually Transmitted Diseases and HIV: Changing Challenges and Opportunities

In the area of sexually transmitted disease and human immunodeficiency virus prevention, major changes have taken place over the past few decades, which have modified the scope and structure of both the challenges and the opportunities facing the field, thereby redefining public health in this domain. In this context, the relevant parameters include: the shift in our understanding of health from the sole provision of diagnostic and treatment services to sick individuals, to the provision of prevention services to well populations with the goal of maximizing wellness; the current global economic crisis and the consequent decline in financial resources available for public health; the related increased emphasis on accountability, efficiency, effectiveness, impact evaluation, and maximization of returns on public health investments; an epidemiologic transition from infectious to chronic diseases; demographic changes in mortality, fertility, and migration with their resultant modifications of the age, sex, and geographic

structure of populations; and significant shifts in sexual norms and behaviors accelerated by the effects of such population drivers as urbanization and globalization. Concurrent with these changes in challenges have been remarkable developments in the tools, technologies, and the science base available to public health and healthcare workers in sexually transmitted disease and human immunodeficiency virus prevention.

At this time, we have efficacious biomedical interventions for the prevention of sexually transmitted infections [8], and during the past few years biomedical interventions including male circumcision, microbicides, pre-exposure chemoprophylaxis, and early anti-retroviral therapy have been shown to effectively prevent acquisition and transmission of HIV [9–14]. However, challenges remain and exert pressure on public health so as to change its definition and scope. One such challenge involves the need for defining combination intervention packages which take into consideration the highly complex interactions among interventions and the context they are introduced into; and the need to maximize the synergies among interventions implemented concurrently while minimizing potential antagonisms among them [15–18]. Other challenges include: the limited arsenal of effective interventions; the difficulty involved in implementing effective prevention interventions at sufficient scale and intensity relative to the need; the scattering of interventions across geographic areas and the resulting inability to realize synergies that multiple interventions in one location could lead to; the insufficient targeting of interventions to key affected populations, especially in concentrated and mixed epidemics; and the lack of linkages between prevention services, between prevention, care and treatment services, and across clinical and community-based settings [19, 20].

These challenges push the boundaries of HIV and STI science. The outcomes that need to be focused on are no longer, solely, individual-level health outcomes, even if those are considered in the aggregate. It is important to attend to rates of transmission and acquisition that take place in populations. The key issues are no longer, solely, those of biomedical interventions to affect biomedical processes or behavioral interventions to change risk behaviors of individuals. STI/HIV scientists now have to consider how much of the biomedical and behavioral interventions need to be employed, in which combinations, at what scale, to which subpopulations, at which time, for what duration. Concurrently, it is essential to figure out which resources (and how much) and which intervention combination will be used for which subpopulation in order to maximize returns on STI/HIV prevention investments.

The Changing Topography of the Science Base

The STI/HIV scientific field has responded to these challenges by issuing new guidance for HIV prevention programs [19] and by introducing use of new scientific paradigms to the field, such as implementation science and program science, to guide the new public health [8, 15]. The financial crises in the early twenty-first century and the resulting efforts to control public spending and debt have exerted growing pressure on traditional funding channels for health globally. Thus, two key issues for the new public health are strategic allocation of limited resources to maximize return on public health investments and the generation of additional resources for prevention [18, 20]. The public health field has responded to the need of generating additional resources by developing new funding mechanisms [20]. Strategic allocation of resources to maximize return on public health investments is the key focus of program science [18]. Cost-effectiveness, cost–benefit, and comparative effectiveness analyses are increasingly used to monitor return on investments.

Increasingly, health care providers are challenged to understand the determinants of health and policies that can influence health [21]. Physicians and nurses are expected to function as advocates for preventive policies in their communities. A new public health approach calls for its workers to move beyond the causes and effects of individuals' health; rather, they need to consider population science, and be well versed in population-level determinants, transmission dynamics, complex interactions, and health systems.

Mathematical modeling, traditionally employed to describe infection transmission dynamics and to predict future behavior of epidemics, is increasingly the methodology the field turns to in support of policy choices and population-level evaluations of intervention effects. Recent examples of this practice include the use of mathematical modeling in the identification and description of combination interventions [22] and in the proposal that universal voluntary HIV testing with immediate antiretroviral therapy may be a viable strategy for eliminating HIV [23–25].

The so-called "prevention cascade" has become a salient focus for many in the operations research area following the realization that, despite availability of efficacious interventions for the prevention of mother-to-child HIV transmission (PMTCT), many in the developing world have had inadequate access to these interventions and scientific understanding of the field performance of the interventions was lacking [26, 27]. This emphasis marked a major shift in STI/HIV prevention science, away from a focus solely on efficacy to one which includes real-world effectiveness and population-level impact [28].

The focus on effectiveness, population-level impact, and thus, issues of coverage and scale-up, has highlighted the importance of health systems in STI/HIV prevention. Health systems strengthening interventions now receive considerable attention at both the programmatic and scientific levels [29]. Moreover, health systems strengthening efforts are now considered to be a specific approach to responding to HIV/AIDS epidemics [30]. Examples include the U.S. public health efforts to integrate STI and HIV programs and to promote public health practices in primary care settings.

The requirement that prevention efforts achieve population-level impact has reactivated methodological debates around best ways of monitoring and evaluating health at the population level and attributing effect to interventions. While some in the field argue for the need for community randomized trials and approximations to RCTs through the use of counterfactuals where RCTs cannot be implemented, others point to the drawbacks of RCTs [31, 32]. The results of these debates will have to take sufficient account of the complexities involved in populations, the interactions that rule cause–effect relationships in complex systems, the importance of the interactions between interventions and the context into which they are introduced, and the interactions among interventions themselves.

Emerging Foci in the New Public Health Science

Several functions, which have traditionally been served by prevention program experts based on past experience, are increasingly becoming the subject of scientific inquiry and analyses. These new foci include analyses of social and sexual networks [33]; analyses of concentrations of morbidity and risk behaviors [34–36]; analyses of targeting of prevention interventions[37]; and potential strategic approaches to expanding coverage, and consideration of the health systems context [38]. These developments suggest public health science is undergoing major change and may look quite different in the coming decade.

Volume Contents

In this book, the authors examine present and anticipated sexual health challenges, their determinants and the populations that are disproportionately affected in a complex world with great inequalities. The book is divided into four sections that together provide an integrated perspective of personal, population, and systems-level aspects of STI/HIV prevention in developed country settings. These chapters are intended to provide a holistic view of the STI/HIV landscape in combination with pragmatic approaches to prevention.

The first section introduces socio-demographic factors and subsequent challenges that influence sexual health in the early part of the twenty-first century as well as societal issues that create parameters affecting the epidemiology of STI and HIV. Topics outside of the traditional social

determinants of health, such as migration patterns and commercial enterprises, are examined to demonstrate more direct implications of these influences. Adimora and Schoenbach describe the social determinants of heterosexual partnering and sexual networks as they relate to STI/HIV with emphasis on the US where STI rates exceed those of other industrialized countries. They argue for a new approach to STI/HIV prevention that addresses social determinants of STIs and other outcomes. Peter White's chapter focuses on disparities in the distribution of STI and HIV in space, time, and by population group, and then explores the causes of these disparities and their implications for interventions. He argues that thinking in terms of populations, not just individuals, is critical to applying the best intervention science. Discussion includes the complex interaction of many factors often elucidated by theoretically based insight from mathematical modeling which allows the testing of hypotheses and guidance of empirical research. From an epidemiological perspective, Butler and Hallett examine the literature on migration and the spread of STIs, particularly HIV. They dissect the operations of migration as both a mechanism that brings infected individuals together with uninfected individuals and a trigger for different types of changes in behavior. While acknowledging data limitations, they suggest the importance of understanding the impact of migration on STI and HIV epidemics so as to identify appropriate interventions. Jolly and Wylie explore characteristics of sexual networks through theories of homophily, heterogeneity and social aggregation, and then describe networks wherein specific STIs and HIV survive. They review social network-inspired prevention strategies and suggest that a social network approach could facilitate analyses of social cohesion and social capital which in turn could positively influence network norms and lower STI rates. The authors conclude that network methods should be considered for routine surveillance and research but note the challenge of not knowing the extent to which their application results in an improvement over previous methods. In their chapter, Wohlfeiler and Kerndt frame their discussion of sexual health in the context of the need to balance achievement of public health with protection of individual rights. They discuss these issues through two examples: patrons of commercial sex venues like bathhouses and sex clubs, and performers in the adult film industry. They argue that public health must work with these nontraditional partners to achieve positive health outcomes in populations vulnerable to STI/HIV infection.

Important considerations for successful implementation of STI/HIV programs constitute the focus of the second section of the book. These chapters address issues critical to ensuring high population-level impact. Chesson and colleagues discuss distribution of funding levels for HIV and STIs in the US and how it relates to burden of disease. In review of key models, they further discuss the association between funding levels and disease incidence and what might happen in either the absence or increase of funding. They conclude with discussion of resource allocation models, the importance of taking cost effectiveness into consideration when making funding decisions, and the potential of public investment in maximizing STD and HIV prevention impact. Peters and colleagues review the current state of knowledge and practice on scaling up and achieving universal coverage of HIV and STD health services as well as what is known about targeting interventions to specific populations. They contend that the concept of scaling up needs to go deeper than the simple notion of quantitative coverage of health services to ensure sustainable effects. Targeting approaches are assessed as ways to improve the effectiveness, equity, and efficiency of health service delivery. In recognizing the worldwide influence of electronic media, Rietmeijer and MacFarlane explore its role in STI/HIV prevention. They provide an overview of the scientific literature that has examined the Internet as an environment for STI/HIV risk, prevention and care, and propose avenues for future research and development of innovation at the interface between electronic media and the prevention and care of STI/HIV. They further suggest the role of new technologies in shaping a new approach to public health. Kevin Fenton's chapter describes the complexities of leadership and governance for prevention and public health

programs describing them as essential building blocks of effective health systems, robust public health responses, and ultimately, effective STI/HIV prevention and sexual health programs in western industrialized settings. He discusses the challenges facing the public health workforce and then critically examines the evolving definitions of leadership within the context of public health, STI/HIV prevention, and sexual health programs. He argues that successful public health systems, including those that support sexual health, require an understanding of the whole health system as well as both political action and technical solutions. The chapter identifies key domains for strengthening leadership for STI/HIV prevention and supports the need to continuously nurture public health leadership as a core component of successful sexual health programs.

The third section focuses on six specific populations disproportionately affected by STI/HIV with special attention to influences of social determinants on their sexual health. Jeanne Marrazzo writes about STD/HIV prevention issues for women, including opportunities such as the HPV vaccine and topical antiretrovirals for HIV. She acknowledges the diversity of impacted women and notes the complexities that underlie women's vulnerability to these infections. The chapter by Needle and colleagues focuses on persons who inject drugs (PWIDs) who constitute an estimated 15.9 million people worldwide and bear a disproportionate burden of STI/HIV. They document consequences and costs of not acting on science-based policies as well as the importance of scaling up comprehensive HIV prevention programs. They move on to examine macro-level, structural determinants of STI/HIV in PWIDs that shape vulnerability, risk, transmission and response to these infections. They conclude with a discussion of challenges that remain in addressing disease in this vulnerable population. Guadamuz and colleagues focus on men who have sex with men (MSM) acknowledging the many variables that operate beyond the level of the individual and influence their disproportionate burden of disease. They discuss a series of complex interrelated domains that impact the efficacy and effectiveness of STI/HIV prevention practice among MSM in the US and suggest that there are opportunities to enhance health promotion programs that integrate multiple levels of intervention and make our research agendas more innovative. In particular, they suggest a new framework for STI/HIV prevention in MSM based on the syndemics theory which acknowledges the interaction of various psychosocial health conditions as enhancers of the harmful effects of each other and together raise risk levels for STI and HIV. Dean and Myles explore how the sexual health of various racial/ethnic groups is influenced by structural and social determinants and provide examples of the impact of key societal systems on the ability of racial and ethnic minorities to achieve optimal sexual health. They discuss systems-based approaches to improve sexual health and reduce rates of STIs among racial and ethnic minorities in the United States.

Focused on adolescents, Fortenberry and Hensel explore an approach to STI prevention that shifts the traditional approaches of risk factor reduction to a construct that emphasizes sexual health. They suggest an approach that supports healthy sexual development while still maintaining attention to adverse outcomes of sexual behaviors such as STIs. Their construct is linked to three key public health indicators: number of recent sex partners; frequency of condom use; and STI. Sexual health, they suggest, is a guiding paradigm for a successful public health approach to STI prevention.

The final section includes a series of critical reviews of recent prevention programs that have addressed STI/HIV prevention from a systems-level perspective. These programs incorporate dimensions beyond the traditional approaches including many represented in this book. Two HIV/AIDS programs are illustrated in the first couple of chapters for the US and Australia. With an historical lens, Valdiserri provides a critical review of programmatic responses to the HIV/AIDS epidemic in the US which help elucidate efforts that have resulted in successful prevention outcomes, deconstruct and analyze attempts that have failed, and continue to refine our knowledge of the various determinants that influence program success and failure. This chapter explores a variety of prevention approaches spanning those that target individuals, focus on communities, or strive to alter the systems that serve individuals, families, and communities at risk for acquiring or transmitting HIV. He demonstrates the complex interplay between people, communities, systems, and circumstances that have and must continue to be considered to address the HIV epidemic. Mindel and Kippax describe Australia's approach to HIV/AIDS through a partnership model that includes government, affected communities, public health, and research institutions. They credit their ongoing success to use of a social public health framework which, when effective, recognizes that people are not only individuals but also members of groups, networks, and collectives. Their analysis includes comparisons with approaches of other developed countries, including the US. The next review by Valentine and DeLisle illustrates lessons learned from the 1999 syphilis elimination campaign in the U.S. which aimed not only to eliminate the disease but also to reduce disparities in sexual health and improve public health capacity. The campaign sought to better address a variety of individual factors and social determinants that sustain the infectious syphilis epidemic by promoting public health interventions at the individual, community, and structural levels. As the campaign did not reach its intended goals, the authors concluded that epidemics can evolve faster than agencies, programs, or research can address them, as was the case with the syphilis elimination campaign in the US. They note challenges at local, state, and federal levels in willingness to adjust strategies when outcomes fall short of expectations. Markowitz and Hariri review the status and impact of the recently recommended HPV vaccine in the U.S. with a focus on its role in prevention of associated outcomes such as cervical cancer. Noting that the addition of this vaccine adds primary prevention strategies to cervical cancer prevention, the authors discuss the opportunities it avails for interaction among traditional and nontraditional disciplines as part of the arsenal of cervical cancer prevention as well as the potential to reduce disparities in cervical cancer morbidity and mortality. They also discuss such challenges as public perceptions, vaccine uptake, high cost and low access issues. The comparison of approaches to Chlamydia control in the US and UK is the topic of the chapter by Low and colleagues. After reviewing the evolution and current state of Chlamydia control efforts in both countries, they raise questions about the real impact of these models in reducing burden of disease, including adverse outcomes, and in turn suggest the need for additional innovations outside the current paradigm to control this pervasive disease.

Given the timely but evolving nature of many of these topics and the challenging context of public health in the twenty-first century, the literature continues to grow as will the public health responses to these pervasive infectious diseases. Moving ahead, our challenge will be to apply what is known, for the populations in greatest need, at a scale and coverage for appropriate impact, with a commitment to learn, improve, and evaluate as we implement. No doubt, new iterations of a "new public health" will continue to be topics of discussion for upcoming generations of public health researchers, policy makers, and practitioners.

References

1. CDC. Sexually transmitted disease surveillance 2010. Atlanta: U.S. Department of Health and Human Services; 2011. http://www.cdc.gov/std/stats10/surv2010.pdf.
2. Chesson HW, Blandford JM, Gift TL, Tao G, Irwin KL. The estimated direct medical cost of sexually transmitted diseases among American youth, 2000. Perspect Sex Reprod Health. 2004;36(1):11–9. http://www.guttmacher.org/pubs/journals/3601104.html.
3. European Centre for Disease Prevention and Control/WHO Regional Office for Europe. HIV/AIDS surveillance in Europe 2010. Stockholm: European Centre for Disease Prevention and Control; 2011. http://ecdc.europa.eu/en/publications/Publications/111129_SUR_Annual_HIV_Report.pdf.
4. Terris M. The changing face of public health. J Public Health. 1959;49:1113–9.
5. Sanders BS. Local health department. Growth or Illusion? Public Health Rep. 1959;74:13–20.
6. Ncayiyana D, Goldstein G, Goon E, Yach D. WHO: New public health and WHO's ninth general program of work: a discussion paper. Geneva: World Health Organization; 1995.
7. Preventing Chronic Disease: the New Public Health. Robert Wood Johnson Foundation. Issue Brief Sept 2011. http://www.allhealth.org/publications/Public_health/Preventing_Chronic_Disease_New_Public_Health_108.pdf
8. Blanchard JF, Aral SO. Program science: an initiative to improve the planning, implementation and evaluation of HIV/sexually transmitted infection prevention programmes. Sex Transm Infect. 2011;87(1):2–3.
9. Gray RH, Kigozi G, Serwadda D, et al. Male circumcision for HIV prevention in men in Rakai, Uganda: a randomized trial. Lancet. 2007;369(9562):657–66.
10. Auvert B, Taljaard D, Lagarde E, et al. Randomized, controlled intervention trial of male circumcision for reduction of HIV infection risk: the ANRS 1265 trial. PLoS Med. 2005;2:e298.
11. Bailey RC, Moses S, Parker CB, et al. Male circumcision for HIV prevention in young men in Kisumu, Kenya: a randomized controlled trial. Lancet. 2007;369:643–56.
12. Abdool Karim Q, Abdool Karim SS, Frohlich JA, et al. Effectiveness and safety of Tenofovir Gel, an antiretroviral microbicide, for the prevention of HIV infection in women. Science. 2010;329(5996)):1168–74.
13. Grant RM, Lama JR, Anderson PL, et al. Preexposure chemoprophylaxis for HIV prevention in men who have sex with men. N Engl J Med. 2010;363(27):2587–99.
14. Cohen MS, Chen YQ, McCauley M, et al. Prevention of HIV-1 infection with early antiretroviral therapy. N Engl J Med. 2011;365(6):493–505.
15. Padian NS, McCoy SI, Abdool Karim SS, et al. HIV prevention transformed: the new prevention research agenda. Lancet. 2011;378(9787):269–78.
16. Aral SO, Lipshutz JA, Douglas JM. Introduction. In: Aral SA, Douglas JM Jr., editors, Lipshutz JA (assoc. editor). Behavioral interventions for prevention and control of sexually transmitted diseases. New York: Springer Science+Business Media, LLC; 2007. p. ix–xix.
17. Hawe P, Shiell A, Riley T. Theorising interventions as events in systems. Am J Community Psychol. 2009;43:267–76.
18. Aral SO, Blanchard J. The Program Science Initiative: improving the planning, implementation and evaluation of HIV/STI prevention programs. Sex Transm Infect. 2012;88(3):157–9.
19. President's Emergency Plan for AIDS Relief (PEPFAR) prevention guidance. http://www.pepfar.gov.
20. Kaiser Family Foundation. Innovative financing mechanisms for Global Health: Overview & Considerations for U.S. Government Participation. U.S. Global Health Policy, Published online: 19 Oct 2011. http://www.kff.org/globalhealth/upload/8247.pdf
21. Monroe JA. Exploring the context. Am J Prev Med. 2011;41(4S3):S155–9.
22. Nagelkerke NJD, Jha P, de Vlas SJ, Korenromp EL, Moses S, Blanchard JF, Plummer FA. Modelling HIV/AIDS epidemics in Botswana and India: impact of

interventions to prevent transmission. Bull World Health Organ. 2002;80:89–96.

23. Williams B, Wood R, Dukay V, et al. Treatment as prevention: preparing the way. J Int AIDS Soc. 2011;14 Suppl 1:S6.

24. Granich RM, Gilks CF, Dye C, DeCock KM, Williams BG. Universal voluntary HIV testing with immediate antiretroviral therapy as a strategy for elimination of HIV transmission: a mathematical model. Lancet. 2009;373:48–57.

25. Granich R, Gupta S, Suthar A, et al. ART in prevention of HIV and TB: update on current research efforts. Curr HIV Res. 2011;9(6):446–69.

26. Stringer EM, Chi BH, Chintu N, et al. Monitoring effectiveness of programmes to prevent mother-to-child HIV transmission in lower-income countries. Bull World Health Organ. http://www.who.int/bulletin/volumes/86/1/07-043117/en/

27. Barker PM, Mphatswe W, Rollins N. Antiretroviral drugs in the cupboard are not enough: the impact of health systems' performance on mother-to-child transmission of HIV. J Acquir Immune Defic Syndr. 2011;56(2):e45–8.

28. Aral SO, Blanchard JF, Lipshutz JA. STD/HIV prevention intervention: efficacy, effectiveness and population impact. Sex Transm Infect. 2008;84(Suppl II):ii1–3.

29. Shakarishvili G, Atun R, Berman P, et al. Converging health systems frameworks: towards a concepts-to-actions roadmap for health systems strengthening in low and middle income countries. Global Health Governance 2010;III(2) http://www.ghgj.org

30. Responding to the HIV/AIDS epidemic through health systems strengthening efforts. http://www.healthsystems2020.org/section/topics/hiv.

31. Thomas J, Curtis S, Smith J. The broader context of implementation science. J Acquir Immune Defic Syndr. 2011;58(1):e19–21.

32. Padian N, Holmes C, McCoy S, et al. Response to letter from Thomas et al critiquing "Implementation science for the US President's Emergency Plan for AIDS Relief". J Acquir Immune Defic Syndr. 2011;58(1):e21–2.

33. Chen MI, Ghani AC. Republished paper: populations and partnerships: insights from metapopulation and pair models into the epidemiology of gonorrhea and other sexually transmitted infections. Sex Transm Infect. 2010;86(Suppl III):iii63–9.

34. Leichliter JS, Chesson HW, Sternberg M, Aral SO. The concentration of sexual behaviours in the USA: a closer examination of subpopulations. Sex Transm Infect. 2010;86(Suppl III):iii45–51.

35. Chesson HW, Sternberg M, Leichliter JS, Aral SO. The distribution of chlamydia, gonorrhea and syphilis cases across states and countries in the USA, 2007. Sex Transm Infect. 2010;86(Suppl III):iii52–7.

36. Chesson HW, Sternberg M, Leichliter JS, Aral SO. Changes in the state-level distribution of primary and secondary syphilis in the USA, 1985–2007. Sex Transm Infect. 2010;86(Suppl III):iii58–62.

37. Tanser F, Bärnighausen T, Cooke GS, Newell M-L. Localized spatial clustering of HIV infections in a widely disseminated rural South African epidemic. Int J Epidemiol. 2009;38(4):1008–16.

38. Aral SO. Defining coverage: the importance of context. Presented at 6th IAS conference on HIV pathogenesis treatment and prevention, Rome, Italy, July 2011.

Part I

Socio-demographic Societal and Supra-Societal Determinants and Influences

Social Determinants of Sexual Networks, Partnership Formation, and Sexually Transmitted Infections

2

Adaora A. Adimora and Victor J. Schoenbach

Social Determinants of Sexually Transmitted Infection

Social factors have long been recognized as important determinants of health [1]. In recent years, social determinants—"the conditions in which people are born, grow, live, work and age, including the health system" (WHO Commission on Social Determinants) [2]—have attracted increasing attention as fundamental causes of disparities in health status between individuals and populations. Although most studies about social determinants address chronic, non-communicable diseases, a recent examination of the social epidemiology literature from 1975 to 2005 found 44 review articles with infectious disease outcomes, with the majority focused on HIV/AIDS [3]. The emphasis on HIV is perhaps not surprising, since HIV and other sexually transmitted infections (STI) are by their nature social diseases. Researchers have recently begun to trace the pathways between social determinants and HIV/ STI [4–7]. The expression of sexuality, a perva-

sive influence in human society, is shaped by society. Social factors of all kinds, including those related to education, occupation, neighborhoods, migration, urbanization, mobility, affluence, media, religion, substance use, incarceration, and technological change, can influence sexual behaviors, partnership formation, and sexual networks, with resultant effects on STI dissemination. This chapter explores some of the primary modern-day social determinants of heterosexual partnering and sexual networks relevant to HIV/STI, particularly in the USA, where STI rates exceed those of all other industrialized countries [8].

Determinants of STI Transmission

Key determinants of the extent of spread of an STI from an infected person to others are the likelihood of transmission during sexual contact, sexual contact rate and sexual network patterns, and duration of infectiousness of an infected person. The likelihood of transmission depends partly on the prevalence of infection in the pool of potential sexual partners [9]. Effective health care, including prompt and appropriate diagnosis and curative treatment, shortens the length of time during which infected people remain infectious. Even treatment that is not curative may reduce infectiousness. Most notably, antiretroviral therapy (ART) for HIV-infected patients decreases their levels of HIV viremia and likely decreases their infectiousness to others, an observation that

A.A. Adimora, M.D., M.P.H. (✉)
Division of Infectious Diseases, UNC School
of Medicine, 130 Mason Farm Road, CB #7030,
Chapel Hill, NC 27599-7030, USA
e-mail: Adimora@med.unc.edu

V.J. Schoenbach, Ph.D.
Department of Epidemiology, UNC Gillings School
of Global Public Health, 2104D McGavran-Greenberg,
CB #7435, Chapel Hill, NC 27599-7435, USA

S.O. Aral, K.A. Fenton, and J.A. Lipshutz (eds.), *The New Public Health and STD/HIV Prevention:*
Personal, Public and Health Systems Approaches, DOI 10.1007/978-1-4614-4526-5_2,
© Springer Science+Business Media New York 2013

has generated enthusiasm for expanded testing and treatment [10]. Other prominent strategies for reducing STI dissemination are use of condoms, which reduce transmission efficiency, and initiatives to reduce contact with infected partners through sex education to discourage early onset of coitus and reduce overall number of sex partners.

Condom Use

Consistent and correct male condom use decreases the risk of STIs (and of pregnancy) [11]. Consistent condom use results in 80% reduction in the incidence of heterosexual HIV transmission [12]. The most common cause of condom failure is lack of use during one or more episodes of intercourse [13]. The proportion of the US women who have ever used a condom has substantially increased during the past two decades. Among the US women respondents in the NSFG 1982, 1995, and 2002 cycles who had ever had sexual intercourse, 52%, 82%, and 90%, respectively, reported ever having used condoms. Among the US women respondents in the 2002 NSFG, aged 15–44 who had ever had sexual intercourse, 92% of non-Hispanic White and non-Hispanic Blacks and 78% of Hispanic women had ever used a male condom. Much smaller proportions (5% of Black women and 1% of Hispanic and non-Hispanic White women) have ever used a female condom [14]. *Consistent* condom use, however, is much less common; for example, in 2002 only 30% of the US men and 25% of the US women reported having used a condom during most recent sexual intercourse. Moreover, of those at risk for HIV because of STD treatment within the past year or high-risk sexual behaviors or drug use, 60% overall (55% men, 68% women) did not use a condom during last intercourse [15].

Health Care

Because treatment of an infected individual may protect current and future sexual partners, health care is a powerful force in STI dynamics. Health care availability and quality are important social determinants of health [16]. Disparities in access to health care are much greater in the United States than in other industrialized countries, and contribute to the dramatic racial and ethnic disparities in rates of chronic diseases and STIs, including HIV [17]. In 2008, 46.3 million people in the US (15.4% of the population) lacked health insurance. Hispanics (32% uninsured), Blacks (19%), and Asian Americans (17%) are considerably more likely to be uninsured than Whites (10%) [18]. Health care reform, finally enacted in 2010, will reduce the number of uninsured persons by about half. However, differences in comprehensiveness of coverage, required co-pays and deductibles, and allowed reimbursement rates (which reduce the number of providers available to patients who rely on Medicaid) will continue to affect actual access to health care services. There are also powerful nonfinancial barriers to access, such as residential segregation, facility hours of operation and location, and availability of transportation. Even when access to care is equivalent, compared to Whites, African Americans are more likely to receive low-quality health care, with resultant increased mortality [17].

Effective health care involves access to medications as well as to services. Access to medications has been a long-standing problem for many patients with chronic health conditions. State AIDS Drug Assistance Programs provide medications to low-income, uninsured people with HIV infection in the US. However, the economic crisis that began in 2007, with the resulting unprecedented demand for program services due to increased unemployment, caused many of these state programs to run out of funding during 2010, rendering them unable to provide medications to eligible clients and placing more than 1,000 people on waiting lists as of May 2010 [19]. In the absence of ART these individuals will be more infectious to people in their sexual network, many of whom are likely also individuals of lower socioeconomic status.

Sex Education

Comprehensive sex education programs have been found to be effective in reducing risky sexual behavior among youth [20]; yet a campaign by religious and political conservatives led to state laws and federal funding restrictions on sex education programming in public schools that presented condoms as effective in preventing STI. A great expansion in federal funding for public school sex education (more than $1.5 billion over nearly 30 years) took place beginning in the 1980s to support abstinence-until-marriage sex education, notwithstanding the lack of data to support its effectiveness in reducing risky behavior [21]. Over 80% of abstinence-only curricula used by grantees of the largest federal abstinence-only initiatives contained false, misleading, or distorted information about reproductive health, including efficacy of condoms for preventing infection [22]. Youth exposed to such programs were significantly less likely to perceive condoms as efficacious for preventing STIs [22]. A recent randomized trial of a theory-based abstinence-only intervention in African-American middle school youth found reduced onset of intercourse at 24 months post randomization compared to a health-promotion control group and no difference in self-reported condom use among sexually active participants. The authors noted, however, that the intervention did not meet federal criteria, was not moralistic, and did not criticize the use of condoms [23].

Sexual Network Patterns and Behaviors Influence STI Rates

In the abstract, the world is a vast network of sexual partnerships and potential partnerships. Most adults are connected to another adult, sometimes more than one, and many have been connected to others in the past. With sufficient interconnectedness, sexual pathogens could spread throughout the entire population. However, most people form relatively few partnerships, typically with people of similar age, race/ethnicity, and socioeconomic class [24]. A small percentage, though, has many partners, including partners with varied social, demographic, and risk characteristics. This proportionately small but relatively more active subset creates interconnected networks that can dramatically affect STI spread.

People's propensity to acquire sexual partners varies by age, gender, marital status, biological influences, psychological characteristics, and personal circumstances [25]. Social, economic, and political factors affect these propensities and also the environment in which they are expressed. Together, individual and social factors determine the number, configuration, and dynamics of sexual partnerships over time, creating the networks that enable STI to propagate.

Long-Term Monogamy

The major institutions that directly govern sexual activity in contemporary society are family, religious institutions, and the legal system [26]. These institutions tend to support and protect long-term heterosexual monogamy over other partnering patterns. To the extent that people remain in long-term monogamous relationships (whether heterosexual or homosexual), sexual acquisition and transmission of infection outside the dyad will not occur.

Historically, most Americans have spent a substantial proportion of their sexually active adult lives in long-term monogamous relationships, which have served as the foundations on which families were created. However, during the latter part of the twentieth century the dominance of this traditional family structure has declined as a result of the rising age at marriage, increasing cohabitation among unmarried young adults, increases in nonmarital childbearing (and decreases in marital childbearing), and rising divorce rates [27]. For example, the percentage of the US women aged 25–29 years who had never married rose from 12% in 1970 to 48% in 2008; the corresponding percentage for men rose from 20% to 61%. Meanwhile, households with unmarried couples have increased, accounting for 4.6% of all households in Census 2000 [28]. Although many cohabiting adults eventually marry their partner, many do not.

Serial Monogamy

The long-term decline in the age of first sexual intercourse has been "one of the best recognized trends in sexual behavior in the USA in the twentieth century," according to Turner et al. (p. 177) [29]. That trend combined with the rising age at marriage has, over time, led to an interval on the order of a decade during which teenagers and young adults are unmarried but sexually active. The sexual partnerships during this period are typically of short term even if monogamous ("serial monogamy"), and their number has grown across successive birth cohorts. For example, for the 1950s birth cohort about 50% of men and 30% of women report having had five or more sexual partners since age 18 [29]. The number of recent partners is smaller: 71% of the US adults aged 18–59 years had only one sex partner during the past year and an additional 12% had no partners (p. 177). However, 39% had more than one partner during the past 5 years (p. 178) [24]. Young adults are the most likely to have multiple recent partners; e.g., 32% of adults aged 18–24 years reported having multiple partners during the past year (p. 177) [24].

The set of all partners an individual has had comprised a sexual network through which a sexually transmitted pathogen can travel or may have traveled. As individuals change partners networks can interconnect. With serial monogamy, however, STI can travel only from past partners through the index person to future partners, not the reverse.

Timing of Partnerships: "The Gap" and Concurrency

Serial monogamy creates much greater opportunity for STI spread than does long-term monogamy. But the transmission potential of serial monogamy is influenced by the length of the interval between sequential partners—or "gap length" [30]. STIs are transmitted only if one partner is infected and contact occurs during the infectious period. Because a number of STIs have a restricted period of maximum infectiousness due to treatment or an immune response, longer monogamous partnerships or longer gaps between partnerships make it more likely that a person infected by a new partner will become less infectious by the time a subsequent partnership begins. More than half of the women reporting serial monogamy in the 1995 National Survey of Family Growth had a gap length shorter than the mean infectivity periods of some bacterial STI. Younger women (aged 15–19) were most likely to experience a short gap [30]. Similarly, more than half (59%) of 18–39-year-old male and female participants in a Seattle telephone survey reported a gap of less than 6 months, a time period within the infectious periods of Chlamydia, gonorrhea, syphilis, HIV, HSV, and HPV [31].

When the date of first intercourse with a new partner comes before the date of last intercourse with a previous partner, the gap length is less than zero. Such overlapping ("concurrent") partnerships add an additional dimension of transmission potential to the partners of the index person, and to their partners' partners in turn. Concurrent partnerships can permit even more rapid spread of an infection throughout a population than the same number of sequential monogamous partnerships for several reasons. First, if a person with concurrent partners becomes infected from one partner, transmission to a concurrent partner can occur without the delay involved in ending the first partnership and beginning a new one (i.e., no protective gap). Second, in sequential monogamy, when a person becomes infected by a new partner, the previous partners are not exposed to the new infection. With concurrent partnerships, however, the continuing contact with partners acquired earlier means that they become (indirectly) exposed to infections acquired from subsequent partners [32].

People who have concurrent partnerships experience the same risk of acquiring STIs as do people who have the same number of partners sequentially, but *partners* of people who have concurrent partnerships have increased risk of acquiring infection. Concurrency has been associated with transmission of Chlamydia, syphilis, and HIV infection [33–35]. Concurrent partnerships are more common among unmarried people, younger people, men, and people whose partners are nonmonogamous [36–38]. More than half (54%) of the adolescents with 2 or more partners in a national survey had concurrent partnerships [39].

Assortative and Dissortative Mixing

Most sexual partnerships are relatively assortative with respect to demographic characteristics, meaning that partners tend to have similar ages, race/ethnicity, educational backgrounds, and religious affiliations [24]. The reason is that sex partners are usually drawn from among the people with whom one comes into contact in social situations. Thus, people's sex partners generally resemble the social composition of their immediate social networks. Laumann et al. describe several mechanisms that increase the likelihood that social situations will bring together people with similar demographic characteristics [24]. First, some settings, such as public schools, community colleges, bars, and churches mainly attract people who live nearby. Because geographic areas are often segregated by race and income, social settings and events that draw from these areas are primarily composed of people who are similar with respect to these characteristics. Second, the social situations (schools, churches, jobs, etc.) themselves bring together people with similar interests and education. Third, social network relationships often bring people to social situations; people may choose to participate in the events because of the people they know. For example, acquaintances and friends refer people for jobs and invite them to parties and cultural events, thereby increasing the homogeneity of the participants. Finally—and most directly—potential partners are often introduced by a mutual acquaintance, an occurrence that increases the likelihood of partnership formation between similar people [24].

Assortative mixing enables STIs to circulate within a demographic stratum, leading to differentials in STI incidence and prevalence across strata. With assortative mixing, higher prevalence in a stratum means that sexual contact will present greater risk of transmission among persons in that stratum than among persons in lower prevalence strata. Dissortative mixing is a behavior with a lower risk of STI acquisition for a person in a high-prevalence subgroup but a higher risk for persons from a lower prevalence subgroup. Mixing that is random (partners are selected in proportion to their population distribution) with respect to a characteristic tends to equalize STI prevalence across groups with and without that characteristic.

Although a number of studies have examined mixing among individuals at high risk for STIs (for example, [40]), fewer have evaluated the extent of mixing in the general population. Dissortative mixing is more common among some populations, such as adolescents: 45% of sexually active adolescents in AddHealth reported partners who were at least 2 years younger or older than them; 42%, 14%, and 15%, respectively, of Latino, White, and Black youth had partners of different race/ethnicity [39]. Among San Francisco adults with two or more sex partners in the preceding year, the prevalence of mixing was substantial, with 40% of respondents reporting partners from at least two age groups or ethnic groups. These "heavy mixers" were significantly more likely to have antibodies to HSV-2 [41]. Mixing across different age groups is associated with HIV infection among young MSM [42, 43]. An analysis of sexual mixing patterns among African Americans in North Carolina revealed relatively discordant sexual mixing—especially among the general population of women—a group whose behavior was otherwise relatively at low risk [44]. For example, only 20% of male, compared to 40% of female, high school graduates had a recent partner who had not finished high school. These results were attributed in part to the low ratio of black men to black women.

"Bridging" occurs when individuals whose partnerships are not exclusively assortative connect networks that are otherwise sexually separate from each other. By connecting these otherwise isolated networks, bridging permits infections to spread between them. The level of bridging is thus a critical population-level parameter. A telephone survey of 18–39-year-old adults in Seattle evaluated the potential for bridging between respondents and their last two partners with respect to greater than 5-year age difference, education, bisexual activity, race, and spatial separation of residences; 74% reported dissortative mixing by at least one of the attributes examined [45]. A 1996 study in Thailand demonstrated that women outside the sex industry were placed at substantial risk for HIV infection by the women's high prevalence of male partners who had sex with commercial sex workers (CSWs) (17%), used condoms inconsistently with both CSWs and their non-CSW partners (73%), and were more likely to be HIV+ (OR 2.2). The study calculated that for every 100 sexually active men, 30 women in the general population had been exposed to HIV in the preceding year [46]. A study in Cambodia identified a substantial minority of men (20.5% of the military, 15.7% of police, and 14.7% of motodrivers) as bridgers who had unprotected sex with both high- and low-risk female sex partners [47].

Racially Segregated Sexual Networks

The long history and continued persistence of racial segregation in the USA has strongly promoted assortative mixing by race, which for African Americans has probably weakened the tendency toward assortative mixing by social stratification characteristics such as education, income, and wealth. Notwithstanding the many changes that have taken place in American society since the mid-twentieth century and the dismantling of the legal framework that enforced racial segregation in housing, employment, schools, and other settings including marriage and adoptions, African Americans and whites often still live, learn, work, worship, socialize, recreate, obtain health care, and retire in largely separate worlds. This de facto segregation is important to the structure of sexual networks, because people tend to choose sex partners from the neighborhoods where they live [48]. Segregation may be especially critical to the networks of young people, given continuing—and

increasing—racial segregation in schools [49, 50]. Concentration of Black people and other ethnic minority populations in urban areas and "white flight" to the suburbs have increased the physical separation of living areas to such an extent that school integration can require transferring children across school district lines. Meanwhile, racial segregation in higher education persists due to the concentration of African Americans in Historically Black Colleges and Universities (HBCUs) (in 2001, HBCUs conferred more than 20% of the bachelor's degrees earned by African Americans) [51] and increased underrepresentation of minorities at flagship institutions in states that banned affirmative action practices [52]. Even in multiracial settings, interracial mixing may be limited.

Racial segregation of sexual networks enables the huge Black–White disparity in STI rates to persist in several ways. Most directly, infections that enter the Black community are less likely to be eliminated because of less access to quality health care, and are more likely to remain within the Black population because of limited interracial sexual mixing. Moreover, the imbalanced sex ratio and other factors discussed above promote sexual network patterns that enhance STI dissemination in the Black population. Furthermore, racially segregated sexual networks provide relative protection to the White population, reducing the immediacy of the STI problem to the population with greater structural power to direct resources and shape public policies to control STI.

Sexual Network Influences from Movement of People and Information

Travel and Migration

Technological advances and economic forces that have occurred during the past 50 years have resulted in unprecedented mobility of the world's population. Sexual contact while traveling, whether for tourism, business, or long-term migration, is relatively common; an estimated 5–50% of short-term travelers have sexual contact, and the proportion is higher among longer term travelers [53]. Among 1,018 US Peace Corps volunteers who reported information on their sexual behavior, 61% reported having at least one sex partner during their stay abroad, and about 40% of sexually active volunteers reported having a local partner [54]. Sexual activity while traveling is most likely to occur among those who are male, young, traveling without a long-term partner, heavy alcohol consumers, users of recreational drugs, traveling for a long time, regular visitors to the same location, or people with other markers for high-risk sexual activity, such as early age at first intercourse, frequent casual sex in the traveler's country of origin, greater number of partners, and history of extramarital sex [55].

Travel frees people from social taboos and norms that inhibit their sexual freedom [53]. Sexual contact while traveling often results in dissortative mixing, as people from one geographic locale interact with those from another setting. Travelers and their sex partners are potentially important bridges between geographically separated populations. Indeed, many of the early HIV cases in North America were linked to a Canadian flight attendant who had numerous sexual contacts while traveling extensively [56]. The role of migrant workers, CSWs, and long-distance truck drivers in the HIV epidemic has been well established [57].

Several factors increase travelers' vulnerability to STIs. Some researchers, for example, note a higher frequency of casual partners and unprotected sex—sometimes because of substance use or unplanned or unexpected sexual opportunities [58–60]. Moreover, male travelers may interact with CSWs whose prevalence of STIs is high, while female business and recreational travelers may have sexual contact with male travelers or local men who have had contact with sex workers [58]. Economic inequality between wealthier tourists and sex workers in the countries they visit promotes exchange of sex.

Migration into the USA from many countries has increased during the past 20 years. The term acculturation refers to the changes that occur in both cultures when two cultures meet [61], but the minority culture usually changes more than

does the mainstream culture [62]. When minority groups acculturate, they tend to adopt the sexual behaviors of the larger culture, as increasing contact with the mainstream group introduces new norms and values [62]. Minnis et al. observed a lower prevalence of some sexual risk behaviors (first sexual intercourse before age 17, multiple partners) among foreign-born Latinas than among both non-Latinas and US-born Latinas [63]. Compared to their US-born counterparts, foreign-born Asian and Latino youth are less likely to use illicit drugs and to participate in sexual risk behaviors [64]. Some researchers have noted an association between increased acculturation and some higher risk sexual behaviors, such as increased partner number [65] and earlier age at first sexual intercourse [66], among more acculturated adult and adolescent Hispanics in the USA [65, 66].

Undocumented immigrants typically do not have a legal right to work and may be forced into the informal economy—often in low-paying service and manufacturing jobs—or, in some cases, commercial sex work. In areas where large number of men migrate alone to send wages home to their families, the resulting unbalanced sex ratios can promote "development of a commercial sex industry to service the unpartnered male population" [67]. Undocumented migrants often have limited access to health care and may be unable to obtain treatment for STIs.

Sex workers themselves may migrate to wealthier countries in order to exchange sex. Moreover, people who migrate because of poverty are at increased risk of engaging in commercial sex work; refugees or undocumented workers may be ineligible for legitimate employment. Sex traffickers transport people—especially women and children—for the express purpose of forced commercial sex. In a literature review of sex trafficking in the USA [68], Schauer and Wheaton envision the possibility that in the next 10 years sex trafficking will replace drug trafficking as the number one international crime. It is estimated that the USA is the second largest international destination (after Germany), receiving 18,000–50,000 women and children/year.

Media

Sociologists recognize the media as among the most significant agents in development of sexual behavior through young adulthood [69]. Popular music adolescents listen to most often is mainly about love, sex, and relationships. At least half of the girls aged 12–15 read magazines, such as *Teen* and *Seventeen*, whose major theme is how girls can make themselves attractive enough to get and hold onto a boy [70]. The media influences people's norms and attitudes. Communication researchers posit that the mass media impacts sexual norms and behavior by framing how people think about sex, displaying and reinforcing a consistent set of sexual and relationship norms, and seldom demonstrating sexually responsible models [71].

Television shows have substantial sexual content, and the amount of this content has increased in recent years. A Kaiser Family Foundation study examined a representative sample of 1,154 shows' broadcast in 2004 and 2005—covering the full range of genres other than daily newscasts, sports events, and children's shows—and determined the prevalence of shows with some type of sexual content [72]. Seventy percent of all shows (and 77% of those broadcast during prime time on the major networks) have sexual content—an increase compared to 56% of all shows in the first study in 1998 and 64% in 2002. 68% of all shows included talk about sex, and 35% of all shows portrayed sexual behaviors. Shows with sexual content had an average of 5.0 sexual scenes per hour, compared to 3.2 scenes in the 1998 study. Prime-time and top teen shows had even more sexual content with, respectively, 5.9 and 6.7 sexual scenes per hour. Among all shows in the sample, sexual intercourse was either depicted or strongly implied in 11%. As a result of the greater percentage of shows with sexual content and their greater average number of sexual scenes per show, the 2005 study found nearly twice the number of sexual scenes in the overall program sample as that observed in 1998, when Kaiser first conducted this study. Nearly half (45%) of the 20 shows most popular with teens include sexual behavior, and an additional 25% include some other kind of sexual content. About one in ten characters involved in sexual intercourse appeared to be teens or young adults. References to safer sex, sexual risks, and sexual responsibilities rarely appeared, and an increase noted in 2002 has not been sustained since then [72].

Despite extensive information about the extent of sexual content on American television, considerably less is known about whether the media's sexual content influences people's sexual behavior [71]. Most research has tended to focus on adolescents. In general, there is agreement among findings that increased exposure to sexual content in media is associated with "more permissive attitudes toward sexual activity, higher estimates of the sexual experience and activity of peers, and more and earlier sexual behavior among adolescents" p. 186 [73]. For example, a survey of 1,011 Black and White middle school students in the Southeastern USA revealed that adolescents who are exposed to more sexual content in the media, "and who perceive greater support from the media for teen sexual behavior, report more sexual activity and greater intentions to engage in sexual intercourse in the near future." [74]. Media influence was significantly associated with sexual behaviors and intentions—even after controlling for the influence of other important sources of socialization, such as family, peers, religion, and school. A longitudinal study of 1,017 middle school students examined whether exposure to sexual content in TV, movies, music, and magazines at baseline during ages 12–14 predicted sexual behavior 2 years later [75]. Although the relationship between media exposure and sexual behavior was not statistically significant among Black youth, White adolescents in the top quintile of sexual content exposure at baseline were more than twice as likely to have had sex by age 14–16 as those in the lowest quintile, even after controlling for baseline sexual behavior and other relevant factors.

Causal inference from observational studies such as the above is problematic, since it seems likely that adolescents with stronger sexual interests for reasons other than their media exposure are both more likely to consume sexual media content and also more likely to become sexually active. However, causal potential can be derived from evidence suggesting that mass media can promote sexual health. For example, mass media can be a positive influence on young women's sexual health and development by providing (1) information on sexuality and sexual health through mainstream magazines, newspapers, and radio and (2) diverse portraits of women and female sexuality that can function as models of sexual behavior [76]. Kaiser Family Foundation surveys of regular viewers who watched the TV series *ER* demonstrated that adults learned about HPV and emergency contraception after watching episodes of shows that contained story lines about these topics [77]. A 3-month safer sex televised public service advertisement campaign to increase safer sexual behavior among at-risk young adults in a Kentucky city resulted in significant increases in condom use, condom use self-efficacy, and behavioral intentions among the target group that viewed the ads compared to the control city [78].

"Entertainment-education" uses media to present educational content in an entertainment format to influence audiences' knowledge, attitudes, and behavior. This format has been used in developing countries and occasionally in the USA and other industrialized countries. Viewers of an entertainment-education soap opera in India reported changes in opinions about family planning and sexual behaviors that resulted from viewing the program, such as deciding to undergo a vasectomy, delaying daughters' age of marriage, and development of more negative attitudes toward dowries [79]. In Nigeria, two of the country's most famous singers, Onyeka Onwenu and King Sunny Ade, released two hit songs and accompanying music videos to promote sexual responsibility. During the music campaign contraceptive use increased from 16% to 26% among the target audience of youth and young adults, aged 15–35 [80].

The Internet

The Internet has profoundly altered many spheres of living including social and sexual networks. It is estimated that there were more than 250 million users in North America and 1.7 billion users in the world in 2009 [81], numbers that are certain to grow from initiatives such as the Federal Communications Commission's National Broadband Plan [82] and Google's experimental fiber network initiative [83]. People go online through computers at home, at work, in libraries, and in recreation facilities, as well as through portable or handheld devices accessing WiFi networks. The proliferation of access channels is expanding the range of people who make use of e-mail, special interest groups, chat rooms, Web surfing, file swapping, and/or social networking tools such as MySpace, Facebook, LinkedIn, Twitter, Flickr, YouTube, and Second Life. Explosive growth of social networking sites and associated Web 2.0 technologies is one of the most dramatic developments in Internet technology [84].

Thanks to social networking sites Americans now publicly disseminate an enormous amount of personal information and images that used to be seen primarily by family and close friends. The ability to find people and to get information about them through the Internet creates numerous opportunities to form social relationships and facilitates the process of becoming acquainted. Not surprisingly, a significant fraction of the population uses the Internet to find sex partners. Features that drive the Internet's popularity for sexual interactions include its accessibility, affordability, acceptability, and opportunities it provides for anonymity, learning about and experimenting with different aspects of sexuality or sexual practices, locating a much larger pool of potential sex partners, and more quickly meeting and communicating with potential partners [85, 86].

A 2005 Pew telephone survey of 3,215 US adults identified 2,252 Internet users [87]. Most (55%) of the single people looking for relationships said it was difficult to meet people in the areas where they lived. Respondents indicated a variety of ways to use the Internet related to sex partners: flirting, online dating Websites, finding an off-line venue like a nightclub or singles event where they might meet someone to date, use of e-mail or instant messaging by a third party who introduced them to a potential date, participation in online groups where they hoped to meet people to date, searching for information about someone they had dated in the past, maintenance of a long-distance relationship, searching for information about someone they were currently dating or were about to meet for a first date, and breaking up with a partner.

Slightly more than one in ten respondents (240) used online dating services. Among these online daters, 64% agreed that online dating helps people find a better match because they have access to a larger pool of people to date, and about half agreed that online dating is easier than other methods. 43% of people who used online dating sites actually followed through with a date, with online romances resulting in a long-term relationship or marriage among 17%. Online daters were younger and more likely to be employed; 18% of all online adults aged 18–29 have visited a dating site, compared to 11% of people aged 30–49, 6% of those aged 50–64, and 3% of those aged 65 or older. Online daters reported that they liked to try new things and tended to be less religious and to have relatively liberal social attitudes with respect to gender roles and gay marriage. Interestingly, the study did not find statistically significant differences in online dating use across race/ethnicity or educational levels.

A Dutch study also found no relationship between online dating and either income or education but found that the most active online daters were older (age 40), perhaps because of the relative difficulty this age group has in finding partners through traditional strategies. Divorced people were much more likely to use dating sites [88]. Interestingly, counter to the hypothesis that people use the Internet to compensate for social deficits in the off-line world, people involved in online dating did not report high levels of dating anxiety. As the Internet has become so widely used, the online and off-line populations have become increasingly alike [88].

Along with new opportunities for finding and connecting with sexual partners, the Internet has created new opportunities for transmitting HIV and other STIs—and also new opportunities for public health control activities [84, 89]. A study of clients at the Denver Public Health HIV testing

site in 1999 and 2000 found that 15.8% had used the Internet to find sex partners, and 65.2% of these clients reported having had sex with a partner they found online [89].

Most of the published research concerning the Internet and sexual risk behaviors has been done among men who have sex with men (MSM), as they were among the first groups to take advantage of this medium to find partners. According to a meta-analysis published in 2006, 40% of MSM used the Internet to look for sex partners [90]. White race/ethnicity, increased age, history of unprotected anal intercourse, multiple anal intercourse partners, and engaging in sexual activity at a sex club or a bathhouse have been associated with meeting sexual partners through the Internet [91]. MSM who sought partners online were more likely to engage in unprotected anal intercourse with male sex partners than were MSM who did not (odds ratio 1.68 [90]). Similarly, a study in a London HIV testing clinic found that both MSM and heterosexuals who used the Internet to find sex partners were significantly more likely to have had high-risk sex with a casual partner than those who did not use the Internet for this purpose. However, people who sought sex through the Internet were just as likely to meet their high-risk casual partners off-line as online, suggesting that people willing to engage in risky behavior were seeking sex via the Internet, rather than engaging in riskier behavior because of the Internet [92]. Thus, the Internet may not be responsible for stimulating high-risk behaviors, since high-risk behavior may simply be a characteristic of those who seek sex online [84]. Nevertheless, whether or not the Internet promotes risky behaviors, it certainly facilitates them, particularly among people already inclined to engage in them.

Use of the Internet to find sex partners facilitates intentional sexual mixing of both assortative and dissortative varieties. Websites open only to members of particular subgroups (e.g., the "The Right Stuff," "Latin Singles") facilitate assortative mixing. But some Websites (e.g., http//www. interracialmatch.com) draw people seeking partners of different cultures, races, and ethnicities. It is not yet clear whether this expanded opportunity for dissortative mixing will lead to a significant change in sexual mixing patterns of Americans [67].

Macrosocial Influences on Sexual Partnering and STI Epidemiology

Individuals' choice of partners and the acceptability of different partnership arrangements are influenced by the social environment. A key environmental variable in this regard is the sex ratio, the importance of which has been noted by Guttentag and Secord [93]. The principles of microeconomics provide a useful model of how the sex ratio (ratio of the number of men to the number of women) influences individual choices. Individual behavior is influenced by perceived costs and benefits of different choices. In a market situation in which people seek to maximize benefits and minimize costs, relatively scarce but desirable resources command higher prices than less desirable or more plentiful resources [94, 95]. When there is a relative shortage of eligible males, such males command a higher "price." Because men in this setting have advantageous alternatives, they are less dependent on any individual female partner. Conversely, women in a low-sex-ratio environment have fewer advantageous alternatives and are therefore more dependent on a given partnership. "Dyadic power" refers to the relative strength of a partner's bargaining position. When desirable males are in relatively shorter supply, their dyadic power enables them to negotiate more favorable "terms of trade," which may include the freedom to have multiple female partners even if the female partners prefer exclusive partnerships [93].

Gender inequality derives not only from men's greater average physical strength and aggressiveness, which carry with them the potential for intimate partner violence, but also from the substantially greater economic rewards and resources they enjoy in most societies. Gender inequality affects sexual behaviors, sexual networks, and STI transmission in a variety of ways. Low sexual relationship power among women is associated with decreased condom use [96]. Lack of economic independence, particularly when combined with a low sex ratio, can persuade some women to begin or maintain relationships they would otherwise end [97]. Non-volitional sex and intimate partner violence increase women's vulnerability to STIs; women who are victims of violence or who live in fear of violence can seldom implement risk reduction measures, such as condom use, reduction in partner numbers, or avoidance of partners with high-risk behaviors [98–100].

Structural Power

The term "structural power" refers to economic, political, and legal power, which augment each other, and enable dominant groups in society to "influence and shape social customs and practices, which in turn are a powerful source of control over people's lives." [93] (p. 26). Structural power is held by those nearer the top of socioeconomic hierarchies and serves to reinforce those hierarchies, as privileged persons protect themselves and limit the scope of action ("agency") of those of lower socioeconomic and/or minority status [101]. Population health is powerfully influenced by these social class gradients [102] both because those at the lower end of the scale lack important resources for health and because their environment and opportunities are shaped by those nearer the top of the distribution of money, resources, and power [2]. Through the pathways of differential economic, political, and legal power and resulting social class gradients, structural power affects not only health but also sexual partnering and ultimately STI epidemiology as well.

Incarceration

Incarceration—a stark application of structural power—disrupts existing partnerships, affecting sexual networks and partnering patterns [5]. When one member of a partnership is incarcerated, the remaining partner may pursue other partnerships to make up for the loss of social and sexual companionship and material contributions. Resumption of the original partnership when the incarcerated partner is released creates a situation of concurrent partnerships. Such "separational concurrency" may be common among people whose partners are frequently incarcerated [103]. Perhaps for this reason, incarceration of a sex partner was a risk factor for concurrent partnerships among young men and women in Seattle and Black men and women from the general population in the southern US [104, 105].

Meanwhile, the partner who is incarcerated may form new, sometimes coercive, sexual connections with a pool of individuals among whom the prevalences of high-risk behaviors, HIV infection, and other STIs are high—in a setting where condoms are typically illegal [106–109]. Inmates may also join gangs and develop new long-term ties with antisocial networks [110]. These new associations may connect individuals who were previously at low risk for HIV infection with subgroups whose HIV prevalence is high, so that when inmates return to the community their new associations may lead to sexual partnerships with higher risk partners. A history of incarceration also reduces one's employment prospects [111], which increases risk of poverty and further destabilizes long-term partnerships [112, 113].

Because of the proportion of people and ethnic groups affected, incarceration also adversely affects the community. The US has the highest incarceration rate in the world [114], with about 1% of all US adults in jail or prison in 2007 [115], and over 3.2% of all adult US residents (7.3 million people) on probation, in jail or prison, or on parole at the end of 2008 [116]. Blacks and Hispanics are disproportionately incarcerated, partly as a reflection of ongoing and pervasive racial bias in sentencing of young Black and Hispanic men [117]. In 2008, 3.2% of all US Black men (and 0.15% of Black women) were in federal or state prisons [118]. Among men 25–29 years old in 2002, 10.4% of Blacks and 2.4% of Hispanics, compared to 1.2% of White men, were in prison [119]. Cumulative risk of prison incarceration for 30–34-year-old men born between 1965 and 1969 was 2.91% for Whites,

compared to 20.5% for Blacks [120]. Incarceration on this scale contributes to high unemployment rates in minority communities, shrinking the proportion of financially viable male partners. Incarceration thus reduces the already low ratio of marriageable men to women [4]. High incarceration rates also can influence community norms and create an environment in which "jail culture is normative," as evidenced by trends in clothing and music [110] (p. 224). These norms are likely to influence sexual behavior and sexual networks. In addition, the heavy reliance on incarceration to control drug and crime problems has stressed state budgets and decreased spending for programs, such as education, that can improve communities and the lives of their residents [115].

Poverty, Income Inequality, and Discrimination

Numerous studies have documented poverty's association with mortality and morbidity, including HIV and other STIs (for example, [121–123]). Evidence indicates that in addition to poverty, income *inequality* is itself harmful to health [124–126]. Increases in income inequality, such as those observed in the US, have been associated with increased STI rates [127, 128]. For many Blacks, racism and discrimination are a constant feature of the contextual landscape, which differs dramatically from that of Whites. Residential segregation by race has been one of the most prominent features of racial discrimination in the US. Marked residential segregation by race persists, particularly in urban areas, and is maintained not only by individual actions but also by long-standing structural mechanisms, such as discrimination by banks and realtors [129]. Segregation concentrates poverty and other deleterious social and economic influences within racially isolated groups and thus increases the risk of socioeconomic failure of the segregated group [129]. Segregation has effects in addition to those mediated by lower individual income. For example, compared with the children of middle-income White families, children of middle-income Black families are more likely to be exposed to violence, poverty, drugs, and teenage pregnancy in the neighborhoods where they live [129].

Poverty and racism affect sexual health directly and through a variety of pathways—typically by decreasing the personal agency of those who are affected and placing them "in harm's way." [130]. For example, following the decline in housing prices that helped precipitate the 2008–2009 recession, prosecutors and other officials in several US cities filed lawsuits against Wells Fargo for targeting subprime mortgages at Blacks and Hispanics compared to Whites with similar incomes [131]. 55% of loans to African Americans, 40% to Hispanics, and 35% to Native Americans were subprime loans—compared to 23% to Whites. Women received less favorable lending terms than men [132]. As a result, disproportionate numbers of minority homeowners have experienced or still face foreclosure. The problem is most acute for people who are both poor and the objects of discrimination. Thus in the US one expects—and sees—worse health among the racial minorities who are most likely to experience both poverty and racial/ethnic discrimination: African Americans, Hispanics, and Native Americans, groups who disproportionately experience other societal hardships as well.

Institutional racism is a key factor underlying the enduring racial disparities in income, education, housing, neighborhood quality, government services, political power, morbidity, and mortality [129, 133–136]. Krieger describes five pathways through which discrimination can harm health [137]. Pathways with direct relevance to sexual networks and spread of STIs include economic and social deprivation, residential segregation, targeted marketing of legal and illegal psychoactive substances, and inadequate health care from health care facilities and from specific providers [137].

Poverty and stresses induced by racism tend to destabilize marriage and other long-term partnerships and behaviors; the poor are less likely to marry and less likely to stay married [112]. Women are more likely to be poor, and poverty can further distort gender roles. Poor women may be more likely to stay in relationships that

increase their risk of STI and are in some cases less able to negotiate safer sexual behaviors, such as condom use. In these ways, poverty and racism can have profound effects on partnering and networks.

Homelessness

Homelessness in the US has dramatically increased in the past 20 years, with an estimated 3.5 million people now experiencing homelessness annually [138]. The number of homeless who are living on the streets of New York City, for example, soared 34% between 2009 and 2010, a phenomenon attributed to the 2008–2009 economic recession [139]. Still others are unstably housed with family or friends. Although estimates of racial/ethnic composition vary by region of the country, the homeless population is estimated to be 42% Black, 39% White, 13% Hispanic, 4% Native American, and 2% Asian [138]. About 26% of homeless people are mentally ill, while 13% are physically disabled, and 2% are HIV infected [138, 140].

Homelessness is strongly associated with HIV infection [141, 142]. The rate of AIDS diagnosis among people admitted to public shelters in the city of Philadelphia was nine times that of the city's general population [142]. Moreover, a longitudinal study revealed a dose–response relationship between housing status and HIV risk behavior, with the homeless demonstrating higher risk than those in unstable housing, and both of these groups at higher risk than people with stable housing [143].

Housing can affect sexual risk behaviors through a variety of pathways. People may trade sex for shelter [143]. Lack of housing may prevent people from keeping condoms accessible [144, 145]. In addition, housing affects the structure of social networks, and social network norms and values influence individuals' risk behaviors [144, 146]. Housing may also affect relationships with sexual partners. Homelessness is associated with exposure to intimate partner violence, which may in turn increase HIV risk behavior; sexual coercion and the threat of violence may prevent women from refusing sexual contact or negotiating condom use [144, 145].

Aidala and Sumartojo note that although much of the literature concerning homelessness and its health risks has focused on the characteristics of individuals that put them at risk for homelessness, housing is a manifestation of social and economic inequalities—and further contributes to these inequalities [147]. The risk of becoming homeless in a given community depends largely upon contextual factors, including employment security, adequacy of social services, government policies, institutional practices, and availability of affordable housing. These factors are for the most part outside the individual's control [147]. For example, foreclosures resulting from the subprime mortgage crisis that contributed to the 2008–2009 recession caused homeowners to lose their dwellings. But an additional cause of the related increase in homelessness in US cities was foreclosures on rental properties. In such foreclosures, tenants may be forced out on short notice, unable to recover their security deposits, and highly vulnerable [140].

Conclusions

Social factors are major determinants of the epidemiology of STI, through both direct and indirect pathways. Causes of STI include lack of preventive knowledge, lack of preventive behavior, lack of prompt and effective health care, and social network patterns that facilitate STI dissemination. Although this chapter has focused on social and sexual networks of heterosexuals, we acknowledge that networks of MSM and men who have sex with men and women are also critically important. Social factors influence availability and access to accurate and useful knowledge about sexuality and STI avoidance, encourage or constrain preventive behavior, facilitate or obstruct access to quality health care, and facilitate some partnerships and obstruct or disrupt others. Causes also include underlying conditions and factors that shape desires and attitudes, alter choices and availability of options, and lead to a multitude of adverse outcomes including

exposure to STI. Communicable infections, especially those that spread person-to-person, are inherently social. Thus it is almost axiomatic that social determinants are the major drivers of STI epidemiology. Over 50 years ago the British epidemiologist Jerry Morris wrote, "Society largely determines health; ill-health is not a personal misfortune due often to personal inadequacy but a social misfortune due, more commonly, to social mismanagement and social failure." [148].

The US needs a new approach to public health—an approach that promotes design and implementation of programs that effectively address the social determinants of STIs and other health outcomes; increasing evidence indicates that such interventions will have the greatest public health impact [149]. This new approach will require researchers and public health practitioners to forge and strengthen collaborations among communities, academia, government, and private sector [150]. These collaborations will be needed not only to develop and implement interventions but also to document that these strategies have favorable cost-effectiveness profiles and to find ways for the program providers to capture the cost savings so that interventions become scalable and sustainable.

References

1. Syme SL, Berkman LF. Social class, susceptibility and sickness. Am J Epidemiol. 1976;104(1):1–8.
2. World Health Organization. Social determinants of health. 2010. http://www.who.int/social_determinants/en/. Accessed 22 Mar 2010.
3. Cohen JM, Wilson ML, Aiello AE. Analysis of social epidemiology research on infectious diseases: historical patterns and future opportunities. J Epidemiol Community Health. 2007;61(12):1021–7.
4. Adimora AA, Schoenbach VJ. Contextual factors and the black-white disparity in heterosexual HIV transmission. Epidemiology. 2002;13(6):707–12.
5. Adimora AA, Schoenbach VJ. Social context, sexual networks, and racial disparities in rates of sexually transmitted infections. J Infect Dis. 2005;191 Suppl 1:S115–22.
6. Lane SD, Rubinstein RA, Keefe RH, et al. Structural violence and racial disparity in HIV transmission. J Health Care Poor Underserved. 2004;15(3):319–35.
7. Blankenship KM, Friedman SR, Dworkin S, Mantell JE. Structural interventions: concepts, challenges

and opportunities for research. J Urban Health. 2006; 83(1):59–72.

8. Lin JS, Whitlock E, O'Connor E, Bauer V. Behavioral counseling to prevent sexually transmitted infections: a systematic review for the U.S. Preventive Services Task Force. Ann Intern Med. 2008;149(7):497–508. W496–99.

9. Anderson RM. Transmission dynamics of sexually transmitted infections. In: Holmes KK, Mardh PA, Sparling PF, et al., editors. Sexually transmitted diseases. 3rd ed. New York City: McGraw-Hill; 1999.

10. Dieffenbach CW, Fauci AS. Universal voluntary testing and treatment for prevention of HIV transmission. JAMA. 2009;301(22):2380–2.

11. Holmes KK, Levine R, Weaver M. Effectiveness of condoms in preventing sexually transmitted infections. Bull World Health Organ. 2004;82(6):454–61.

12. Weller S, Davis K. Condom effectiveness in reducing heterosexual HIV transmission. Cochrane Database Syst Rev. 2002(1):CD003255.

13. Steiner MJ, Cates Jr W, Warner L. The real problem with male condoms is nonuse. Sex Transm Dis. 1999;26(8):459–62.

14. Mosher WD, Martinez GM, Chandra A, Abma JC, Willson SJ. Use of contraception and use of family planning services in the United States: 1982–2002. Adv Data. 2004;350:1–36.

15. Anderson JE, Mosher WD, Chandra A. Measuring HIV risk in the U.S. population aged 15–44: results from Cycle 6 of the National Survey of Family Growth. Adv Data. 2006(377):1–27.

16. CSDH. Closing the gap in a generation: health equity through action on the social determinants of health. Final report of the Commission on Social Determinants of Health. Geneva: World Health Organization; 2008.

17. Smedley BD, Stith AY, Nelson AR, editors. Unequal treatment: confronting racial and ethnic disparities in health care. Washington, DC: National Academies Press; 2003.

18. DeNavas-Walt C, Proctor BD, Smith JC. Income, poverty, and health insurance coverage in the United States: 2008. Washington, DC: U.S. Census Bureau; 2009.

19. National Alliance of State and Territorial AIDS Directors. The ADAP watch: May 21, 2010. 2010. http://www.nastad.org/Docs/Public/ InFocus/2010521_ADAP%20Watch%20update%20 -%205.21.10.pdf. Accessed 14 Mar 2010.

20. Card JJ, Lessard L, Benner T. PASHA: facilitating the replication and use of effective adolescent pregnancy and STI/HIV prevention programs. J Adolesc Health. 2007;40(3):275.e1–14.

21. Trenholm C, Devaney B, Fortson K, Quay L, Wheeler J, Clark M. Impacts of four title V, section 510 abstinence education programs final report April 2007. Princeton, NJ: Mathematica Policy Research, Inc.; 2007.

22. United States House of Representatives Committee on Government Reform – Minority Staff Special Investigations Division. The content of federally funded abstinence-only education programs. Washington, DC, United States House of Representatives Committee on Government Reform. 2004. http://oversight.house.gov/documents/ 20041201102153-50247.pdf. Accessed 8 Mar 2008.

23. Jemmott 3rd JB, Jemmott LS, Fong GT. Efficacy of a theory-based abstinence-only intervention over 24 months: a randomized controlled trial with young adolescents. Arch Pediatr Adolesc Med. 2010;164(2):152–9.

24. Laumann EO, Gagnon JH, Michael RT, Michaels S. The social organization of sexuality. Chicago: The University of Chicago Press; 1994.

25. Meschke LL, Zweig JM, Barber BL, Eccles JS. Demographic, biological, psychological, and social predictors of the timing of first intercourse. J Res Adolesc. 2000;10(3):315–8.

26. DeLamater J. The social control of sexuality. Annu Rev Sociol. 1981;7:263–90.

27. Miller BC, Heaton TB. Age at first sexual intercourse and the timing of marriage and childbirth. J Marriage Fam. 1991;53(3):719–32.

28. Simmons T, O'Connell M. Married-couple and unmarried-partner households: 2000, census 2000 special reports. U.S. Census Bureau. 2003. http:// www.census.gov/prod/2003pubs/censr-5.pdf. Accessed 20 May 2010.

29. Turner CF, Danella RD, Rogers SM. Sexual behavior in the United States 1930–1990: trends and methodological problems. Sex Transm Dis. 1995;22(3):173–90.

30. Kraut-Becher JR, Aral SO. Gap length: an important factor in sexually transmitted disease transmission. Sex Transm Dis. 2003;30(3):221–5.

31. Foxman B, Newman M, Percha B, Holmes KK, Aral SO. Measures of sexual partnerships: lengths, gaps, overlaps, and sexually transmitted infection. Sex Transm Dis. 2006;33(4):209–14.

32. Morris M, Kretzschmar M. Concurrent partnerships and transmission dynamics in networks. Soc Net. 1995;17:299–318.

33. Koumans E, Farley T, Gibson J, et al. Characteristics of persons with syphilis in areas of persisting syphilis in the United States: sustained transmission associated with concurrent partnerships. Sex Transm Dis. 2001;28:497–503.

34. Potterat J, Zimmerman-Rogers H, Muth S, et al. Chlamydia transmission: concurrency, reproduction number, and the epidemic trajectory. Am J Epidemiol. 1999;150:1331–9.

35. Adimora AA, Schoenbach VJ, Martinson FE, et al. Heterosexually transmitted HIV infection among African Americans in North Carolina. J Acquir Immune Defic Syndr. 2006;41(5):616–23.

36. Adimora A, Schoenbach V, Bonas D, Martinson F, Donaldson K, Stancil T. Concurrent sexual partnerships among women in the United States. Epidemiology. 2002;13:320–7.

37. Adimora AA, Schoenbach VJ, Doherty IA. Concurrent sexual partnerships among men in the United States. Am J Public Health. 2007;97(12):2230–7.

38. Adimora AA, Schoenbach VJ, Taylor EM, Khan MR, Schwartz RJ. Concurrent partnerships, nonmonogamous partners, and substance use among women in the United States. Am J Public Health. 2011;101(1): 128–36.

39. Ford K, Sohn W, Lepkowski J. American adolescents: sexual mixing patterns, bridge partners, and concurrency. Sex Transm Dis. 2002;29(1):13–9.

40. Aral SO, Hughes J, Stoner B, et al. Sexual mixing patterns in the spread of gonococcal and chlamydial infections. Am J Public Health. 1999;89:825–33.

41. Catania JA, Binson D, Stone V. Relationship of sexual mixing across age and ethnic groups to herpes simplex virus-2 among unmarried heterosexual adults with multiple sexual partners. Health Psychol. 1996;15(5):362–70.

42. Service S, Blower SM. HIV transmission in sexual networks: an empirical analysis. Proc R Soc Lond B Biol Sci. 1995;260(1359):237–44.

43. Hurt CB, Matthews DD, Calabria MS, et al. Sex with older partners is associated with primary HIV infection among men who have sex with men in North Carolina. J Acquir Immune Defic Syndr. 2010;54(2):185–90.

44. Doherty IA, Schoenbach VJ, Adimora AA. Sexual mixing patterns and heterosexual HIV transmission among African Americans in the southeastern United States. J Acquir Immune Defic Syndr. 2009;52(1): 114–20.

45. Spicknall IH, Aral SO, Holmes KK, Foxman B. Sexual networks are diverse and complex: prevalence of relationships bridging population subgroups in the Seattle Sex Survey. Sex Transm Dis. 2009;36(8): 465–72.

46. Morris M, Podhisita C, Wawer MJ, Handcock MS. Bridge populations in the spread of HIV/AIDS in Thailand. AIDS. 1996;10(11):1265–71.

47. Gorbach PM, Sopheab H, Phalla T, et al. Sexual bridging by Cambodian men: potential importance for general population spread of STD and HIV epidemics. Sex Transm Dis. 2000;27(6):320–6.

48. Zenilman JM, Ellish N, Fresia A, Glass G. The geography of sexual partnerships in Baltimore: applications of core theory dynamics using a geographic information system. Sex Transm Dis. 1999;26(2):75–81.

49. Orfield G, Gordon N. Schools more separate: consequences of a decade of resegregation. Cambridge, MA: Harvard University; 2001.

50. Orfield G, Lee C. Racial transformation and the changing nature of segregation. Cambridge, MA: The Civil Rights Project at Harvard University; 2006.

51. Provasnik S, Shafer LL. Historically black colleges and universities, 1976 to 2001 (NCES 2004-062). Washington, DC, US Department of Education, National Center for Education Statistics. 2004. http://nces.ed.gov/pubs2004/2004062.pdf. Accessed 20 May 2010.

52. Long MC. Affirmative action and its alternatives in public universities: what do we know? Public Adm Rev. 2007;67(2):315–30.

53. Matteelli A, Carosi G. Sexually transmitted diseases in travelers. Clin Infect Dis. 2001;32(7):1063–7.

54. Moore J, Beeker C, Harrison JS, Eng TR, Doll LS. HIV risk behavior among Peace Corps Volunteers. AIDS. 1995;9(7):795–9.

55. Richens J. Sexually transmitted infections and HIV among travellers: a review. Travel Med Infect Dis. 2006;4(3–4):184–95.

56. Shilts R. And the band played on. New York: St. Martin's Press; 1987.

57. Carswell JW, Lloyd G, Howells J. Prevalence of HIV-1 in East African lorry drivers. AIDS. 1989;3(11): 759–61.

58. Abdullah AS, Ebrahim SH, Fielding R, Morisky DE. Sexually transmitted infections in travelers: implications for prevention and control. Clin Infect Dis. 2004;39(4):533–8.

59. Hawkes S, Hart GJ, Johnson AM, et al. Risk behaviour and HIV prevalence in international travellers. AIDS. 1994;8(2):247–52.

60. Abdullah AS, Fielding R, Hedley AJ. Travel, sexual behaviour, and the risk of contracting sexually transmitted diseases. Hong Kong Med J. 1998;4(2): 137–44.

61. Redfield R, Linton R, Linton R, Herskovits MJ. Memorandum on the study of acculturation. Am Anthropol. 1936;38:149–52.

62. Berry JW. Immigration, acculturation, and adaptation. Appl Psychol. 1997;46(1):5–34.

63. Minnis AM, Padian NS. Reproductive health differences among Latin American- and US-born young women. J Urban Health. 2001;78(4):627–37.

64. Hussey JM, Hallfors DD, Waller MW, Iritani BJ, Halpern CT, Bauer DJ. Sexual behavior and drug use among Asian and Latino adolescents: association with immigrant status. J Immigr Minor Health. 2007;9(2):85–94.

65. Ford K, Norris AE. Urban Hispanic adolescents and young adults: relationship of acculturation to sexual behavior. J Sex Res. 1993;30(4):316–23.

66. Upchurch DM, Aneshensel CS, Mudgal J, McNeely CS. Sociocultural contexts of time to first sex among Hispanic adolescents. J Marriage Fam. 2001;63(4): 1158–69.

67. Aral SO, Ward H. Modern day influences on sexual behavior. Infect Dis Clin North Am. 2005;19(2): 297–309.

68. Schauer EJ, Wheaton EM. Sex trafficking into the United States: a literature review. Crim Justice Rev. 2006;31(2):146–69.

69. Gagnon J, Simon W. Sexual conduct: the social sources of human sexuality. Chicago: Aldone; 1973.

70. Brown JD, Halpern CT, L'Engle KL. Mass media as a sexual super peer for early maturing girls. J Adolesc Health. 2005;36(5):420–7.

71. Brown JD. Mass media influences on sexuality. J Sex Res. 2002;39(1):42–5.

72. Kunkel D, Eyal K, Finnerty K, Biely E, Donnerstein E. Sex on TV: a Kaiser Family Foundation report. Menlo Park, CA: Kaiser Family Foundation; 2005.

73. Rich M. Sex screen: the dilemma of media exposure and sexual behavior. Pediatrics. 2005;116(1):329–31.
74. L'Engle KL, Brown JD, Kenneavy K. The mass media are an important context for adolescents' sexual behavior. J Adolesc Health. 2006;38(3):186–92.
75. Brown JD, L'Engle KL, Pardun CJ, Guo G, Kenneavy K, Jackson C. Sexy media matter: exposure to sexual content in music, movies, television, and magazines predicts black and white adolescents' sexual behavior. Pediatrics. 2006;117(4):1018–27.
76. Ward LM, Day KM, Epstein M. Uncommonly good: exploring how mass media may be a positive influence on young women's sexual health and development. New Dir Child Adolesc Dev. 2006;112:57–70.
77. Brodie M, Foehr U, Rideout V, et al. Communicating health information through the entertainment media. Health Aff. 2001;20(1):192–9.
78. Zimmerman RS, Palmgreen PM, Noar SM, Lustria ML, Lu HY, Lee Horosewski M. Effects of a televised two-city safer sex mass media campaign targeting high-sensation-seeking and impulsive-decision-making young adults. Health Educ Behav. 2007;34(5):810–26.
79. Papa M, Singhal A, Law S, et al. Entertainment-education and social change: an analysis of parasocial interaction, social learning, collective efficacy, and paradoxical communication. J Commun. 2000;50:31–55.
80. Brown WJ, Fraser BP. Celebrity identification in entertainment-education. In: Singhal A, Cody MJ, Rogers EM, Sabido M, editors. Entertainment-education and social change: history, research, and practice. Mahwah, NJ: Lawrence Erlbaum Associates; 2004.
81. Internet World Stats. Internet world stats: usage and population statistics. 2009. http://www.internetworldstats.com/stats.htm. Accessed 21 Jan 2011.
82. Stelter B, Wortham J. Effort to widen U.S. Internet access sets up battle. The New York Times. 2010. http://www.nytimes.com/2010/03/13/business/media/13fcc.html?emc=eta1. Accessed 21 Jan 2011.
83. Google. Think big with a gig: our experimental fiber network. The Official Google Blog. 2010. http://googleblog.blogspot.com/2010/02/think-big-with-gig-our-experimental.html. Accessed 20 May 2010.
84. Rietmeijer CA, McFarlane M. Web 2.0 and beyond: risks for sexually transmitted infections and opportunities for prevention. Curr Opin Infect Dis. 2009;22(1):67–71.
85. Ross MW, Rosser BR, Stanton J. Beliefs about cybersex and Internet-mediated sex of Latino men who have Internet sex with men: relationships with sexual practices in cybersex and in real life. AIDS Care. 2004;16(8):1002–11.
86. McFarlane M, Bull SS, Rietmeijer CA. Young adults on the Internet: risk behaviors for sexually transmitted diseases and HIV(1). J Adolesc Health. 2002;31(1):11–6.
87. Madden M, Lenhart A. Online dating. Washington, DC, Pew Internet and American Life Project. 2006.
http://www.pewinternet.org/Reports/2006/Online-Dating.aspx?r=1. Accessed 9 Jan 2010.
88. Valkenburg PM, Peter J. Who visits online dating sites? Exploring some characteristics of online daters. Cyberpsychol Behav. 2007;10(6):849–52.
89. McFarlane M, Bull SS, Rietmeijer CA. The Internet as a newly emerging risk environment for sexually transmitted diseases. JAMA. 2000;284(4):443–6.
90. Liau A, Millett G, Marks G. Meta-analytic examination of online sex-seeking and sexual risk behavior among men who have sex with men. Sex Transm Dis. 2006;33(9):576–84.
91. Garofalo R, Herrick A, Mustanski BS, Donenberg GR. Tip of the Iceberg: young men who have sex with men, the Internet, and HIV risk. Am J Public Health. 2007;97(6):1113–7.
92. Bolding G, Davis M, Hart G, Sherr L, Elford J. Heterosexual men and women who seek sex through the Internet. Int J STD AIDS. 2006;17(8):530–4.
93. Guttentag M, Secord P. Too many women: the sex ratio question. Beverly Hills: Sage; 1983.
94. Baumeister RF, Vohs KD. Sexual economics: sex as female resource for social exchange in heterosexual interactions. Pers Soc Psychol Rev. 2004;8(4):339–63.
95. Becker GS. The economic approach to human behavior. Chicago: The University of Chicago Press; 1976.
96. Pulerwitz J, Amaro H, De Jong W, Gortmaker SL, Rudd R. Relationship power, condom use and HIV risk among women in the USA. AIDS Care. 2002;14(6):789–800.
97. Adimora AA, Schoenbach VJ, Martinson FE, Donaldson KH, Fullilove RE, Aral SO. Social context of sexual relationships among rural African Americans. Sex Transm Dis. 2001;28(2):69–76.
98. Kalmuss D. Nonvolitional sex and sexual health. Arch Sex Behav. 2004;33(3):197–209.
99. El-Bassel N, Gilbert L, Wu E, Go H, Hill J. HIV and intimate partner violence among methadone-maintained women in New York City. Soc Sci Med. 2005;61(1):171–83.
100. Maman S, Campbell J, Sweat MD, Gielen AC. The intersections of HIV and violence: directions for future research and interventions. Soc Sci Med. 2000;50(4):459–78.
101. Aral SO. Understanding racial-ethnic and societal differentials in STI. Sex Transm Infect. 2002;78(1):2–4.
102. Marmot MG. Status syndrome: a challenge to medicine. JAMA. 2006;295(11):1304–7.
103. Gorbach PM, Stoner BP, Aral SO, Whittington WLH, Holmes KK. "It takes a village": understanding concurrent sexual partnerships in Seattle, Washington. Sex Transm Dis. 2002;29(8):453–62.
104. Manhart LE, Aral SO, Holmes KK, Foxman B. Sex partner concurrency: measurement, prevalence, and correlates among urban 18-39-year-olds. Sex Transm Dis. 2002;29(3):133–43.
105. Adimora AA, Schoenbach VJ, Martinson F, Donaldson KH, Stancil TR, Fullilove RE. Concurrent sexual partnerships among African Americans in the rural south. Ann Epidemiol. 2004;14(3):155–60.

106. Heimberger TS, Chang HG, Birkhead GS, et al. High prevalence of syphilis detected through a jail screening program. A potential public health measure to address the syphilis epidemic. Arch Intern Med. 1993;153(15):1799–804.
107. Cohen D, Scribner R, Clark J, Cory D. The potential role of custody facilities in controlling sexually transmitted diseases. Am J Public Health. 1992;82(4):552–6.
108. Wolfe MI, Xu F, Patel P, et al. An outbreak of syphilis in Alabama prisons: correctional health policy and communicable disease control. Am J Public Health. 2001;91(8):1220–5.
109. Spaulding A, Lubelczyk RB, Flanigan T. Can unsafe sex behind bars be barred? Am J Public Health. 2001;91(8):1176–7.
110. Freudenberg N. Jails, prisons, and the health of urban populations: a review of the impact of the correctional system on community health. J Urban Health. 2001;78(2):214–35.
111. Butterfield F. Freed from prison, but still paying a penalty: ex-convicts face many sanctions. The New York Times. 2002: A18.
112. Ross H, Sawhill I. Time of transition: the growth of families headed by women. Washington, DC: The Urban Institute; 1975.
113. Hoffman S, Holmes J. Husbands, wives, and divorce. In: Duncan G, Morgan J, editors. Five thousand American families – patterns of economic progress. Ann Arbor, Michigan: Institute for Social Research; 1976. p. 23–75.
114. Walmsley R. World prison population list. 8th ed. London, King's College London International Centre for Prison Studies. 2009. http://www.kcl.ac.uk/depsta/law/research/icps/downloads/wppl-8th_41.pdf. Accessed 23 Jan 2011.
115. The Pew Charitable Trusts. One in one hundred: behind bars in America in 2008. Washington, DC, The Pew Charitable Trusts. 2008. http://www.pewcenteronthestates.org/uploadedFiles/One%20in%20100.pdf. Accessed 2 Mar 2008.
116. Bureau of Justice Statistics. Total correctional population. 2010. http://bjs.ojp.usdoj.gov/index.cfm?ty=tp&tid=11. Accessed 15 Mar 2010.
117. Kansal T, Mauer M. Racial disparity in sentencing: a review of the literature. Washington, DC, The Sentencing Project. 2005. http://www.sentencingproject.org/doc/publications/rd_sentencing_review.pdf. Accessed 15 Mar 2010.
118. Bureau of Justice Statistics. Prisoners in 2008. 2009. http://bjs.ojp.usdoj.gov/index.cfm?ty=pbdetail&iid=1763. Accessed 15 Mar 2010.
119. Butterfield F. Study finds 2.6% increase in U.S. prison population. The New York Times. July 28, 2003: A12.
120. Pettit B, Western B. Mass imprisonment and the life course: race and class inequality in U.S. incarceration. Am Sociol Rev. 2004;69(2):151–69.
121. Ellerbrock TV, Lieb S, Harrington PE, et al. Heterosexually transmitted human immunodeficiency virus infection among pregnant women in a rural Florida community. N Engl J Med. 1992;327(24):1704–9.
122. Zierler S, Krieger N, Tang Y, et al. Economic deprivation and AIDS incidence in Massachusetts. Am J Public Health. 2000;90(7):1064–73.
123. St. Louis ME, Conway GA, Hayman CR, Miller C, Petersen LR, Dondero TJ. Human immunodeficiency virus infection in disadvantaged adolescents. Findings from the US Job Corps. JAMA. 1991; 266(17):2387–91.
124. Lochner K, Pamuk E, Makuc D, Kennedy BP, Kawachi I. State-level income inequality and individual mortality risk: a prospective, multilevel study. Am J Public Health. 2001;91(3):385–91.
125. Lynch JW, Kaplan GA, Pamuk ER, et al. Income inequality and mortality in metropolitan areas of the United States. Am J Public Health. 1998;88(7):1074–80.
126. Kaplan GA, Pamuk ER, Lynch JW, Cohen RD, Balfour JL. Inequality in income and mortality in the United States: analysis of mortality and potential pathways. BMJ. 1996;312(7037):999–1003.
127. Aral SO. The social context of syphilis persistence in the southeastern United States. Sex Transm Dis. 1996;23(1):9–15.
128. Holtgrave DR, Crosby RA. Social capital, poverty, and income inequality as predictors of gonorrhoea, syphilis, chlamydia and AIDS case rates in the United States. Sex Transm Infect. 2003;79(1):62–4.
129. Massey DS, Denton NA. American apartheid: segregation and the making of the underclass. Cambridge, MA: Harvard University Press; 1993.
130. Farmer PE, Nizeye B, Stulac S, Keshavjee S. Structural violence and clinical medicine. PLoS Med. 2006;3(10):e449.
131. Powell M. Memphis accuses Wells Fargo of discriminating against blacks. The New York Times. December 30, 2009.
132. Times TNY. Mortgages and minorities. The New York Times. December 9, 2008.
133. Jones CP. Levels of racism: a theoretic framework and a gardener's tale. Am J Public Health. 2000; 90(8):1212–5.
134. Farmer P. Infections and inequalities: the modern plagues. Berkeley and Los Angeles, CA: University of California Press; 1999.
135. Dao J. Ohio town's water at last runs past a color line. The New York Times. February 27, 2004: A1.
136. Wilson WJ. Truly disadvantaged: the inner city, the underclass, and public policy. Chicago: The University of Chicago Press; 1987.
137. Krieger N. Embodying inequality: a review of concepts, measures, and methods for studying health consequences of discrimination. Int J Health Serv. 1999;29(2):295–352.
138. National Coalition for the Homeless. How many people experience homelessness? 2009. http://www.nationalhomeless.org/factsheets/How_Many.html. Accessed 19 Mar 2009.
139. Bosman J. Number of people living on New York streets soars. The New York Times. 19 Mar 2010.

140. The United States Conference of Mayors. Hunger and homelessness survey: a status report on hunger and homelessness in America's cities – a 25-city survey. 2008. http://usmayors.org/pressreleases/documents/hungerhomelessnessreport_121208.pdf. Accessed 19 Mar 2010.

141. Corneil TA, Kuyper LM, Shoveller J, et al. Unstable housing, associated risk behaviour, and increased risk for HIV infection among injection drug users. Health Place. 2006;12(1):79–85.

142. Culhane DP, Gollub E, Kuhn R, Shpaner M. The co-occurrence of AIDS and homelessness: results from the integration of administrative databases for AIDS surveillance and public shelter utilisation in Philadelphia. J Epidemiol Community Health. 2001; 55(7):515–20.

143. Aidala A, Cross JE, Stall R, Harre D, Sumartojo E. Housing status and HIV risk behaviors: implications for prevention and policy. AIDS Behav. 2005;9(3): 251–65.

144. Weir BW, Bard RS, O'Brien K, Casciato CJ, Stark MJ. Uncovering patterns of HIV risk through multiple housing measures. AIDS Behav. 2007;11(6 Suppl):31–44.

145. El-Bassel N, Gilbert L, Rajah V, Foleno A, Frye V. Fear and violence: raising the HIV stakes. AIDS Educ Prev. 2000;12(2):154–70.

146. el-Bassel N, Schilling RF. Social support and sexual risk taking among women on methadone. AIDS Educ Prev. 1994;6(6):506–13.

147. Aidala AA, Sumartojo E. Why housing? AIDS Behav. 2007;11(6 Suppl):1–6.

148. Marmot M. Early pioneers of epidemiology. Lancet. 2007;370(9602):1819–20.

149. Frieden TR. A framework for public health action: the health impact pyramid. Am J Public Health. 2010;100(4):590–5.

150. Sumartojo E, Doll L, Holtgrave D, Gayle H, Merson M. Enriching the mix: incorporating structural factors into HIV prevention. AIDS. 2000;14 Suppl 1:S1–2.

Epidemiology of STI and HIV: An Overview of Concentration and Geographical and Temporal Dispersion

Peter J. White

Introduction

There is marked variation in the burden of disease due to STI and HIV that is experienced by different communities, and this burden changes over time. There is enormous variation in the burden of HIV both between countries [1] and within countries, with some groups (e.g., MSM, IDU) affected much more heavily than others. Even within risk groups there can be considerable variation. For this reason, it is argued that "Planning an intervention to prevent [HIV] infections … should be guided by local epidemiological and socioeconomic conditions … [including] risk behaviour, attitudes to risk, prevalence of cofactor STIs, stage of the HIV epidemic, existing health services." [2].

In public health, it is increasingly understood that risk factors for many diseases, including noninfectious ones, operate not simply at the individual level [3, 4]. For sexually transmitted infections, this has been recognized for some time: individuals' risk of acquiring an STI depends not only upon their sexual behavior but also on that of their partner(s) and those partner(s)' partners, and so on. A monogamous individual can be at significant risk of acquiring infection from his or her only sexual partner if that partner has other sexual partners—whose behavior, in turn, affects the infection risk of that partner. Therefore, a pattern of behavior (e.g., not using condoms) may be risky in one context but not in another. This means that we need to think in terms of populations, not just individuals. This is much harder both to conceptualize and to study, because interactions are complex, and many factors need to be measured to gain an understanding of a situation. These complex interactions mean that mathematical modeling is important in providing theoretical insight into the roles that different factors may play, testing hypotheses, and guiding empirical research. This chapter describes disparities in the distribution of STI and HIV in space, time, and by population group, and then explores the causes of these disparities and the implications for interventions.

Measurement of Disparities

Data on STI/HIV burden come from both surveillance systems and surveys, typically either population based or of clinic patients [5]. A common visual representation of heterogeneity in distributions is the Lorenz curve, with its associated measure, the Gini coefficient. The Lorenz curve plots the cumulative distribution of a characteristic

P.J. White (✉)
Modelling & Economics Unit, Health Protection Agency, London, UK

MRC Centre for Outbreak Analysis and Modelling, Department of Infectious Disease Epidemiology, Imperial College London, School of Public Health, Norfolk Place, London, W2 1PG, UK
e-mail: p.white@imperial.ac.uk

S.O. Aral, K.A. Fenton, and J.A. Lipshutz (eds.), *The New Public Health and STD/HIV Prevention: Personal, Public and Health Systems Approaches*, DOI 10.1007/978-1-4614-4526-5_3,

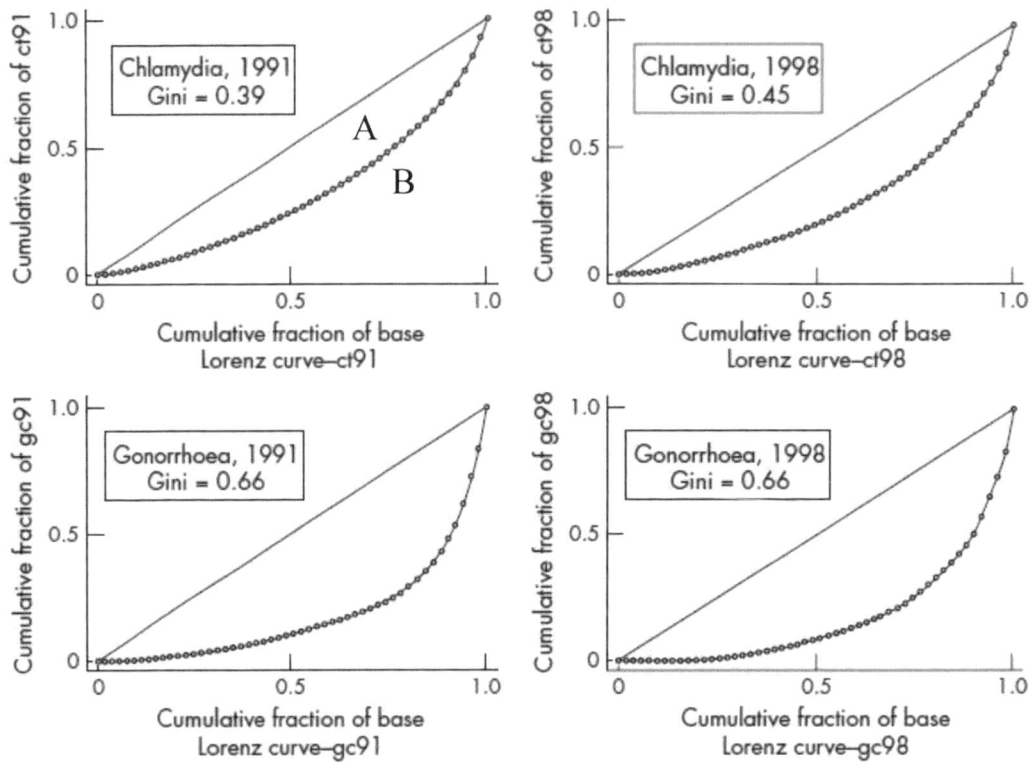

Fig. 3.1 Examples of Lorenz curves and Gini coefficients. Lorenz curves showing the variability in the age-adjusted incidence rates of chlamydia and gonorrhea at the level of the postal forward sortation area in Manitoba, 1991 and 1998. The value of the Gini coefficient is A/(A+B), where A and B are the areas indicated in the top-left graph. From [35] Elliott LJ, Blanchard JF, Beaudoin CM, Green CG, Nowicki DL, Matusko P, Moses S. Geographical variations in the epidemiology of bacterial sexually transmitted infections in Manitoba, Canada. Sex Transm Infect. 2002;78:i139–44

(e.g., disease burden) across the population being considered. If there is an even distribution (perfect equality) then the "curve" is a straight diagonal line running from bottom-left to top-right. If there is perfect inequality (all of the characteristic of the population is possessed by one person) then the curve is horizontal until the far-right edge of the graph, at which point it rises sharply (see Fig. 3.1 for an example). The Gini coefficient is the proportion of the area under the diagonal line of perfect equality that lies between the line of perfect equality and the Lorenz curve: a Gini coefficient of 0 corresponds to perfect equality; 1 corresponds to perfect inequality (Fig. 3.1).

For example Kerani et al. [6] examined the distribution of STIs in King County, WA, finding that syphilis was the most concentrated (Gini coefficient 0.68), followed by gonorrhea (0.57), Chlamydia (0.45), and herpes (0.26).

In many countries there are marked disparities in the burden of STIs in different groups. In the USA, STI burdens vary across states [7–9], within states [8], and within cities [10]; by ethnic groups [9, 11, 12] and socioeconomic status; and between MSM and heterosexuals [9]. A UK study found that in the city of Leeds black people had a 1.6–17-fold higher risk of infection than whites (depending on the STI), whilst for Asians the relative risk was as low as 0.1 of that of whites [13]. However, it is important to note that there are disparities within broadly defined risk groups, e.g., MSM [14].

Temporal Trends and Spatial Patterns

There is often marked variation over time, both at national and local levels and within particular communities, in the burden of a particular STI, not just in the case of an emerging infection like HIV but also in endemic infections like syphilis and gonorrhea. These variations occur due to a variety of factors, including successful public health interventions, and changes in population behavior.

The general pattern of reported STD diagnoses in the USA in the latter part of the twentieth century was an increase during the 1960s, followed by a decline or plateau [15]. Gonorrhea and syphilis declined in the late 1980s and 1990s—a pattern which was seen in many developed countries, including the UK (Fig. 3.2) [16]. However, over the last 10–15 years, many declining trends have reversed. Syphilis has increased in the USA and reemerged markedly in the UK [17]. It has been suggested that changes in sexual risk behavior in the 1980s and 1990s following the discovery of HIV and awareness of AIDS mortality may have contrib-

uted not only to slowing rates of HIV spread below what they otherwise would have been [18] but also to reductions in transmission of other STIs, including syphilis [19] and gonorrhea [16]. The extent to which such behavior change was a spontaneous response to the HIV epidemic or brought about by behavioral interventions is unclear.

HIV Temporal Patterns

The first cases of the disease that was to become "AIDS" were observed in MSM in California and reported in CDC's Morbidity and Mortality Weekly Report in 1981 [20], which was quickly followed by a report of cases of Kaposi's sarcoma [21]. We now know that HIV infection was already widespread globally when it was first detected; the typically long incubation period before developing characteristic disease meant that infection was able to spread for some time before becoming apparent. Phylogenetic analysis has suggested that HIV-1 emerged in equatorial west Africa in 1931 [22] before spreading in

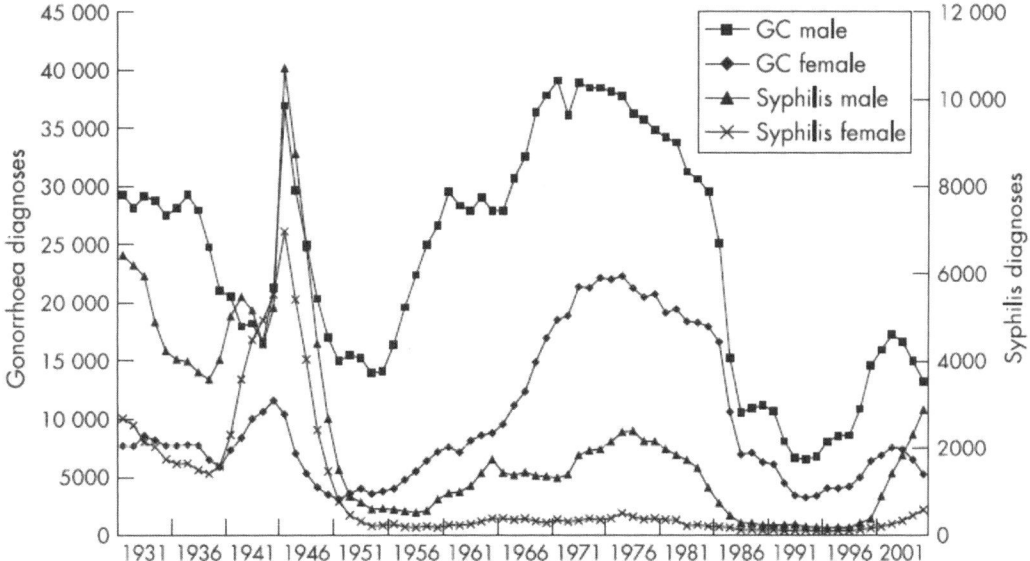

Fig. 3.2 Trends in gonorrhea and syphilis notifications in England and Wales, 1925–2005. Note the different axes. From [16] Ward H. Prevention strategies for sexually transmitted infections: importance of sexual network structure and epidemic phase. Sex Transm Infect 2007; 83(suppl 1): i43–9

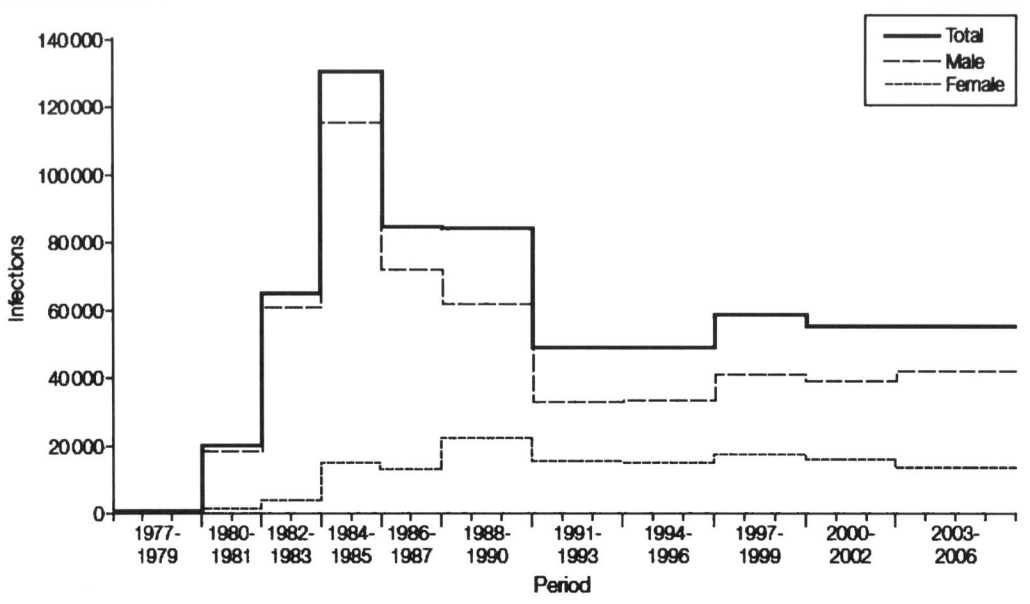

Tick marks denote beginning and ending of a year. The model specified periods within which the number of HIV infections was assumed to be approximately constant.

Fig. 3.3 Estimated HIV incidence in the USA, 1977–2006. From [26] Hall HI, Song R, Rhodes P, Prejean J, An Q, Lee LM, Karon J, Brookmeyer R, Kaplan EH, McKenna MT, Janssen RS; HIV Incidence Surveillance Group. Estimation of HIV incidence in the United States. JAMA. 2008 Aug 6;300(5):520–9

Africa and then globally but very heterogeneously. Later analysis suggested that HIV had been circulating in the USA for around 12 years before it was first recognized in 1981 [23].

Following the discovery of HIV, the pandemic progressed rapidly in the general population in parts of Africa, but elsewhere transmission tended to be concentrated in particular risk groups (e.g., injecting drug users, highly active MSM, sex workers and clients) [24, 25]. Epidemics can exhibit very rapid growth in their initial phases, where there is a relatively large supply of susceptible individuals available to become infected. HIV was discovered whilst the pandemic was in this phase, which in the case of HIV can last for decades due to the long incubation period. As infection spreads and the susceptible population is depleted, infection spreading slows. Often, the initial growth of the epidemic was rapid, because the highest-risk individuals tend to interact with other high-risk individuals.

In developed countries HIV initially affected MSM and IDU as well as commercial sex workers and their clients before becoming more widespread in the heterosexual population. However, there is relatively little transmission in heterosexuals although there are marked disparities between different groups. The historical pattern of HIV incidence in the USA has been recently reported [9, 26], finding that overall incidence peaked in the mid-1980s before declining to historic low levels in the early 1990s and then rising slightly up to the mid-2000s (Fig. 3.3). Rapid community responses from MSM to reduce risk behavior were effective in reducing HIV incidence [18], although transmission rates remained disproportionately high, and may have increased during the HAART era, due to decline in concern about HIV because of the availability of effective treatment.

Increasingly HIV has been spreading amongst the heterosexual population in developed

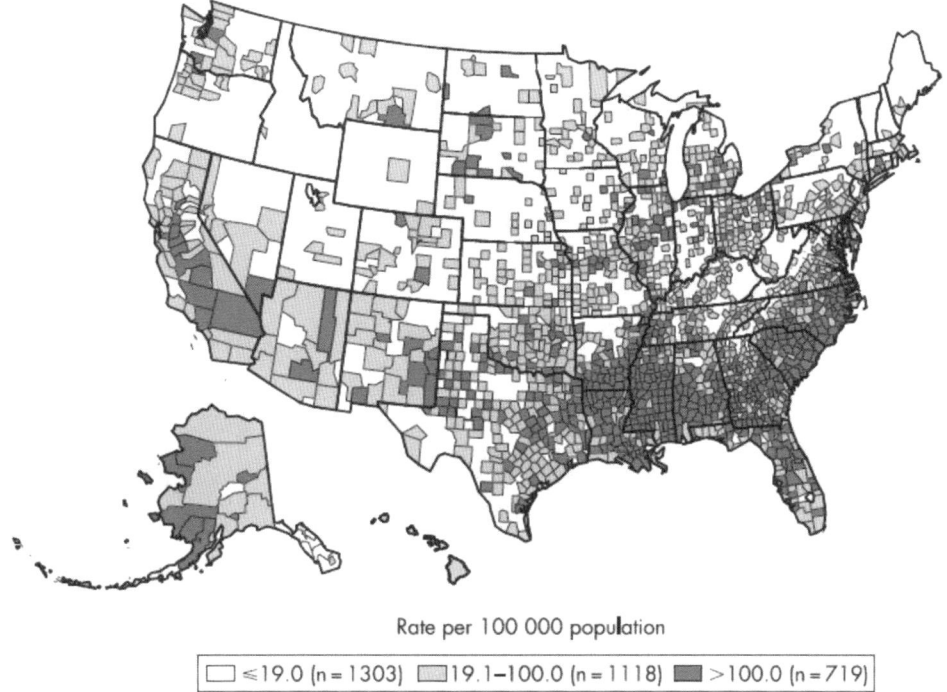

Rate per 100 000 population

☐ ≤19.0 (n = 1303)   ▦ 19.1–100.0 (n = 1118)   ■ >100.0 (n = 719)

Fig. 3.4 Geographic heterogeneity in the distribution of gonorrhea in the USA. Gonorrhea rates by county in the USA, 2005. From [15] Sevgi O Aral, Kevin A Fenton, and King K Holmes. Sexually transmitted diseases in the USA: temporal trends. Sex Transm Infect 2007; 83: 257–66

countries, particularly in Europe [27], although highest transmission rates remain amongst MSM [25, 28]. Currently in the UK, the majority of prevalent HIV infections are imported, mostly from sub-Saharan Africa [29]. Although rare, there is some transmission in the UK from imported infections, including in sexual partnerships involving disassortative mixing by ethnic group [30]. Transmission amongst IDU occurs through sharing of needles and is effectively combated by provision of sterile needles, which has resulted in a marked decline in the incidence of HIV in IDU where it has been used successfully (e.g., the UK), although this intervention is controversial in some countries [31].

Spatial Distributions

The spatial distribution of STI burden is heterogeneous (see Fig. 3.4 for an example). Rothenberg [32] found that gonorrhea in Upstate New York was highly concentrated with a relative risk in core areas being up to 40 times that of background rates. Core areas were shown to have "high population density, low socioeconomic status and a male to female case ratio of one or lower." The same author, with others, found that syphilis was tightly clustered spatiotemporally in urban areas of New York state, and more dispersed in rural areas [33]. Potterat et al. [34] also found gonorrhea to be highly clustered.

Different STIs differ in the extent of their spatial heterogeneity. A common pattern is that syphilis is the most geographically concentrated, followed by gonorrhea, whilst chlamydia, genital herpes, and genital warts are much more widespread [6, 8, 13, 35, 36].

Furthermore, the disease foci tend to overlap, indicating that risk behaviors relevant to different STIs are (unsurprisingly) correlated, and that there is a geographic focus of risk behavior [37, 38]. Additionally, whilst the dispersal of infection may ebb and flow over time, the location of disease foci tends to be stable [37, 38], although not in all cases. For example, a spatiotemporal analysis of syphilis in Baltimore, MD, found that between 1994 and 2002, during which time an epidemic increased and then declined, two spatial clusters persisted throughout (with transmission intensity increasing and then declining) and a third transient cluster arose and then disappeared [39].

Epidemic Phases

Wasserheit and Aral [40] proposed a general conceptual framework in the temporal evolution of infection spreading (Fig. 3.5), beginning with an early growth phase (Phase I), followed by hyperendemicity (Phase II), decline (Phase III), and endemism (Phase IV). Typically, the syndrome and pathogen are identified in the growth phase, followed by interventions beginning in the hyperendemic phase (which the authors split into II and II', pre- and post-commencement of interventions). Important components of interventions are the development of tests for the pathogen and effective treatments. Progression of the epidemic through these phases is accompanied by changes in the distribution of infection in the population due to the impacts of interventions, changes in population behavior, and other factors. The dynamic nature of STI/HIV epidemiology means that it is necessary to remain vigilant for changes in the distribution of infection risk and to ensure that public health responses remain appropriate [16, 40, 41].

Of course there are additional complexities in reality. For example, in the USA, syphilis has exhibited repeated epidemic cycles, although the reasons for these cycles are debated: some have proposed sociological factors, whilst others have suggested that the cause is partial immunity [42]. In the UK, there was a marked decline in gonorrhea during the 1980s and early 1990s, followed by a marked increase and subsequent fall [16]. Changes in sexual risk behavior are likely to have been the major factor, with failure of treatment services to meet demand in the early 2000s likely having exacerbated the problem [43].

In both the USA and the UK there have been marked increases in syphilis incidence, following a period when it was hoped that elimination was imminent [16]. Schumacher et al. [44] found that in Baltimore the increase in incidence was associated with an increase in MSM and young women with large numbers of recent sex partners.

Theoretical Framework: Insights from Modeling

Mathematical modeling plays a key role in the conceptual understanding of the epidemiology of infectious diseases and interventions against them [45–49]. Pioneering STI modeling work was prompted by concerns about increases in gonorrhea in the USA [50–54]. Development of models promotes clarity of thinking in the description of processes through defining and characterizing the component parts of the system and the nature of their interactions. Creating a model that is *mathematical* allows rigorous analysis and comparison with data, for example to determine whether a proposed cause of a particular outcome could have had an effect of sufficient magnitude to be a sufficient explanation (e.g. see Hallett et al. [55]). Although mathematical modeling requires specialist skills, the design and analysis of models should be a multidisciplinary activity, as modeling synthesizes evidence from many disciplines including sociology, epidemiology, and clinical medicine.

For an infectious agent to persist in its host population 'chains' of transmission from person to person must be sustained. Of course, many transmission chains terminate because the infected person does not pass on the infection before they cease to be infectious, due to recovery (through natural immunity or treatment), or death (or leaving the relevant population).

The criterion for persistence of an infection is that the *reproduction number*—the average number of transmission events occurring from an infected individual—be at least 1 so that on average infection is passed on to at least one person before the index infected individual ceases to be

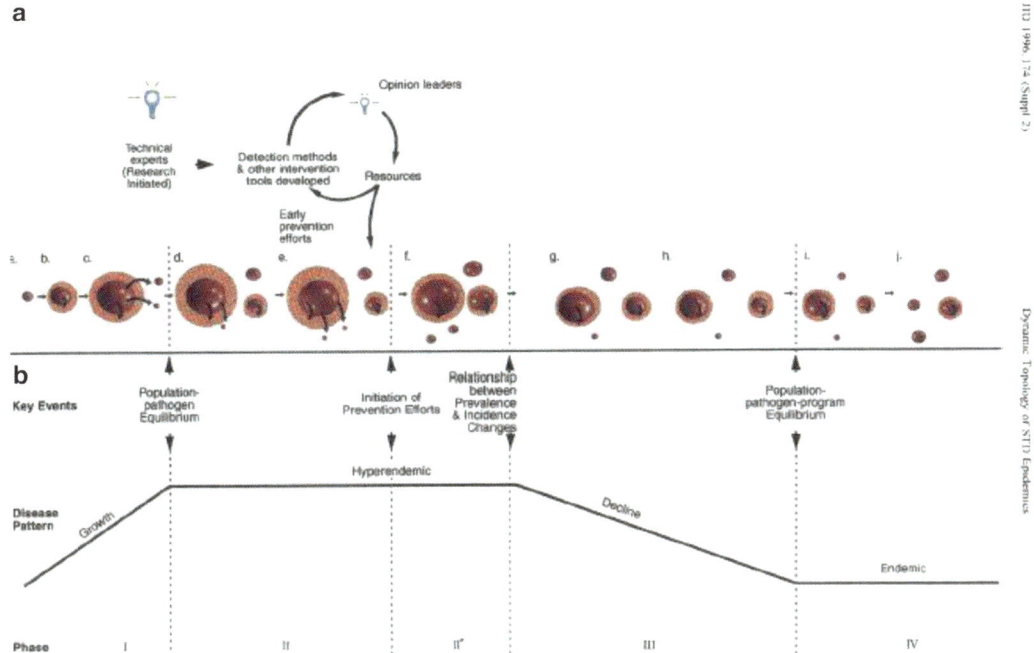

Fig. 3.5 The concept of epidemic phases of sexually transmitted diseases. (**a**) "Natural" and "controlled" history of STD epidemics from the perspective of changes over time in subpopulations in which spread and maintenance sexual networks are located. Dense spheres depict subpopulations containing spread networks, while mottled "halos" represent subpopulations containing maintenance networks. Arrows that link spheres with halos or with new spheres represent bridge populations. This population-level, host-focused perspective emphasizes the importance of program interventions and social networks as determinants of the epidemiology of STDs. (**b**) "Natural" and "controlled" history of STD epidemics from the perspective of changes over time in disease patterns, highlighting key events that mark transitions into new phases of epidemic. This population-level, pathogen-focused perspective is complementary to that in (**a**), and each disease phase corresponds to a stage in the evolution of sexual networks and subpopulations that are central to STD transmission. From [40] The dynamic topology of sexually transmitted disease epidemics: implications for prevention strategies. J Infect Dis. 1996;174(Suppl 2): S201–13

infectious [45, 50]. Mathematically, the reproduction number is the product of the average infectious period of an infected person and the rate of transmission to others during the infectious period. This rate of transmission from the infectious person depends upon the rate of potentially infectious contacts with others (in the case of STI, having a sexual partnership with someone susceptible to infection) and the probability of transmission upon contact. It is clear that the average rate of sexual partnership formation is too low for most STIs to persist in most populations *if everyone exhibited average behavior* [56]. For example, gonorrhea typically has a short infectious period, and transmission requires that someone infected with it has sex with an uninfected partner during that short period. Therefore, persistence of STI in the population depends upon the presence of individuals with above-average rates of sexual partner acquisition, making it vital to account for the variation in rates of sexual partner acquisition, not just average rates.

Recognizing heterogeneity in risk behavior introduces another complication: the need to consider patterns of sexual mixing within the population [57–62]. Sexual mixing is the extent to which individuals with particular characteristics choose as sexual partners individuals with particular characteristics. Persistence of infection in the population requires *sustained* person-to-person transmission. This requires not only that the average infected person has sufficient other sexual partners during their infectious period that at least one of them becomes infected, but also that the person(s) who become(s) infected also has/have sufficient other sexual partners during the infectious period for further transmission to occur.

The *core group* for an STI is that part of the population which allows the infection to persist in the population [32, 52, 63]. Members of the core group have both relatively high rates of sexual partner acquisition, and tend to select as sexual partners others who have relatively high rates of sexual partner acquisition. The size of the core group depends upon the infectious agent and the characteristics of the population [56, 57]. Gonorrhea and syphilis have relatively short infectious periods, so their persistence requires individuals who have very high rates of sexual partner acquisition, resulting in a typically small core group. On the other hand, Chlamydia and HIV have much longer infectious periods, so their core group tends to be much larger (although still a minority of the population). Consistent with these tendencies, a study in Seattle found that 50% of clinic patients with gonorrhea also had Chlamydia, whilst only 10% of patients with Chlamydia also had gonorrhea [64], meaning that Chlamydia was much more widespread in the population than gonorrhea. Furthermore, core groups are expected to be concentric [65]. For example, a spatial analysis of diagnoses of Chlamydia, gonorrhea, syphilis, and HIV in Wake County, North Carolina [36], found that all four infections had a spatial focus, and that they were overlapping.

Strictly, the minimum partner acquisition rate required for sustained transmission of infection depends not only upon the duration of the infectious period but also the infectivity [56]: the greater the mathematical product of the infectious period and transmission probability per contact, the lower the minimum partner acquisition rate required to sustain infection in the population.

It is important to note that factors such as the transmission probability in a sexual partnership and duration of infection are not "fixed" characteristics of each particular pathogen but have

behavioral components to them and hence can vary between population groups, and over time, including in response to education campaigns and changes in provision of healthcare. Specifically, the transmission probability depends upon the number of potentially infectious sex acts in a partnership, which depends upon the frequency of sex acts not protected by condom use, and the duration of the partnership (or the infectious period, whichever ends first). The infectious period also has a behavioral component: infected individuals who obtain successful treatment have their infectious period shortened. Individuals might not seek care at all, or only seek care after a prolonged period, due to lack of knowledge of STIs or due to barriers in their access to care. Changing social circumstances can result in the size of the core group and its membership changing [40].

It is important to emphasize that whilst the core group is necessary for infection to persist in the population, infection is not confined to the core group: many individuals who are outside the core group can acquire infection as it spreads from the core group into the general population [32]. There can also be transmission within the general population, so it is not necessary to have sex with a member of the core group to acquire infection. However, transmission within the general population is too inefficient for chains of transmission to be maintained indefinitely, so those infection chains eventually terminate.

The prevalence of an STI in a population depends upon multiple interacting factors, including the frequency distribution of rates of sexual partner acquisition, the degree of interaction between the core group and the general population (e.g., see Gamett and Anderson [57]), the patterns of condom use (which reduce the probability of transmission per sexual contact), and the rate of treatment of infection (which reduces the infectious period for treatable infections).

Mathematical modeling shows that the degree of sexual mixing between high-risk and low-risk individuals in the population can have a major impact on the prevalence of an STI like gonorrhea, which has a short infectious period, but much less impact on the prevalence of Chlamydia, which has a much longer infectious period.

The degree of mixing can be varied from *assortative* (i.e., "like with like," where high-risk individuals only choose as partners other high-risk individuals and low-risk individuals only choose as partners other low-risk individuals) to *random* (where the choice of sexual partners is proportionate to the proportion of all sexual partnerships that occur in the population). When mixing is assortative, infection is confined to the high-risk individuals (because it cannot persist in the low-risk individuals) and so the prevalence of infection at the population level is low: a relatively large proportion of the high-risk individuals are infected but they represent a small proportion of the whole population. If mixing is made slightly less assortative, then the overall prevalence of infection increases because infection can now "leak out" from the core group into the low-risk general population (which is much larger than the core group). If mixing is made slightly less assortative still then the overall prevalence of infection can rise further. However, there can come a point when making mixing even less assortative produces a fall in the overall prevalence and if mixing is sufficiently random then infection fails to persist and prevalence drops to zero. The reason for this is that as mixing is made more random, increasingly infection is transmitted not to high-activity individuals who are likely to "pass it on;" but to low-risk individuals who are unlikely to infect others, due to their low rate of sexual partner acquisition.

Treating curable STIs reduces the infectious period, meaning that the partner acquisition rate required to sustain transmission is increased, thus reducing the size of the core group, as well as reducing the prevalence of infection. Both suppressive therapy for incurable STIs (e.g., HSV, HIV) and use of condoms reduce the transmission probability per contact, meaning that more contacts are required on average for transmission to occur, which also has the effect of reducing the size of the core group.

It is important to emphasize that characterizing mixing patterns is more complex than just considering partners' rates of sexual partner change. Other factors include sex, age, ethnicity, other physical characteristics, socioeconomic status, membership of particular social networks, religion, geographic location, etc. (However, studies are of course limited in what information can feasibly be collected.) Age-mixing patterns are important determinants of STI risk [66]. There is marked variation in sexual activity with age, with teens and younger adults having the highest rates of sexual partner acquisition. For curable STIs with short infectious periods, the risk of being currently infected is associated with recent risk behavior, and prevalence is highest in the most sexually active age groups and declines with age as sexual activity declines. For incurable STIs, such as HIV, the risk of being currently infected depends upon the individual's entire history of risk behavior, and prevalence increases with age. Sexual partnerships between young women and older men was found to be an important risk factor for HIV acquisition in Zimbabwe, with infection being passed back from an older generation to a younger one [67].

Bridging

A particular type of mixing pattern that is important in some contexts is bridging between high- and low-risk groups by another group, e.g., clients of sex workers form a bridge between the sex workers and the regular partners of the clients. Johnson et al. [68] report, "HIV infection risk among pregnant women in Lima [Peru] depends largely on their male partners' risk behaviors. Even monogamous women had very large sexual networks." Morris et al. [69] found that in Thailand there were high rates of exposure of women to HIV from male partners who were clients of sex workers. In the USA, Adimora et al. [70] found that having a nonmonogamous sexual partner was an HIV risk for individuals who were otherwise at low risk. Studies such as these emphasize that individuals' risk of acquiring infection depends upon not only their behavior but also that of their partner(s)—and, in turn, their partners. Another example is that sex workers who are also IDU can bridge between IDU who are not sex workers and sex workers who are not IDU.

Bisexual men can bridge between MSM who only have sex with men, and heterosexual women [11, 71]. This may be particularly important in social groups where homosexuality is particularly stigmatized, resulting in MSM having female partners—who believe that their partner only has sex with women, and may even believe their partner to be monogamous [11]—whilst also having male partners "on the down low."

Networks of Sexual Partnerships

Infectious disease can be conceptualized as spreading through a network of contacts between individuals. Detailed investigation of the networks of contacts between individuals through which infections spread is an area of growing interest in infectious disease epidemiology, and has been long-studied in sexually transmitted infections, with a seminal paper by Klovdahl having been published more than a quarter of a century ago [72]. (Of course, contact tracing to identify potentially infected individuals for treatment, rather than study of network characteristics, had already been established for some considerable time).

As mentioned in the section on *Bridging*, the behavior of one's sexual partners has a potentially greater influence on one's STI risk than one's own behavior. The behavior of one's partners is a determinant of one's position in the sexual partnership network. There has been a considerable amount of empirical and theoretical work on the importance of networks of sexual contacts in STI transmission, seeking to identify those network characteristics that are associated with high disease burdens [66, 73–75]. As described succinctly by Morris et al., "At the population level, [an infectious agent's] epidemic potential is determined by underlying network connectivity. Connectivity is influenced by many factors, including: the dynamics of partnership formation, dissolution, and sequencing; population mixing by demographic and behavioral attributes; and geographic clustering and access" [76]. For general reviews of the study of networks see references [77–79].

Complexity of Studying Networks and Individual-Level Analysis

Analysis of networks rather than individuals or population groups involves a very large step up in complexity of data collection and analysis. This is because the sexual partnership, rather than the individual, is the primary sampling unit [66], which is challenging for both empirical investigation (not least because many partnerships are transient) and statistical analysis, requiring development of new methods. The theoretical modeling and data analysis described thus far in this chapter has been at aggregate level, with individuals being categorized and represented by descriptive statistics. This is true even where populations are stratified by sex, activity class (according to rates of sexual partner change), age group, etc.: each particular stratum or subgroup has a characteristic (mean) value for each of its parameters, so at the population level a particular characteristic has a discrete, rather than continuous, distribution. In compartmental models, the population is divided into categories representing different infection states as appropriate to the natural history of the infection being modeled (e.g., uninfected and susceptible, latently infected, symptomatic and infectious, asymptomatic and infectious, immune). These infection states may also be stratified by age, sex, activity, class, etc. The model tracks the aggregate number of individuals in each of these categories and how these numbers change over time as an epidemic progresses and interventions are introduced.

By contrast, network analysis, whether empirical study or by computer simulation, is an individual-level analysis. This is appealing in terms of realism, but is inevitably costly in terms of resources, both for empirical or theoretical study. In an individual-based model (IBM), each individual in the population is tracked as a separate entity within the computer's memory, which means that individual partnerships are also tracked individually, recording when they start and end, with whom they occur, how frequently sex acts (and potentially which types of act) occur in that partnership, how frequently condoms are used, etc. Additionally, individual characteristics like rates of sexual partner change in the population can have continuous, rather than discrete, distributions; spreading of multiple infections and interactions between them can be more readily modeled; and the life histories of individuals can be tracked.

However, these more-realistic models are considerably harder to analyze, and collecting the detailed data needed to estimate parameters is challenging. Typically it is difficult to gain algebraic insight into how the model behaves, so instead of being able to calculate where threshold changes in behavior will occur, one has to explore parameter space by varying parameters and looking for changes in the model's behavior. This requires a lot of computation and, unfortunately, even with modern computers, simulations take considerable time to run and require the use of efficient coding techniques. An IBM considers individuals, and since events that change the status of individuals (e.g. infection, recovery, starting or ending a partnership) are probabilistic, stochasticity (randomness) has to be incorporated into the model. This means that each "run" of the model will produce a different result, even with the same input parameters. Therefore, for a given set of input parameters, the model has to be "run" multiple times. In addition, each "run" of an IBM takes considerably longer than a corresponding "run" of a compartmental model. (Stochastic effects are also a problem for empirical study: they cause "noise" which makes it harder to determine whether an apparent pattern is real or just due to random chance).

Uses of Modeling

Despite the technical challenges, important progress in our understanding of STI-transmission networks has come through computer modeling [76, 80–86]. Modeling can guide empirical research by determining what network characteristics might be important (e.g., concurrency [76, 80, 81]), and examining the potential impact of biases in empirical data [83, 84].

A neat example of the use of computer modeling to examine the importance of network structure that results from different contact patterns of individuals is the study by Ghani and Aral [86]. This study examined the effect on the prevalence of gonorrhea and HSV2 of different patterns of interaction between sex workers and their clients and the impact of the relative size of the sex-worker population (fewer sex workers would mean that each had on average more encounters with clients). They found that the size of the sex-worker population was the most important determinant of prevalence, and that if clients tended to use multiple sex workers rather than being a regular client of one sex worker then prevalence tended to increase.

However, it is important to realize that computer modeling studies demonstrate the importance of particular network characteristics *conditional upon the model being correct*. There is a need for more and better empirical evidence to test modeling results. Unfortunately, obtaining this evidence is challenging, due to the requirement for very detailed data.

Alternative Theoretical Modeling Approaches

The complexity of modeling large networks of sexual contacts has motivated the development of alternative, simpler, theoretical modeling approaches [87]. These may offer important insights through being more tractable than a "fully specified" network simulation, and also have the advantage of not requiring detailed empirical network data to parameterize and test them.

Chen et al. [88] applied a meta-population modeling approach—a modification of compartmental modeling in which the population is made up of linked subpopulations—to gonorrhea in the UK to address the question of how it persists at low prevalence. They found that the complexity of a fully specified individual-level contact network is not needed to model the concentration of infection in "distinct subpopulations, with much higher incidence rates in young people, some ethnic minorities and inner city subpopulations" and the "contextual risk experienced by members of at-risk subpopulations." They propose, "that the epidemiology of gonorrhoea is largely driven by subpopulations with higher than average concentrations of individuals with high sexual risk activity."

An alternative modeling approach is to use pair models in which the interaction between individuals is modeled at the level of the partnership but partnerships are tracked not individually but in terms of their aggregate number [89–94]. That is, the model tracks the aggregate number of partnerships between a pair of uninfected individuals (which have no transmission risk); an uninfected individual and an infectious individual; a pair of infectious individuals; an infectious individual and an immune individual, etc. This approach provides an approximation to a network structure, and works best for a homogeneous network, although some approximations for heterogeneous networks have been developed [90, 92, 93].

One application of the pair modeling approach has been to examine the importance of gaps between monogamous sexual partnerships and overlapping (concurrent) partnerships, where the gap between the end of one partnership and the start of a subsequent one is negative [95]. For curable STIs if the gap between partnerships is too long then transmission of infection will not occur because an infected individual will have recovered from infection before the opportunity for onward transmission occurs. Analysis of UK data found that "gonorrhea is sustained by the presence of a small group of individuals with short gap lengths and medium length partnerships. Interventions targeted at this group are more effective than those targeted at individuals with high numbers of sexual partners but longer gap lengths." Other studies have found that it is common for gaps between partnerships to be short enough to allow transmission of STIs [96].

Empirical Studies of Networks

Empirical data collection for sexual partnership networks is labor-intensive, time-consuming, and costly because of the need to sample sexual partnerships rather than individuals. Commonly, networks are imputed from egocentric data collected from a sample of individuals: survey respondents are asked about their numbers of sexual partners over periods of time and the characteristics of (typically a sample of) those partners. However, the partners themselves are usually not traced, and instead a computer algorithm is used to calculate networks whose structures are as consistent as possible with the data. Unfortunately, egocentric data provide an incomplete specification of the sexual contact network, so multiple hypothetical networks can be consistent with the available data.

Importantly, egocentric data do not give information on the presence or absence of cycles (loops of contacts which may promote rapid infection transmission around the loop but not beyond it), size of components (i.e., clusters of linked individuals), the extent of long-range connectedness of the network (a few long-range links can result in a short path length between many individuals, promoting rapid spread of infection), and other important characteristics [66]. Obtaining this more-detailed information requires contact tracing or a census of the network. (Although note that it has been suggested that it may be possible to develop algorithms to impute network structure reasonably reliably from egocentric data [66]—see below.)

Contact tracing is a routine intervention against STIs, which is feasible because of the discrete nature of sexual contact, which occurs with a relatively small number of usually identifiable individuals. Through this process it is possible in principle to construct the entire sexual network of contacts. However, in practice this rarely happens because it is very labor-intensive, and it is usually not possible to identify all links in the network. Unfortunately, a small proportion of missing links can radically alter the apparent structure of the network and its apparent connectedness: a network that appears to be sparsely connected may actually be much more highly interconnected. A few highly connected people can greatly shorten the average path length between individuals, resulting in a "small world" network, in which there can be effective rapid widespread transmission of infection.

The links which are most likely to be missed may be the most important from the point of view of the connectivity of the network: casual partners are more likely not to be identified or found, and those partners may be more likely to be highly connected. (Although highly connected individuals may be more likely to be traced because there are more partnerships through which they may be traced, if many of the partnerships are not elucidated then the high degree of connectedness of the individual would not be apparent).

However, the picture is further complicated by the fact that short-term casual partnerships typically have fewer sex acts than longer term partnerships and have higher rates of condom use, meaning that there is less likely to be transmission of infection if one of the partners is infected (although an individual with many partners is more likely to be infected)—although for infections like gonorrhea, which are short-term and relatively highly infectious, relatively few sex acts per partnership can still result in a substantial transmission risk, and indeed a high partner acquisition rate (or concurrent partnerships) is required for its transmission.

One way of dealing with missing links is to include venues for meeting partners, especially casual ones, in social network analyses [34, 97]. The importance of this was demonstrated by Jolly and colleagues [98], who found that augmenting traditional contact tracing data with data on social venues where sexual partnering occurred joined eight of the largest network components, creating a component of 89 individuals. An additional cause of missing links is the time period considered: if a longer period were considered then apparently separate network components may indeed have been linked [99].

Insights into Transmission Networks from Genetic Analysis of Pathogens

The problem of missing links can also be addressed using genetic analysis of pathogen specimens, which is increasingly providing insights into transmission networks. Genetic analysis offers powerful insights into the networks and dynamics of infection in a way that just looking at the distribution of infection in a population cannot. It can be performed in conjunction with contact tracing data or in the absence of such data, using just diagnostic specimens from patients. Broadly, genetic analysis can be divided into genotyping and nucleotide sequence analysis. Genotyping involves analyzing sections of the pathogen genome (which may be done "directly" through nucleotide sequencing or "indirectly" through techniques such as restriction-fragment length polymorphism) to assign the isolate to a category. Nucleotide sequence analysis involves sequencing large portions of the genome, or even the whole genome, and offers much more detailed data, enabling construction of "transmission trees" in which it is possible to infer the timing of a transmission events and, to some extent, the presence of "missing links" and who may have infected whom within the dataset.

A multidisciplinary research study in the UK examined the benefits of combining contact tracing and gonorrhea-typing data [100]. The authors applied genotyping in conjunction with contact tracing to compare gonorrhea transmission in the cities of Sheffield and London. They found that endemic transmission was relatively more important in Sheffield than in London, which has a much more transient population [101]. Two clusters accounted for half of the cases in Sheffield. A subsequent study using a higher resolution typing system in London identified 21 strains of gonorrhea circulating in distinct transmission networks [102]. Transmission networks involving MSM (7 strains) and heterosexuals (14 strains) tended to be separate, with a very small amount of "bridging" via bisexual men. Additionally, individuals infected with a particular strain had similar behavioral and demographic characteristics, including ethnicity. This study found that despite the incidence of gonorrhea being 16 times higher in those of black ethnicity compared to whites, there was no significant difference in the numbers of partners reported in the 3 months preceding diagnosis [103]. Of the 21 strains identified, 13 were widespread across London but eight were geographically clustered in areas of high incidence [103]. The authors note, "This geographical clustering is particularly apparent among heterosexual men and women. Unlike similar studies in the United States [6, 32, 104, 105], this geographical clustering of cases does not relate strongly to measures of social deprivation but reflects the ethnic makeup of the different areas of London. Those areas with a high proportion of people of black African or black Caribbean ethnicity experience the highest incidence of gonorrhoea." [103].

A gonorrhea genotyping study in Amsterdam [106] found 11 clusters of at least 20 patients, 7 of which were 81–100% MSM, 3 of which were 87–100% heterosexual, and 1 contained roughly equal numbers of MSM, and heterosexual males and females. There was variation amongst clusters in behavioral characteristics, including use of the Internet to find sexual partners. Fifty-two individuals (7% of the sample) had infections with different strains at different anatomical sites, indicating high-risk behavior.

Wylie, Jolly, and collaborators have studied transmission of Chlamydia in sexual contact networks in Manitoba, Canada [99, 107, 108]. They found that contact tracing and genotyping data gave concordant results [107]. Using genotyping data to identify transmission clusters it was found that they were socio-demographically, and often geographically, distinct [108]. Additionally, they report that genotyping and geographic data can indicate potential connections—"missing links" between unlinked individuals [108].

Choudhury et al. [102] recommend, "Molecular methods should be combined with exhaustive contact tracing, but … where contact tracing is more difficult, [detailed genotyping] can provide valuable additional data on endemic networks and outbreaks … The rapid identification of new strains spreading in subpopulations—i.e. early epidemic phase—should inform intensified partner notification and outreach at risk venues in an attempt to prevent strains becoming endemic. Similarly, knowledge of the distribution of endemic—i.e. later epidemic phase—strains across the city could be used to target health promotion and enhanced case finding."

Whilst contact tracing data are valuable in understanding transmission patterns, pathogenic genetic analysis alone can also provide important insights. Phylogenetic analysis of the nucleotide sequence of HIV has been informative about its evolutionary history and temporal global spread [22, 23], and the details of its transmission through local sexual partnership networks [109]. A study of HIV in MSM in the UK reported that [110] there are at least six large transmission chains, each beginning with a separate introduction into the UK (although of course there will have been more introductions than this), and that there was decline in the transmission rate in the early 1990s, which the authors attribute to behavior change, as it predates the HAART era. Lewis et al. [109] found that HIV spreading in MSM in London occurred in several clusters, and that a quarter of transmission events occurred within 6 months of infection. HIV transmission through heterosexual sex in the UK is very low, although molecular evidence shows that there is some transmission from imported infections, including in sexual partnerships involving disassortive mixing by ethnic group [30]. Unfortunately, many HIV infections are still being diagnosed late [111, 112]. As well as resulting in a poorer prognosis for the individual, and the possibility of unknowing transmission to partners, this reduces the timeliness of insights from phylogenetic analyses for informing current prevention efforts.

Different Networks for Different Infections

Importantly, whilst STIs spread through the population via the sexual partnership network, different infections "see" a different network structure (which is why their distributions vary: [56, 99, 113–116]), determined by the timing of formation and dissolution of sexual partnerships, and the duration and infectivity of infection. The "gap length" between sexual partnerships is an important determinant of transmission risk and network connectivity [95, 96]. An individual who has gonorrhea for a month will likely expose fewer sexual partners to that infection than if they had Chlamydia for a year. Indeed, if the gap length is long enough then the infected individual may have recovered prior to having sex with another person and hence there may be no risk of trans-mission. (Additionally, individuals with symp-tomatic infection may reduce their sexual contacts whilst those with asymptomatic infection would likely not change their behavior.) Therefore, the potential transmission network for an infection (where links between individuals consist of sex-ual partnerships in which transmission could have occurred) is a subset, specific to the particu-lar infection, of the sexual partnership network (where links between individuals consist of sex-ual partnerships which occurred) of the popula-tion. The actual transmission *network* for the infection (where links between individuals con-sist of sexual partnerships in which transmission occurred) will be a subset of the potential trans-mission network, since not all potential transmis-sion events actually occur, because transmission is a probabilistic process. This means that when empirically elucidating a sexual partnership net-work the timing and duration of partnerships are critical. Indeed, sexual partnership networks are dynamic, with partnerships forming and dissolv-ing, so links between individuals through which infection may spread "appear" and "disappear." However, not all studies take this into account but, for simplicity, assume a "static" network in which all links are present simultaneously.

Characteristics of Networks Associated with High Burden of Disease and Phases of Epidemics

There has been particular interest in sexual part-nership network structures associated with a high STI burden, and how changes in network struc-ture are associated with phases of epidemics [16, 38, 40, 117]. Early work on gonorrhea [32, 34] found that their transmission was associated with highly connected networks of individuals, many of whom had multiple partners, resulting in large network components—that is, core groups. Later studies have confirmed these findings for syphilis and gonorrhea [33, 105, 118]. It is less clear if this is the case for longer term infections such as Chlamydia and herpes, a substantial proportion of which may be asymptomatic, which are typically found to be more dispersed and more prevalent.

Comparing the network structures found through contact tracing, Potterat et al. [117] suggest that the endemic phase of an epidemic is associated with linear, dendritic network components in which individuals have relatively few partnerships connecting them to others, whilst the epidemic phase is associated with highly connected individuals including loop structures, which they argue lead to rapid spread of infection. (In a network with loop structures there are multiple paths along which infection can spread, whilst in a linear structure, failure to spread along one link means that no individuals "downstream" of that link could become infected.) However, the endemic phase networks pertained to Chlamydia whilst the epidemic phase networks pertained to gonorrhea. Ward [16] cautions that this "needs further explora-tion because similar data could also be produced by different sampling and organism-specific characteristics." However, consistent with Potterat et al., Friedman et al. [119] also found that membership of a cyclic network structure compared with being a member of a dendritic structure was a risk factor for HIV infection amongst IDU.

Whilst it is clearly the case that sexual part-nership network connectivity determines the risk of infection entering the network and the subse-quent extent of infection spreading, and that changes in network connectivity can lead to changes in epidemic phase, it is important to rec-ognize that the effects of changes in network con-nectivity are nonlinear. Increases in component sizes have relatively little effect until a relatively few additional links join components together, causing a large increase in component size, facil-itating rapid transmission [38]. This is because if no one in a network component is infected then there is no infection risk to any member but as additional links form and increase the component size the risk of infection entering the component increases. Whilst a small incremental increase in connectivity is associated with a large increase in infection risk when the critical threshold level of connectivity is crossed, a small decremental change taking network connectivity back below that critical threshold produces a large reduction in infection risk.

Potterat [38] suggests, "It may be that there are only a few dozen neighborhoods in the United States … that … act as Strategic STD Reserves, as it were, for the observed focal hyperendemicity of bacterial STD," and that epidemics occur when the connectivity of the wider population with these reservoir populations crosses a critical threshold. Wylie et al. [99] had previously suggested, "Gonorrhea endemicity … may depend on a balance between short term persistence within several key areas where intra-community networks are sufficiently large to permit short term, localized persistence, coupled with a slower influx and spread to other geographic areas." This accords with the meta-population view of STI epidemiology [88]. Potterat et al. [117] argue that "a few months spent obtaining quality contact tracing data can provide a reliable network configuration that suggests epidemic phase," and is a superior approach to interpretation of case-reports through surveillance systems, which is made difficult by changes in diagnostic tests, testing patterns, care-seeking behavior, etc., meaning that it can take years to determine "true" epidemic trends.

Scale-Free Networks

The suggestion that sexual partnership networks may be scale-free [120] gave rise to concern because it was argued that this means that the reproduction number is infinite and therefore infection can never be eliminated. However, it is unlikely that sexual partnership networks are in fact scale-free [66, 121]. It is worth noting that the Liljeros et al. [120] analysis was of egocentric data, which give only partial information on network structure. The mechanism of network formation that produces a scale-free network is *preferential attachment*: the more partners one has the more attractive one becomes by virtue of having so many partners and the more partners one is likely to acquire in the future. Whilst this may well be the case for Websites, where the more links a Website has the more likely it is to be found and linked-to by others, whether this mechanism really operates in human sexual

partnerships is questionable. Furthermore, the number of sexual partners one can have can only span a finite range, whereas to produce a scale-free network requires that some individuals have very high numbers of partners.

Concurrency

As described above, core groups comprising relatively few highly interconnected individuals have been found to play an important role in the spreading of STIs, particularly those with relatively short infectious periods such as gonorrhea and syphilis, through creating highly interconnected networks. However, a highly connected sexual partnership network may arise without any individuals in the network being particularly highly connected themselves—i.e., without there being a core group. This can arise through individuals having only a few sexual partners, but in concurrent sexual partnerships (where there is a negative gap length between partnerships). It is not necessary to have a few very highly connected individuals to have a highly connected network.

It has been argued that a key characteristic of behavior that underlies a large amount of the variation in the burden of STIs and HIV in different populations is the prevalence of concurrency: individuals being in more than one sexual partnership simultaneously [122]. This can lead to rapid transmission of infection through the network of sexual partnerships, because the infection can be acquired from one partner and rapidly passed to the other(s). A large amount of theoretical analysis of concurrency has been done by Morris and collaborators [66, 80, 81]. In a recent analysis they report that their modeling analysis found that small differences in the prevalence of concurrency can lead to large differences in the prevalence of infection [76]. A number of empirical studies have found an association between a higher prevalence of concurrency and a higher burden of disease [123–126]. Concurrency may be particularly important for infections with a short duration, such as gonorrhea, because they have limited time to spread from an infected individual. It may also be important for the spread of

HIV via primary infection [127] because primary HIV infection (PHI) is characterized by high infectivity for a short period, which potentially allows it to spread very rapidly through a highly connected network of even short-term contacts.

However, there is uncertainty over the importance of concurrency in the dynamics of STIs and the extent to which it may underlie disparities [128, 129], and more empirical evidence is required. Unfortunately, collecting the detailed information required is very demanding, as discussed below. The challenge is that concurrency is not a risk factor for acquisition of infection by the individual with concurrent partners, but rather it is a risk factor for rapid transmission following acquisition—that is, it is a population-level characteristic [66].

Future Analysis of Networks

To evaluate the importance of network characteristics such as concurrency in the transmission of infection we need to measure the extent of those network characteristics in population-based surveys in multiple settings and measure how much STI risk is associated with them. The challenge is that each population study, which involves collecting detailed data at considerable expense, constitutes only a single data point [66], because the unit of analysis is the population, as we are analyzing population-level characteristics. This makes it difficult to generalize because there are relatively few of these data points.

As detailed elucidation of networks is not feasible in routine public health surveillance or in routine population-based surveys, such as Demographic & Health Surveys, "Standardised measures of the extent and nature of sex work within populations and the size and nature of the interactions among core groups, bridge populations, and the general population would help both research efforts and programmatic activities" [130]. Developing such measures is challenging [131], but would greatly increase the number of "data points" that are available to inform analyses of the importance of population-level network characteristics. It is important to obtain data from representative population-based surveys, to examine the sexual partnership network and to complement studies of transmission networks which come from studies of patients.

Morris et al. [66] suggest that network structures may in fact be largely determined by simple rules and that mixing patterns and the extent of concurrency—which can be obtained from egocentric data—may explain most of the variation in networks. If this is indeed the case then it would be a boon for epidemiological understanding guiding public health interventions. However, a considerable amount of work is required to empirically elucidate multiple different networks in order to robustly quantitatively formulate the network-formation rules and then to validate the inferred networks.

Analysis of pathogen genetic data is likely to become an important technique for sexual partnership network analysis, as genetic analysis becomes increasingly routine in diagnostic testing and hence the data becomes increasingly available at minimal additional cost. Combined with enhanced routine surveillance datasets there are exciting prospects for improved understanding and more effective interventions.

Watts [77] powerfully makes the argument for multidisciplinary research in the field of networks, noting that whilst the analytic methods are necessarily highly mathematical, "many of the core ideas—not just applications—[have] come from sociology." He notes that there is a "rapidly emerging and highly interdisciplinary synthesis of new analytical techniques, enormously greater computing power, and an unprecedented volume of empirical data."

Synthesis: Causes of Disparities

There are complex causes of disparities in health outcomes, resulting from multiple interacting factors. Clearly, individual STI risk is not explained only by individual characteristics. Context is important: *having multiple sexual partners is only an infection risk if those partners are infected themselves; conversely, being monogamous does not protect one from infection if one's partner is not monogamous (or has an infection from a previous partnership).* An analysis of ethnic variations in sexual behavior and STI risk in the UK found that although the general trend was for those groups who reported greater numbers of sexual partners to be at greater risk of acquiring an STI, variations in individual-level sexual behavior alone were insufficient to explain infection risk disparities across ethnic groups [132]. The authors conclude that there is "a need for targeted and culturally competent prevention interventions."

"Context" is a complex combination of multiple interacting factors, and multilevel approaches are needed to understand STI risk. Aral [41] categorizes such factors as social structures, environmental influences, lifestyle influences, and physiological influences. The context can also change over time due to social or economic changes or changes in epidemic phase. Individual infection risk is determined by an interaction between individual behavioral factors and population-level factors, chiefly the prevalence of infection in the population group from which one selects one's sexual partner(s).

This section focuses on examples of important interacting factors and how they contribute to disparities in the STI and HIV burden. Examples include social factors affecting populations of African and Caribbean heritage in the USA and the UK, biological factors affecting men who have sex with men, and the variety of factors that may underlie the burden of HIV in populations in sub-Saharan Africa.

Complexity

Infectious disease transmission is a highly nonlinear system—that is, there are complex interactions between components of the system, which means that there is not a simple proportional relationship between a particular causal factor and the outcome in terms of disease burden. In one context, varying a causal factor (e.g., condom use) by a particular amount may make little difference to disease outcomes, whilst in another context a variation of that same amount may have a large impact.

Interacting factors can amplify each other's effects, so relatively small differences between groups in rates of sexual partner change, mixing patterns, or access to care can in combination result in large disparities in disease burden. Hogben and Leichliter [133] review the interplay of social factors such as segregation, access to health care, socioeconomics, and correctional experiences with sexual networks and STI risk. Additionally, biological interactions can occur between STIs. This has been most closely examined for HIV [134–136]: some STIs increase the infected individuals' susceptibility to acquiring HIV (if they are HIV negative), or can increase their HIV infectivity (if they are HIV positive). Fox et al. synthesize current evidence to calculate a "risk score" for HIV transmission in HIV-discordant partnerships [137].

Furthermore, there are often threshold effects ("tipping points"): in some circumstances, small differences in behavior can translate into large differences in disease burden if those differences cause a threshold to be crossed. Examples of threshold effects that have been discussed above are the minimum partner acquisition rate required for an infection to persist, and the critical level of sexual partnership network connectivity to lead to an epidemic. Another example of a threshold effect was explored by White et al. [43], using a model to examine the impact of clinic treatment capacity on the incidence of gonorrhea. Where capacity is inadequate, there is a vicious circle in which failure to treat infections promptly allows infection to spread, maintaining a high incidence of infection and maintaining the inadequacy of care. Increasing capacity sufficient to break out of this vicious circle enters a virtuous circle in which prompt treatment of infection averts transmission, reducing incidence and reducing the need for treatment—thus saving money as well as improving health. Importantly, breaking out of the vicious circle requires that the increase in treatment rates crosses a threshold for gaining control of infection spreading. Once control is gained, it can be maintained by keeping treatment rates above the (lower) threshold for losing control; if this does not occur then the vicious circle is reentered and a substantial increase in treatment rates is required to reestablish control.

The model shows that there can be a very large disparity in the burden of disease when infection is under control compared with when it is not, solely due to this effect.

Sexual Partnership Networks Are not the Only Networks that Are Important

Whilst sexual partnership networks alone are complicated, they are not the only networks that have an impact on sexual health—and, indeed, other aspects of health. Sexual behavior and sexual network structures are influenced by the social, demographic, cultural, and political context. Hence, there are in fact multiple interrelated and interacting networks that affect spreading of STIs. Information affecting knowledge, attitudes, and behaviors spreads through social networks [3, 138–143]. Sexual partners may be found through social networks [60, 144]. These interactions can exacerbate inequalities between population groups by increasing the assortativeness of STI risk. Rothenberg [145] presents hypotheses regarding interactions between network structures and other risk factors.

Spatial Heterogeneity

The marked spatial heterogeneity in STI burden is due to spatial heterogeneities in the multiple interacting factors associated with STI burden and sexual partner choice, including knowledge, attitudes, and behaviors; access to care; socioeconomic status; education; and ethnicity. Additionally, sexual partnerships often involve individuals who live close together, at least in high-burden areas. Early work on gonorrhea by Rothenberg [32] reported, "Contact investigation data suggest that sexual contact tends to exhibit geographic clustering"; Potterat et al. [34] reported "residential proximity" of risk groups, and a later study by Zenilman et al. [105] found that sexual partners in core transmission areas tended to live just a few hundred meters from each other.

A Disproportionately Affected Group: Black People in the USA and the UK

African Americans tend to experience a higher burden of STI and HIV than whites in the USA [11, 112]. This disparity also exists in the UK [13, 132]. In both countries these disparities are not explained by individual-level factors alone [132, 146]. Aral et al. point out that [146] whilst "white Americans acquire STIs predominantly when they engage in high-risk behaviours, African Americans acquire them through low-risk behaviours because prevalence of infection in the population is high." Tillerson et al. [11] report, "Black women are no more likely to have unprotected sex, have multiple sexual partners, or use drugs than women of other racial/ethnic groups [but] … are more likely to have risky sex partners and STDs."

Potterat [38] comments, "There remains the need to develop a more valid picture of just what it is about the conformation of sexual networks in high prevalence neighborhoods which contributes to disproportionate STD transmission risk in different ethnic groups." Laumann and Youm [147] suggest that an important factor underlying the higher burden of bacterial STI in black Americans is that there is more mixing between low-risk individuals and high-risk individuals within the African-American community than in other communities.

A modeling analysis of data from south-east London in the UK found that the much higher incidence of gonorrhea in those of black Caribbean ethnicity than black African and white ethnic groups was due to high rates of sexual partner change by a small minority of the black Caribbean population, combined with a tendency of members of all groups to choose sexual partners of the same ethnicity [148]. The authors say, "profound differences in gonorrhoea rates between ethnic groups can be explained by modest differences in a limited number of sexual behaviours and mixing patterns."

The review by Adimora and Schoenbach [149] found that a number of contextual factors were important in the USA, including "poverty, discrimination, … illicit drug use …, ratio of men to women, incarceration rates, and racial segregation, [and the] influence sexual behavior and sexual networks." The authors concluded that "exclusive emphasis on individual risk factors and determinants is unlikely to … significantly decrease HIV rates among blacks" and that multidisciplinary research is required to develop effective interventions. This is echoed by Kraut-Becher et al. [150] who conclude that future research that examines "the interaction of several factors is more likely to produce effective public health interventions and reductions in HIV transmission." For concise descriptions of interacting contextual factors affecting STIs and HIV in African Americans see references [146, 150].

It has been suggested that the "down low" phenomenon—bisexual black men having illicit male sex partners of which their female sex partners are unaware—contributes to the disparity in the burden of STI and HIV in black populations by bridging between MSM and heterosexual women whose individual behavior is low-risk [70]. However, the importance of this phenomenon has been questioned [151], with the authors suggesting that it is not unique to black populations, although others have suggested that black men are less likely to disclose to female partners that they also have sex with men [11].

Multiple studies report that in the USA incarceration is associated with STI risk [146, 149, 152, 153]. High incarceration rates, along with high rates of mortality due to disease and violence [146], in African-American men produce a low ratio of men to women. This promotes concurrency of sexual partnerships amongst non-incarcerated men, which in turn promotes higher rates of infection transmission. Concurrency has been found to be correlated with STI prevalence (e.g., references [126, 154]), and Morris et al. [76] suggest that relatively small differences in the prevalence of concurrency in different ethnic groups in the USA may explain large disparities in disease burden.

In a network-modeling analysis of egocentric data from the Add Health study [76] Morris and coauthors argue that racial disparities are due to a combination of two factors: (1) assortative partner choice by ethnic group (most people choose partners of the same ethnic group, most of the time: 95% of partnerships were racially concordant in the dataset) and (2) African Americans having more partnership concurrency than whites. Importantly, rates of concurrency were only slightly higher in African Americans but resulted in a much greater burden of disease because it created a much more highly interconnected network, facilitating more rapid and more widespread transmission of infection. Concurrency is also postulated as the explanation for the high burden of HIV in much of sub-Saharan Africa (see below).

A Disproportionately Affected Group: Men Who Have Sex with Men

Men who have sex with men typically experience a higher burden of disease from STI and HIV than heterosexuals living in the same setting. Dougan et al. [25] reported, "Twenty-five years after the first case of AIDS was reported, gay and bisexual men remain the group at greatest risk of acquiring HIV in the United Kingdom."

Superficially, this disparity may be apparently explained by individual-level risk factors: on average, MSM have more sexual partners than heterosexuals, and the variance in the numbers of sexual partners tends to be greater for MSM: i.e., the proportion of MSM reporting having large numbers of sexual partners is greater than the corresponding proportion for heterosexuals. However, an analysis by Goodreau and Golden [155] that neatly demonstrates the power of mathematical modeling to determine whether a postulated causal factor could have an effect of sufficient magnitude to explain a particular outcome shows that individual-level behavior alone does not explain the large discrepancy in disease burden. Goodreau and Golden [155] found that a key factor is the higher transmission probability of penile–anal intercourse compared with penile–vaginal intercourse. Additionally, unlike heterosexuals, MSM can be "versatile" with regard to sex-role—i.e., the same individual can be both receptive (which has a higher risk of acquisition of HIV) and insertive (which has a higher risk of HIV transmission). The study reports, "The US heterosexual population would only experience an epidemic comparable to MSM if the mean partner number of heterosexual individuals was increased several fold over that observed in population-based studies of either group. In order for MSM to eliminate the HIV epidemic, they would need to develop rates of unprotected sex lower than those currently exhibited by heterosexual individuals in the United States. In this model, for US heterosexual individuals to have a self-sustaining epidemic, they would need to adopt levels of unprotected sex higher than those currently exhibited by US MSM."

An additional factor contributing to the disproportionate STI burden in MSM may be the fact that a homosexual network can be more clustered (and hence have more potential paths for transmission) than a heterosexual network: whilst MSM could be connected in a closed-loop cycle of three individuals, the smallest possible closed-loop in a heterosexual network is four individuals.

HIV Burden in Africa

There has been a lot of debate about why the burden of HIV is so much greater in some African countries, which have "generalized" epidemics with high prevalence in the heterosexual population, than elsewhere. A study by Lopman et al. in Zimbabwe [156] found that individual-level proximate determinants explained very little of the risk of HIV acquisition, and they comment "in this generalized epidemic there is little difference in readily identifiable characteristics of the individual between those who acquire infection and those who do not." A variety of explanations for the exceptional burden of HIV in generalized epidemics in Africa have been offered, and it may be the case that a combination of factors are responsible, including higher rates of sexual partner change; age-differentials in sexual partnerships [67]; "epidemiological synergy" in which STIs promote the transmission of HIV [134–136] (so a high prevalence of STIs accelerates the

spread of HIV); epidemiological synergy due to malaria [157]; and a higher prevalence of concurrent sexual partnerships [158]. Variation in the burden of disease between African countries and between different communities in those countries may be due at least in part to differences in the prevalence of male circumcision [159], which randomized control trials have found to reduce susceptibility of males to HIV acquisition by 60% [160–162], and which modeling analysis suggests may reduce transmission of HIV from men to women by 46% [163]. Other factors that may be important are differences in sexual behavior (including different responses to awareness of HIV), differences in access to care, and differences in government policies, laws (e.g., concerning homosexual behavior or commercial sex), and social attitudes about HIV.

Conclusion and Practical Applications of Insights

We need a better understanding of STI epidemiology and the causes of disparities to enable us to intervene effectively to reduce the burden of STIs and HIV and reduce inequality. Having established the complexity of STI epidemiology and the causes of disparities, how much information do we need to gather from a particular setting to guide effective actions? Effective action requires that we correctly identify the key factors driving STI transmission *that can be impacted by cost-effective interventions*. If we are not able to affect a particular factor significantly—at least, without excessive cost—then clearly it is not a suitable target for intervention.

To design effective interventions we need to know the importance of different factors in driving STI transmission, how much those factors can be impacted by interventions, at what cost, over what timescale, and in which groups. This means that we need to have a better understanding about causes. Many factors have been found to be associated with disparities, but many of them may be correlates rather than underlying causal factors. Complexities of sexual behavior mean that getting an understanding of a particular situation requires detailed characterization. We need to know not just mean rates and variances in numbers of partners over time but also such characteristics as mixing patterns, gap lengths between partnerships or concurrency (including the number of concurrent partners), condom use (with different partners), and access to care. It is challenging to collect detailed data routinely. Social network analysis approaches have led to important insights into STI/HIV epidemiology, but nevertheless simpler approaches continue to have value due to the empirical and technical challenges of network analysis. Indeed, many modelers who use network models also use simpler models: the appropriate model to use depends upon the question being asked and the data available to parameterize the model.

Key to improving understanding is having more data on more settings to determine the generalizability of current findings. This in turn requires the development of indicators that are practicable to measure on a large scale in multiple settings. These indicators would also be used for public health monitoring that complements the existing surveillance systems to guide timely interventions that are appropriate to the epidemic phase [16, 40, 41], and to evaluate the effectiveness of those interventions.

Elucidation of detailed network structure to inform on the epidemic phase to guide public health action has been advocated [117], but network elucidation for STI public health monitoring is not the norm and is not likely to become so, particularly in an era of budget cuts. At present, typically only around half of sexual partners of index-case patients are notified for purposes of infection management, and many of those are contacted by the index patient, rather than clinical staff. Finding partners of partners is rare outside of a research study. If Morris et al. [66] are correct that network structure can be inferred from a few simple measures collected from egocentric sampling then monitoring network structure becomes much more feasible—once the inferential rules have been determined. Of course, detailed research is required to validate putative indicators and determine if the information they yield is worth the cost of obtaining the data, but indicators

are likely to include behavioral and network measures such as rates of partnership turnover, gap length between partnerships, prevalence of non-monogamy, numbers of concurrent partners, and mixing patterns. An alternative approach may be to use genetic analysis of pathogen isolates, which is becoming routine as the technology becomes ever cheaper. Coupled with enriched routine surveillance data, pathogen genetic analysis may offer a cheap means of realizing Potterat et al.'s vision of monitoring network structure.

Alongside an improved understanding of the epidemiology we need to develop implementation science: i.e., we also need a better understanding of how to intervene effectively. This includes developing better tools to assess interventions. Aral et al. [15] commented that "evaluation of the population level impact of STD prevention programmes is still limited." Crucially, *it also involves incorporating evaluation into the design of interventions, and ensuring that the necessary data are collected prospectively.* Aral et al. [15] report, "The lack of a comprehensive, standardised and consistent measurement and reporting system for risk behaviours and programme activities further complicates evaluation concerns. Implementation science … is in the very early stages of development. Consequently, many questions central to planning and implementation of prevention programmes—including when to implement particular interventions, who to target, how much coverage is required to have a population level impact, how much coverage is achievable, what incremental impact can be expected from the addition of a particular intervention to the intervention mix and at what point diminishing marginal returns set in—often remain unanswered."

The roll-out of interventions such as Chlamydia screening, expedited partner therapy, male circumcision (to reduce HIV acquisition and transmission), ART for HIV, and routinized universal HIV testing provides an opportunity to measure the effectiveness of interventions at scale—provided evaluation is incorporated into the roll-out planning, such as using a stepped-wedge trial design. Unfortunately, these opportunities are usually not taken.

The spatiotemporal scales and complexity of dynamic interactions in infectious disease epidemiology mean that evaluating public health interventions in a randomized controlled trial framework is challenging, costly, time-consuming, and often simply not possible. Even when such trials can be carried out, there remain questions about generalizability of both positive and negative findings to settings outside the trial, including applying the intervention in the same location under "real-world" rather than "research" conditions [55]. A key problem is that even relatively large-scale trials are typically much smaller than the full-scale intervention, and are carried out for a short period (especially relative to the dynamics of long-term infections like HIV). Also, it is not practicable to measure the contributions and interactions of different intervention components through a factorial trial design with multiple arms and replicates. Mathematical modeling can be used to assess the effectiveness of "real-world" interventions that have been applied at full scale by comparing the observed outcome with a model-derived counterfactual, and can be used to examine the relative contributions of different components of interventions to the outcome [55].

How to Intervene?

Another key question is the scale of intervention required: its coverage, intensity, and duration. Unfortunately, the non-linearities of infection transmission dynamics complicate decision-making because they mean that the benefit of an intervention is almost never proportional to its scale—doubling the size of the intervention usually does not simply double the benefit. Indeed, it is often the case that a small intervention produces little population-level benefit, but increasing the size of the intervention produces disproportionately large increase in the population-level benefit (by averting transmission), until a point is reached where there is little further incremental benefit to be gained by further scaling-up. An example of this is described by White et al. [43]. Also, effects of interventions are usually time-varying.

The nonlinear and time-varying interactions inherent in infectious disease epidemiology mean that mathematical modeling has an important role to play in helping to determine what scale of intervention is required [43, 159] and over what timescale outcomes should be expected: it is important not to assess too soon and draft an incorrect conclusion that an intervention has not been effective. Furthermore, combinations of interventions are often necessary, particularly against HIV. Non-linearities mean that when interventions are combined their effect together is almost never additive. That is, the whole is almost never equal to the sum of the parts: there are usually synergies (greater-than-additive effects) or redundancies (less-than-additive effects) [164].

An important use of modeling is examining uncertainty. Typically, it is not obvious what the most (cost-)effective intervention would be. For example, Garnett et al. [165] found that "Both reducing numbers of sex partners and increasing condom use can lower [STI]… incidence … Unfortunately, there is no simple and general rule that will allow the efficiency of interventions to be calculated."

Targeting

A key consideration for interventions against STI/HIV is whether to have a targeted or a generalized intervention. The impact of targeting a core group of high-risk individuals will depend upon the importance of the core group in the persistence of infection. Provided it can be done effectively, targeting core groups is likely to have more of an impact on syphilis and gonorrhea than on Chlamydia or herpes, which are much more widespread. This is why Chlamydia screening is typically a generalized intervention, with eligibility determined by age. Overlapping core groups for different STIs mean that a geographically targeted intervention may be effective against multiple infections [36, 37]. (However, in settings where persistence may be due to widespread low-degree concurrency then there is not in fact a core group to be targeted.) Where targeting is used, the selection of the target population needs to be cognizant of transmission dynamics. Chen et al. [95] argue, "gonorrhea is sustained by the presence of a small group of individuals with short gap lengths and medium length partnerships. Interventions targeted at this group are more effective than those targeted at individuals with high numbers of sexual partners but longer gap lengths."

There has been debate over the importance of PHI (primary HIV infection) in HIV transmission, and whether interventions targeted at it could be effective. The importance of PHI will vary temporally and according to circumstances. In a nascent epidemic the majority of infections will be recently acquired whereas in a mature epidemic HIV-positive individuals will be in all stages of infection, and so the relative importance of PHI will decline over time. Recent modeling studies have found that all stages of HIV infection play a significant role in transmission [166, 167]. Nevertheless, frequent testing of high-risk individuals to detect PHI may have a role to play in prevention of transmission through highly interconnected networks [127, 168]. Targeting may be a more efficient use of scarce resources than a generalized intervention, but not if the costs of targeting exceed the savings, or if targeting is not practicable. Targeting may also be counterproductive if it is stigmatizing and discourages the target groups from participating in the intervention. Although the distribution of HIV in the USA is highly heterogeneous, "routinizing" of testing the entire population in a variety of healthcare settings is advocated [112]. In the UK, it has been recommended that there should be universal testing of the population living in geographic areas with diagnosed HIV prevalence exceeding 1 per 1,000 persons [169, 170].

Network Interventions

Our growing understanding of networks can inform effective interventions [141]. Of course, contact tracing from infected STI clinic patients is a "network" intervention against STIs that predates the field of social network analysis. It is used to identify individuals who are at elevated risk of having acquired infection (because they have been in contact with an infected person) and who may be potentially at high risk of transmitting it. Individuals who are highly connected in the sexual partnership network may be effective targets for education, as reducing their number of sexual partners may greatly reduce network connectivity. Highly connected individuals are more likely to acquire infection, meaning that treatment clinics may be an effective means of reaching them, and providing an opportunity for intervention.

Contact tracing has the problem of missing links, for which alternative network approaches may compensate. Valencia et al. [171] reported, "It is possible to identify theoretically high-risk commercial sex clients from the network perspective using simple data collection and categorization approaches." Venues associated with high-risk activity or acquisition of infection may be effective targets for interventions [34, 97, 98]. Wohlfeiler and Potterat [172] argue for interventions: "Helping gay and bisexual men make more informed choices about their partners and fragmenting networks" and that "Network-level interventions are particularly well suited for places such as commercial sex venues and Internet sites where gay and bisexual men meet new sexual partners."

Another potential intervention aimed at reducing network connectivity is to encourage behavior change to reduce sexual partnership concurrency in settings where it is important. It has been argued that a small reduction in the prevalence of concurrency could greatly reduce the burden of disease in African Americans [76]. (Also, even for individuals who do not have concurrent partners, a short gap length between partnerships facilitates transmission [95, 96] and an increase in gap length may potentially reduce the burden of disease in populations.) However, there is uncertainty over the importance of concurrency in different settings, and it is likely that the importance of concurrency varies between settings and varies over time within settings (e.g., see Eaton et al. [127]). Furthermore, it is not clear to what extent interventions can alter rates of concurrency.

Social networks can be used to educate and attempt to change social norms, particularly in high-risk groups where the social and transmission networks may be closely related [141]. New technology presents new challenges, by affecting social networks and norms and through directly affecting sexual contact networks through "dating" Websites and more dynamic cell-phone-based technology such as Grindr (http://www.grindr.com). However, these technologies also provide new tools to study networks and better understand behavior, and they potentially provide new intervention approaches, using social media to disseminate health-promotion messages to alter knowledge, attitudes, behaviors, and social norms.

In the last few decades, we have come a long way in our understanding of STI/HIV epidemiology, as well as the interacting factors associated with epidemic phase, dynamic spatiotemporal distributions, and disparities in disease burden. However, there is much still to be learned, particularly in the field of intervention science: we need to prioritize translating knowledge into effective action. Additionally, the complex dynamics of social and sexual behavior and of infection transmission mean that we need better tools for real-time monitoring of behavior and transmission to improve vigilance and to adapt to ever-changing health needs.

References

1. UNAIDS. AIDS epidemic update. 2009. ISBN 978 92 9173 832 8.
2. Grassly NC, Garnett GP, Schwartländer B, Gregson S, Anderson RM. The effectiveness of HIV prevention and the epidemiological context. Bull World Health Organ. 2001;79:1121–32.
3. Christakis NA, Fowler JH. Connected: the surprising power of our social networks and how they shape our lives. Little, Brown and Company; 2009. ISBN-10: 0316036145; ISBN-13: 978-0316036146.
4. Nudge: improving decisions about health, wealth, and happiness. Yale University Press; 2008. ISBN-10: 0300122233; ISBN-13: 978-0300122237.
5. Hoover K, Bohm M, Keppel K. Measuring disparities in the incidence of sexually transmitted diseases. Sex Transm Dis. 2008;35(12):S40–4. doi:10.1097/OLQ.0b013e3181886750.
6. Kerani RP, Handcock MS, Handsfield HH, et al. Comparative geographic concentrations of 4 sexually transmitted infections. Am J Public Health. 2005;95:324–30.
7. Semaan S, Sternberg M, Zaidi A, Aral SO. Social capital and rates of gonorrhea and syphilis in the United States: spatial regression analyses of state-level associations. Soc Sci Med. 2007;64:2324–41.
8. Chesson HW, Sternberg M, Leichliter JS, Aral SO. The distribution of chlamydia, gonorrhoea and syphilis cases across states and counties in the USA, 2007. Sex Transm Infect. 2010;86 Suppl 3:iii52–7.
9. Lansky A, Brooks JT, DiNenno E, Heffelfinger J, Hall HI, Mermin J. Epidemiology of HIV in the United States. J Acquir Immune Defic Syndr. 2010;55:S64–8.
10. Jennings J, Carriero FC, Celentano D, Ellen JM. Geographic identification of high gonorrhea transmission areas in Baltimore, Maryland. Am J Epidemiol. 2005;161:73–80.
11. Tillerson K. Explaining racial disparities in HIV/AIDS incidence among women in the U.S.: a systematic review. Stat Med. 2008;27:4132–43. doi:10.1002/sim.3224.
12. Klevens RM, Diaz T, Fleming PL, Mays MA, Frey R. Trends in AIDS among hispanics in the United States, 1991–1996. Am J Public Health. 1999;89(7):1104–6.
13. Monteiro EF, Lacey CJN, Merrick D. The interrelation of demographic and geospatial risk factors between four common sexually transmitted diseases. Sex Transm Infect. 2005;81:41–6. doi:10.1136/sti.2004.009431.
14. Macdonald N, Elam G, Hickson F, Imrie J, McGarrigle CA, Fenton KA, Baster K, Ward H, Gilbart VL, Power RM, Evans BG. Factors associated with HIV seroconversion in gay men in England at the start of the 21st century. Sex Transm Inf. 2008;84:8–13.
15. Aral SO, Fenton KA, Holmes KK. Sexually transmitted diseases in the USA: temporal trends. Sex Transm Infect. 2007;83:257–66.
16. Ward H. Prevention strategies for sexually transmitted infections: importance of sexual network structure and epidemic phase. Sex Transm Infect. 2007;83 Suppl 1:i43–9.
17. Simms I, Fenton KA, Ashton M, et al. The re-emergence of syphilis in the United Kingdom: the new epidemic phases. Sex Transm Dis. 2005;32:220–6.
18. Stall RD, Hays RB, Waldo CR, Ekstrand M, McFarland W. The Gay '90s: a review of research in the 1990s on sexual behavior and HIV risk among men who have sex with men. AIDS. 2000;14 Suppl 3:S101–14.
19. Chesson HW, Dee TS, Aral SO. AIDS mortality may have contributed to the decline in syphilis rates in the United States in the 1990s. Sex Transm Dis. 2003;30(5):419–24.

20. Centers for Disease Control. Pneumocystis pneumonia – Los Angeles. MMWR Morb Mortal Wkly Rep. 1981;30:250–2.

21. Centers for Disease Control. Kaposi's sarcoma and Pneumocystis pneumonia among homosexual men – New York City and California. MMWR Morb Mortal Wkly Rep. 1981;30:305–8.

22. Korber B, Muldoon M, Theiler J, Gao F, Gupta R, Lapedes A, Hahn BH, Wolinsky S. Timing the ancestor of the HIV-1 pandemic strains. Science. 2000;288:1789–96.   doi:10.1126/science.288.5472.1789.

23. Gilbert MT, Rambaut A, Wlasiuk G, Spira TJ, Pitchenik AE, Worobey M. The emergence of HIV/AIDS in the Americas and beyond. Proc Natl Acad Sci USA. 2007;104:18566–70.

24. Hughes G, Porter K, Gill ON. Indirect methods for estimating prevalent HIV infections: adults in England and Wales at the end of 1993. Epidemiol Infect. 1998;121:165–72.

25. Dougan S, Evans BG, Macdonald N, Goldberg DJ, Gill ON, Fenton KA, Elford J. HIV in gay and bisexual men in the United Kingdom: 25 years of public health surveillance. Epidemiol Infect. 2008;136:145–56.

26. Hall HI, Song R, Rhodes P, Prejean J, An Q, Lee LM, Karon J, Brookmeyer R, Kaplan EH, McKenna MT, Janssen RS, HIV Incidence Surveillance Group. Estimation of HIV incidence in the United States. JAMA. 2008;300(5):520–9.

27. Atun RA, McKee M, Coker R, Gurol-Urganci I. Health systems' responses to 25 years of HIV in Europe: inequities persist and challenges remain. Health Policy. 2008;86:181–94.

28. White PJ, Ward H, Garnett GP. Is HIV out of control in the UK? An example of analysing patterns of HIV spread using incidence-to-prevalence ratios. AIDS. 2006;20:1898–901.

29. Prost A, Elford J, Imrie J, Petticrew M, Hart GJ. Social, behavioural, and intervention research among people of sub-Saharan African origin living with HIV in the UK and Europe: literature review and recommendations for intervention. AIDS Behav. 2008;12:170–94.

30. Aggarwal I, Smith M, Tatt ID, Murad S, Osner N, Geretti AM, Easterbrook PJ. Evidence for onward transmission of HIV-1 non-B subtype strains in the United Kingdom. J Acquir Immune Defic Syndr. 2006;41(2):201–9.   doi:10.1097/01.qai.0000179430.34660.11.

31. Stancliff S. Syringe access and HIV incidence in the United States. JAMA. 2008;300(20):2370.

32. Rothenberg RB. The geography of gonorrhea: empirical demonstration of core group transmission. Am J Epidemiol. 1983;117:688–94.

33. Rothenberg RB, Sterk C, Toomey KE, et al. Using social network and ethnographic tools to evaluate syphilis transmission. Sex Transm Dis. 1998;25:154–60.

34. Potterat JJ, Rothenberg RB, Woodhouse DE, Muth JB, Pratts CI, Fogle JS. Gonorrhea as a social disease. Sex Transm Dis. 1985;12:25–32.

35. Elliott LJ, Blanchard JF, Beaudoin CM, Green CG, Nowicki DL, Matusko P, Moses S. Geographical variations in the epidemiology of bacterial sexually transmitted infections in Manitoba, Canada. Sex Transm Infect. 2002;78:i139–44.

36. Law DG, Serre ML, Christakos G, Leone PA, Miller WC. Spatial analysis and mapping of sexually transmitted diseases to optimise intervention and prevention strategies. Sex Transm Infect. 2004;80:294–9. doi:10.1136/sti.2003.006700.

37. Fichtenberg CM, Ellen JM. Moving from core groups to risk spaces. Sex Transm Dis. 2003;30(11):825–6.   doi:10.1097/01.OLQ.0000097141.29899.7F.

38. Potterat JJ. Sexual network configuration of sexually transmitted diseases hyperendemicity as harbinger of epidemicity. Sex Transm Dis. 2009;36(1):49–50.

39. Law DG, Bernstein K, Serre ML, Schumacher C, Leone PA, Zenilman JM, Miller W, Rompalo AM. Modeling a syphilis outbreak through space and time using the Bayesian maximum entropy approach. Ann Epidemiol. 2006;16(11):797–804.

40. Wasserheit JN, Aral SO. The dynamic topology of sexually transmitted disease epidemics: implications for prevention strategies. J Infect Dis. 1996;174 Suppl 2:S201–13.

41. Aral SO. Determinants of STD epidemics: implications for phase appropriate intervention strategies. Sex Transm Infect. 2002;78:i3–13.

42. Grassly NC, Fraser C, Garnett GP. Host immunity and synchronized epidemics of syphilis across the United States. Nature. 2005;433:417–21. doi:10.1038/nature03072.

43. White PJ, Ward H, Cassell JA, Mercer CH, Garnett GP. Vicious and virtuous circles in the dynamics of infectious disease and the provision of health care: gonorrhea in Britain as an example. J Infect Dis. 2005;192:824–36.

44. Schumacher CM, Ellen J, Rompalo AM. Changes in demographics and risk behaviors of persons with early syphilis depending on epidemic phase. Sex Transm Dis. 2008;35:190–6.

45. Infectious diseases of humans: dynamics and control. Oxford University Press, New York; 1991. 768pp. ISBN-10: 0198545991; ISBN-13: 978-0198545996.

46. Grassly NC, Fraser C. Mathematical models of infectious disease transmission. Nat Rev Microbiol. 2008;6:477–87.

47. Garnett GP. An introduction to mathematical models in sexually transmitted disease epidemiology. Sex Transm Infect. 2002;78:7–12.

48. Mishra S, Fisman DN, Boily M-C. The ABC of terms used in mathematical models of infectious diseases. J Epidemiol Community Health. 2011;65:87–94. doi:10.1136/jech.2009.097113.

49. White PJ, Enright MC. Mathematical models in infectious disease epidemiology. In: Cohen J, Powderly WG, Opal SM, editors. Infectious diseases, 3rd ed. Elsevier; 2010. p. 70–75. ISBN-10: 0323045790; ISBN-13: 978-0323045797.

50. Cooke KL, Yorke JA. Some equations modelling growth processes and gonorrhea epidemics. Math Biosci. 1973;16:75–101.

51. Lajmanovich A, Yorke JA. A deterministic model for gonorrhea in a nonhomogeneous population. Math Biosci. 1976;28(3–4):221–36. doi:10.1016/0025-5564(76)90125-5.

52. Yorke JA, Hethcote HW, Nold A. Dynamics and control of the transmission of gonorrhea. Sex Transm Dis. 1978;5(2):51–6.

53. Hethcote HW, Yorke JA, Nold A. Gonorrhea modeling: a comparison of control methods. Math Biosci. 1982;58(1):93–109.   doi:10.1016/0025-5564(82)90053-0.

54. Hethcote HW, Yorke JA. Gonorrhea transmission dynamics and control, lecture notes in biomathematics, vol. 56. Berlin: Springer; 1984. 105pp. ISBN 0-387-13870-6.

55. Hallett TB, White PJ, Garnett GP. The appropriate evaluation of HIV prevention interventions: from experiment to full scale implementation. Sex Transm Infect. 2007;83(Suppl I):i55–60.

56. Brunham RC, Plummer FA. A general model of sexually transmitted disease epidemiology and its implications for control. Med Clin North Am. 1990;74:1339–52.

57. Garnett GP, Anderson RM. Factors controlling the spread of HIV in heterosexual communities in developing countries: patterns of mixing between different age and sexual activity classes. Philos Trans R Soc Lond B. 1993;342:137–59.

58. Anderson RM, Gupta S, Ng W. The significance of sexual partner contact networks for the transmission dynamics of HIV. J Acquir Immune Defic Syndr. 1990;3:417–29.

59. Aral SO, Hughes JP, Stoner B, Whittington W, Handsfield HH, Anderson RM, Holmes KK. Sexual mixing patterns in the spread of gonococcal and chlamydial infections. Am J Public Health. 1999;89(6):825–33.

60. Aral SO. Patterns of sex partner recruitment and types of mixing as determinants of STD transmission. Venereology. 1995;8:240–2.

61. Gupta S, Anderson RM, May RM. Networks of sexual contacts: implications for the pattern of spread of HIV. AIDS. 1989;3:807–17.

62. Blower SM, McLean AR. Mixing ecology and epidemiology. Proc R Soc Lond B Biol Sci. 1991;245(1314):187–92.

63. Brunham RC. Core group theory: a central concept in STD epidemiology. Venereology. 1997;10:34–9.

64. Golden MR, Whittington WLH, Handsfield HH, Hughes JP, Stamm WE, Hogben M, Clark A, Malinski C, Helmers JRL, Thomas KK, Holmes KK. Effect of expedited treatment of sex partners on recurrent or persistent gonorrhea or chlamydial infection. N Engl J Med. 2005;352:676–85.

65. Garnett GP. The geographical and temporal evolution of sexually transmitted disease epidemics. Sex Transm Infect. 2002;78(Suppl):i14–9.

66. Morris M, Goodreau S, Moody J. Chapter 7: sexual networks, concurrency, and STD/HIV. In: Holmes KK, Sparling PF, Stamm WE, Piot P, Wasserheit JN, Corey L, Cohen MS, editors. Sexually transmitted diseases. 4th ed. McGraw-Hill Medical; 2008. p. 109–126. ISBN-10: 0071417486; ISBN-13: 978-0071417488.

67. Gregson S, Nyamukapa CA, Garnett GP, Mason PR, Zhuwau T, Caraël M, Chandiwana SK, Anderson RM. Sexual mixing patterns and sex-differentials in teenage exposure to HIV infection in rural Zimbabwe. Lancet. 2002;359(9321):1896–903.

68. Johnson KM, Alarcon J, Watts DM, Rodriguez C, Velasquez C, Sanchez J, Lockhart D, Stoner BP, Holmes KK. Sexual networks of pregnant women with and without HIV infection. AIDS. 2003;17:605–12.

69. Morris M, Podhisita C, Wawer MJ, Hancock MS. Bridge populations in the spread of HIV/AIDS in Thailand. AIDS. 1996;10(11):1265–71.

70. Adimora AA, Schoenbach VJ, Martinson FE, et al. Heterosexually transmitted HIV infection among African Americans in North Carolina. J Acquir Immune Defic Syndr. 2006;41:616–23.

71. Hightow LB, Leone PA, Macdonald PD, McCoy SI, Sampson LA, Kaplan AH. Men who have sex with men and women: a unique risk group for HIV transmission on North Carolina College campuses. Sex Transm Dis. 2006;33(10):585–93.

72. Klovdahl AS. Social networks and the spread of infectious diseases. Soc Sci Med. 1985;21(11):1203–16.

73. Doherty IA, Padian NS, Marlow C, Aral SO. Determinants and consequences of sexual networks as they affect the spread of sexually transmitted infections. J Infect Dis. 2005;191 Suppl 1:S42–54.

74. Morris M, editor. Network epidemiology: a handbook for survey design and data collection (international studies in demography). Oxford University Press, New York; 2004. 252pp. ISBN-10: 0199269017; ISBN-13: 978-0199269013.

75. Kretzschmar M. Sexual network structure and sexually transmitted disease prevention – a modeling perspective. Sex Transm Dis. 2000;27(10):627–35.

76. Morris M, Kurth AE, Hamilton DT, Moody J, Wakefield S, Handcock M, for The Network Modeling Group. Concurrent partnerships and HIV prevalence disparities by race: linking science and public health practice. Am J Public Health. 2009;99(6):1023–31.

77. Watts DJ. The "new" science of networks. Annu Rev Sociol. 2004;30:243–70.

78. Luke DA, Harris JK. Network analysis in public health: history, methods, and applications. Annu Rev Public Health. 2007;28:69–93.

79. Smith KP, Christakis NA. Social networks and health. Annu Rev Sociol. 2008;34:405–29.

80. Morris M, Kretzschmar M. Concurrent partnerships and transmission dynamics in networks. Soc Net. 1995;17:299–318.

81. Morris M, Kretzschmar M. Concurrent partnerships and the spread of HIV. AIDS. 1997;11:641–8.

82. Ghani AC, Swinton J, Garnett GP. The role of sexual partnership networks in the epidemiology of gonorrhea. Sex Transm Dis. 1997;24(1):45–56.

83. Ghani AC, Donnelly CA, Garnett GP. Sampling biases and missing data in explorations of sexual partner networks for the spread of sexually transmitted diseases. Stat Med. 1998;17(18):2079–97.

84. Ghani AC, Garnett GP. Measuring sexual partner networks for transmission of sexually transmitted diseases. J R Stat Soc A Stat Soc. 1998;161: 227–38.

85. Ghani AC, Garnett GP. Risks of acquiring and transmitting sexually transmitted diseases in sexual partner networks. Sex Transm Dis. 2000;27(10): 579–87.

86. Ghani AC, Aral SO. Patterns of sex worker-client contacts and their implications for the persistence of sexually transmitted infections. J Infect Dis. 2005; 191:S34–41.

87. Chen MI, Ghani AC. Populations and partnerships: insights from metapopulation and pair models into the epidemiology of gonorrhoea and other sexually transmitted infections. Sex Transm Infect. 2010;86(6):433–9.

88. Chen MI, Ghani AC, Edmunds WJ. A metapopulation modelling framework for gonorrhoea and other sexually transmitted infections in heterosexual populations. J R Soc Interface. 2009;6:775–91.

89. Keeling MJ, Rand DA, Morris AJ. Correlation models for childhood epidemics. Proc Roy Soc ser B. 1997;264:1149–56.

90. Keeling MJ. The effects of local spatial structure on epidemiological invasions. Proc Roy Soc ser B. 1999;266:859–67.

91. Bauch CJ, Rand DA. A moment closure model for sexually transmitted disease transmission through a concurrent partnership network. Proc Roy Soc ser B. 2000;267:2019–27.

92. Eames KTD, Keeling MJ. Modeling dynamic and network heterogeneities in the spread of sexually transmitted disease. Proc Natl Acad Sci USA. 2002;99:13330–5.

93. Eames KTD, Keeling MJ. Monogamous networks and the spread of sexually transmitted diseases. Math Biosci. 2004;189:115–30.

94. Ferguson NM, Garnett GP. More realistic models of sexually transmitted disease transmission dynamics: sexual partnership networks, pair models, and moment closure. Sex Transm Dis. 2000;27:600–9.

95. Chen MI, Ghani AC, Edmunds J. Mind the gap: the role of time between sex with two consecutive partners on the transmission dynamics of gonorrhea. Sex Transm Dis. 2008;35:435–44.

96. Kraut-Becher JR, Aral SO. Gap length: an important factor in sexually transmitted disease transmission. Sex Transm Dis. 2003;30(3):221–5.

97. Day S, Ward H, Ghani AC, Bell G, Goan U, Parker M, Claydon E, Ison C, Kinghorn G, Weber J. Sexual histories, partnerships and networks associated with the transmission of gonorrhoea. Int J STD AIDS. 1998;9:666–71.

98. De P, Singh AE, Wong T, Yacoub W, Jolly AM. Sexual network analysis of a gonorrhoea outbreak. Sex Transm Infect. 2004;80:280–5. doi:10.1136/sti.2003.007187.

99. Wylie JL, Jolly AM. Patterns of chlamydia and gonorrhea infection in sexual networks in Manitoba, Canada. Sex Transm Dis. 2001;28(1):14–24.

100. Day S, Ward H, Ison C, Bell G, Weber J. Sexual networks: the integration of social and genetic data. Soc Sci Med. 1998;47(12):1981–92.

101. Ward H, Ison CA, Day SE, Martin I, Ghani AC, Garnett GP, Bell G, Kinghorn G, Weber JN. A prospective social and molecular investigation of gonococcal transmission. Lancet. 2000;356:1812–7.

102. Choudhury B, Risley CL, Ghani AC, et al. Identification of individuals with gonorrhoea within sexual networks: a population-based study. Lancet. 2006;368:139–46.

103. Risley CL, Ward H, Choudhury B, et al. Geographical and demographic clustering of gonorrhoea in London. Sex Transm Infect. 2007;83:481–7.

104. Krieger N, Waterman PD, Chen JT, et al. Monitoring socioeconomic inequalities in sexually transmitted infections, tuberculosis, and violence: geocoding and choice of area-based socioeconomic measures— the public health disparities geocoding project (US). Public Health Rep. 2003;118:240–60.

105. Zenilman JM, Ellish N, Fresia A, et al. The geography of sexual partnerships in Baltimore: applications of core theory dynamics using a geographic information system. Sex Transm Dis. 1999;26:75–81.

106. Kolader M-E, Dukers NHTM, van der Bij AK, Dierdorp M, Fennema JSA, Coutinho RA, Bruisten SM. Molecular epidemiology of Neisseria gonorrhoeae in Amsterdam, The Netherlands, shows distinct heterosexual and homosexual networks. J Clin Microbiol. 2006;44(8):2689–97. doi:10.1128/JCM.02311-05.

107. Cabral T, Jolly AM, Wylie JL. *Chlamydia trachomatis* omp1 genotypic diversity and concordance with sexual network data. J Infect Dis. 2003;187(2):279–86. doi:10.1086/346048.

108. Wylie JL, Cabral T, Jolly AM. Identification of networks of sexually transmitted infection: a molecular, geographic, and social network analysis. J Infect Dis. 2005;191:899–906.

109. Lewis F, Hughes GJ, Rambaut A, Pozniak A, Leigh Brown AJ. Episodic sexual transmission of HIV revealed by molecular phylodynamics. PLoS Med. 2008;5:e50. doi:10.1371/journal.pmed.0050050.

110. Hué S, Pillay D, Clewley JP, Pybus OG. Genetic analysis reveals the complex structure of HIV-1

transmission within defined risk groups. Proc Natl Acad Sci. 2005;102(12):4425–9. doi:10.1073/pnas.0407534102.

111. Chadborn TR, Baster K, Delpech VC, Sabin CA, Sinka K, Rice BD, Evans BG. No time to wait: how many HIV-infected homosexual men are diagnosed late and consequently die? (England and Wales, 1993–2002). AIDS. 2005;19(5):513–20.

112. Fenton KA. Changing epidemiology of HIV/AIDS in the United States: implications for enhancing and promoting HIV testing strategies. Clin Infect Dis. 2007;45:S213–20.

113. Stoner BP, Whittington WL, Hughes JP, Aral SO, Holmes KK. Comparative epidemiology of heterosexual gonococcal and chlamydial networks – implications for transmission patterns. Sex Transm Dis. 2000;27(4):215–23.

114. Klovdahl AS, Potterat JJ, Woodhouse DE, Muth JB, Muth SQ, Darrow WW. Social networks and infectious disease: the Colorado Springs study. Soc Sci Med. 1994;38:79–88.

115. Rothenberg RB, Hoang TDM, Muth SQ, Crosby R. The Atlanta Urban Adolescent Network Study: a network view of STD prevalence. Sex Transm Dis. 2007;34(8):525–31.

116. De Rubeis E, Wylie JL, Cameron DW, Nair RC, Jolly AM. Combining social network analysis and cluster analysis to identify sexual network types. Int J STD AIDS. 2007;18:754–9.

117. Potterat JJ, Muth SQ, Rothenberg RB, Zimmerman-Rogers H, Green DL, Taylor JE, Bonney MS, White HA. Sexual network structure as an indicator of epidemic phase. Sex Transm Infect. 2002;78:i152–8.

118. Rothenberg RB, Kimbrough L, Lewis-Hardy R, Heath B, Williams OC, Pradyna T, Johnson D, Schrader M. Social network methods for endemic foci of syphilis: a pilot project. Sex Transm Dis. 2000;27(1):12–8.

119. Friedman SR, Neaigus A, Jose B, Curtis R, Goldstein M, Ildefonso G, Rothenberg RB, Des Jarlais DC. Sociometric risk networks and risk for HIV infection. Am J Public Health. 1997;87:1289–96.

120. Liljeros F, Edling CR, Amaral LAN, et al. The web of human sexual contacts. Nature. 2001;411(6840):907–8. doi:10.1038/35082140.

121. Jones JH, Handcock MS. Sexual contacts and epidemic thresholds. Nature. 2003;423(6940):605–6. doi:10.1038/423605a.

122. Hudson CP. Concurrent partnerships could cause AIDS epidemics. Int J STD AIDS. 1993;4:249–53.

123. Potterat JJ, Zimmerman-Rogers H, Muth S, et al. Chlamydia transmission: concurrency, reproduction number, and the epidemic trajectory. Am J Epidemiol. 1999;150:1331–9.

124. Koumans E, Farley T, Gibson J, et al. Characteristics of persons with syphilis in areas of persisting syphilis in the United States: sustained transmission associated with concurrent partnerships. Sex Transm Dis. 2001;28:497–503.

125. Jennings J, Glass B, Parham P, Adler N, Ellen JM. Sex partner concurrency, geographic context, and adolescent sexually transmitted infections. Sex Transm Dis. 2004;31(12):733–9. doi:10.1097/01.olq.0000145850.12858.87.

126. Adimora AA, Schoenbach VJ, Doherty IA. Concurrent sexual partnerships among men in the United States. Am J Public Health. 2007;97:2230–7.

127. Eaton JW, Hallett TB, Garnett GP. Concurrent sexual partnerships and primary HIV infection: a critical interaction. AIDS Behav. 2010;15(4):687–92. doi:10.1007/s10461-010-9787-8.

128. Aral SO. Partner concurrency and the STD/HIV epidemic. Curr Infect Dis Rep. 2010;12:134–9. doi:10.1007/s11908-010-0087-2.

129. Kretzschmar M, White RG, Caraël M. Concurrency is more complex than it seems. AIDS. 2010;24:313–5.

130. Aral SO, Blanchard JF. Phase specific approaches to the epidemiology and prevention of sexually transmitted diseases. Sex Transm Infect. 2002;78(Suppl):i1–2.

131. UNAIDS Working Group on Measuring Concurrent Sexual Partnerships. HIV: consensus indicators are needed for concurrency. Lancet. 2009;375:621–2.

132. Fenton KA, Mercer CH, McManus S, et al. Ethnic variations in sexual behaviour in Great Britain and risk of sexually transmitted infections: a probability survey. Lancet. 2005;365:1246–55.

133. Hogben M, Leichliter JS. Social determinants and sexually transmitted disease disparities. Sex Transm Dis. 2008;35(12):S13–8. doi:10.1097/OLQ.0b013e31818d3cad.

134. Wasserheit JN. Epidemiologic synergy – interrelationships between human-immunodeficiency-virus infection and other sexually-transmitted diseases – (Reprinted from AIDS and Womens Reproductive Health, CH 5, 1992). Sex Transm Dis. 1992;19:61–77.

135. Fleming DT, Wasserheit JN. From epidemiological synergy to public health policy and practice: the contribution of other sexually transmitted diseases to sexual transmission of HIV infection. Sex Transm Inf. 1999;75:3–17.

136. Corbett EL, Steketee RW, ter Kuile FO, et al. HIV-1/AIDS and the control of other infectious diseases in Africa. Lancet. 2002;359:2177–87. doi:10.1016/S0140-6736(02)09095-5.

137. Centola D. The spread of behavior in an online social network experiment. Science. 2010;329:1194–7. doi:10.1126/science.1185231.

138. Fox J, White PJ, Weber J, Garnett GP, Ward H, Fidler S. Quantifying sexual exposure to HIV within an HIV serodiscordant relationship: development of an algorithm. AIDS. 2011;25:1065–82.

139. Centola D, Willer R, Macy M. The Emperor's Dilemma: a computational model of self-enforcing norms. Am J Sociol. 2005;110(4):1009–40.

140. Christakis NA, Fowler JH. The collective dynamics of smoking in a large social network. N Engl J Med. 2008;358:2249–58.

141. Friedman SR, Bolyard M, Mateu-Gelabert P, Goltzman P, Pawlowicz MP, Singh DZ, Touze G, Diana Rossi D, Maslow C, Sandoval M, Flom PL. Some data-driven reflections on priorities in AIDS network research. AIDS Behav. 2007;11:641–51. doi:10.1007/s10461-006-9166-7.

142. Rogers EM. Diffusion of innovations. 3rd ed. New York: Free Press; 1983.

143. Smith AMA, Subramanian SV. Population contextual associations with heterosexual partner numbers: a multilevel analysis. Sex Transm Infect. 2006; 82:250–4.

144. Youm Y, Laumann EO. Social network effects on the transmission of sexually transmitted diseases. Sex Transm Dis. 2002;29:689–97.

145. Rothenberg R. Maintenance of endemicity in urban environments: a hypothesis linking risk, network structure and geography. Sex Transm Infect. 2007;83:10–5. doi:10.1136/sti.2006.017269.

146. Aral SO, Adimora AA, Fenton KA. Understanding and responding to disparities in HIV and other sexually transmitted infections in African Americans. Lancet. 2008;372:337–40.

147. Laumann EO, Youm Y. Racial/ethnic group differences in the prevalence of sexually transmitted diseases in the United States: a network explanation. Sex Transm Dis. 1999;26:250–61.

148. Turner KME, Garnett GP, Ghani AC, Sterne JAC, Low N. Investigating ethnic inequalities in the incidence of sexually transmitted infections: mathematical modelling study. Sex Transm Infect. 2004;80:379–85. doi:10.1136/sti.2003.007575.

149. Adimora AA, Schoenbach VJ. Social context, sexual networks, and racial disparities in rates of sexually transmitted infections. J Infect Dis. 2005;191 Suppl 1:S115–22.

150. Kraut-Becher J, Eisenberg M, Voytek C, Brown T, Metzger DS, Aral S. Examining racial disparities in HIV: lessons from sexually transmitted infections research. J Acquir Immune Defic Syndr. 2008;47 Suppl 1:S20–7.

151. Ford CL, Whetten KD, Hall SA, Kaufman JS, Thrasher AD. Black sexuality, social construction, and research targeting 'The Down Low' ('The DL'). Ann Epidemiol. 2007;17:209–16.

152. Pouget ER, Kershaw TS, Niccolai LM, Ickovics JR, Blankenship KM. Associations of sex ratios and male incarceration rates with multiple opposite-sex partners: potential social determinants of HIV/STI transmission. Public Health Rep. 2010;125 Suppl 4:70–80.

153. Khan MR, Miller WC, Schoenbach VJ, Weir SS, Jay S, Kaufman JS, Wohl DA, Adimora AA. Timing and duration of incarceration and high-risk sexual partnerships among African Americans in North Carolina. Ann Epidemiol. 2008;18:403–10.

154. Adimora AA, Schoenbach VJ. Contextual factors and the black-white disparity in heterosexual HIV transmission. Epidemiology. 2002;13(6):707–12.

155. Goodreau SM, Golden MR. Biological and demographic causes of high HIV and sexually transmitted disease prevalence in men who have sex with men. Sex Transm Infect. 2007;83:458–62.

156. Lopman B, Nyamukapa C, Mushati P, Mupambireyi Z, Mason P, Garnett GP, Gregson S. HIV incidence in 3 years of follow-up of a Zimbabwe cohort — 1998–2000 to 2001–03: contributions of proximate and underlying determinants to transmission. Int J Epidemiol. 2008;37:88–105. doi:10.1093/ije/dym255.

157. Abu-Raddad LJ, Patnaik P, Kublin JG. Dual infection with HIV and malaria fuels the spread of both diseases in sub-Saharan Africa. Science. 2006;314:1603–6. doi:10.1126/science.1132338.

158. Mah TL, Halperin DT. Concurrent sexual partnerships and the HIV epidemics in Africa: evidence to move forward. AIDS Behav. 2010;14(1):11–6.

159. UNAIDS/WHO/SACEMA Expert Group on Modelling the Impact and Cost of Male Circumcision for HIV Prevention. [Hankins C, Hargrove J, Williams B, Abu Raddad L, Auvert B, Bollinger L, Dorrington R, Ghani A, Gray R, Hallett T, Kahn JG, Lohse N, Nagelkerke N, Porco T, Schmid G, Stover J, Weiss H, Welte A, White P, White R.] Male circumcision for HIV prevention in high HIV prevalence settings: what can mathematical modelling contribute to informed decision making? PLoS Med. 2009; 6(9): e1000109. doi:10.1371/journal.pmed.1000109.

160. Auvert B, Sobngwi-Tambekou J, Cutler E, Nieuwoudt M, Lissouba P, Puren A, Taljaard D, et al. Randomized, controlled intervention trial of male circumcision for reduction of HIV infection risk: the ANRS 1265 Trial. PLoS Med. 2005;2:e298.

161. Bailey RC, Moses S, Parker CB, Agot K, Maclean I, Krieger JN, et al. Male circumcision for HIV prevention in young men in Kisumu, Kenya: a randomised controlled trial. Lancet. 2007;369:643–56.

162. Gray RH, Kigozi G, Serwadda D, Makumbi F, Watya S, Nalugoda F, Kiwanuka N, et al. Male circumcision for HIV prevention in men in Rakai, Uganda a randomised trial. Lancet. 2007;369:657–66.

163. Hallett TB, Alsallaq RA, Baeten JM, Weiss H, Celum C, Gray R, Abu-Raddad L. Will circumcision provide even more protection from HIV to women and men? New estimates of the population impact of circumcision interventions. Sex Transm Infect. 2011;87:88–93. doi:10.1136/sti.2010.043372.

164. Dodd PJ, White PJ, Garnett GP. Notions of synergy for combinations of interventions against infectious diseases in heterogeneously mixing populations. Math Biosci. 2010;227:94–104. doi:10.1016/j.mbs.2010.06.004.

165. Garnett GP, White PJ, Ward H. Fewer partners or more condoms? Modelling the effectiveness of STI

prevention interventions. Sex Transm Infect. 2008;84(Suppl II):i4–11.

166. Hollingsworth TD, Anderson RM, Fraser C. HIV-1 transmission, by stage of infection. J Infect Dis. 2008;198:687–93.

167. Abu-Raddad LJ, Longini IM. No HIV stage is dominant in driving the HIV epidemic in sub-Saharan Africa. AIDS. 2008;22:1055–61.

168. Fox J, White PJ, Macdonald N, Weber J, McClure M, Fidler S, Ward H. Reductions in HIV transmission risk behaviour following diagnosis of primary HIV infection: a cohort of high-risk men who have sex with men. HIV Med. 2009;10:432–8. doi:10.1111/j.1468-1293.2009.00708.x.

169. HIV testing – new guidelines call for wider testing. London, UK. 2008. http://www.hpa.org.uk/NewsCentre/NationalPressReleases/2008 PressReleases/ 080918HIVTestingNewGuidelines callforwidertesting/.

170. Health Protection Agency. Time to test for HIV: expanded healthcare and community HIV testing in England. Interim report. London, UK. 2010.

171. Remple VP, Patrick DM, Johnston C, Tyndall MW, Jolly AM. Clients of indoor commercial sex workers: heterogeneity in patronage patterns and implications for HIV and STI propagation through sexual networks. Sex Transm Dis. 2007;34(10):754–60. doi:10.1097/01.olq.0000261327.78674.cb.

172. Wohlfeiler D, Potterat JJ. Using gay men's sexual networks to reduce sexually transmitted disease (STD)/human immunodeficiency virus (HIV) transmission. Sex Transm Dis. 2005;32(10):S48–52. doi:10.1097/01.olq.0000175394.81945.68.

Migration and the Transmission of STIs

4

Ailsa R. Butler and Timothy B. Hallett

Introduction

Historically migration has been associated with the spread of ideas, artifacts, knowledge, and, less favorably, disease. This last, dramatically witnessed with the importation in the fifteenth century of small pox to the New World, resulted in dire consequences for the indigenous population [1]. A few hundred years later, small pox was introduced to Australia both in 1780 and 1870, and was a major cause of Aboriginal deaths [2]. With such grave effects it is perhaps no wonder that migration has been intuitively associated with spread of diseases through communities and that migrants are associated or even "blamed" for the spread of disease. More recently, there are reports of South Africans blaming migrants from Zimbabwe for spreading HIV [3, 4]. In any population, the spread of infectious disease depends on the rate of contact between susceptible and infectious individuals [5] and migration provides an important mechanism by which that can continue to happen. However with a sexually transmitted infection (STI) it is not movement and mixing alone but also changes in sexual behavior concomitant with migration that determine the impact on the potential level of disease spread.

In this chapter, we aim to examine the literature on migration on the spread of STIs, particularly HIV, from an epidemiological perspective to dissect the operations of migration as a mechanism of bringing infected individuals together with uninfected individuals and migration as a trigger for different types of changes in behavior. In the "Background" section, we begin by describing global patterns of migration and quantifying the volume of interest in this topic over time to illustrate the breadth and character of research in this area. Next we describe some of the early major studies that have documented a powerful association between migration and STIs at the individual and population levels and comment on the influence of biological properties of STIs and the epidemic context. In the "Review" section we define three distinct routes by which migration can influence epidemics—determining spatial distribution; affecting connectivity sexual partner networks; and directly influencing individuals' risk behavior—and illustrate these with examples drawn from our review of the literature.

A.R. Butler (✉) • T.B. Hallett
Department Infectious Disease Epidemiology,
Imperial College London, School of Public Health,
St. Mary's Campus, Norfolk Place,
London W2 1PG, UK
e-mail: abutler@imperial.ac.uk

Background

In 2006 3% (192 million) of the world's population were classified as international migrants; this has grown from 82 million in 1970 and 175

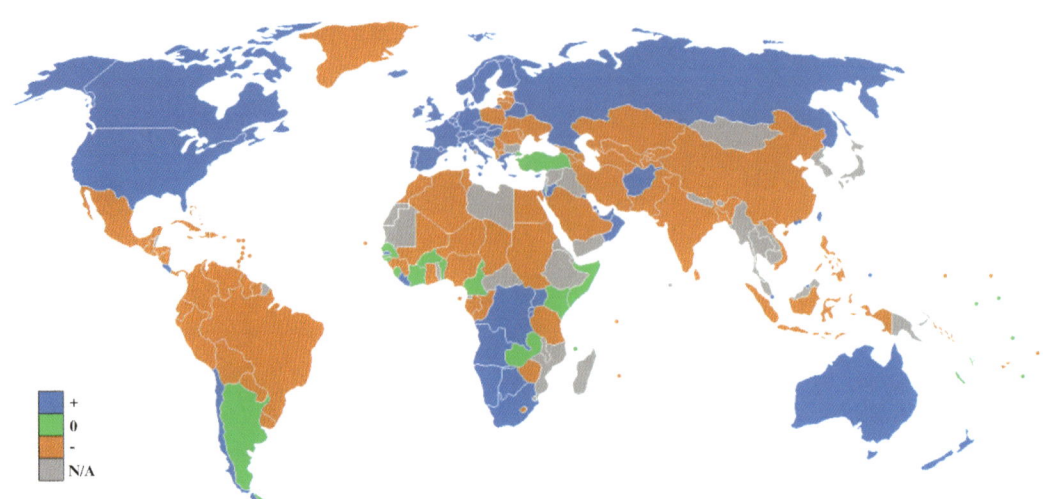

Fig. 4.1 Net migration rate showing positive, negative, and 0, based on CIA factbook data, 2006. http://www.cia.gov/cia/publications/factbook/fields/2112.html; http://en.wikipedia.org/wiki/File:Net_migration_rate_world.PNG

million in the year 2000 [6]. International migrant is defined by the United Nations as any person who changes his or her country of usual residence (long term for at least 1 year, short term for more than 3 months and less than 1 year). The predominant reason for migration is for economic improvement and most migrants travel from developing to developed countries [7]. In the year 2000 60% of the world's migrants lived in the more developed regions and 40% in the less developed regions [8]. International migration patterns are both cyclical and highly fluid. Unemployment, socioeconomic instability, political unrest, and unequal distribution of resources are all important issues that sustain mobility and represent common factors in both voluntary and forced migration [9]. The map shows the net emigration and immigration of countries across the world (Fig. 4.1).

Countries where the largest number of migrants originated from in 2006 were China, India, and the Philippines; the countries that received the most migrants were the USA, Russia, Germany, Ukraine, and France [7]. The International Organization for Migration (IOM) estimates that in the European Union 8.8%

(64 million) of the population is made up of migrants. Most of the world's migrants live in Europe, Asia, and North America [8].

Africa has seen a decline in its share of international migrants from 12% in 1970 to 9% in 2000 [10]. The percentage of the world's population that is made up of international migrants is increasing over time, Fig. 4.2a. As can also be seen in Fig. 4.2a there is a steep increase in the level of international migrants as a percentage of the population in North America, and a less steep rise in Oceania. In Africa however international migrants as a percentage of the population have decreased. The number of international migrants by region over time is given in Fig. 4.2b. Overall numbers have increased for every area; this is most pronounced for North America, Europe, and Asia.

The volume of interest in migration and HIV and STIs over time was explored by looking at the number of publications in each area collected on PubMed, an electronic archive of biomedical and life sciences journal literature. The number of publications on "migration and HIV/AIDS" or "migration and STIs" has increased over time at a rapid rate (Fig. 4.3a). In recent years, there have been approximately 160 new publications per

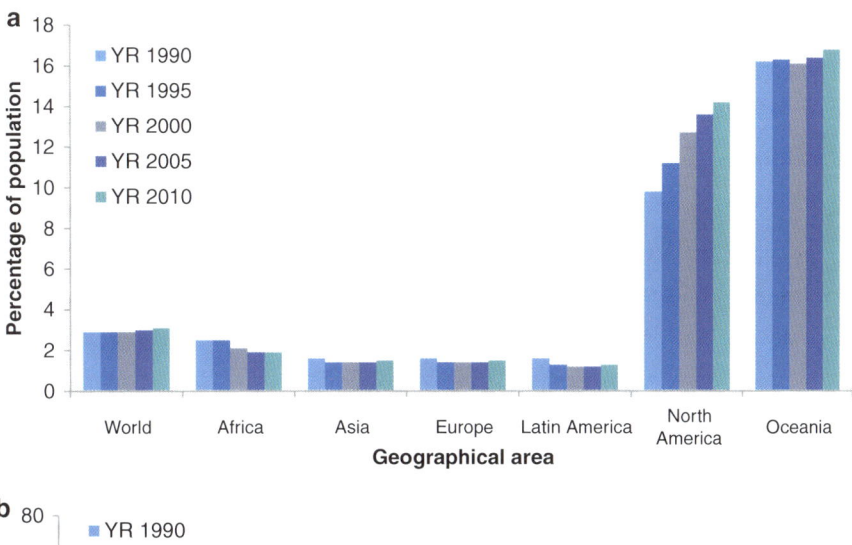

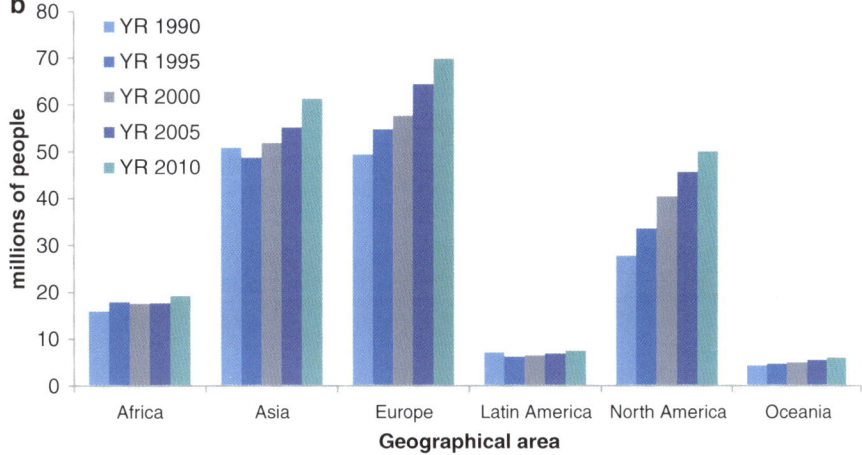

Fig. 4.2 (**a**) Estimated international migrants as a percentage of the total population over time from 1990 to 2010 by geographical area at mid-year (UN DP). (**b**) Estimated number of international migrants at mid-year over time from 1990 to 2010 by geographical area (UN DP)

year. The start of the steady rise in papers looking at migration and STIs/HIV seems to date from the emergence of HIV in the 1980s until 2007, although we also note that the differential coverage of this archive to journal articles published before the mid-1990s could generate a bias. The majority of publications focused on "migration and HIV/AIDS" rather than "migration and STIs" (Fig. 4.3b) and only a very small proportion of the literature on migration and STIs was made up of papers on other STIs. For this reason many of the examples cited here focus on HIV. There were more publications on syphilis or chlamydia than on gonorrhea.

From this review, it is clear that, from the very earliest works, there have been recurrent themes concerning the interaction between HIV and migration that we will briefly illustrate. These include how STIs have spread from urban to rural areas, the particular role of truck drivers in spreading HIV in sub-Saharan Africa, and the persistence of remarkable associations

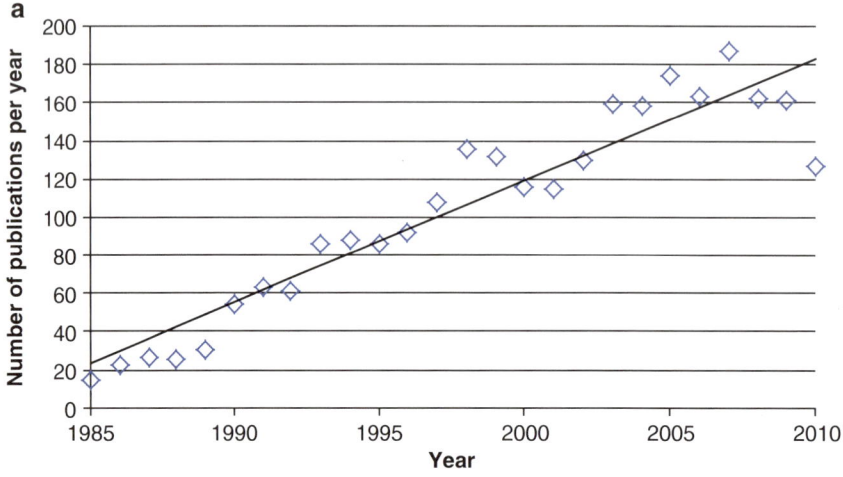

Fig. 4.3 (**a**) Number of publications on migration and HIV/AIDS, 1985-2010; (**b**) distribution of publications on migration and HIV/STIs by topic. Search limited to title and abstract. Source: *PubMed*

between the distribution of disease and proximity to main roads.

HIV infections in rural parts of a country have often been found to be linked to epidemics in urban centers through migration. Many early studies have identified travel and migration as risk factors for HIV [11–15]. In rural Zaire, for example, the risk factors found for HIV in a 1986 study included residence outside the area (immigrants) and greater than average number of sexual partners [16]. In rural Malawi, Glynn et al. [17] found a large proportion of HIV cases in recent immigrants to the district and in those who had been absent from the district. In Kisesa, north

west Tanzania, those who moved into the ward had a higher HIV prevalence than those who had lived in the ward all their lives [18].

Studies of HIV prevalence have consistently indicated that HIV has spread along the trucking routes of East and Central Africa and then into the rural areas [19]. Long-distance lorry drivers are a quintessential mobile population, who move through many disparate communities and are likely to have particular risk behaviors for acquisition and transmission of STIs [20]. As early as 1991–1992 a study found 26% of long-distance lorry drivers and their assistants working between Kenya and Zaire to be HIV positive [21]. Significant associations were found between HIV seropositivity and being employed in long-distance driving for more than 11 years [21].

A set of studies have also long reported that living near roads is associated with a substantially elevated risk of HIV and STI infection. Colvin et al. [22] looked at the prevalence of HIV and other STIs in a rural community in the Lesotho highlands and found that all cases of HIV occurred in villages along the only main road in the area. Similar observations have been found in small studies in many other African countries [15, 23, 24]. Tanser et al. [25] measured HIV prevalence in rural South Africa through anonymous surveillance among pregnant women stratified by local village clinic. With large sample sizes, they found a close correlation between proximity of homesteads to primary or secondary roads and HIV prevalence.

At the individual level, Nunn et al. [12] found that change of residence was strongly associated with an increased risk of HIV infection in the rural Masaka district of Uganda, and the authors concluded that this was due to the more risky sexual behavior among those who moved. Importantly, 70% of those joining the area came from the same administrative district and almost all from similar rural areas (only 11% came from Kampala city where seroprevalence rates were known to be higher). Similar findings were reported in Tanzania [13]. This work suggests that the act of migration itself puts migrants at high risk of acquiring HIV and this fuels transmission within rural areas. This pattern contrasts with the notion that migrants only import infection from distant high-prevalence communities. These broad considerations have led us to attempt to assemble an organizing framework for the influence of migration on STI epidemics that we describe below.

Review

Epidemiologically, migration can do three distinct things to STI epidemics. Firstly, it can determine the spatial distribution of the infection including seeding new populations, importation and exportation of infections to locations, and, indirectly, determining epidemic persistence. Secondly, it can affect the connectivity of the sexual network, prevent local saturation because of movement to new populations (new susceptibles), and bridge gaps between geographically separate network components (connecting different sexual networks). Thirdly, the migration event can directly influence levels of individual risk behavior either directly (own risk behavior) or indirectly (others behavior), and can either increase or decrease risk. Each of these processes will be discussed.

Population Mobility Determines Spatial Distribution of Infection

First we will look at the role of population movement in seeding infection to networks. Early in the spread of HIV in South Africa, transmission seemed to be fuelled by migrants connecting high- and low-prevalence areas through frequent movement from homesteads to the area of work [26]. Many early HIV cases were linked directly to migrant workers [27, 28]. A decade later, migrant men were still 2.4 times more likely to be HIV infected compared to nonmigrant men [29, 30]. More recently, migrants from high endemic countries have seeded new HIV outbreaks among heterosexuals in low-endemic countries [31]. Molecular studies have shown importation of heterosexual HIV infections from high-endemic countries (subtype B and non-B strains) to low-endemic countries, as in the case of the Netherlands [32].

At the beginning of the HIV epidemic in Mexico all cases involved people who had previously lived in the USA [32, 33], suggesting that returning migrants were effectively importing HIV. Migrants would have acquired HIV in the USA through connecting to the US network of contacts, of which they would otherwise not have been a part. The migrants were not particularly at high risk of acquiring infection (they reported high condom use and only a small fraction became infected [34]), and the cases of infection more likely reflect the much higher levels of HIV in circulation in the USA than in Mexico at that time. In some cases migrants will have lower HIV prevalence than the national HIV prevalence. For example, Zimbabwean migrants to the UK actually have a lower HIV prevalence than the national level in Zimbabwe [35], which may reflect how opportunities to migrate to the UK are correlated with lowered risks of infection acquisition.

The relative contribution of migration to epidemics may also be influenced by epidemic phase. Voeten et al. [36] found that association between recent in-migration status of individuals and HIV prevalence varied according to year. Across 28 sub-Saharan African countries, the authors found that, for both men and women, the association was strongest between 1985 and 1994, slightly weaker between 1995 and 1999, and was not seen from 2000 onward. These findings suggest that as epidemics become established across a country, migration becomes less important in driving its spatial distribution and that in matured generalized epidemics, migration does not put individuals at substantially higher risk than others.

Patterns of movement, and lack of movement, in populations can determine the geographic distribution of infection. In particular, limited levels of migration can allow for skewed spatial distribution of disease [37, 38] whereas more extensive movement and mixing would tend to generate an even distribution of disease. For example, in China, where recent economic growth has led to mass migration of rural workers to cities, reported syphilis cases have increased tenfold over the past decade. The greatly increased population density in cities could be reflected in much tighter concentrations of STI distribution in cities, which could be exacerbated by, for instance, drawing sex workers to cities and inadequate provision of STI treatments, which could further accelerate infection spread there.

Lastly, movement can actually enable the persistence of endemic infections in some populations where otherwise they would naturally fade out. To see this, investigators have used the framework of "meta-populations"—populations that consist of many small, interconnected, discrete subpopulations [39]. In each small subpopulation (that could represent a small isolated village), a "fragile" infection (such as a bacterial STI) may become extinct as the number of susceptible individuals falls below a critical threshold. However, in other subpopulations which may be larger, may have different patterns of risk, or are at a different point in epidemic phase, the infection may currently persist and so migration to the first subpopulation can supply new infections. This is known as the "rescue" effect in the ecological literature, and this phenomenon could explain why real extinction events are rarer than might be expected [37]. Thus, although local epidemics can go extinct, across the whole meta-population, the disease persists. For some pathogens, where cyclical changes in prevalence are part of the natural epidemiological dynamic—like syphilis [40]—subpopulations would need to be out of phase with each other for the rescue effect to work. Interestingly, while increased migration promotes the strength of the rescue effect, it can also "synchronize" subpopulation epidemics, undermining the same. It has been proposed that in the USA, increased transport links could be responsible for the progressive "synchronization" of cyclical syphilis epidemic [40].

Population Mobility Promotes Extended Transmission Through Communities

The second organizing theme is that movement of people can connect geographically and socially separated sexual networks and promote extended transmission of disease through communities in ways that would not otherwise be possible. Geographically separated communities can be easily linked by migrants travelling back and forth. For example, Mexican women may be infected when their husbands return from the USA [34, 41]. Also the seasonal migration of Mexicans between the USA and their rural hometowns in Mexico may contribute to the transmission of HIV through Mexico [42]. Migrants not only bring infection to a new location (as in the previous section), but also they join networks together that can exhibit different properties and propensity for epidemics overall.

Circular migration, whereby individuals repeatedly return to the same location, is a special and particularly important case of bridging networks, as it affords quasi-continuous connection between two places and two sexual networks.

For circular migration, the frequency of oscillation is an important determinant of the extent of the connectivity between networks. Epidemiologically, it may be expected that frequent return trips secure the connection between disparate networks, affording a temporal intermingling of sex acts with different partners in different places (sexual partner concurrency) [43, 44], and increasing the chance of a partner being exposed shortly after the migrant is newly infected (which carries a much higher chance of transmission in the case of HIV) [45]. Indeed, much of the literature which considers migration and HIV transmission links frequent returns home with an increased risk of spreading disease to the rural area. In a mathematical model of HIV transmission in rural South Africa, Coffee et al. [26] showed that an epidemic can grow much larger when high-risk behavior among migrants was linked to the frequent return of migrants.

More frequent returns home could lead to less connectivity with another network, which would reduce the influence of migration. Indeed in some studies, migrants returning home more frequently have less risk of outside partnerships: Collinson [46] found that the majority of men working not too far away from their homes on game parks or commercial farms reported fewer partners than resident men or long-distance migrants (who returned home only once or twice per year). Infrequent returns home could, of course, weaken the link with the "home" network through, among other factors, a reduction in the coital frequency with a main stable partner [26]. If transmission in that partnership decreases, the expected extra population-level risk of transmission associated with the concurrent sex partners could be negated.

During the apartheid era in South Africa, a cyclical pattern of migration developed in which migrants travelled back and forth to work sites [26]. Circular migration in South Africa was aptly described by Wilson when he explained, "Nowhere else in the world has an industrial economy employed for so long such a high proportion of oscillating migrants in its labour force" [47]. As John Hargove considered, the reason for the particularly high HIV prevalence rates in southern Africa was less the fault of "roads" per se [along which infection could spread] but "Rhodes," Cecil John Rhodes the nineteenth century mining magnate who recruited men from all over southern Africa to work in the South African mines [48]. Migration patterns did not alter after apartheid as expected. Instead temporary migration was seen to increase, and the participants got younger and the proportion of female temporary migrants grew [46].

Movement can also be thought of as providing a "mixing" mechanism for the population and mixing prevents "saturation" of infection—that is, when the rate of new infections in a group is reduced because much of the population is already infected. Sex workers (SW) who stay in one location may rapidly infect a small set of regular clients, but they could infect far more if they move to new communities and are continually in contact with new clients. One modeling study demonstrated how different patterns of contact between SW and their clients can influence the persistence of STIs [49]. Using model simulations they found that persistence of either short- (e.g., gonorrhea) or long (e.g., HSV-2)-duration infection was more likely if clients visited many different SWs than the same SW. Movement of either the client or the SW had the effect of making different SW to client contact more likely.

The Effect of Population Mobility on Levels of Individual Risk Behavior

A third organizing theme for the interaction between migration and STI transmission is that the migration event itself can trigger changes in individual risk behavior both directly (changes in one's own behavior) and indirectly (i.e., a change in the behavior of a partner of a migrant).

It can be difficult to distinguish behavioral changes caused by migration events from selection effects caused by the individuals that are the most likely to be infected also being the most likely to migrate. Epidemiologically, however, the effects are distinct. Behavior changes caused by migration generate within-individual variation in risk behavior and generation of risk behavior. Individuals who are more likely to be infected and also more likely to migrate only shape the way in which sexual partner networks in communities become connected (discussed previously).

First, migration can lead to increased opportunity for sexual behavior that increases the risk of disease transmission. Magis-Rodriguez et al. [33] found that changes in sexual behavior occurred during migration, including increased number of sexual partners for men, that could be attributed to loneliness or less family contact to influence behavior. Magis-Rodriguez et al. [33] found in terms of sexual practices that Mexican migrants had more sexual partners as well as greater use of injected medicines and drugs when away from home. However, they also tended to use a condom in their most recent partnership. Coffee et al. [50] also found that urban migration patterns were linked to an increase in risky sexual behavior with migrants more likely to report high number of partners. Of course, this does not uniformly happen: in a rare prospective study of migrants, those migrating from rural to urban areas in Zimbabwe did not report higher levels of sexual risk behavior, or HIV, than residents either before or after they moved [51]. In a review of studies examining migration and HIV in India, Rai [52] found a mixture of associations: although some studies did report a higher HIV prevalence among migrant workers suggesting increases in risk within those individuals that move, other studies detected no trend, and in one study in India [53] migrants' behavior showed less risk during migration.

Migration can also trigger behavior changes among those who do not themselves migrate. Female partners of migrating men, for instance, were more likely to be infected from an external partner than women with non-migrating partners [30, 54].

It has been argued that it is not the process of migration itself but rather the situations people find themselves in once they have migrated (e.g., poor living and working conditions and diminished status rendering them more vulnerable to health and social problems) that are the root cause of increased risks of acquiring or transmitting infection [52]. Individual migrants in transit stations (i.e., border towns and port cities, areas where mobile populations congregate) in Central America and Mexico as described by Bronfman et al. [41] experienced a deficiency of public services, repeated human rights violations, violence, poverty, and corrupt authorities. Within this social context, transactional sex, sex for survival, rape, and nonprofessional commercial sex occurred in conditions that lowered prevention practices such as condom use and increased the risk of STI transmission [41]. In some transit stations over 60% of the women who migrated had forced sexual intercourse at some point on their journey. Studies have indicated that the most effective interventions at reducing the influence of migration on STI epidemics might include provision of more sanitary and comfortable accommodation for migrant workers that allowed them to bring their families with them and a change in employment conditions bringing them up to standards similar to those of other workers [46, 50, 52]. This echoed the point made by Hargrove [48] in relation to southern Africa, and is, in part, the motivation, for programs such as "Corridors of Hope," which has been set up by USAID and partner governments and organizations to promote practical collaboration along southern Africa's major transport corridor linking South Africa, Zimbabwe, and Zambia. In South Africa, coresident married migrant farmers did not have increased risk after migration as there was a protective effect on risk behavior if couples moved together [26, 50]. However the provision of good family accommodation may not be enough to make many migrants bring their families. Furthermore, the strong cultural attachment to ancestral land and cheaper cost of living often mean that wives and children would remain in their rural homes.

In 2001 the relationship between HIV/AIDS and migration was recognized by the UN in paragraph 50 of the United Nations General Assembly Special Session (UNGASS) declaration. The UN urged member states to implement strategies that would facilitate access to HIV/AIDS prevention programs for migrants and mobile workers, including the provision of information on health and social services [9]. The development of the HIV epidemic outside the European Union (EU) is, via movement of people, one of the key determinants of the epidemic within the EU [55]. Assisting low-income countries with high levels of HIV can be viewed as a prevention strategy as well as a humanitarian policy.

Although evidence now links HIV spread to human mobility, little policy development has focused on the relationship between migration and HIV/AIDS. The IOM has shown that ill-adapted migration policies are behind many of the social factors that increase the health risk of mobile populations. Most policy is focused on restrictive measures and protectionist approaches. In 2003, over 60 countries in the world required foreigners to be tested for HIV before being allowed entry, often using a positive test result to block entry [9]. Such practices are believed to contribute to illegal and undocumented migration and can deter migrants from making use of prevention services. Migration should be seen as a public health issue. Migrant uptake and access to prevention treatment and care services need to be monitored to ensure that these services are used and for services to be "migrant-friendly," for example with non-stigmatizing approaches and a respect to confidentiality [9]. The prevention and control programmes need to adapt to meet changing needs.

National policy responses that address prevention, care, and support throughout the migration process become part of an empowerment approach that improves an individual's legal, social, economic, and health status. Specific recommendations include creating a safe blood supply in areas of high population movement, making condoms easily available, supplying materials for universal precaution, providing HIV/AIDS prevention and counseling services, and increasing access to safe injection supplies and health services that include reproductive health matters [9].

The IOM further recommends strategies that link efforts between originating, transit, and destination countries; twinning programs that foster cross border collaboration; integrating HIV/AIDS programs into other services for migrants; conducting outreach to undocumented migrants that directs risk reduction towards the behavior and not the migrant; involving migrant communities in advocating for public policy that ensures migrants fundamental right to health and social services; and a definition of Main Categories of Migrants [6].

One would expect that whilst programs that did not include interventions for migrants to be treated would be less effective, programs with interventions designed to assess the needs of migrants would be more effective. At-risk groups such as sex workers, MSM, and IDUs that migrate require specific intervention programs in order to target these key populations. Vissers et al. [56] used a mathematical model to investigate the impact on HIV incidence of two interventions, condom promotion and health education aimed at partner reduction, and found that if mobile groups did not participate then the effectiveness of both interventions could be reduced by 40%. Thus, a lack of consideration of migration would have weakened the intervention, whilst an active targeting of mobile populations has the potential to greatly increase the effectiveness of such campaigns.

Conclusion

This chapter aimed to describe how migration can influence the spread of STIs. This topic has attracted substantial attention growing remarkably over the last 20 years, although the focus has been predominantly on HIV and much less on other STIs. From the earliest studies, a picture has emerged of a strong but multifaceted and sometimes contradictory interaction between migration and STI/HIV epidemiology that keys into processes acting at the individual, community, and wider population levels. We have tried to describe distinct mechanisms for this interaction in an organizing framework. We have illustrated the theory with empirical examples whilst acknowledging that existing data are often insufficient to attribute a particular observation to one factor rather than another. In this regard further work based on longitudinal data would provide a valuable addition to our understanding.

It is important to understand how migration can affect STI and HIV epidemics so that we can better match intervention responses to the local epidemic context. Further translational work evaluating real interventions for migrants will be required. Failing to fully understand how migration influences an epidemic is to not recognize a potentially important epidemic driver and to perhaps miss a highly leveraged point of intervention.

Acknowledgements We thank Profs Simon Gregson and Geoff Garnett for useful discussion and the Qatar National Research Foundation (ARB, TBH) and The Wellcome Trust (TBH) for funding support.

References

 1. Fenner F. Small pox and its eradication. History of international public health. Geneva: World Health Organisation; 1988.
 2. Glynn IGJ. The life and death of small pox. Cambridge: Cambridge University Press; 2004.
 3. Kapp C. South Africa failing people displaced by xenophobia riots. Lancet. 2008;371(9629):1986–7.
 4. Valji N. Creating the nation: the rise of violent xenophobia in the new South Africa. York: Centre for the Study of Violence and Reconciliation, York University; 2003.
 5. Hamer WH. Epidemic disease in England. Lancet. 1906;1:733–9.
 6. International Organisation for MIgration. http://www.iom.int. 2011. Accessed 2011.
 7. ECDC. Migrant health: background note to the ECDC report on migration and infectious diseases in the EU. In: Control ECfDPa, editor. 2009.
 8. United Nations Population Division. International migration. 2002. Accessed May 2011.
 9. Interagency Coalition on AIDS and Development. International migration and HIV/AIDS. 2011. Accessed 2011.
10. Trends in total migrant stock: the 2003 revision. United Nations, Department for Economic and Social Affairs, Population Division. 2003.
11. Nunn AJ, Kengeya-Kayondo JF, Malamba SS, Seeley JA, Mulder DW. Risk factors for HIV-1 infection in adults in a rural Ugandan community: a population study. AIDS. 1994;8(1):81–6.
12. Nunn AJ, Wagner HU, Kamali A, Kengeya-Kayondo JF, Mulder DW. Migration and HIV-1 seroprevalence in a rural Ugandan population. AIDS. 1995;9(5):503–6.
13. Barongo LR, Borgdorff MW, Mosha FF, et al. The epidemiology of HIV-1 infection in urban areas, roadside settlements and rural villages in Mwanza Region, Tanzania. AIDS. 1992;6(12):1521–8.
14. Serwadda D, Wawer MJ, Musgrave SD, Sewankambo NK, Kaplan JE, Gray RH. HIV risk factors in three geographic strata of rural Rakai District, Uganda. AIDS. 1992;6(9):983–9.
15. Killewo J, Nyamuryekunge K, Sandstrom A, et al. Prevalence of HIV-1 infection in the Kagera region of Tanzania: a population-based study. AIDS. 1990;4(11):1081–5.
16. Nzilambi N, De Cock KM, Forthal DN, et al. The prevalence of infection with human immunodeficiency virus over a 10-year period in rural Zaire. N Engl J Med. 1988;318(5):276–9.
17. Glynn JR, Ponnighaus J, Crampin AC, et al. The development of the HIV epidemic in Karonga District, Malawi. AIDS. 2001;15(15):2025–9.
18. Boerma JT, Urassa M, Nnko S, et al. Sociodemographic context of the AIDS epidemic in a rural area in Tanzania with a focus on people's mobility and marriage. Sex Transm Infect. 2002;78 Suppl 1:i97–105.
19. Bwayo J, Plummer F, Omari M, et al. Human immunodeficiency virus infection in long-distance truck drivers in east Africa. Arch Intern Med. 1994;154(12):1391–6.
20. Bwayo JJ, Omari AM, Mutere AN, et al. Long distance truck-drivers: 1. Prevalence of sexually transmitted diseases (STDs). East Afr Med J. 1991;68(6):425–9.
21. Mbugua GG, Muthami LN, Mutura CW, Oogo SA, Waiyaki PG, Lindan CP, Hearst N. Epidemiology of HIV infection among long distance truck drivers in Kenya. East Afr Med J. 1995;72(8):515–8.
22. Colvin M, Sharp B. Sexually transmitted infections and HIV in a rural community in the Lesotho highlands. Sex Transm Infect. 2000;76(1):39–42.
23. Wawer MJ, Serwadda D, Musgrave SD, Konde-Lule JK, Musagara M, Sewankambo NK. Dynamics of spread of HIV-I infection in a rural district of Uganda. BMJ. 1991;303(6813):1303–6.
24. Soderberg S, Temihango W, Kadete C, et al. Prevalence of HIV-1 infection in rural, semi-urban and urban villages in southwest Tanzania: estimates from a blood-donor study. AIDS. 1994;8(7):971–6.
25. Tanser F, Lesueur D, Solarsh G, Wilkinson D. HIV heterogeneity and proximity of homestead to roads in rural South Africa: an exploration using a geographical information system. Trop Med Int Health. 2000;5(1):40–6.
26. Coffee M, Lurie MN, Garnett GP. Modelling the impact of migration on the HIV epidemic in South Africa. AIDS. 2007;21(3):343–50.
27. Ramjee G, Karim SS, Sturm AW. Sexually transmitted infections among sex workers in KwaZulu-Natal, South Africa. Sex Transm Dis. 1998;25(7):346–9.

28. Abdool Karim Q, Abdool Karim SS, Singh B, Short R, Ngxongo S. Seroprevalence of HIV infection of HIV infection in rural South Africa. AIDS. 1992;6:1535–9.

29. Lurie MN, Williams BG, Zuma K, et al. The impact of migration on HIV-1 transmission in South Africa: a study of migrant and nonmigrant men and their partners. Sex Transm Dis. 2003;30(2):149–56.

30. Lurie MN, Williams BG, Zuma K, et al. Who infects whom? HIV-1 concordance and discordance among migrant and non-migrant couples in South Africa. AIDS. 2003;17(15):2245–52.

31. Xiridou M, van Veen M, Coutinho R, Prins M. Can migrants from high-endemic countries cause new HIV outbreaks among heterosexuals in low-endemic countries? AIDS. 2010;24(13):2081–8.

32. Op de Coul EL, Coutinho RA, van der Schoot A, et al. The impact of immigration on env HIV-1 subtype distribution among heterosexuals in the Netherlands influx of subtype B and non-B strains. AIDS. 2001;15(17):2277–86.

33. Magis-Rodriguez C, Gayet C, Negroni M, et al. Migration and AIDS in Mexico: an overview based on recent evidence. J Acquir Immune Defic Syndr. 2004;37 Suppl 4:S215–26.

34. Magis-Rodriguez C, Lemp G, Hernandez MT, Sanchez MA, Estrada F, Bravo-Garcia E. Going North: Mexican migrants and their vulnerability to HIV. J Acquir Immune Defic Syndr. 2009;51 Suppl 1:S21–5.

35. Gregson S, Gonese E, Hallett TB, et al. HIV decline in Zimbabwe due to reductions in risky sex? Evidence from a comprehensive epidemiological review. Int J Epidemiol. 2010;39(5):1311–23.

36. Voeten HA, Vissers DC, Gregson S, et al. Strong association between in-migration and HIV prevalence in urban sub-Saharan Africa. Sex Transm Dis. 2010;37(4):240–3.

37. Hanski I. Metapopulation ecology. Oxford: Oxford University Press; 1999.

38. Chen XS. One stone to kill two birds. Bull World Health Organ. 2009;87(11):814–5.

39. Levins SA. Dispersion and population interactions. Am Nat. 1974;108:207–28.

40. Grassly NC, Fraser C, Garnett GP. Host immunity and synchronized epidemics of syphilis across the United States. Nature. 2005;433(7024):417–21.

41. Bronfman MN, Leyva R, Negroni MJ, Rueda CM. Mobile populations and HIV/AIDS in Central America and Mexico: research for action. AIDS. 2002;16 Suppl 3:S42–9.

42. Bastos FI, Caceres C, Galvao J, Veras MA, Castilho EA. AIDS in Latin America: assessing the current status of the epidemic and the ongoing response. Int J Epidemiol. 2008;37(4):729–37.

43. Morris M, Kretzschmar M. Concurrent partnerships and the spread of HIV. AIDS. 1997;11(5):641–8.

44. Watts CHM, May RM. The influence of concurrent partnerships on the dynamics of HIV/AIDS. Maths Biosci. 1992;108(1):89–104.

45. Hollingsworth TD, Anderson RM, Fraser C. HIV-1 transmission, by stage of infection. J Infect Dis. 2008;198(5):687–93.

46. Collinson MA. Striving against adversity: the dynamics of migration, health and poverty in rural South Africa. Glob Health Action. 2010;3.

47. Wilson F. Minerals and migrants: how the mining industry has shaped South Africa. Proceedings of the American Academy of Arts and Sciences. 2001; 130:99–122.

48. Hargrove JW. Migration, mines and mores: the HIV epidemic in Southern Africa. In: Centre of Excellence in Epidemiological Modelling and Analysis. Stellenbosch University, South Africa; 2007.

49. Ghani AC, Aral SO. Patterns of sex worker-client contacts and their implications for the persistence of sexually transmitted infections. J Infect Dis. 2005;191 Suppl 1:S34–41.

50. Coffee MP, Garnett GP, Mlilo M, Voeten HA, Chandiwana S, Gregson S. Patterns of movement and risk of HIV infection in rural Zimbabwe. J Infect Dis. 2005;191 Suppl 1:S159–67.

51. Mundandi C, Vissers D, Voeten H, Habbema D, Gregson S. No difference in HIV incidence and sexual behaviour between out-migrants and residents in rural Manicaland, Zimbabwe. Trop Med Int Health. 2006;11(5):705–11.

52. Rai T. Exploring the relationship between circular labour migration and HIV vulnerability in India. London: Imperial College; 2010.

53. International Institute for Population Studies and Macro International. National family health survey 3 (2005–6) (NFHS-3) Main report. Mumbai, India: International Institute; 2007.

54. Kishamawe C, Vissers DC, Urassa M, et al. Mobility and HIV in Tanzanian couples: both mobile persons and their partners show increased risk. AIDS. 2006;20(4):601–8.

55. ECDC. HIV infection in Europe: 25 years into the epidemic. In: Control ECfDPa, editor. Technical report ed. Stockholm.

56. Vissers DC, DeVlas SJ, Bakker R, Urassa M, Voeten HA, Habbema JD. The impact of mobility on HIV control: a modelling study. Epidemiol Infect. 2011; 2011:1–9.

Sexual Networks and Sexually Transmitted Infections; "The Strength of Weak (Long Distance) Ties"

Ann M. Jolly and John L. Wylie

Introduction

Social networks are natural social units of people (nodes, actors) linked directly or indirectly to others by interaction, affections, associations or relationships and, for the purposes of this chapter, sexual intercourse. Sexual networks through which sexually transmitted pathogens are transmitted form the centre of this review of sexual networks. The fundamental concept of a social network is that the collection of links (paths or edges) and nodes forms an entity far greater than the sum of its parts [1], including interdependent norms, members, organisation and culture.

Considering a sexual network in which *Neisseria gonorrhoeae*, *Treponema pallidum*, *Chlamydia trachomatis* or HIV circulate exclusively and independently of one another, may be somewhat artificial. Technically, these and other pathogens can spread from any infected individual to any susceptible people with whom he or she has

unprotected sex and thence to another generation of sex partners within a sexual network. Therefore, sexually transmitted infections (STIs) should spread through networks of varying structures, as long as they contain infectious people and unprotected sexual intercourse takes place. However, empirical work on STI networks [2, 3], and basic epidemiological data [4, 5], has provided evidence that networks harbouring gonorrhoea differ from those which harbour chlamydia, which again differ from those harbouring HIV, suggesting that different networks have specific innate properties suited to specific organisms. Specific structures of different networks with identical number of contacts, links between them, the same type and number of sexual relationships, and the same variation in sex partners between dyads (sexual activity classes) were elucidated by Klovdahl et al. in a hypothetical graph (Fig. 5.1) [6]. Not only are the number of people who had three sex partners the same in each graph, but so are the number of links also, such that people with three partners had contact with people with only one partner in both graphs. However, a pathogen may pass from one end of the graph to the other in one component by only one route, whereas in the other transmission it is made possible simultaneously by three routes. Thus the authors show that the structure of a network has implications for pathogen transmission through different routes of transmission over and above those described by its basic numeric properties, such as the number of links or the number of nodes, and even the pairing of degree combinations.

With apologies to Dr. Mark Granovetter.

A.M. Jolly, Ph.D. (✉)
Centre for Communicable Disease and Infection Control,
Infectious Disease Emergency Preparedness Branch,
Public Health Agency of Canada, AL 0603B,
Tunney's Pasture, Room 3438 100 Eglantine Driveway,
Ottawa, ON, Canada K1A 0K9
e-mail: Ann_M_Jolly@phac-aspc.gc.ca

J.L. Wylie, Ph.D.
Cadham Provincial Laboratory,
750 William Avenue, Winnipeg, MB, Canada, R3C 3Y1

S.O. Aral, K.A. Fenton, and J.A. Lipshutz (eds.), *The New Public Health and STD/HIV Prevention:*
Personal, Public and Health Systems Approaches, DOI 10.1007/978-1-4614-4526-5_5,
© Springer Science+Business Media New York 2013

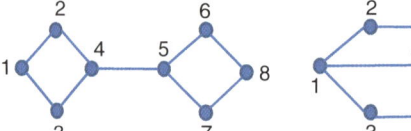

Fig. 5.1 Two graphs, each with an equal number of people represented by dots, and relationships represented by lines, where transmission of infection through relationships is facilitated in the second graph because the structure of relationships makes passage easier, rather than in the first where transmission through the network relies on individuals 5 and 6. Adapted from Klovdahl AS, Potterat JJ, Woodhouse D, Muth J, Muth S, Darrow WW. HIV infection in an urban social network: a progress report. Bulletine Methodologie Sociologique 1992;36:24–33

In a seminal paper in 1996 [7], Wasserheit and Aral elucidated a theory that STI epidemiology of different sexually transmitted pathogens changes over time in response to control strategies, and to changes in behaviours of the hosts. They hypothesise that due to increased STI prevention efforts, pathogens can survive only in members of social and sexual networks who have unprotected sex with higher number of sex partners, and less access to effective sexual health care than other populations. The current review builds on that evolutionary approach, exploring the common characteristics of sexual networks using network theories of homophily, heterogeneity, and social aggregation. Then we will review specific differences in the networks which seem essential for the survival of gonorrhoea, chlamydia, syphilis, viral STI, and HIV in sociometric networks where data for more than one generation of sex partners are available. There will be less emphasis on egocentric data, usually collected from one individual with proxy data on his or her sex partners and, in some instances, from first-generation sex partners themselves. Findings from molecular analysis of pathogens within couples or networks will be integrated into pathogen-specific network reviews. Finally, as many social network-inspired prevention strategies are similar for different pathogens, these are reviewed in the final section of the paper, in a more general context.

Sexual Networks, Transmission Networks and Disease Networks

It is important to differentiate here between (1) a sexual network where members have intercourse with each other, some of whom may or may not have an STI; (2) a network which definitely contains members infected and transmitting an STI (transmission and infection network); and (3) a network in which members have symptoms, diagnoses and possibly long-term symptomatic infections (disease network). In the first case, the network can be viewed as a complete network containing all sexual intercourse between all couples in a network, linking them all directly or indirectly through a third person to each other. Of course in reality this is subject to incomplete reporting, omitting and forgetting, but basically the network depicts a subset of all recalled coital links. A transmission network is a subset of the sexual network, containing only those named as sex partners, and likely exposed, by infected people, some of whom may actually be uninfected, but who nevertheless were potentially infected and who should be tested. Ideally, a transmission network is directed, with the arrows denoting who infected whom. However, due to the asymptomatic nature of many STIs, it is challenging in many cases to determine the direction of transmission. For this reason, unless one has specific data to the contrary, transmission networks have been graphed as undirected. It should be noted here that the process of contact tracing or respondent nomination is not a proxy for transmission; it may indeed be synchronised with the onset of symptoms, but by no means should be taken for granted that because person A named person B, C, and D that person A is the transmitter, and persons B, C, and D are the susceptibles who were infected subsequently.

Defining a transmission network implies identification of actual transmission events within a sexual network. A number of techniques are useful in determining transmission, such as careful documentation of dates of first and last intercourse; use of condoms; type of sex, vaginal/penile, anal/penile and/or oral/penile; recording and listing of symptoms for those unfamiliar with them, dates of onset, specimen collection, test results, accuracy of test method; and finally confirming strain concordance [8, 9]. For diseases such as syphilis, transmission direction may be easier to ascertain than HIV or chlamydia for example, as the disease in individuals can be staged by symptoms appearing at different times, although the presence of HIV may cause acceleration or atypical disease and should be taken into account [10].

Last, a disease network is again a subset of the transmission network, containing only those individuals who have symptoms. For many STIs this is an impractical approach to graphing and investigation, as many are asymptomatic for the whole course (chlamydia) or a part of the course (HSV) in a high proportion of people, or the infection may have a long, mostly asymptomatic incubation period (HIV). Nevertheless, the first sexual network which provided definite proof of an infectious source of AIDS contained only those men who had symptoms, so disease networks cannot be discounted [1, 11].

Methods of Collecting Sexual Network Data

Contact Tracing

Two most commonly used methods of collecting sexual network data from individuals have been (a) contact tracing or partner notification and (b) variations of snowball sampling, such as chain link sampling or respondent-driven sampling. The first and oldest of these is contact tracing or partner notification in which index individual has a positive laboratory test for a notifiable sexually transmitted pathogen which is recognised in the public health legislation of the region as being amenable to intervention. The person's name, birth date, gender and other relevant identifying and locating information are recorded such that he or she can be contacted by public health staff

who then interviews the person with the goals of education on risk reduction, confirming adequate treatment, and management of sex partners to or from whom the STI may have been transmitted [12]. If a sex partner is found to be positive, he or she becomes an "index" case and the process is reiterated, until no new positive partners are found. In this way, a sexual network is sampled with an intentional bias towards interviewing only those who are infected.

There are three ways in which partner notification is conducted: provider referral, contracting and self-referral. First, the public health nurse can elicit the names, identifying and locating information of sex partners of the client for the infectious period, since just before symptom onset, or in the absence of symptoms, usually 3 months before the current diagnosis date [13, 14]. Then the nurse or disease investigation specialist (DIS) will notify the partner, without divulging the name of the index case, that he or she has been exposed to an STI and encourage him or her to present for testing and examination. The client may wish to notify his or her own partners, in which case the nurse or the DIS may still note the partner information, with the proviso that if the partner(s) has not presented for care within a certain period of time, the public health officer will do so (contracting). Last, in many jurisdictions, the names and locating information of sex partners are not recorded by public health staff and the patient is solely responsible for notifying his or her own partners (self-referral). This last method is considered to be the least effective with the fewest number of clients examined [15], as is partner notification attempted by untrained physicians [16]. It is important to note that partner notification practices and effectiveness [17] differ depending on infecting pathogen [15] such that median numbers of clients newly brought to treatment and those newly diagnosed of all those elicited are highest for gonorrhoea and chlamydia, a little lower for syphilis and lowest of all for HIV.

Evaluating the completeness of network data generated by contact tracing has been done mostly by Brewer, who found that people forget 14–25% of sex partners from the past 2 years, elicited during two interviews spaced 1 week and 3 months apart [18, 19]. About 40% were forgotten if one imputed the number of partners over 2 years from a period of recent partner recruitment. However the number of partners forgotten was moderately correlated with the number reported ($r=0.67$), even in people who had many or very few number of recent partners, which is of interest when examining the number of partners and network structure required for different pathogens. Reassuringly, sex partners remembered did not differ significantly from those forgotten, by demographic characteristics, such as sexual orientation; type of partnership; positive or negative feelings towards partners and network characteristics, such as frequency of contact. Forgetting partners leads, of course, to an underreporting of partners; lower number of links between partners (density), and smaller network size, which in turn results in fewer nominations; examinations and lower number of infected clients brought to treatment.

Re-interviewing patients, reading back lists of already nominated partners, prompting the client to recall more partners, using memory cues such as identifying important events and relating those to partners can significantly improve the number of patients nominated and thus the number of those brought to treatment [19]. Ethnographic enquiries, participant observation and other methods commonly used by sociologists have been found to be useful in STI investigations [9, 20], not only for eliciting more partner data but also for refining a general understanding of the social context in which STI occurs. Early evaluations of social network-enhanced contact tracing have revealed between 30% and 100% additional cases diagnosed compared with traditional contact tracing only for syphilis and HIV infection, justifying the adoption and evaluation of these additional methods, which are being incorporated into guidelines on source investigations [13, 14, 21].

Mathematical models of simulated populations have also been used to evaluate the completeness and biases in contact investigations within transmission networks [22]. Three methods of estimating the frequency of number of partners in a network were tested: (1) asking participants to estimate the number of partners which their partners may have; (2) snowball sample participants by selecting certain people initially and sampling a proportion of progressive generations of sex partners and (3) contact tracing, where initial index cases who have confirmed infection are selected, and they are encouraged to notify their partners, or have public health do so. While all three methods resulted in an underestimation of both sex partners and the links between them, contact tracing resulted in the least bias, especially when applied to a high proportion of cases and provided the least underestimation of component sizes.

Respondent-Driven Sampling

This method is more frequently used in research rather than for routine disease investigation, where a small number of "seeds" (initial participants) are selected to begin the study. In principle, it is not necessary to choose a representative group of seeds (e.g., covering all ethnic groups), as the nature of RDS ensures that any bias in seed selection is overcome by the sampling design. However, in practice using seeds that differ in their ethnicity, gender and geographic location within a city minimises the number of waves of recruitment required [23]. Initial participants (seeds) are selected from a population who are then provided with cards or tokens on which the unique number of the seed is recorded along with the study recruitment phone number, to give to friends who may fall into the study target group, and who may be interested in participating. When the friends present with the card, they are entitled to participate in the study and are compensated for their time and effort. In many situations the initial respondent is compensated for each new person he or she recruits. Ideally, in sampling a sexual network, the respondents would refer all sexual partners or friends who may benefit from an STI test within a given time period, who again would refer all of their sex partners in turn such that sequential waves of enrolment occur and anonymous linked chains of study participants are created [24–26]. RDS is a relatively new form of chain-referral network sampling designed to overcome many of the problems typically associated with chain-referral methods, including the generation of a non-probability sample. Mathematical evaluations of RDS showed that probability samples can be generated using this method, facilitating the use of conventional statistics to analyse the results [27] http://www.respondentdrivensampling.org/, thus correcting for biases in sampling to reflect the target population.

Sexual Network Data

One of the first detailed descriptions of sexual networks containing gonorrhoea was published in 1985, a product of the traditional work of DIS combined with innovative analysis. The Colorado Springs study by Potterat and Rothenberg et al. was unique in that it contained most, if not all, of the main themes of STI epidemiology for the foreseeable future and will form the basis for our discussions in this review [28]. In that study, from 6 months of data, there were six "lots" or components which contained 20% of all cases. Components include all people connected directly by one link or indirectly by many links, denoting sexual intercourse. In this study, the small minority of six components contained 20% of all the cases. The fact that they contained a disproportionate number of cases presages later network analysis of similar groups, as did the small number of social venues where sex partners met (pick up joints). Of 300 venues available only six were frequented by 51% of the cases. This study was ground-breaking not only as an initial description of a sexual network containing gonorrhoea constructed without the benefit of modern network software, but also because the investigators identified (1) the fact that many in fact most of the people in the study chose sexual partners who were similar to themselves—homophily; (2) that a relatively small group generated a disproportionately high number of infections—heterogeneity and (3) the small number of common "pick up" joints through which a majority of the at-risk population could be reached—social aggregation.

Homophily

Homophily in social networks is a well-known phenomenon whereby people with similar demographic, behavioural and personal characteristics are more likely to form bonds with people similar to them, summarised in the adage, "birds of a feather flock together". The mechanism for this is that a close friendship between A and B will limit the time spent between A and another friend C, unless it is spent with both C and B simultaneously. This enhances all three friendships, or if a link between C and B does not yet exist, the common relationship with A is likely to generate an acquaintance if not a friendship [29]. Such ties not only reinforce relationships but also limit them, as documented by many sociological studies, controlling the information people receive, the experiences they undergo, the attitudes they form and the behaviours they adopt [30].

Geographic Homophily

The initial description of how "like mixes with like" was in the form of contiguous census tract areas in which cases of gonorrhoea were clustered [28]. Fifty-one percent of cases were from four census tracts in the core downtown area of Colorado Springs; 5 other adjacent tracts accounted for 21% more of the cases, and the remaining 10 cases were in peripheral census tracts. Sixty-five percent of all relationships containing one core person were with another core person. Fifty percent of people who came from periphery had a partner also from the periphery, while the minority partnered with people from the core or adjacent census tracts. Although a residence in an area defined post hoc by the proportion of gonorrhoea cases is a proxy for sociodemographic and other behavioural factors, this early analysis presaged later work.

As STI incidence decreased, targeting of whole neighbourhoods [31] was not as efficient as it had been in previous years [32]. Wylie and Jolly showed that central member of the largest component containing people infected with gonorrhoea and chlamydia lived in one instance outside the city of Winnipeg, and in another, outside the high-incidence or "core" area of Winnipeg but both were essential in transmitting infection to persons inside and outside the area [2]. A certain amount of geographic heterogeneity (addressed below), like homogeneity, is an important element of sustained transmission, as demonstrated in a study of distances between sex partners [33].

Ethnic Homophily

Correlated with geographic clustering is ethnic homophily, due to the fact that ethnic groups tend to cluster in certain neighbourhoods, although some people choose to have sex with someone outside their own ethnic group. The most conclusive research was a study measuring how likely it is that a person with two partners a year chooses a partner demographically and behaviourally similar to him- or herself [34]. Also measured was homophily in sex partners' ethnic backgrounds, ages and education levels, known to be important sociologically. Homophily was highest amongst African-American women who reported that 91.8% of their partners were African-American men, while 52% of partners of African-American men were of the same ethnic background. Consistent with this, 56% of White women reported White partners, and 84% of White men reported White female partners. Eighty-three percent of men who were 19 years or younger reported partners in the same age range, 64% in the 20–29-year age group had partners within the same age group and 53% of people had partners above the age of 30. While people tended to pick partners with similar number of partners as themselves, the concordance was not as striking as more observable social groupings. These authors also showed that mixing within a population defined by low prevalence within all segments of subpopulations such as those defined by age, education, ethnic backgrounds and number of partners is an essential component of STI transmission in the population.

Thorough studies of geographic epidemiology of STI [4, 5, 31–33, 35, 36] have shown high STI rates in inner-city, low-income, minority populations, without good access to health care. These papers emphasise the need to focus prevention efforts on relatively small, geographically well-identified populations which contain a large proportion of STI cases. While precise descriptions of person, place and time with a view to intervention are cornerstones of epidemiology and good public health practice, they may be only proxy measures of the ultimate causes of concentrations of STI. Social networks have been cited in some of these papers as being the root of the concentration of STI, as people recruit sex partners in some cases from social networks [37], determined by cost of housing and confined by geographic space [38], particularly in less affluent communities where transport is relatively costly.

Age Homophily

An early indication of homophily in age-based sexual networks was contained in a study which showed that syphilis in adult males was associated with crack cocaine, while diagnoses with gonorrhoea were in much younger men who had similar number of sex partners, but were less likely to use crack and were also much less likely to have syphilis. Further analysis of young men who did use crack showed that they were still far more likely to have gonorrhoea and far less likely to have syphilis than older men, which reinforced the fact that they and the young women they had sex with were in different sexual networks or at least distant from each other [39]. This early work was confirmed later by Jennings et al. [40] who showed that approximately 75% of men have sex with women who are less than 2 years older or younger than themselves. More recent studies in specific populations such as those with chlamydia and gonorrhoea in an STD clinic found that the majority of men and women select partners within their own age categories, <19; 20–29 and >29, indicating that sexual partnerships were formed within the context of social relationships where aggregation by age is common [34]. Other research into sex partners of people using dyadic data shows similar patterns [2, 41].

Heterogeneity

The second interesting phenomenon in the 1985 Colorado Springs paper was that although the people who originally tested positive for gonorrhoea had similar number of partners as others in different components, a small group of them and their partners linked in one component had the highest number of infectious days or "force of infectivity", allowing exposure to many more partners over a longer period of time. The finding that a small number of people affect gonorrhoea epidemiology on a large scale had been theorised earlier by Yorke and Hethcote who discovered that when screening for gonorrhoea was introduced in the United States, the detection of an additional 10% of gonococcal infections in women resulted in a 20% decrease of infections in the years immediately following [42]. This gave rise to the theory that a subpopulation must exist to maintain an epidemic of gonorrhoea, in which the incidence is so high that 20% of all new infections are pre-empted by the susceptible already being infected. Reinfection with gonorrhoea was estimated to occur twice annually in this population. In 1991 Brunham unified empirical data with mathematical theory when he posited that for an infection to be sustained in such a small subpopulation (given sufficient number of partners to whom infection could be transmitted), productive chains of transmission must exist, therefore linking members together directly or indirectly through a network of sexual relationships [43].

The importance of this heterogeneity in numbers of sex partners in addition to duration of infectiousness was emphasised in a landmark study in 2001 by Liljeros and Stanley. They noticed the peculiar shape of the number of reported lifetime sex partners reported in population-based samples of men and women from Sweden, to which they fit a power law [44]. A true power law is analogous to by far the majority of people being between 4 and 7 ft tall, while the minority are spread out over the next two or three orders of magnitude with a minute proportion being over 4,000 ft tall, which clearly does not represent reality. However, the number of flights leaving major cities across the globe may well satisfy this distribution, with many cities such as Cape Town, South Africa, having lower number of flights, and places such as London, England, having greater number. Although the fit of their model and precise definitions and generating

functions of scale-free distributions have been hotly debated [45, 46], the fact remained that a small proportion of highly active people with number of partners in the thousands or tens of thousands are likely to be efficient transmitters of gonorrhoea and other sexually transmitted pathogens, who affect the transmission and the epidemiology of STIs disproportionately through their networks. Following closely on the first study, Schneeberger published a similar analysis of empirical data [45, 46], which stimulated a focus on new methods by which to describe the non-random process by which sex partners are recruited [46–48], and the resulting skewed frequency distribution of numbers of partners [49]. Assumptions in the traditional compartmental model (a) of homogeneity, even when populations are divided into classes denoting the number of sex partners, and (b) of randomness in which an individual has the same probability of coming into contact with any other individual in the population regardless of demographic, physical proximity or disease status are insufficient in allowing for heterogeneity, and the interdependence of one individual's disease status on that of his or her neighbours remains problematic. Last, the fact that people generally have a finite number of sex partners whom they can infect and be infected by, means that random mixing of sexual partners within compartments is invalid, as when the number of sex partners infected rises, the number of potential susceptibles decreases.

The range in numbers of sex partners which people from samples of the general population report may not resemble that of populations with confirmed STI, or of contacts of people with STI, simply because the latter generally have more sex partners, at least enough to sustain transmission than those populations in which STI are not transmitted. Second, the number of sex partners may not be recorded—only those who have enough locating data to allow contact tracing to take place, therefore underestimating the total number of partners. Allowing for various biases, it is clear that York and Hethcote's 1978 concept of the population incidence of gonorrhoea being made up of an average of two rates, one in the core where the prevalence is about 20% and where a significant proportion of infections are transmitted to those who were previously infected [42] and the rate in the remainder of the STI-susceptible population with fewer number of partners in which new infections were seldom pre-empted, presages both the current empirical and theoretical data.

Ethnic Heterogeneity

Discussions of initial investigations of ethnic differences and partnerships between people of two different backgrounds have also evolved. People who have sex with people from a different ethnic group can potentially serve as conduits for pathogen transmission where the disease incidence between the two groups differs substantially. Inter-ethnic partnerships are associated with higher risk of disease [34, 50, 51] and exposure to higher number of partners [50]. In a study of women attending an STD clinic in Tennessee [52], sexual behaviour for Black and White women was similar. However, the prevalence of infection in Black women was 36.7% when compared with 27.1% in White women. The likely reason for higher rates in Black women was that their chance of having sex with an infected man was higher due to his having high number of partners (see below for why this pairing pattern may occur). This illustrates the point that even in the absence of sexual network data, using only the number of partners of each case can lead to incorrect assumptions of disease risk, and that mixing matrices based on the number of partners may also be inadequate to describe a pattern which relies on race and not just sexual activity class. Also, the fact that Blacks have, and have had, historically higher rates of STIs, and that they form a marginalised group in American society [52–54], is important to one's understanding of the risk of gonorrhoea in Black women attending an STD clinic in Tennessee.

A comparison of networks containing gonorrhoea and chlamydia revealed disproportionately large number of cases in African Americans in Colorado Springs, USA, and First Nations (North American Indians) in Winnipeg, Canada [55]. Both populations formed only 7% and 3% of the population but bore 34% and 18% of the number of cases, respectively, which raises interesting questions concerning the structure of these networks and whether similar structures may exist in all minority populations which bear disproportionately higher burdens of illness. In the absence of empirical network data, Laumann and Youm [56] have provided a network explanation for consistently higher rates of STI in African Americans. They demonstrated that, like in the earlier study by Quinn, while many African Americans have comparable number of partners to their White counterparts, more African Americans have partners who have many more partners. This was confirmed empirically in a household sample of respondents living in a high-incidence, minority neighbourhood who were asked to nominate up to six people with whom they had had sex in the last 3 months [50, 57]. The partners of African-American women were more likely to have many partners than those of Caucasian women. In addition many more partnerships take place between African Americans only, whereas a higher proportion of Whites and Hispanics have sex with African Americans, thus concentrating the infections within minority communities. In a notable example, 92% of African-American women reported having sex with African-American men, but only half of the African-American men reported sex with partners from their own ethnic background [34].

Geographic Heterogeneity

While a certain amount of homophily within sexual networks defined by geography and socioeconomic characteristics is ideal for targeting certain populations, intervention with *only* the residents of that area only would ignore important routes of infection into the community. The existence of people who have sex with others from another region—spatial bridgers—in itself may be an adaptation to a geographic, ethnic, language-specific or age group-targeted approach, in that relationships which elude the intervention are best "fitted" for survival as they are less likely to be detected and thus chains of transmission less likely to be interrupted. Sexual partnerships have been documented in a Canadian province between people living in communities 500 or more km

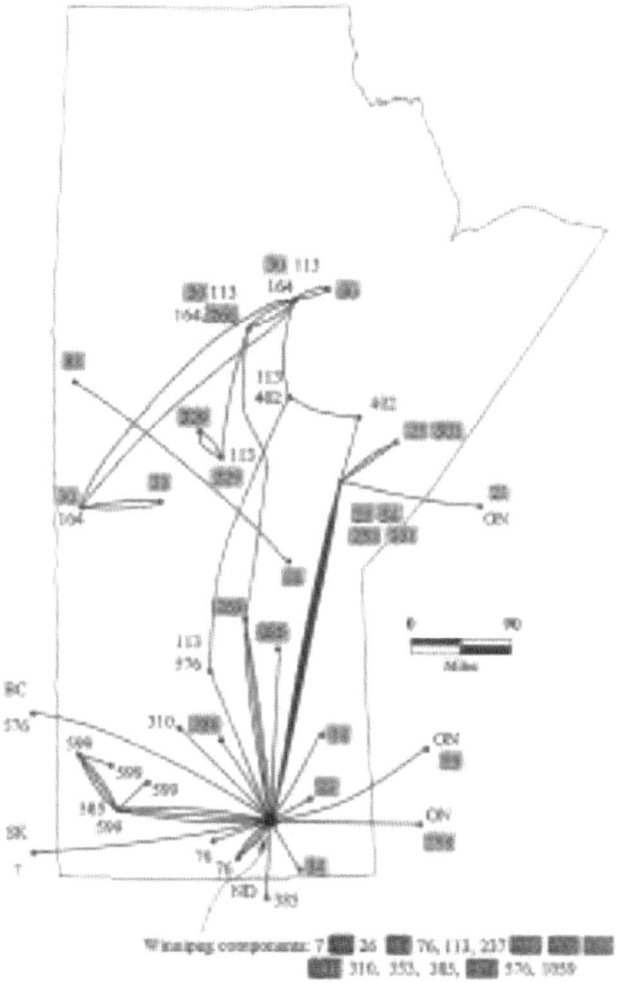

Fig. 5.2 Overview of potential transmission routes in the province of Manitoba, Canada. Individual points represent cities, towns or aboriginal reserves. The largest point in southern Manitoba represents Winnipeg. Lines represent sexual contacts between individuals in different geographic locations. The number of lines between points represents the number of sexual contacts identified. The exception is the thick line between Winnipeg and northern Manitoba. This line represents approximately 25 sexual contacts. Numbers at each of the points represent components of the graphs and provide a means to trace the extent to which geographic bridges occur within that component. Shaded numbers indicate components containing both gonorrhoea and chlamydia. Clear numbers are chlamydia-only components, BC, SK, ON and ND represent network connections to British Columbia, Saskatchewan, Ontario and North Dakota, respectively. Some community locations have been altered slightly for visual clarity. The locations of sexual northern communities with small populations have also been altered. Reprinted with the permission of the Editor, Sexually Transmitted Diseases from Wylie JL, Jolly A. Patterns of chlamydia and gonorrhea infection in sexual networks in Manitoba, Canada. *Sex Transm Dis*. 2001;28(1):14–24

apart with only water and ice road access [58] (Fig. 5.2); across the United States [59] (Fig. 5.2) and internationally [1] (Fig. 5.3), [60] (Fig. 5.4), where people from inside the community have sex with those from far away [50, 61–63], forming a conduit through which infection can pass.

Recently, a graph of places where male sex workers who also used drugs, had previously worked prior to coming to Houston had many of the cities in common with the above two maps [59]. The importance of people who have sex partners from their own geographic area and

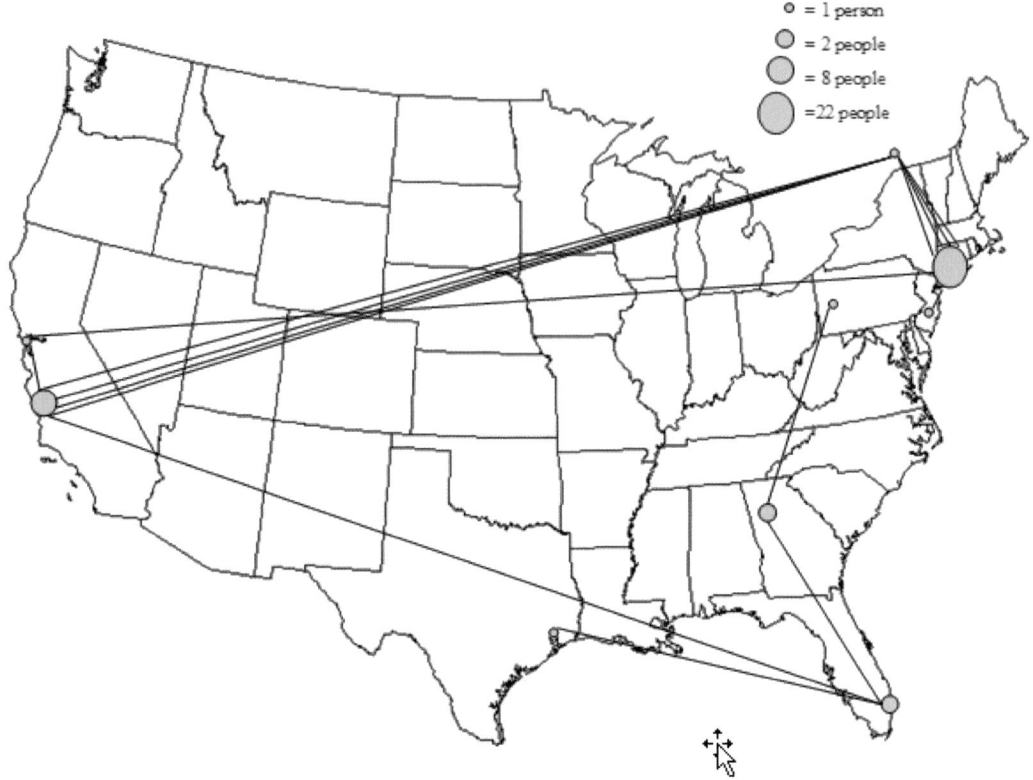

Fig. 5.3 Geographic graph of the first 40 cases of AIDS, by city residence. Where only state information was available, nodes were placed at the capitals of that state. Adapted from Auerbach DM, Darrow WW, Jaffe HW, Curran JW. Cluster of cases of the Acquired Immune Deficiency Syndrome; patients linked by sexual contact. Am J Med. 1984;76:487–492

outside it, though small in number (5–8%) [61, 63], is not to be underestimated. "Bridging" is an essentially social/sexual network mechanism by which well-defined communities revealed in epidemiological investigations with disproportionately large burdens of STI transmit to the remainder of the lower risk more general population.

In addition to the challenges of effectively managing patients and their partners across jurisdictional boundaries, spatial bridgers have been found to have more sex partners compared with residents who have sex with people from within their communities in Ontario, Canada [64], as well as higher HIV rates and increased amounts of drug injecting in Houston, Texas [59]. Although data analysed from Sweden revealed no demographic, laboratory test or socio-economic differences between individuals with long-distance

relationships and those without, concurrency and numbers of sex partners were not measured [61]. The higher risk nature of people who have sex with people both within and outside of their own communities is supported to some extent by descriptions of exogenous higher income, highly educated males, who have higher number of sex partners than men from King County, Washington, consistent with a profile of sex work clients [33, 63].

Spatial bridgers seem to have higher risk behaviours and infection levels than do people who have sex with members of their own geographic region and form effective conduits for transmission. Further investigation is needed into networks containing extra regional relationships in order to establish causes such as individual personality traits such as extroversion, adventurer and leadership roles within networks, and most

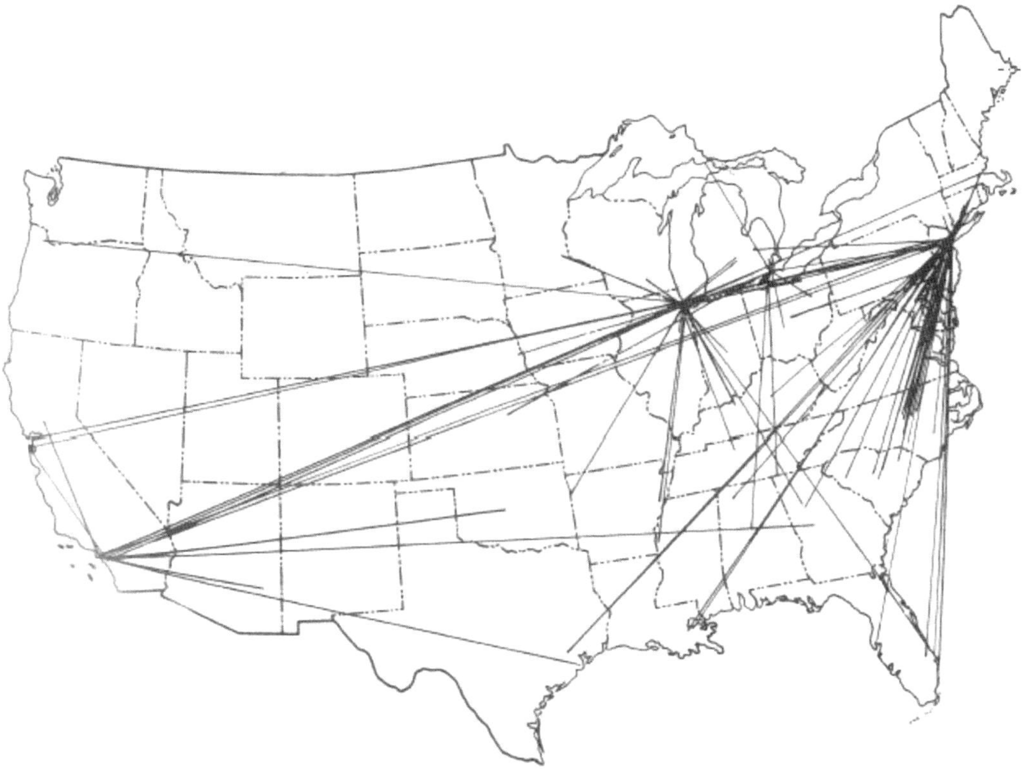

Fig. 5.4 Residence of out-of-city sex contacts named by syphilis patients in cities of 1,000,000 or more population March 1962 (for distances of more than 50 miles). From Donohue JF. Problems posed by population mobility in control of syphilis. In: Proceedings of the world forum on syphilis and other trepanematoses. Atlanta, GA: U.S. Department of Health, Education and Welfare; 1964:38

important, the existence of economic networks where sex is exchanged for money, goods or shelter.

Heterogeneity in Age

Disparities in age have also been associated with higher risk behaviours. Jennings et al. [40] showed that approximately 25% of men have sex with women who are more than 2 years older or younger than themselves. These men were more likely to have had more sex partners in the past 2 months; engaged in commercial sex, been drunk at least once a week in the last 3 months, used drugs including alcohol and marijuana, or sex with someone who used drugs or alcohol at last intercourse. On multivariate analysis only the partners' taking drugs or alcohol at last sex was associated with age bridging. A more recent and noteworthy account of the effects of disparate ages within sexual networks has been in HIV networks in Africa, where the tendency of much older men to partner with younger women has accelerated the spread of HIV into younger, lower prevalence sexual networks, and increased the epidemic size by continually infecting new generations of susceptibles [65–67]. Sociometric network data have revealed wide age ranges within components due to the presence of some members who are 10 or more years older than the mean age. These older members are the equivalent of "spatial bridgers" who form a conduit between populations with different rates, adversely affecting the epidemiology of HIV, and HSV2. In another empirical study young African Americans who had sex with people 2 or more years older or younger than themselves were more likely also to have sex with people outside of their social network [68–70].

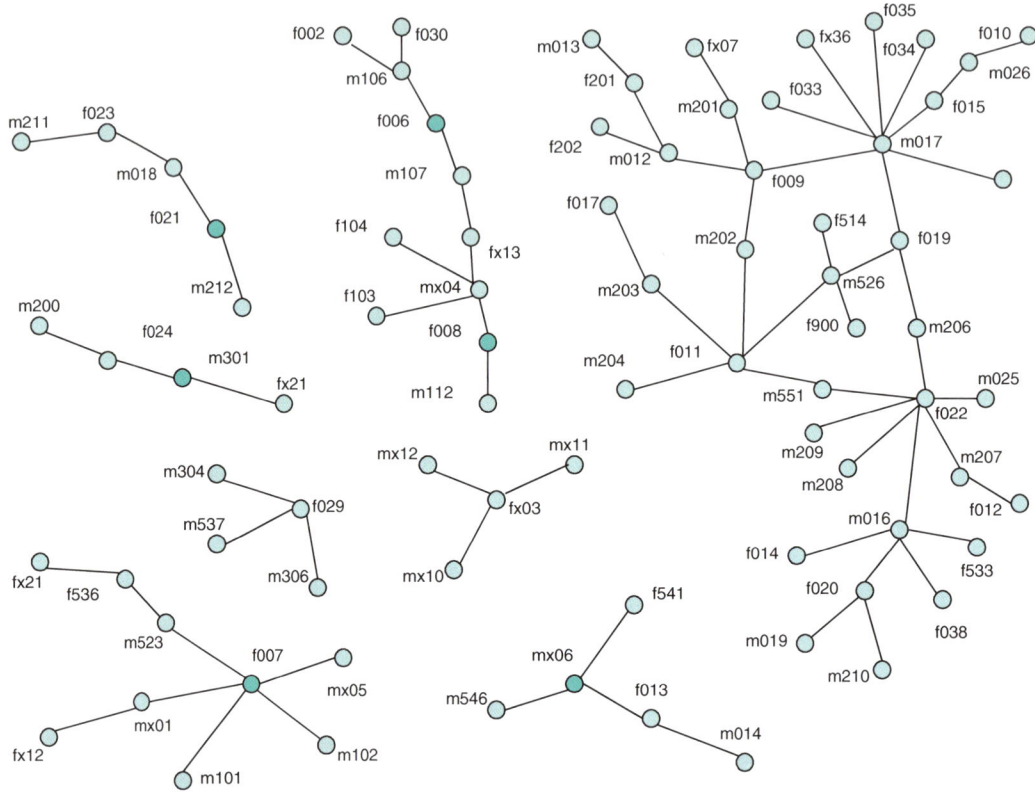

Fig. 5.5 Graph of sexual networks of four or more people revealed by contact tracing cases from January 1999 to December 2001 during a gonorrhoea outbreak

Social Aggregation

The third major finding in the 1985 Colorado Springs paper on gonorrhoea was that although 529 people named 1,009 places which they frequented to "pick up" sex partners, only six places accounted for common establishments frequented by 51% of all cases [28]. The importance of a large number of people clustering around a relatively small number of common social venues was re-emphasised in the sexual network analysis of a gonorrhoea outbreak involving 182 people in Alberta, Canada, carried out simultaneously with a traditional epidemiological case–control study [71]. The case–control study, in which controls were drawn from those with medical visits to the local health centres who did not have a laboratory diagnosis for gonorrhoea nor had been named as contacts, demonstrated that risk

behaviours, such as numbers of partners, and risk markers such as age, were not associated with infection. However, those who had frequented a certain bar which was a known "pick up joint" were more likely to be infected than those who had attended different bars or none at all. Construction of the sexual networks of all cases and contacts revealed a giant component of 39 individuals (21% of the cases and contacts). All clients with gonorrhoea were linked to the bar, and then by sexual intercourse to their corresponding network members, resulting in a bipartite network of one place (the bar) and 89 people representing 49% of the entire population of cases and contacts. Identifying central locations such as this can be immensely helpful in targeting prevention efforts such as urine or point-of-care testing, condom distribution and educational messages (Figs. 5.5 and 5.6).

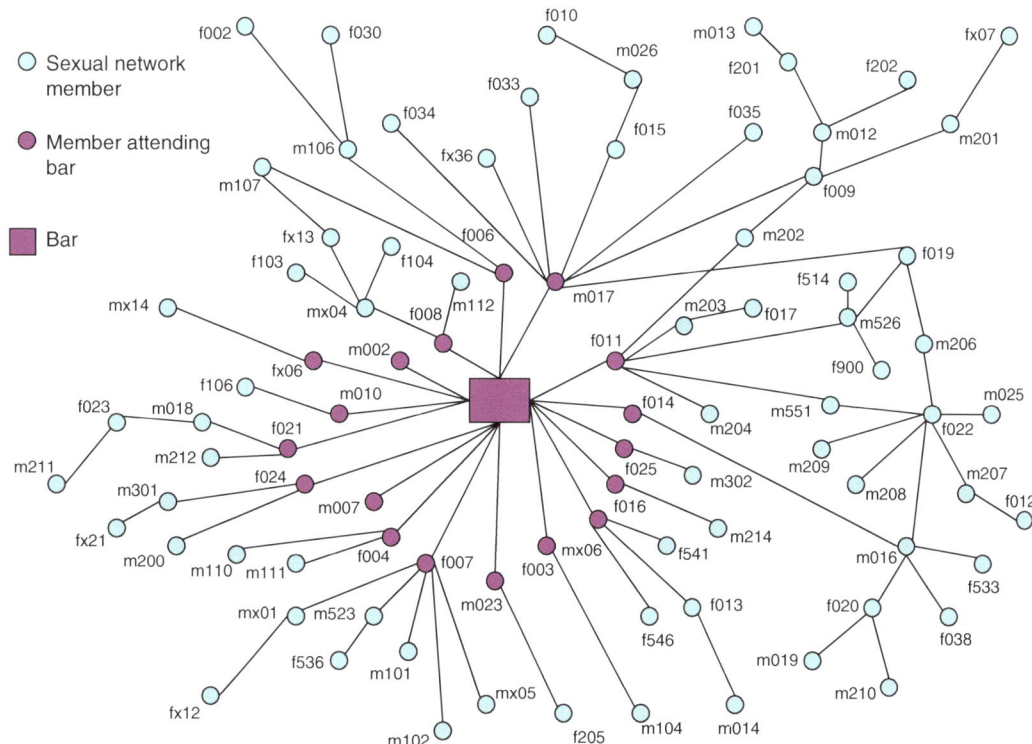

Fig. 5.6 Network members ($n=89$) viewed by their connection to a bar associated with gonorrhoea acquisition. A prefix to the identifier of "m" denotes a male, while "f" denotes a female sex partner. Bar patrons possessed significantly higher centrality measures compared to non-patrons. Adapted from Sexually Transmitted Infections; De P, Singh AE, Yacoub W, Jolly AM. Sexual network analysis of a gonorrhoea outbreak. Sexually Transmitted Infections 2004;80:280–285

In conclusion, assortative sexual mixing patterns between age groups, ethnic groups and geographic areas are proxy indicators of social aggregation—the primary driving factor in our choices of both social and sexual associates, and an essential part of an ecological niche for STIs. Another essential part are the disassortative or heterogeneous associations inherent in the structure of sexual networks, which transmit pathogens from higher to lower incidence regions of the network and enhance the resilience of both against local change. We have attempted to show here that social and sexual network affiliations are reasonable explanations for geographic, ethnic and age mixing patterns. Mixing between people with different numbers of partners is an inherent structural characteristic within a social or a sexual network, the implications of which cannot be totally accounted for by dyadic data or partner mixing matrices alone. Measuring only the number of partners each person has cannot fully explain two graphs with differing capacities for spread despite identical number of nodes and links [6]. Likewise, epidemiologists [71] have demonstrated that information centrality and not numbers of partners is associated with gonorrhoea exposure in an outbreak. Last, physicists [47, 72, 73] have elucidated naturally occurring graphs which are highly connected, yet extraordinarily resistant, to random disturbances of links or nodes. Thus, scientists from three different disciplines have shown that the entire network and its structure cannot be reduced to the number of sex partners of each member without considerable loss of meaning.

While the first part of the paper focussed on general themes and common results found in most sexual networks, the remainder of the paper is dedicated to aspects of pathogen-specific networks.

Pathogen-Specific Networks

In this section we review the distinctive characteristics of the networks in which specific pathogens circulate as these may be key to the
pathogen's survival. At the start of each section
we give a brief review of the molecular epidemiology of pathogens with respect to transmission
within networks. This molecular focus is on how
variation in the genetic characteristics within a
species can be used to identify different "types"
or strains within that species. In turn, analysing
the transmission dynamics of these individual
strains can provide a richer understanding of
transmission dynamics within a network. In general, pathogen strains in people who have had
direct sexual contact have shown concordance.
This is particularly true of bacterial STI where
strain types are more stable over time, but even
with HIV infection, couples have closely related
types of virus. It should be noted that particularly
in viral transmission, the time since HIV infection and strain typing is crucial, in that current
partners may not have similar strain types to
those partners with whom the index case was
having sex in previous years. Another primary
consideration is that of selecting an appropriate
gene from the organism. There is a balance
between selecting a gene or genes with sufficient
variation such that two infected people who have
not had sex will have a greater probability of
being discordant than those who are infected and
have had sex. Likewise, a gene which is highly
variable and changes randomly as an adaptation
to the human immune system may not be concordant in two infected people who have had sex,
even though they were tested within a few days
of each other. Last, it must be noted that just
because people share a common strain of a bacterium, this does not always indicate a direct sexual
relationship. However, if one assumes that one
individual infected another and the strains are
discordant, this is a very specific indication that
even though they may have had sex, the index
case could not have infected that particular sex
partner.

Gonorrhoea and Chlamydia

There are only a small number of articles which
describe sexual networks containing gonorrhoea,
reflecting not only the small number of scientists
working with social networks and infectious diseases but also the number who have access to
experienced, knowledgeable and meticulous and
public health or research staff. The advantages
and validity of contact tracing as a method for
collecting sexual network data of people with
gonorrhoea have been confirmed consistently
with a variety of old and new typing systems.
Wylie et al. demonstrated that reported partnerships of people infected with *N. gonorrhoea* were
consistent with serotypes of gonorrhoea, and by
pulsed field gel electrophoresis (PFGE), but not
by typing of the *opa* gene [74]. The *opa* gene
encodes an outer membrane protein of the gono-
coccus and as such the protein is exposed to the
human immune system. The variability observed
in this protein is believed to be one of the means
by which a gonococcal cell can evade the host
immune system. This variability arises from
genetic variability within the *opa* gene itself and
it is this variability that is the basis for designat-
ing different strains based on *opa* gene type.
Since the gene is responding to the human
immune system, typing methods based on this
gene may therefore be subject to more variability
than the other two methods. However, it was
used successfully by Ward, Day and Ison in an
analysis of gonorrhoea-infected sexual network
members in Sheffield and London [75]. Later on,
validation of contact tracing data in early work
was confirmed by sequencing the porB gene [76],
and by NG-Mast which includes porB and TbpB
[77, 78]. While gene sequencing is not a sensitive discriminating method by which to detect
unreported relationships between people, it is
very specific. Concordant strains between the
majority of partners have been validated, with
only a small minority of strain discordant partners. This small minority were usually a result of
multiple partnerships of both individuals in a
short space of time.

Table 5.1 Transmission efficiency (β), durations (D) and partner change rates (c) for select sexually transmitted pathogens

Agent	Transmission efficiency β at one intercourse	Duration of infectiousness in years D	c
N. gonorrhoea	0.22–0.32 [84]	0.5 absence of control	2.27–1.56
		0.15 with screening and PN [85]	0.68–0.47
C. trachomatis	0.10 [86]	0.83 absence of control [87]	
T. pallidum (multiple intercourses)	0.09 at 30 days	0.5 absence of control	
	0.28 at 90 days	0.25 with control [89]	
	0.63 recently exposed [88]		
HIV	0.0001–0.0023	1.00 [91]	
	0.0041 in the presence of ulcer [90]		

Microbiological analysis of sequences of chlamydia and contact tracing show good convergence [79, 80]. The most common recently used method to distinguish chlamydia types is to sequence *omp1* which encodes the major outer membrane protein (MOMP). Due to stability of *omp1* one can use the sequencing results to confirm that contact tracing actually follows transmission routes with high specificity but not sensitivity. Where it may be of most help is assessing infection source in the case of discordant gene types by ruling out transmission if the sequences are discordant, and searching for others.

To form a viable eco-niche for gonorrhoea the number of susceptible people infected by each infectious person must be greater than one, on average. Mathematical ecologists have contributed a valuable heuristic device by which some minimum requirements may be defined [42, 81, 82]. There needs to be sufficient number of sexual partners in at least some of the networks to transmit infection with a high enough probability during the duration of the infectious period of gonorrhoea. Given the effort and human error in defining most of these estimates, few empirical data are available. As gonorrhoea is one infection for which more data exist than for many others it is a useful template for analysis, which is extendible to other STIs for which less data are available. Table 5.1 gives some basic parameters [83].

The infectious period for gonorrhoea starts at the earliest 1 day before the onset of symptoms, during the last day of the incubation period, and ends when the person is treated (which could be incidental) or when the infection spontaneously resolves (about 6 months). As many studies have reported substantial number of patients who continue to have sex despite frank symptoms [3], it is wise to assume that not all those who have symptoms will seek treatment immediately, or ever. The transmission probability per intercourse has been reported as 0.25 using positive cultures from infected cases exposed to the contact population in which the rate was estimated [84] and 0.32, using strain-specific methods where each person in the couple had confirmed gonorrhoea (Apedaile, unpublished). This relatively high transmission probability compared with that of chlamydia at 0.10 may make up for the shorter duration of infection which may be truncated by symptoms appearing within 5–7 days in about 65% of males, leading the client to seek treatment. Also it is much more likely to be transmitted in a short-term sexual relationship than some other pathogens, with lower transmission probabilities but long duration times, thereby "favouring" transmission by casual, anonymous and commercial sex. It is likely also that those people who prefer short-term casual sexual relationships have time to recruit more sex partners.

In 2001, Wylie and Jolly used laboratory and sexually transmitted disease notifiable disease registry data to clearly define specific networks in which gonorrhoea and/or chlamydia were present, in Manitoba, Canada [2]. They examined the 23 largest networks of 10 or more people. Two basic types of networks were identified: radial, in which a few members had five to 13 partners linked together by the majority who had only

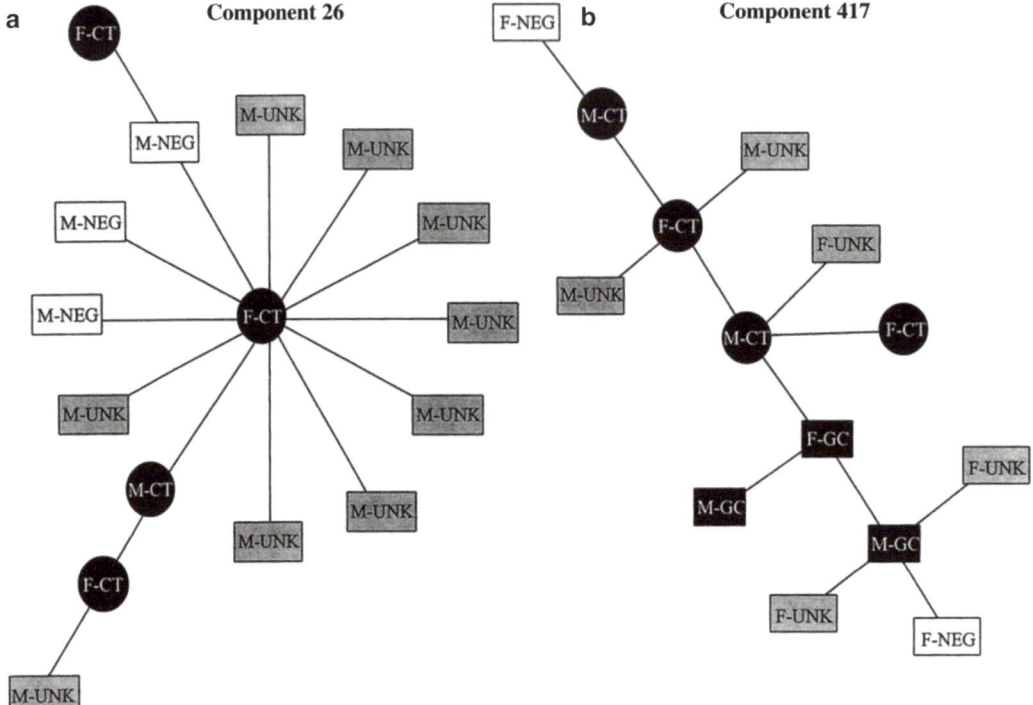

Fig. 5.7 Examples of radial (**a**) and linear components (**b**) identified in Manitoba by network analysis. Each *square* and *circle* represents an individual, with *squares* denoting gonorrhoea, *circles* chlamydia and both together coinfection. "M" within the *square* or the *circle* denotes males and "F", females. *Grey rectangles* represent unnamed contacts, and *solid black shapes* represent confirmed cases of infection. Reprinted with permission of the Editor, Sexually Transmitted Diseases, from Wylie JL, Jolly AM. Sexually Transmitted Diseases 2001; 14–24

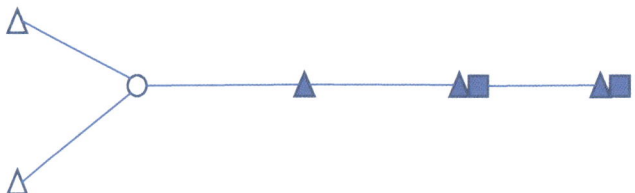

Fig. 5.8 A network from a sampling study in Winnipeg, Manitoba, of all reported cases of gonorrhoea and chlamydia and their contact. The *circles* represent individuals who were not tested or who tested negative. The *triangles* show infection with chlamydia and the *squares* show people with gonorrhoea. The person represented by the *solid triangle* was selected by random sampling, and the other *two solid shapes* represent individuals with chlamydia and gonorrhoea coinfection who also had repeated infections over a 7-month period. Adapted from Wylie JL, Jolly AM. Sexually Transmitted Diseases 2001; 14–24

between one and three partners, and linear, in which degree centrality was not as varied, and people were linked through only one to four partners (Figs. 5.7 and 5.8). Comparison of the two types of networks revealed that the 16 linear networks contained individuals with gonorrhoea, and 10 of those contained individuals infected with both gonorrhoea and chlamydia. Members of linear components were more likely to be North American Indians (First Nations), have positive test results and come from different geographic locations. The higher proportion of First

Nations people diagnosed with gonorrhoea, and correspondingly with chlamydia and gonorrhoea coinfection, was quantified in a later publication [58], and definitively in 2007 [3], where a cluster analysis of STI in the Manitoba population demonstrated three distinct types of networks, two of which had lower degree centralisation (variation in degree) denoting linear networks. They were composed of predominantly First Nations people from rural Manitoba. Members of these networks were also more likely to have gonorrhoea, and coinfection with chlamydia, which was more likely to have been laboratory confirmed when compared with the largest cluster of primarily urban, Caucasian, chlamydia-infected networks. Higher proportions of ethnic minorities have also been reported within gonorrhoea networks in the United States [63] as well as higher proportions of bridgers when compared with chlamydia networks.

The lower median number of partners in the gonorrhoea components in Manitoba compared with chlamydia networks seems counter-intuitive, as many earlier studies characterised individuals with chlamydia as having higher education and income levels, and lower risk profiles [4, 5, 32, 92]. However, a study comparing sociometric gonorrhoea and chlamydia networks in which partner elicitation was standardised at 3 months prior to diagnosis showed that people with gonorrhoea did have more sex partners both in the past year and past 3 months. In network terms, this would result in more star-shaped or radial structures, and is consistent with the short duration time for gonorrhoea, and the relatively high transmission probability, required for successful diffusion of gonorrhoea in a network [51]. Also associated with higher number of partners is concurrency [93], as it allows for more partners to be recruited in a short time frame. In the Manitoba study, the lower number of named partners of people with gonorrhoea may have been due to the shorter time over which people are infectious due to higher likelihood of the onset of symptoms, prompting many to seek care. Chlamydia infections are more likely to be asymptomatic and when diagnosed are routinely interviewed for

partners within the last 3 months [94]. The differences in findings at 3 months and a whole year also suggest that gonorrhoea transmission within a network has a significantly shorter "lifespan" than does chlamydia.

The fact that the majority of gonorrhoea networks, if not all of them, harbour chlamydia also suggests that the network structure for gonorrhoea forms a viable ecological niche for both pathogens. This is supported by the fact that the giant components of bacterial STI networks often contain both pathogens [2, 3, 17, 55, 71, 95–97]. While it is likely that giant components result from expending more effort in contact tracing for clients with both notifiable infections compared to only one [17], and with correspondingly higher number of partner nominations, locations, tests and treatment, it is also clear that the giant components are a minimum estimate of network completeness and connectivity, and in reality the giant component is much larger and more densely linked. Therefore, it is possible that smaller components containing individuals with only gonorrhoea are fragments of de facto giant components, an artificial result of incomplete partner reporting. This is supported by the morphology of networks containing only gonorrhoea [2], which appear similar to that of the periphery of the giant components, with linear branches of one to four partners per client (Fig. 5.7). In one study, a giant component contained higher concentrations of coinfected people with the highest reproductive rates of 0.97 in coinfected non-repeaters, and 1.41 in repeaters [98] compared with people who had either gonorrhoea or chlamydia only. It is logical to hypothesise that the smaller, seemingly disconnected gonorrhoea components are "fed" by similar regions in all STI networks.

The absence of chlamydia in some components, or regions of them, is likely due to STI management practice guidelines which recommend treatment be given for chlamydia on the diagnosis of gonorrhoea given the high rates of coinfection [13, 99]. This is supported by the epidemiological studies which show higher socioeconomic status of individuals infected with chlamydia, and more diverse geographical range, associated with screening incidence rather than true occurrence of infection. The reality is that these demographic characteristics reflect (a) those who are screened and tested positive, which in turn indicates good access to preventive care, and/or (b) those who are well educated and able to attend clinics for annual or biannual physical examinations at which STI screening is recommended.

Age differences in people with chlamydia and gonorrhoea reflect the propensity of *C. trachomatis* for columnar epithelial cells, which are more exposed in the cervices of younger women due to ectopy, lack of immunity [100] and, of course, their choice of partners who are of similar ages. The average age of people infected with gonorrhoea is higher and due to homophily, network members also are older. Many of the differences between networks affected by the two pathogens can be explained by homophily, whether geographic, demographic and behavioural.

Syphilis and HIV

Contact tracing for syphilis is the most long-standing intervention to prevent infection [101]. Testing for syphilis usually involves indirect methods detecting non treponemal antibodies, and those which detect treponemal antibodies in sera. Microscopy of swabs of the chancres in primary syphilis reveals treponemae, but this test is restricted to those sites in the early stage of the disease. Recent advances in amplification technology have prompted scientists to amplify three genes for detection, diagnosis and typing with limited results, especially in sera samples. Only half the samples from ulcerative swabs in one study were appropriate for sequencing, although no between-couple comparisons were done [102]. Due to the difficulty in obtaining good amplified DNA from sera during the secondary and latent periods, the short period and limited number of chancre sites for swabs during the primary period, and the early stage of syphilis sequencing science, contact tracing has not yet been confirmed or refuted by treponemal sequencing.

In contrast, much work has been done with HIV, although the results and their implications are complex due to the clonal nature of the infection, and the long asymptomatic period which delays testing. However, a study of a network of people transmitting and contracting HIV was correlated with phylogenetic data spanning a decade [103]. Two regions of viral DNA were used in the analysis, p17 *gag* and *env* V3, and common methods of constructing the trees, neighbour joining (used in the gonorrhoea sequencing above), Fitch–Margoliash and maximum likelihood methods, gave the most accurate trees, while the use of data from both regions resulted in greater accuracy than either one alone or different methods of phylogenetic tree construction [104]. Due to the rapid changes in this virus over time and within and between people, additional appropriate regions can be selected and analysed to reflect transmission networks accurately.

The first sexual network of men with AIDS linked by sexual intercourse [11] (Fig. 5.8) resembled some of the early networks of syphilis, which spanned the whole of the United States and parts of Europe (Fig. 5.4) [60]. After a long decrease, syphilis has been on the increase in the developed world since the late 1990s [105], due in part, to the reduction in funding devoted to it [63, 106]. Major outbreaks have usually involved men who have sex with men (MSM) [107–111], and sex workers who exchange injection drugs or money for sex [112–114]. Occasionally, recent outbreaks have been in diverse populations not usually associated with syphilis transmission, such as a group of middle class young women from suburban Atlanta who hosted sex parties with African-American and White men on alternate weekends (Fig. 5.9) [114], and another group of predominantly First Nations heterosexual adults, many of whom used alcohol (http://www.wrha.mb.ca/healthinfo/preventill/files/Syphilis_080604.pdf). Sexual networks of MSM and those in which sex is exchanged directly for money or drugs seem to provide the most common environment for syphilis transmission, evinced by a great variation in the number of partners, some with very high number of partners and concurrent sex partners. Less traditional sexual networks such as those in Atlanta are remarkable in that they also had unusually high number of partners and concurrency and one

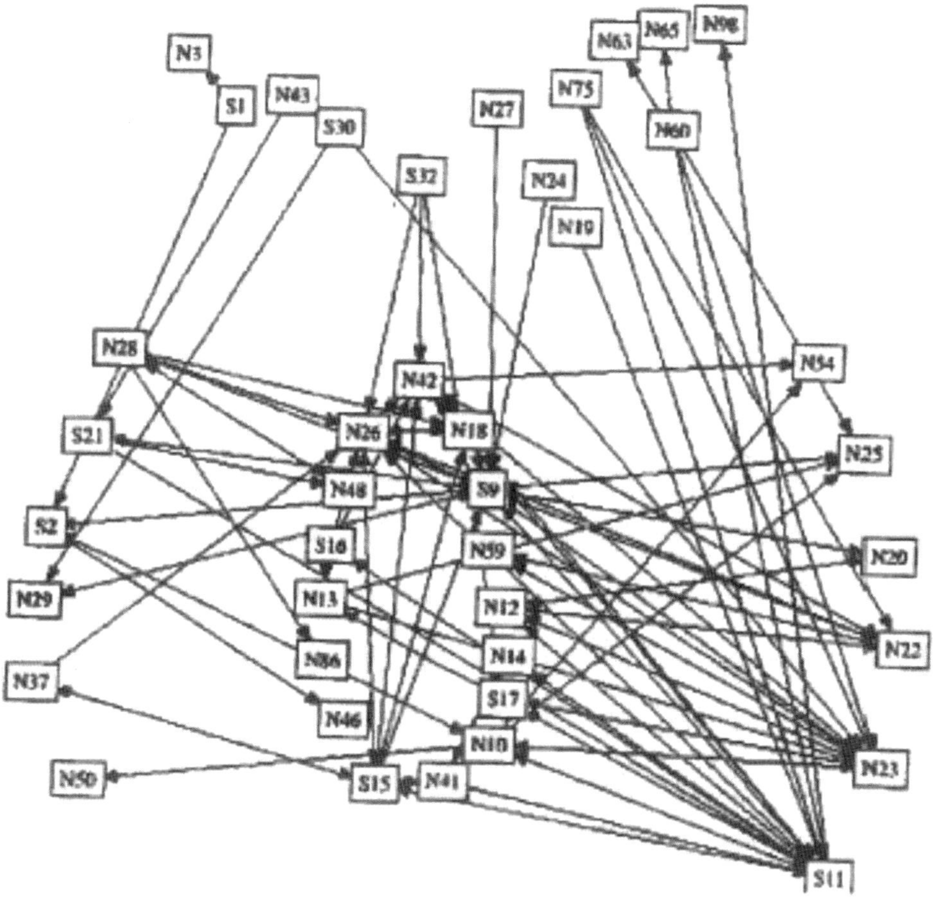

Fig. 5.9 Reprinted with permission from the Editor, Sexually Transmitted Diseases, from Rothenberg RB, Sterk C, Toomey KE, et al. Using social network and ethnographic tools to evaluate syphilis transmission. Sex Transm Dis. 1998;25(3):154–160

other essential feature—they contained some network members from other socially distant networks.

As syphilis was a relatively rare infection in 1996, transmission outside of traditional MSM, sex work and IDU populations was enabled only by bridging, achieved only if networks contained members from diverse groups in which syphilis is endemic. This importance of sex partners who travel long distances was recognised in 1962 (Fig. 5.3, above). This is consistent with recent findings from a cluster analysis of sexual networks in which all of the syphilis cases were found in one cluster, characterised by network members bridging all geographic regions of Manitoba [3]. The existence of social or geo-graphic "long distance" links may be indicative of prevention programs successfully eradicating infection from certain populations such that inci-dence in other populations in which control mea-sures are relaxed becomes more critical. As above, these long distance or heterogeneous links are all the more effective for transmission due to associ-ations with other high-risk behaviours [59, 64].

A second feature of the syphilis networks is their density; that is, a high proportion of connec-tions of all that are possible exist—higher than those in gonorrhoea or chlamydia graphs. The graphs of the young women who initiated sex parties in Atlanta and the other from Fulton County, Atlanta, demonstrate a plethora of cliques and cores, areas in the graph where there are

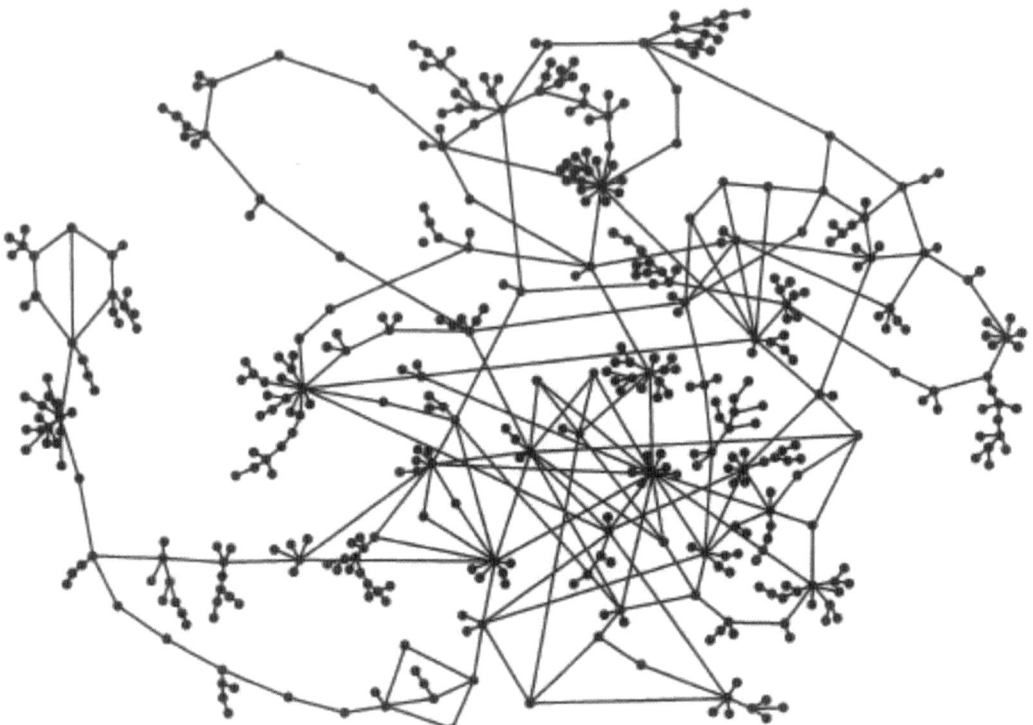

Fig. 5.10 Graph of the largest component in gang-associated STD outbreak, Colorado Springs 1989–1991, $n=410$. Reprinted with permission from the Editor, Sexually Transmitted Infections from Potterat JJ, Phillips-Plummer L, Muth SQ, et al. Risk network structure in the early epidemic phase of HIV transmission in Colorado Springs. Sexually Transmitted Infections. 2002;78(Suppl 1):I159–I163

more connections between people than in other areas. Interestingly, a graph of penicillinase-producing *N. gonorrhoeae* outbreak in a gang showed similar features, and did contain two cases of early syphilis (Fig. 5.10) [95]. Although more sparsely connected, networks of clients with syphilis in Vancouver, British Columbia, show similar multiple connections between people [20], rather than the linear graphs of chlamydia and gonorrhoea. The sparseness may be a result of unreported or anonymous partnerships, as a later paper on this outbreak revealed 88 or 6% repeated infections [115]. It is legitimate to argue that these graphs are highly connected given the fact initial rises in the number of cases stimulated deeper investigations, resulting in higher number of connections being found. However, it is equally valid to hypothesise that

the networks with connections marked currently by syphilis transmission were as dense as previously, and required only occasional long distance or heterogeneous bridges to funnel the infection into a viable network. In conclusion, it appears that in order for syphilis to be endemic, higher number of sexual connections are required than those for gonorrhoea or chlamydia maintenance alone.

Two of the earliest graphs of sexual networks of people with HIV are similar in one respect; they contain people surrounded by many sexual contacts like star bursts. They also contain loops or enclosed circles known as bicomponents in which each person within the subgroup is connected to at least two others, and if one of the members is removed, the linked component does not break apart. In other words, superfluous members

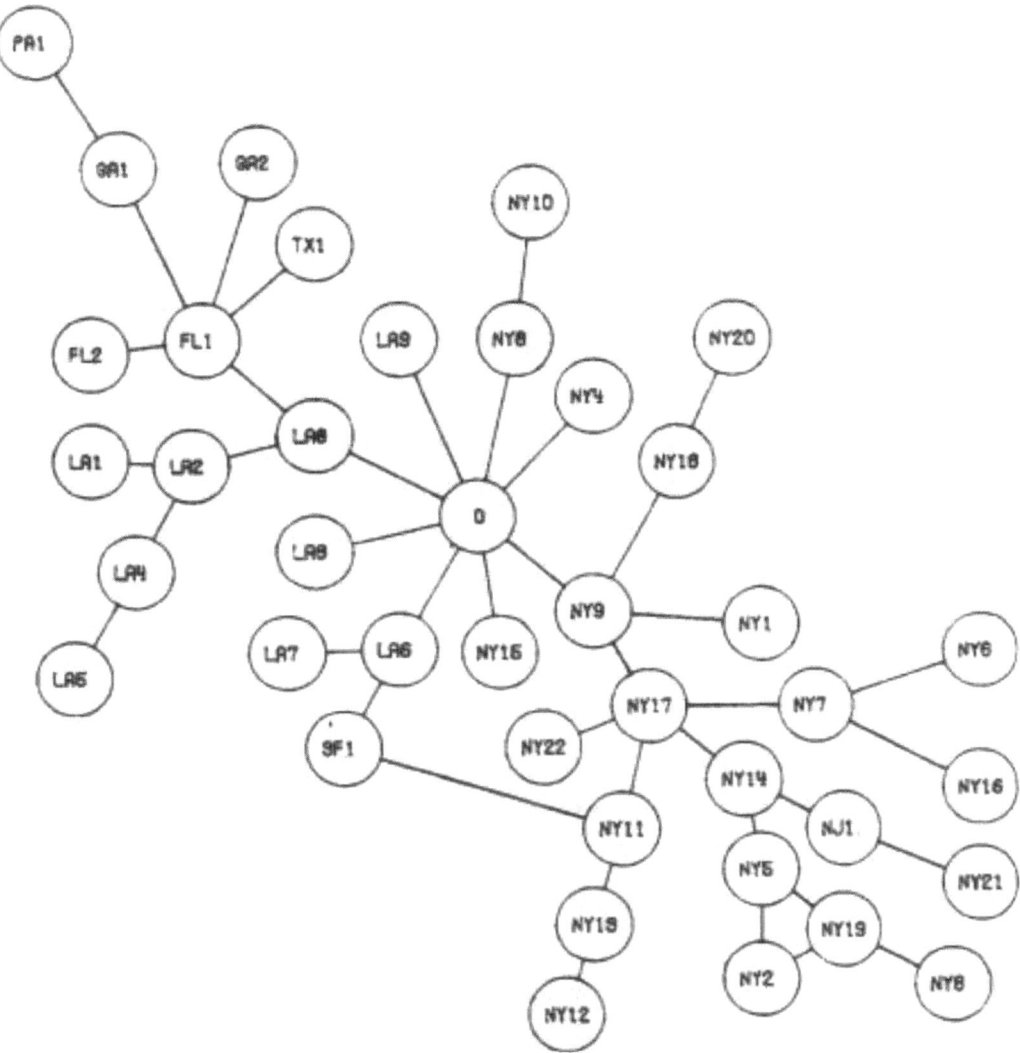

Fig. 5.11 Graph of the sexual links of the first 40 cases of AIDS showing an enclosed loop of NY11, NY17, NY9, 0, LA6 and SF1 reprinted with permission of the Editor, Social Science and Medicine, from Klovdahl AS. Social networks and the spread of infectious diseases: the AIDS example. Social Science and Medicine 1985; 21(11):1203–1216

within a bicomponent supply each member with at least one extra source of infection, rendering the transmission path robust to intervention. It is remarkable that even in 1982, early on in the AIDS epidemic, a path of six links enclosing six men from New York, San Francisco and Los Angeles who had direct and indirect sexual contact with each other and displayed symptoms of HIV infection was able to be identified (Fig. 5.11) [11]. At the time it was estimated that the population at risk comprised 2,500,000 male Americans between the ages of 15 and 54 who were homosexual [1]. These loops were all the more evident in a small group of MSM from Iceland [116], due to the isolated nature of the island and low population (Fig. 5.12), but are still present in later graphs.

The presence of the radial structures of high-degree males is explained by the finding that in the first group of men from North America, the highest number of sex partners reported was 1,560 per year (range 10–1,560), with the average

SEXUAL NETWORKS OF MALE HOMOSEXUALS IN ICELAND

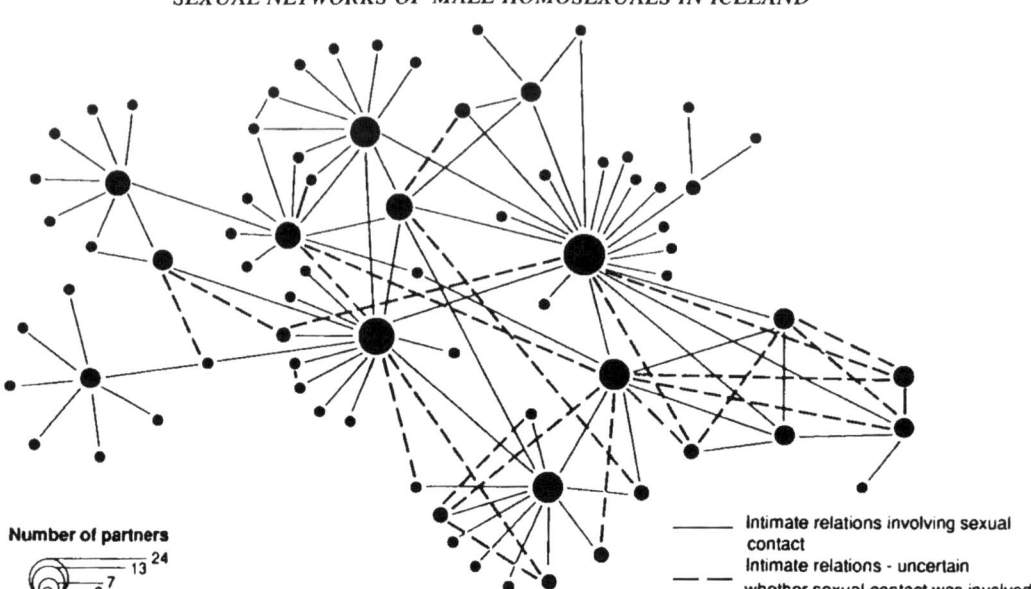

Fig. 5.12 Sexual network of a male homosexual network in Iceland, showing enclosed loops. Reprinted with permission of the Editor, Journal of Acquired Immune Deficiency Syndrome from Haraldsdottir S, Gupta S, Anderson RM. Preliminary studies of sexual networks in a male homosexual community in Iceland. Journal of Acquired Immune Deficiency Syndromes 1992;5(4): 374–81

being 227 [1]. This was an early indication of the heterogeneity in partner choice needed to first introduce HIV into a population, which then could be sustained by the densely linked networks containing a number of circular structures. Population-based data collected much later and analysed using methods from physics and mathematics confirmed the important role of such people with very high number of partners in transmission.

Similar to the relatively rare syphilis infections, HIV is uncommon in many populations infected with chlamydia and gonorrhoea in the developed world. Therefore, new HIV infections within sexual networks are mostly exogenous, whether by virtue of geography, demography, culture or behaviour. This was demonstrated in Figs. 5.3 and 5.4 above, and elucidated in a recent paper showing cities in which male sex workers had worked prior to working in Houston, Texas, Fig. 5.13 [59]. The male sex workers who had worked in multiple cities were also more likely to be HIV positive, three times more likely to inject drugs and had double the number of sex partners than male sex workers who worked in Houston only. Higher number of partners and rates of anal intercourse were also reported in people who bridged small, remote aboriginal Canadian communities [64], and in men who arrange to have unprotected sex with other men through Internet Websites [117].

Syphilis networks and HIV networks are similar in that they contain people with large number of sex partners, they contain circular bicomponents with more than one independent transmission route between people [118, 119] and they contain sex partners from distant locations. These characteristics converge to form viable ecological niches for both pathogens, as both are relatively rare, and both have low transmission probabilities. Of course, once both are extant in a network, the ulcerative nature of syphilis potentiates HIV infection, while the assault of HIV on the immune system exacerbates syphilis infection and may prolong syphilis infectiousness [120].

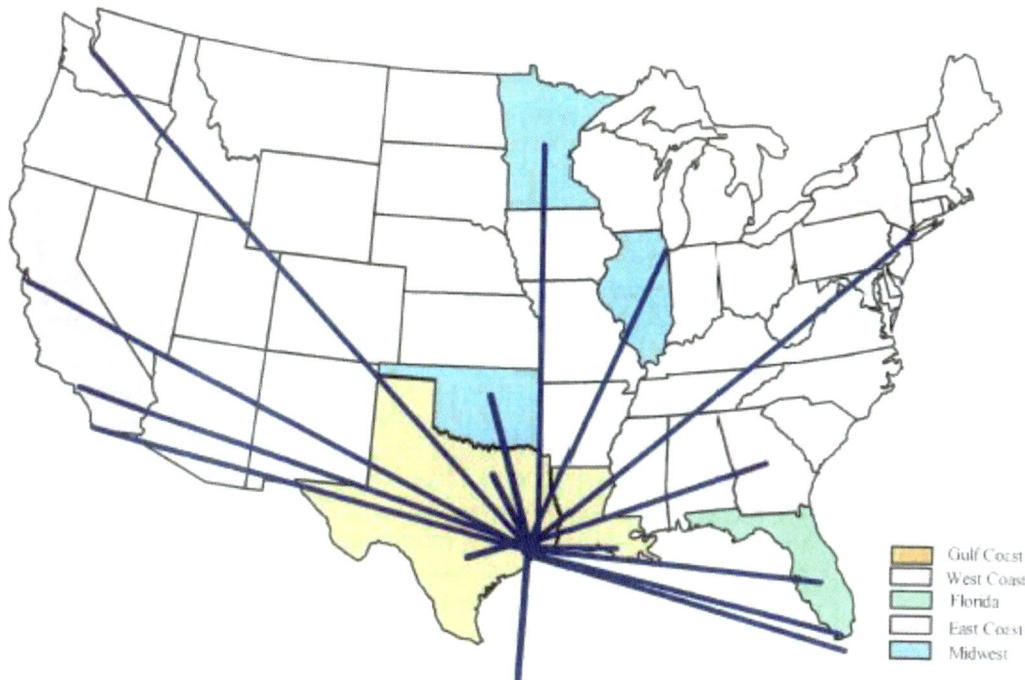

Fig. 5.13 Cities where male sex workers (MSWs) had traded sex for money before coming to Houston. A *line* indicates a bridge between cities. At least one MSW traded sex for money in each of the two cities connected by the lines. Reprinted with permission of the Editor, Journal of Urban Health from Williams ML, Atkinson J, Klovdahl A, Ross MW, Timpson S. Spatial bridging in a network of drug-using male sex workers. Journal of Urban Health: Bulletin of the New York Academy of Medicine 2005;82:i35–i41

Prevention and Networks

The traditional method of contact tracing to interrupt the chain of STI transmission has been in use in various jurisdictions at least since the 1940s and longer in others [101]. In essence it is a form of network sampling in which the infection or transmission network is sampled such that only those contacts or network members who have positive laboratory results are interviewed for their contacts. The emphasis, therefore, is on people with infection and on locating and eliciting their contacts so that they can be examined, tested and treated. Interestingly, the concept of a sexual network was referenced in early work by mathematical modellers who pointed out that greater emphasis should be placed on the identification of contacts with whom the case had had sex just prior to the onset of symptoms (upstream contacts), rather on those who are infected by the index case (downstream contacts) [42]. This concept is important, as it is more likely that the upstream contact is an effective transmitter as he or she has infected one person already—the current case—whereas the ability of the subsequent contacts to spread infection is unknown.

Enhancement of traditional contact tracing using social network methods provides public health staff with various advantages. The first of these is a more client-friendly approach such as that used by sociologists and anthropologists which is fundamentally more interactive than that employed by medical staff which is more clinical, objective and more socially alien. Social scientists have traditionally collected information from people by means of observation, ethnographies and open-ended questionnaires, all of which are more varied and scientifically rigorous than the questionnaires used in contact tracing

[121, 122]. Social network methods are focussed on the entire component rather than on each individual, and on the social context in which the sex is taking place. There is more emphasis placed on interviewing, testing or treating the contacts epidemiologically as they may be equally likely, if not more likely, to transmit infection as the cases [123], and last, a focus on the whole network has the added benefit of being more aware of the presence of coinfections circulating. Less obvious advantages of social network-enhanced interviewing include more careful designation of source and spread cases; characterisation and relationship building with groups at risk of STI; continual evaluation of network membership, risk behaviours, infections and relationships over time and increased opportunities for community-based involvement in interventions [124]. Evaluations of network-enhanced partner notification compared with traditional partner notification have revealed additional people with infections which traditional methods would not have identified, as under the methods section, above.

Venue-Specific Interventions

The early work identifying "lots" of people infected with gonorrhoea and their contacts and the common "pick up joints" patronised by the majority has been confirmed by more recent data, and valuable opportunities for education, testing and treating at those locations have also been identified. Despite the apparent ease of launching interventions in this way, studies evaluating such prevention strategies are rare if not non-existent. The most significant barrier to these initiatives may be establishing trust and gaining permission from the owner of the establishment, though in some cases this has been surprisingly forthcoming [125]. It is important for some establishments, including bathhouses, commercial sex establishments, bars and Internet sites, that the owner's business depends on returning clients and their well-being is therefore of concern.

Network Interventions

Interventions with networks of individuals as a group have been evaluated in some settings. In an outbreak of syphilis in Vancouver's population of injection drug users and sex workers an attempt to pre-empt further infections was made by distributing azithromycin (1.8–1.2 g according to weight) to people in the affected area of the city, with additional doses distributed to associates and sex partners [126]. This strategy was intended to reach otherwise unaccessible people at risk in the network, by increasing trust in having people in the affected community deliver the medication, and by its anonymity, which due to the taboo and often illegal nature of exchanges in the area may be welcome. Although reported safe sex practices and knowledge of syphilis had increased in participants when they responded to an evaluation a year later, compared with eligible non-participants, the rebound in incidence of syphilis was greater than expected as infection filtered back into the population. This is consistent with known geographic links with people in northern British Columbia and in the Yukon, the adjacent northern territory, and undisclosed links with infected people, which resulted in a 6% repeat infection rate [115].

More commonly used network interventions involve including leaders or members of a peer group who receive training in intervention and then deliver it, in some manner, within their own networks. Work with peer networks of injection drug users in reducing the risk of infection from injection and sex is likely more efficient and possibly more effective than traditional peer interventions [127]. This approach was tried in Romany people in Bulgaria and in MSM in Russia and Bulgaria and evaluated [128, 129]. Both interventions used sociological methods to identify leaders, who then were trained and conducted HIV prevention by counselling, discussing and offering advice on HIV prevention. After the intervention, participants were more willing to discuss risk reduction, perceptions of network norms of safer sex became more positive and reports of condom use increased.

Future Directions

Network methods, whether used in case contact investigations, outbreak investigations and in analytic approaches to both routine surveillance and research, are intuitively appealing because of a common immediate grasp of the network graphs. The increasing shortage of funding devoted to public health, the globalisation of STIs and their resurgence may be addressed well by network methods. For example, the traditional case–control study in an STI outbreak is unintuitive in that the selection of controls with equal opportunity for exposure is problematic, as is the possibility that they may also become infected. These two challenges render the case–control study labour intensive and costly, while the network approach is strategic in that it focuses attention on both cases and contacts, and the routes by which people become infected. Also, the international spread of LGV has demonstrated the transmission of STI over a vast area such that localised approaches which disregard transmission routes may be less successful than in the past. Last, the changing eco niches which harbour STI have grown in response to screening and treatment in recommended groups, as recognised by Wasserheit and Aral. [7]. The discovery of STI in groups not usually affected again calls for a network approach focussed on specific people and the routes of transmission into and out of those non-traditional groups and reaffirms findings of those ideas.

What remains a challenge is to define more specifically the extent to which network analysis application results in an improvement over previous methods [9]. One of the most important of these is the evaluations of network enhanced contact tracing effectiveness and efficiency, both routinely and during an outbreak. It is to be noted that in some jurisdictions contact tracing interviews have attenuated over time, and many for the bacterial STI are interviews conducted over the phone, which may not give a true reflection of a good baseline for contact tracing. In such settings it is possible that the value network-enhanced contact tracing may be overestimated. However, contact investigations can be amended to include the network approach, both in the interview process and in content, with little additional work over and above traditional methods.

Evaluations of the network methods against "routine practice" can therefore be biased, as much of the improvement may be ascribed to thorough and more complete organisation and delivery of contact interviews, resulting in a higher percentage of contacts interviewed and better and more accurate data from that. A second challenge is the complicated nature of study design and replicability. As contact tracing practices differ so much in jurisdictions and also for different pathogens, what added advantage network investigation brings also varies, though consistent improvements in the number of contacts interviewed, tested and brought to treatment should satisfy most that it is effective. This observational approach is not counted amongst the highest standards of evidence, though it is impossible and may be unethical to perform a randomised clinical trial. First, this kind of intervention is susceptible to changes in social context, which goes against the sterile objectivity of the clinical trial. Second, it is serving largely a vulnerable, marginalised population which by its nature has never typically been well accepted in mainstream institutions such as hospitals. Third, an adequate sampling frame from which to draw a representative random sample of marginalised people seldom exists, and fourth, if a sample is recruited, the chances that the individuals are acquainted with each other and may even have encouraged each other to participate are high, thus compromising the requirement for independent observations.

In order to minimise bias and adhere to high standards of proof, outcome evaluations based on the number of patients nominated, tested and brought to treatment should be conducted alongside process evaluations of the amounts of time spent on interviews: timeliness of interviews after receipt of positive laboratory tests, completeness of data and interviewee opinion of the process. As drug use, sex work and culture of vulnerable people differ between jurisdictions, comparing network-enhanced contact tracing with traditional

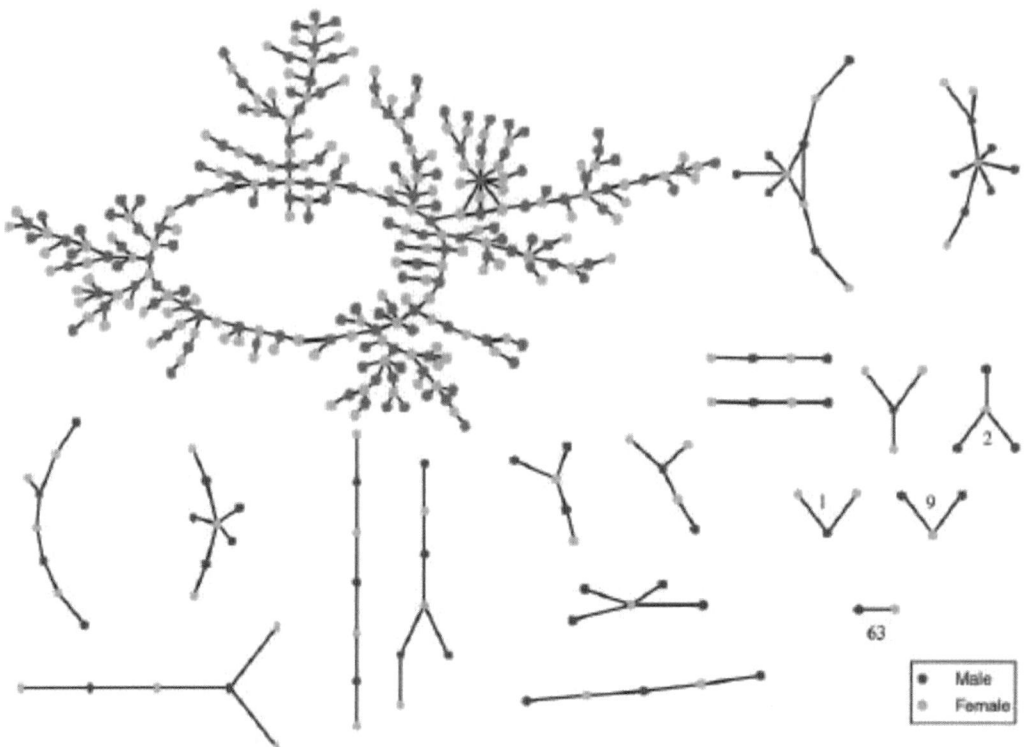

Fig. 5.14 Romantic and sexual network of high school students of a school in a midsize town in the United States Midwest. Reprinted with permission of the editor American Journal of Sociology, from Bearman, PS, Moody J, Stovel K. Chains of affection: the structure of adolescent romantic and sexual networks. American Journal of Sociology 2004;110:44–91

methods in two different areas may not yield accurate results, so before and after studies may be more suitable. Yet another complication involves the efficiency of public health workers initially spending large amount of time within disadvantaged neighbourhoods. Once staff have identified key informants, the places where people assemble and the general rhythm of life, these may aid immensely in future interventions and inquiries as to changes in drug choices, sex work, availability of injecting equipment and outbreaks. This last is not easily quantifiable, but no less important.

Research into networks has already come far, and future research is bound to reveal new and relevant information. One of the most immediate of the network questions, which has already been partly addressed, is how STI networks differ from those of people without STI. The sexual network of high school students (Fig. 5.14) and another of

adults on Likoma Island, Malawi (Fig. 5.15), are the sole examples of a sexual network within a general, relevant population, collected without STI as the motivation. From the high school example it does seem possible that sexual networks of those who are uninfected may resemble those who are, although only for some pathogens such as chlamydia. The implication for prevention is that should chlamydia be able to survive in typical adolescent networks, careful thought may have to be given in intervening the structure of the network, but routine screening, peer education and treatment of key people may be more effective than mass interventions. The second network from Africa demonstrates that the structure and density associated with HIV, syphilis, chlamydia and gonorrhoea can exist in the absence of high rates of these infections. In this example, bicomponents contained people with

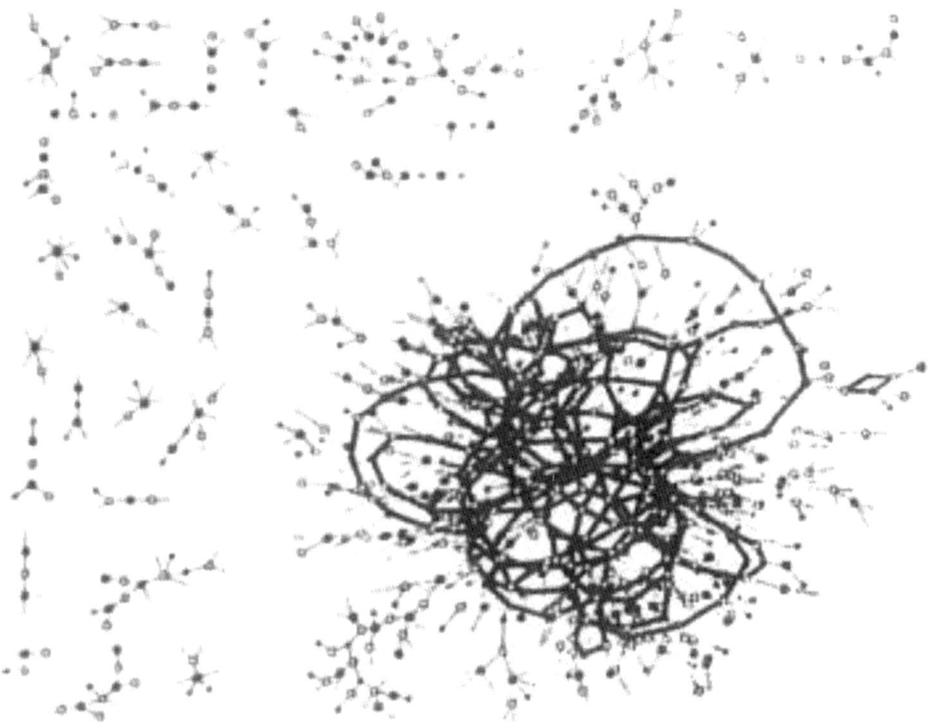

Fig. 5.15 Components of the Likoma sexual networks of size six and larger. *Circles* represent individuals. *Lines* represent sexual partnerships between individuals. *Black circles*: male survey respondents; *grey circles*: female survey respondents. *Larger circles* represent network members who were interviewed during the sexual network survey and who were sexually active during the recall period ($n=896$). *Smaller circles* represent network members who were found within the village rosters but were not interviewed because they were outside the sampling frame of this study (all young adults aged 18–35 years and their spouses living in the seven sample villages). The *subset of lines* not connecting two circles represent partnerships with individuals we were not able to identify in rosters of potential partners. The *subset of thicker lines* represent partnerships within bicomponents that are between network member who are connected by more than one independent pathway within the sexual network. This *graph* represents the full network of individuals identified during this study, over a 3-year recall period. Reprinted with permission of the Editor of AIDS, from Helleringer, S, Kohler H-P. Sexual network structure and the spread of HIV in Africa: evidence from Likoma Island, Malawi. AIDS 2007;21:2323–2332

lower rates of infection than smaller components or other regions of the giant components, indicating a possible protective structure. Higher infection rates in smaller components separate from the main population was also observed in Colorado Springs [130] (Fig. 5.16). However, far more examples of sexual networks in far more diverse contexts are needed before definitive, generalisable statements can be made.

Research concerning the diffusion processes of different STI may also help in our understanding of STI epidemics. Specifically, the properties of the agent itself may affect diffusion, as does the network itself. As time passes, the interaction between the agent, network and prevention strategies evolves which again affects each of the above. Some work has been done in networks evolving over time [114], though much more needs to be done to explain the roles of individuals with repeat STI, those who do not seek treatment, asymptomatic carriers, members of circular, ring-shaped bicomponents and those with many and possibly concurrent partners who facilitate pathogen spread within a network. Facilitating this work is the advancement in strain typing methods which can be used to more accurately

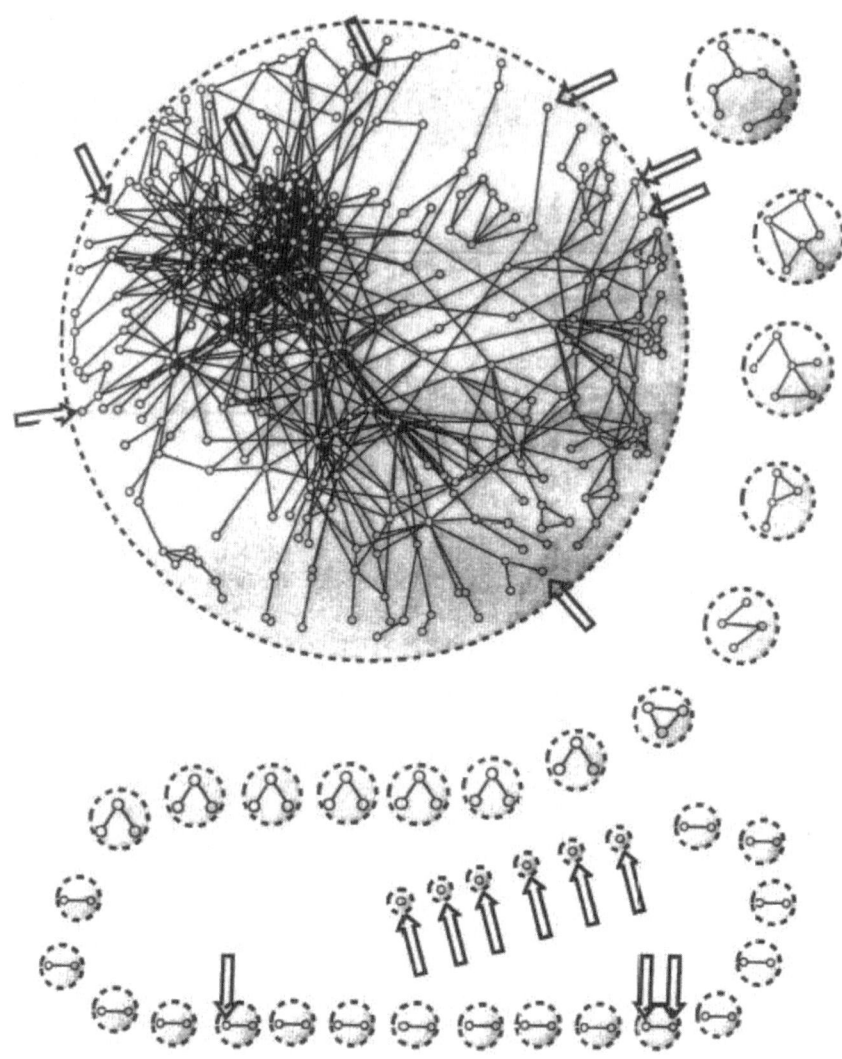

Fig. 5.16 Social network of close personal friends; sexual and drug sharing partners with whom participants shared lodging or food. This diagram shows by the *arrows* those respondents who were HIV positive located for the most part on the periphery of the network. Reprinted with the permission of the Editor, Sociological Focus, from Darrow WW, Potterat JJ, Rothenberg RB, Woodhouse DE, Muth SQ. Using knowledge of social networks to prevent human immunodeficiency virus infections: The Colorado Springs study. Sociological Focus 1999;32(2): 143–158

mark the route of a pathogen through a transmission network.

Geographic analyses of networks have also more to divulge, especially as they influence network formation. Concentrations of inner-city minority populations with historically high STI rates influence the dynamics of network formation so that there is a continuing relationship between likelihood of people meeting their neighbours and formation of an STI network. After introduction into a network, shared practices, beliefs and norms may serve to perpetuate STIs over and above individuals' choices. Using a social network approach may facilitate analyses of social cohesion and social capital which positively influence network norms and lower STI rates.

Last, a deeper understanding of personalities, roles, risk perception and norms of networks may aid in the understanding of people who bridge different ethnic, geographic and age groups, with those who have many more sex partners than their associates. While these encounters may mark higher risks for STI transmission, these same people may be ideal leaders in reaching others to disseminate interventions.

In conclusion, successful sexually transmitted pathogens are those which not only adapt and infect the host but also those that adapt to the whole reservoir—a changing network of humans and control measures. Incidental infection of a single host is simply a "polling" event which is only truly effective if the pathogen can pass further into a network where it can remain endemic. It follows then, that in the changing networks, where we have reached the point of diminishing returns through mass screening, we should focus more precisely on those network structures which complement pathogen characteristics, facilitating their spread. For syphilis and HIV, network density seems to be one of the keys to transmission, as are lower number of partners (degree centrality) and bicomponents in chlamydia and gonorrhoea networks. When these structures are observed in the routine follow-up of STIs, proactive screening for existing and other STIs, outreach and more specific investigation of the context in which the sex occurs will be helpful. In addition, people central to the network can be re-interviewed and offered testing either at the first sign of reintroduction of a pathogen or routinely. Consistent, regular contact with health care providers, whether in clinics or in an outreach setting, can only help build good interactive relationships between clients and health care staff. The advantage of these more precise, locally based approaches is that some of the treatment and testing pressure on pathogens is removed, slowing the evolution of resistance and loss of genes required for testing.

Acknowledgement The authors thank Ms. Aristea Kokkinos for her precise and painstaking help with the references.

References

1. Klovdahl AS. Social networks and the spread of infectious diseases: the AIDS example. Soc Sci Med. 1985;21(11):1203–16.
2. Wylie JL, Jolly A. Patterns of chlamydia and gonorrhea infection in sexual networks in Manitoba, Canada. Sex Transm Dis. 2001;28(1):14–24.
3. De Rubeis E, Wylie JL, Cameron DW, Nair RC, Jolly AM. Combining social network analysis and cluster analysis to identify sexual network types. Int J STD AIDS. 2007; 18(11):754–59. http://ijsa.rsm-journals.com/cgi/reprint/18/11/754; http://dx.doi.org/10.1258/095646207782212234.
4. Zimmerman HL, Potterat JJ, Dukes RL, et al. Epidemiologic differences between chlamydia and gonorrhea. Am J Public Health. 1990;80(11): 1338–42.
5. Rice RJ, Roberts PL, Handsfield HH, Holmes KK. Sociodemographic distribution of gonorrhea incidence: implications for prevention and behavioral research. Am J Public Health. 1991;81:1252–8.
6. Klovdahl AS, Potterat J, Woodhouse D, Muth J, Muth S, Darrow WW. HIV infection in an Urban Social Network: a progress report. Bull Methodol Sociol. 1992;36:24–33.
7. Wasserheit JN, Aral SO. The dynamic topology of sexually transmitted disease epidemics: implications for prevention strategies. J Infect Dis. 1996;174(2): S201–13.
8. Potterat JJ, Meheus A, Gallwey J. Partner notification: operational considerations. Int J STD AIDS. 1991; 2(6):411–5.
9. Rothenberg R. The transformation of partner notification. Clin Infect Dis. 2002;35(2):S138–45. http://dx.doi.org/10.1086/342101.
10. Karp G, Schlaeffer F, Jotkowitz A, Riesenberg K. Syphilis and HIV co-infection. Eur J Intern Med. 2009;20(1):9–13. doi:10.1016/j.ejim.2008.04.002.
11. Auerbach DM, Darrow WW, Jaffe HW, Curran JW. Cluster of cases of the acquired immune deficiency syndrome; patients linked by sexual contact. Am J Med. 1984;76:487–92.
12. Rothenberg RB, Potterat JJ, Holmes KK, Mardh P, Sparling PF, et al., editors. Strategies for management of sex partners; sexually transmitted diseases. Vol. 2. New York: McGraw-Hill; 1990. p. 1081–86.
13. Canadian guidelines on sexually transmitted infections. Ottawa, ON: Public Health Agency of Canada; 2006.
14. Sexually transmitted diseases treatment guidelines, 2006. MMWR Morb Mortal Wkly Rep. 2006;55 (RR-11):1–100.
15. Brewer DD. Case-finding effectiveness of partner notification and cluster investigation for sexually transmitted diseases/HIV. Sex Transm Dis. 2005; 32(2):78–83.

16. Langille DB, Shoveller J. Partner notification and patient education for cases of Chlamydia trachomatis infection in a rural Nova Scotia health unit. Can J Public Health. 1992;83(5):358–61.

17. Rasooly I, Millson ME, Frank JW, et al. A survey of public health partner notification for sexually transmitted diseases in Canada. Can J Public Health. 1994;85 Suppl 1:S48–52.

18. Brewer DD, Webster CM. Forgetting of friends and its effect on measuring friendship networks. Soc Net. 1999;21:361–73.

19. Brewer DD, Garrett SB, Kulasingam S. Forgetting as a cause of incomplete reporting of sexual and drug injection partners. Sex Transm Dis. 1999;26(3): 166–76.

20. Ogilvie G, Knowles L, Wong E, et al. Incorporating a social networking approach to enhance contact tracing in a heterosexual outbreak of syphilis. Sex Transm Infect. 2005;81(2):124–7.

21. Annan T, Evans B, Hughes G. Guidance for managing STI outbreaks and incidents. London, UK: Health Protection Agency; 2008:12.

22. Ghani AC, Donnelly CA, Garnett GP. Sampling biases and missing data in explorations of sexual partner networks for the spread of sexually transmitted diseases. Stat Med. 1998;17(18):2079–97.

23. Ramirez-Valles J, Heckathorn DD, Vázquez R, Diaz RM, Campbell RT. From networks to populations: the development and application of respondent-driven sampling among IDUs and Latino gay men. AIDS Behav. 2005;9(4):387–402. http://dx.doi.org/10.1007/s10461-005-9012-3.

24. Heckathorn DD. Respondent-driven sampling: a new approach to the study of hidden populations. Soc Probl. 1997;44(2):174–99. http://dx.doi.org/10.1525/sp.1997.44.2.03x0221m.

25. Heckathorn DD. Respondent-driven sampling II: deriving valid population estimates from chain-referral samples of hidden populations. Soc Probl. 2002;49(1):11–34. http://dx.doi.org/10.1525/sp.2002.49.1.11.

26. Abdul-Quader AS, Heckathorn DD, Sabin K, Saidel T. Implementation and analysis of respondent driven sampling: lessons learned from the field. J Urban Health. 2006;83(1 Suppl):1–5. http://dx.doi.org/10.1007/s11524-006-9108-8.

27. Salganik MJ, Heckathorn DD. Making unbiased estimates from hidden populations using respondent-driven sampling. Sunbelt Social Network Conference, Cancun, Mexico; 2003.

28. Potterat JJ, Rothenberg RB, Woodhouse DE, Muth JB, Pratts CI, Fogle JS. Gonorrhea as a social disease. Sex Transm Dis. 1985;12(1):25–32.

29. Granovetter M. The strength of weak ties. Am J Sociol. 1973;78(6):1360–80.

30. McPherson M, Smith-Lovin L, Cook JM. Birds of a feather: homophily in social networks. Annu Rev Sociol. 2001;27(1):415–44. http://dx.doi.org/10.1146/annurev.soc.27.1.415.

31. Blanchard JF, Moses S, Greenaway C, Orr P, Hammond GW, Brunham RC. The evolving epidemiology of chlamydial and gonococcal infections in response to control programs in Winnipeg, Canada. Am J Public Health. 1998;88(10):1496–502.

32. Rothenberg RB. The geography of gonorrhea. Am J Epidemiol. 1983;117:688–94.

33. Rothenberg R, Muth SQ, Malone S, Potterat JJ, Woodhouse DE. Social and geographic distance in HIV risk. Sex Transm Dis. 2005;32(8):506–12. http://dx.doi.org/10.1097/01.olq.0000161191.12026.ca.

34. Aral SO, Hughes JP, Stoner B, et al. Sexual mixing patterns in the spread of gonococcal and chlamydial infections. Am J Public Health. 1999;89(6): 825–33.

35. Rothenberg R. The relevance of social epidemiology in HIV/AIDS and drug abuse research. Am J Prev Med. 2007;32(6 Suppl 1):S147–53. http://dx.doi.org/10.1016/j.amepre.2007.02.007.

36. Bush KR, Henderson EA, Dunn J, Read RR, Singh A. Mapping the core: chlamydia and gonorrhea infections in Calgary, Alberta. Sex Transm Dis. 2008;35(3):291–97. http://ovidsp.ovid.com/ovidweb.cgi?T=JS&NEWS=N&PAGE=fulltext&AN=0 0007435-200803000-00015&D=ovftj. 10.1097/OLQ.0b013e31815c1edb.

37. Laumann EO, Gagnon JH, Michael RT, Michaels S. The social organization of sexuality: sexual practices in the United States. Chicago, IL: University of Chicago Press; 1994. p. 750.

38. Wallace R, Fullilove MT, Flisher AJ. AIDS, violence and behavioral coding: information theory, risk behavior and dynamic process on core-group socio-geographic networks. Soc Sci Med. 1996;43(3): 339–52.

39. Ellen JM, Langer LM, Zimmerman RS, Cabral RJ, Fichtner R. The link between the use of crack cocaine and the sexually transmitted diseases of a clinic population. A comparison of adolescents with adults. Sex Transm Dis. 1996;23(6):511–6.

40. Jennings JM, Luo RF, Lloyd LV, Gaydos C, Ellen JM, Rietmeijer CA. Age-bridging among young, urban, heterosexual males with asymptomatic *Chlamydia trachomatis*. Sex Transm Infect. 2007;83(2):136–41. http://dx.doi.org/10.1136/sti.2006.023556; http://sti.bmj.com/cgi/content/abstract/83/2/136.

41. Foulkes HB, Pettigrew MM, Livingston KA, Niccolai LM. Comparison of sexual partnership characteristics and associations with inconsistent condom use among a sample of adolescents and adult women diagnosed with Chlamydia trachomatis. J Womens Health (Larchmt). 2009;18(3):393–99. http://search.ebscohost.com/login.aspx?direct=true&db=cin20&AN=2010222653&site=ehost-live.

42. Yorke JA, Hethcote HW, Nold A. Dynamics and control of the transmission of gonorrhea. Sex Transm Dis. 1978;5(2):51–6.

43. Brunham RC. The concept of core and its relevance to the epidemiology and control of sexually transmitted diseases [editorial]. Sex Transm Dis. 1991;18(2):67–8.

44. Liljeros F, Edling CR, Amaral LAN, Stanley HE, Aberg Y. The web of human sexual contacts. Nature. 2001;411(6840):907–8. http://dx.doi.org/10.1038/35082140.

45. Schneeberger A, Nat R, Mercer CH, et al. Scale-free networks and sexually transmitted diseases: a description of observed patterns of sexual contacts in Britain and Zimbabwe. Sex Transm Dis. 2004;31(6):380–7.

46. Eames KTD, Keeling MJ. Monogamous networks and the spread of sexually transmitted diseases. Math Biosci. 2004;189(2):115–30.

47. Newman M. Power laws, Pareto distributions and Zipf's law. Contemp Phys. 2005;46(5):323–51. http://www.informaworld.com/10.1080/00107510500052444.

48. Chan DYC, Hughes BD, Leong AS, Reed WJ. Stochastically evolving networks. Phys Rev E. 2003;68(066124):066124-4–24.

49. Britton T, Nordvik MK, Liljeros F. Modelling sexually transmitted infections: the effect of partnership activity and number of partners on R0. Theor Popul Biol. 2007;72(3):389–99.

50. Gorbach PM, Drumright LN, Holmes KK. Discord, discordance, and concurrency: comparing individual and partnership-level analyses of new partnerships of young adults at risk of sexually transmitted infections. Sex Transm Dis. 2005;32(1):7–12.

51. Stoner BP, Whittington WL, Hughes JP, Aral SO, Holmes KK. Comparative epidemiology of heterosexual gonococcal and chlamydial networks: implications for transmission patterns. Sex Transm Dis. 2000;27(4):215–23.

52. Quinn RW, O'Reilly KR, Khaw M. Gonococcal infections in women attending the venereal disease clinic of the Nashville Davidson County Metropolitan Health Department, 1984. South Med J. 1988;81:851–4.

53. Moran JS, Aral SO, Jenkins WC, Peterman TA, Alexander ER. The impact of sexually transmitted diseases on minority populations. Public Health Rep. 1989;104(6):560–5.

54. Zenilman JM. Gonorrhea, chlamydia and the sexual network: pushing the envelope. Sex Transm Dis. 2000;27(4):224–5.

55. Jolly AM, Muth SQ, Wylie JL, Potterat JJ. Sexual networks and sexually transmitted infections: a tale of two cities. J Urban Health. 2001;78(3):433–45.

56. Laumann EO, Youm Y. Racial/ethnic group differences in the prevalence of sexually transmitted diseases in the United States: a network explanation [see comments]. Sex Transm Dis. 1999;26(5):250–61.

57. Fichtenberg CM, Muth SQ, Brown B, Padian NS, Glass TA, Ellen JM. Sexual network structure among a household sample of urban African American

58. Jolly AM, Moffatt MEK, Fast MV, Brunham RC. Sexually transmitted disease thresholds in Manitoba, Canada. Ann Epidemiol. 2005;15(10):781–8. http://dx.doi.org/10.1016/j.annepidem.2005.05.001.

59. Williams ML, Atkinson J, Klovdahl A, Ross MW, Timpson S. Spatial bridging in a network of drug-using male sex workers. J Urban Health. 2005;82:i35–42. http://jurban.oupjournals.org/.

60. Donohue JF. Problems posed by population mobility in control of syphilis. In: Proceedings of the world forum on syphilis and other trepanematoses. Atlanta, GA: U.S. Department of Health, Education and Welfare; 1964:38.

61. Nordvik MK, Liljeros F, Osterlund A, Herrmann B. Spatial bridges and the spread of chlamydia: the case of a County in Sweden. Sex Transm Dis. 2007;34(1):47–53. http://dx.doi.org/10.1097/01.olq.0000222722.79996.4b.

62. Wylie JL, Cabral T, Jolly AM. Identification of networks of sexually transmitted infection: a molecular, geographic, and social network analysis. J Infect Dis. 2005;191(6):899–906. http://dx.doi.org/10.1086/427661.

63. Kerani RP, Golden MR, Whittington WLH, Handsfield HH, Hogben M, Holmes KK. Spatial bridges for the importation of gonorrhea and chlamydial infection. Sex Transm Dis. 2003;30(10):742–9.

64. Calzavara LM, Bullock SL, Myers T, Marshall VW, Cockerill R. Sexual partnering and risk of HIV/STD among Aboriginals. Can J Public Health. 1999;90(3):186–91.

65. Brunham RC, Cheang M, McMaster J, Garnett G, Anderson R. Chlamydia trachomatis, infertility, and population growth in sub-Saharan Africa [see comments]. Sex Transm Dis. 1993;20(3):168–73.

66. Boily MC, Brunham RC. The impact of HIV and other STDs on human populations. Are predictions possible? [published erratum appears in Infect Dis Clin North Am 1994 Jun;8(2):xi-xii]. Infect Dis Clin North Am. 1993;7(4):771–92.

67. Anderson RM, Ng TW, Boily MC, May RM. The influence of different sexual-contact patterns between age classes on the predicted demographic impact of AIDS in developing countries. Ann N Y Acad Sci. 1989;569:240–74.

68. Ellen JM, Brown BA, Chung S, et al. Impact of sexual networks on risk for gonorrhea and chlamydia among low-income urban African American adolescents. J Pediatr. 2005;146(4):518–22. http://dx.doi.org/10.1016/j.jpeds.2004.11.023.

69. Morris M, Zavisca J, Dean L. Social and sexual networks: their role in the spread of HIV/AIDS among young gay men. AIDS Educ Prev. 1995;7(5 Suppl):24–35.

70. Service SK, Blower SM. HIV transmission in sexual networks: an empirical analysis. Proc R Soc Lond B Biol Sci. 1995;260(1359):237–44.

71. De P, Singh AE, Wong T, Yacoub W, Jolly AM. Sexual network analysis of a gonorrhoea outbreak. Sex Transm Infect. 2004;80(4):280–5.

72. Watts DJ, Strogatz SH. Collective dynamics of 'small-world' networks. Nature. 1998;393(6684):440–2.

73. Barabasi AL, Bonabeau E. Scale-free networks. Sci Am. 2003;288(5):60–9.

74. Wylie JL, Maclean I, Brunham R, Craig C, Jolly AM. Gonorrhea types and sexual networks in Manitoba, Canada. Sunbelt XIX International Sunbelt Social Network Conference. 1999.

75. Ward H, Ison CA, Day SE, et al. A prospective social and molecular investigation of gonococcal transmission. Lancet. 2000;356(9244):1812–7.

76. Liao M, Bell K, Gu WM, et al. Clusters of circulating *Neisseria gonorrhoeae* strains and association with antimicrobial resistance in Shanghai. J Antimicrob Chemother. 2008;61(3):478–87.

77. Martin IM, Ison CA, Aanensen DM, Fenton KA, Spratt BG. Rapid sequence-based identification of gonococcal transmission clusters in a large metropolitan area. J Infect Dis. 2004;189(8):1497–505.

78. Fredlund H, Falk L, Jurstrand M, Unemo M. Molecular genetic methods for diagnosis and characterisation of Chlamydia trachomatis and Neisseria gonorrhoeae: impact on epidemiological surveillance and interventions. APMIS. 2004;112(11–12): 117–84.

79. Falk L, Lindberg M, Jurstrand M, Backman A, Olcen P, Fredlund H. Genotyping of *Chlamydia trachomatis* would improve contact tracing. Sex Transm Dis. 2003;30(3):205–10.

80. Cabral T, Jolly AM, Wylie JL. *Chlamydia trachomatis omp1* genotypic diversity and concordance with sexual network data. J Infect Dis. 2003;187(2):279–86. http://dx.doi.org/10.1086/346048.

81. Anderson RM. Wasserheit JN, Aral SO, Holmes KK, Hitchcock PJ, editors. The transmission dynamics of sexually transmitted diseases: the behavioral component; Research issues in human behavior and sexually transmitted diseases in the AIDS era. Vol Ist. Washington, DC: American Society for Microbiology; 1991:38–60.

82. Anderson RM, May RM. Infectious diseases of humans; dynamics and control. Vol 1st. Oxford, England: Oxford University Press; 1992:234.

83. Brunham RC, Plummer FA. A general model of sexually transmitted disease epidemiology and its implications for control. Med Clin North Am. 1990;74(6):1339–52.

84. Holmes KK, Johnson DW, Trostle HJ. An estimate of the risk of men acquiring gonorrhea by sexual contact with infected females. Am J Epidemiol. 1970;91(2):170–4.

85. Hook EW, Handsfield HH, Holmes KK, Mardh P, Sparling PF, et al. editors. Gonococcal infections in the adult; sexually transmitted diseases. Vol 2nd. Toronto: McGraw-Hill Information Services Co; 1992:149–65.

86. Stigum H, Magnus P, Bakketeig LS. Effect of changing partnership formation rates on the spread of sexually transmitted diseases and human immunodeficiency virus. Am J Epidemiol. 1997; 145(7):644–52.

87. McCormack WM, Alpert S, McComb DE, Nichols RL, Semine DZ, Zinner SH. Fifteen month follow-up study of women infected with Chlamydia trachomatis. N Engl J Med. 1979;300(5):123–5.

88. Garnett GP, Aral SO, Hoyle DV, Cates W, Anderson Jr RM. The natural history of syphilis. Implications for the transmission dynamics and control of infection [see comments]. Sex Transm Dis. 1997;24(4): 185–200.

89. Schroeter et al. Therapy for incubating syphilis: effectiveness of gonorrhea treatment. JAMA. 1971;218(5):711. http://jama.ama-assn.org/cgi/reprint/218/5/711. Accessed 6 May 2010.

90. Gray RH, Wawer MJ, Brookmeyer R, et al. Probability of HIV-1 transmission per coital act in monogamous, heterosexual, HIV-1-discordant couples in Rakai, Uganda. Lancet. 2001;357(9263): 1149–53.

91. Renton AM, Whitaker L, Riddlesdell M. Heterosexual HIV transmission and STD prevalence: predictions of a theoretical model. Sex Transm Infect. 1998;74(5):339–44.

92. Rothenberg R. Change your friends. Addiction. 2006;101(7):913–4, discussion 914.

93. Potterat JJ, ZimmermanRogers H, Muth SQ, et al. *Chlamydia* transmission: concurrency, reproduction number, and the epidemic trajectory. Am J Epidemiol. 1999;150(12):1331–9.

94. Communicable Disease Control. Manitoba health. Sexually transmitted disease control. Winnipeg, Manitoba; 1997.

95. Potterat JJ, Muth SQ, Rothenberg RB, et al. Sexual network structure as an indicator of epidemic phase. Sex Transm Infect. 2002;78 Suppl 1:I152–8.

96. Jolly AM, Wylie JL. Sampling individuals with large sexual networks – an evaluation of four approaches. Sex Transm Dis. 2001;28(4):200–7.

97. Potterat JJ, Muth SQ, Rothenberg RB. Sexual network structure as an indicator of epidemic phase. Sex Transm Infect. 2002;78 Suppl 1:I152–8.

98. Jolly AM, Wylie JL. Gonorrhoea and chlamydia core groups and sexual networks in Manitoba. Sex Transm Infect. 2002;78 Suppl 1:I145–51.

99. CDC. Sexually transmitted diseases treatment guidelines – 2002. MMWR Morb Mortal Wkly Rep. 2002;51:1–80.

100. Schachter J, Stephens RS. Biology of Chlamydia trachomatis. In: Holmes KK, Sparling PF, Stamm WE, et al., editors. Sexually transmitted diseases. 4th ed. New York, NY: McGraw Hill; 2008. p. 555–74.

101. Iskrant AP, Kahn HA. Statistical indices used in the evaluation of syphilis contact investigation. J Vener Dis Inf. 1948;29(1):1–6.

102. Martin I, Gu W, Yang Y, Tsang R. Macrolide resistance and molecular types of Treponema pallidum causing primary syphilis in Shanghai, China. Clin Infect Dis. 2009;49(4):515–21. http://dx.doi.org/10.1086/600878.

103. Leitner T, Escanilla D, Franzen C, Uhlen M, Albert J. Accurate reconstruction of a known HIV-1 transmission history by phylogenetic tree analysis. Proc Natl Acad Sci USA. 1996;93(20):10864–9.

104. Paraskevis D, Magiorkinis E, Magiorkinis G, et al. Phylogenetic reconstruction of a known HIV-1 CRF04_cpx transmission network using maximum likelihood and Bayesian methods. J Mol Evol. 2004;59(5):709–17. doi:10.1007/s00239-004-2651-6.

105. European Centre for Disease Prevention and Control. Annual epidemiological report on communicable diseases in Europe. 2009:69–71.

106. Brown WJ, U.S. Department of Health, Education and Welfare, Public Health Sevice, Communicable Disease Center, editors. The first step toward eradication. In: Proceedings of the World Forum on Syphilis and other Trepanematoses. Atlanta: U.S. Department of Health, Education and Welfare; 1964:21–5.

107. Primary and secondary syphilis – United States 2002. MMWR Morb Mortal Wkly Rep. 2003;52(46):1117–20.

108. Knapper CM, Roderick J, Smith J, Temple M, Birley HDL. Investigation of an HIV transmission cluster centred in South Wales. Sex Transm Infect. 2008;84(5):377–380.   http://dx.doi.org/10.1136/sti.2008.030536.

109. Northern Ireland, Department of Health and Social Security. Syphilis outbreak. Communicable Diseases Monthly Report (Northern Ireland). 2001;10(9):1–3.

110. Leber A, MacPherson P, Lee BC. Epidemiology of infectious syphilis in Ottawa: recurring themes revisited. Can J Public Health. 2008;99(5):401–5. http://www.cpha.ca.

111. Jayaraman GC, Read RR, Singh AE. Characteristics of individuals with male-to-male and heterosexually acquired infectious syphilis during an outbreak in Calgary, Alberta, Canada. Sex Transm Dis. 2003;30(4):315–9.

112. Patrick DM, Rekart ML, Jolly A, et al. Heterosexual outbreak of infectious syphilis: epidemiological and ethnographic analysis and implications for control. Sex Transm Infect. 2002;78(1):164–9.

113. 2004 Canadian sexually transmitted infections surveillance report. Can Commun Dis Rep. 2007;33S1:1–69.

114. Rothenberg RB, Sterk C, Toomey KE, et al. Using social network and ethnographic tools to evaluate syphilis transmission. Sex Transm Dis. 1998;25(3):154–60.

115. Ogilvie G, Taylor D, Moniruzzaman A, et al. A population based study of infectious syphilis rediagnosis in British Columbia, 1995–2005. Clin Infect Dis. 2009;48(11):1554–58.   http://dx.doi.org/10.1086/598997.

116. Haraldsdottir S, Gupta S, Anderson RM. Preliminary studies of sexual networks in a male homosexual community in Iceland. J Acquir Immune Defic Syndr. 1992;5(4):374–81.

117. Adam BD, Husbands W, Murray J, Maxwell J. Circuits, networks, and HIV risk management. AIDS Educ Prev. 2008;20(5):420–34.

118. Rothenberg R. Commentary – how a net works – implications of network structure for the persistence and control of sexually transmitted diseases and HIV. Sex Transm Dis. 2001;28(2):63–8.

119. Potterat JJ, Phillips-Plummer L, Muth SQ, et al. Risk network structure in the early epidemic phase of HIV transmission in Colorado Springs. Sex Transm Infect. 2002;78 Suppl 1:I159–63.

120. Walter T, Lebouche B, Miailhes P, et al. Symptomatic relapse of neurologic syphilis after benzathine penicillin G therapy for primary or secondary syphilis in HIV-infected patients. Clin Infect Dis. 2006;43(6):787–90.

121. Brewer DD. Supplementary interviewing techniques to maximize output in free listing tasks. Field Methods. 2002;14(1):108–18. doi:10.1177/1525822 X02014001007.

122. Brewer DD, Garrett SB, Rinaldi G. Free-listed items are effective cues for eliciting addition items in semantic domains. Appl Cognitive Psychol. 2002:343–58.

123. Zimmerman-Rogers H, Potterat JJ, Muth SQ, et al. Establishing efficient partner notification periods for patients with chlamydia. Sex Transm Dis. 1999;26(1):49–54.

124. Rothenberg R, Narramore J. The relevance of social network concepts to sexually transmitted disease control. Sex Transm Dis. 1996;23(1):24–9.

125. Remple VP, Patrick DM, Johnston C, Tyndall MW, Jolly AM. Clients of indoor commercial sex workers: heterogeneity in patronage patterns and implications for HIV and STI propagation through sexual networks. Sex Transm Dis. 2007;34(10):754–60.

126. Rekart ML, Patrick DM, Chakraborty B, et al. Targeted mass treatment for syphilis with oral azithromycin. Lancet. 2003;361(9354):313–4. doi:10.1016/S0140-6736(03)12335-5.

127. Broadhead RS, Heckathorn DD, Weakliem DL, et al. Harnessing peer networks as an instrument for AIDS prevention: results from a peer-driven intervention. Public Health Rep. 1998;113 Suppl 1:42–57.

128. Amirkhanian YA, Kelly JA, McAuliffe TL. Identifying, recruiting, and assessing social networks at high risk for HIV/AIDS: methodology, practice, and a case study in St Petersburg, Russia. AIDS Care. 2005;17(1):58–75. http://search.ebscohost.com/login.aspx?direct=true&db=cin20&AN=20094 01955&site=ehost-live.

129. Kelly JA, Amirkhanian YA, Kabakchieva E, et al. Prevention of HIV and sexually transmitted diseases in high risk social networks of young Roma (Gypsy) men in Bulgaria: randomised controlled trial. BMJ. 2006;333(7578):1098–1101.   http://search.ebscohost.com/login.aspx?direct=true&db=cin20&AN=2 009350637&site=ehost-live.

130. Darrow WW, Potterat JJ, Rothenberg RB, Woodhouse DE, Muth SQ. Using knowledge of social networks to prevent human immunodeficiency virus infections: the Colorado Springs Study. Sociol Focus. 1999;32(2):143–58.

Personal Risk and Public Impact: Balancing Individual Rights with STD and HIV Prevention

6

Dan Wohlfeiler and Peter R. Kerndt

Introduction

Society frequently has to strike a balance between assuring individuals their maximum level of freedom and assuring a set of conditions that benefit the health of the public.

In the United States, which holds individual rights to be a core value in multiple realms, attempts made to place any limitations on those rights can quickly come up against strong opposition. Mandating vaccines, restricting cigarette smoking in public places, levying alcohol taxes, requiring automobile drivers to wear seatbelts and prohibiting them from driving while holding a cell phone, requiring motorcyclists to wear helmets, and restricting gun use are all examples of how society has struggled to balance individual rights and the public's health.

Achieving a balance between promoting public health and protecting individuals' rights in the most personal and intimate realm of human behavior—sexuality—has been especially difficult. Furthermore, the very nature of sexuality, being passionate, intimate, and often extremely private, makes it all the more difficult to have policy debates which are open, rational, and scientific.

The mission of public health is to "fulfill society's interest in assuring conditions in which people can be healthy." [1]. However, it has been particularly challenging to address those conditions which may affect individuals' sexual behaviors and risk. While considerable attention has been paid to studying and understanding social determinants [2], many of the interventions for reducing transmission of Human Immunodeficiency Virus (HIV) and other Sexually Transmitted Diseases (STDs) operate at the individual and, increasingly, the biomedical level. This is in marked contrast to other fields of public health, such as tobacco, injury, and nutrition where intervening on social determinants and environmental factors is central to public health strategies.

In this chapter, we describe how STD and HIV preventionists have navigated several important areas of conflict as they have sought to reduce transmission in this highly charged policy arena.

We will examine two specific conflicts. In the first, we will examine efforts to balance society's interest in reducing transmission and healthcare costs against the rights of patrons attending legal establishments, such as bathhouses and sex clubs, also known as commercial sex venues (CSVs). In this example, we will illustrate how these efforts become even more complex when they involve the rights of a minority community—the gay

D. Wohlfeiler (✉)
California DPH STD Control Branch,
850 Marina Bay Parkway, Building P, 2nd Floor,
Richmond, CA 94804, USA
e-mail: dan.wohlfeiler@cdph.ca.gov

P.R. Kerndt
LA County Department of Public Health,
2615 South Grand Avenue, Room 500, Los Angeles,
CA 90007, USA

S.O. Aral, K.A. Fenton, and J.A. Lipshutz (eds.), *The New Public Health and STD/HIV Prevention: Personal, Public and Health Systems Approaches*, DOI 10.1007/978-1-4614-4526-5_6,
© Springer Science+Business Media New York 2013

community—which has historically had fewer rights than the majority. While these venues play a less important role epidemiologically than they did at the beginning of the HIV epidemic, their history holds important lessons for both surveillance and prevention efforts. In the second, we will address efforts to balance the rights of performers in the adult film industry to be protected from exposure to sexually transmitted infections, versus the rights of the industry to operate freely to maximize profits.

Finally, we will suggest implications for future prevention efforts, including surveillance and selection of interventions.

Commercial Sex Venues

Gay men and lesbians have long suffered discrimination, and the fight for equal rights was framed, very early on, as a fight for individual rights. Even the name of one of the earliest gay rights organizations—the Society for Individual Rights, founded in the early 1960s in San Francisco—reflected this orientation [3].

Living openly was extremely rare until the 1970s, when gay men and lesbians began to create open communities in many cities in the United States and Western Europe. With this newfound freedom came the ability to find new partners easily. STDs quickly reached epidemic proportions among gay men. However, treatment was often readily accessible and for many STDs, successful. Furthermore, there were few pressures from either inside or outside the gay community to reduce risk behavior or STD transmission [4].

In 1977, San Francisco elected the first openly gay public official, Harvey Milk, only to lose him to assassination by a former city official a year later [5]. As the gay community was beginning to acquire some levels of acceptance and political clout, HIV was already spreading throughout the gay community. In the early 1980s, 10–15,000 gay men in San Francisco were becoming infected with HIV each year [6]. And unlike other STDs, HIV—still unnamed and with often fatal consequences—called into question the community's newfound freedoms. One of the freedoms most

debated was the right of individuals to meet new sexual partners, especially in CSVs.

Early epidemiologic studies indicated that HIV (although the virus was not yet identified) was being transmitted through sexual contact, as well as attendance at bathhouses [7]. Later studies showed similar associations between infection and bathhouse attendance [8, 9].

Debates about bathhouses have been covered extensively [10–12]. Some called for closing bathhouses altogether; others defended them as a fundamental right. Some gay community leaders held themselves up as examples, announcing that they had reduced their number of partners and their attendance at bathhouses and similar venues [13]. While the conflicts between the community, bathhouse owners, and health departments have been well documented elsewhere, what we believe important to call attention to here are the different approaches taken by public health, and even schisms within the field, that CSVs brought to light.

Even individual public health professionals experienced this conflict. In 2006, a gay public health official removed himself from a national advisory board of a project seeking to help health departments address the optimal roles for health departments to take when it came to CSVs, including bathhouses and Internet sites [14]. He did so out of a belief that any governmental regulation of bathhouses would be unacceptable despite studies that showed their potential risks to attendees. "We as gay men have fewer rights than other communities," he said. "So if we want the right to go into bathhouses and have sex there, any way we want, we should have that right." Similarly, many of the program staff within community-based HIV-prevention organizations have had major differences of opinion regarding how to balance individual freedoms and public health. Those who have defended bathhouses as important venues to reach high-risk populations and as valuable community institutions have drawn little criticism from within the gay community, with several notable exceptions [15, 16]. Critics of the notion of absolute freedom, including the right to go to bathhouses, have been notably rare from inside the gay community, again with some notable exceptions [17].

Three different cities have taken dramatically different approaches to reducing risk in CSVs. The different models reflect different levels of responsibility for reducing transmission for patrons, venue owners, and public health. Today, San Francisco venues have rules prohibiting unprotected anal sex. Clubs must obtain verbal consent from patrons to follow the rules and are expected to enforce them through monitoring. No private rooms are allowed, thus making it easier to enforce. This model grants a shared responsibility for reducing the risk to both individual patrons and business owners.

Los Angeles requires clubs to obtain a permit, pay an annual fee, and allow unannounced inspections by public health department inspectors. This fee helps offset the costs to health departments associated with inspecting the venues. In order to obtain a permit, a CSV must provide free condoms and lubricant, allow testing, obtain patron waivers, post notices concerning the risks of STD/HIV, and have rules prohibiting unprotected anal sex and alcohol and drug use. However, Los Angeles has allowed these establishments to have private rooms, which makes enforcement impossible. In this model, most responsibility for behavior change falls to the individual, although business owners are responsible for some HIV/STD screening costs.

Current regulations mandate that CSVs in Los Angeles fund trained personnel to offer voluntary HIV/STD testing and risk reduction counseling 20 h a week during peak business hours with the health department providing and bearing the testing costs in the public health laboratory. Currently, however, this policy only reaches a relatively small number of individuals. For example, in 2009 at eleven CSVs with an annual attendance estimated to be 600,000 five years earlier [18], only approximately 2,000 rapid HIV tests, 300 chlamydia and gonorrhea tests, and less than 100 syphilis tests were conducted during the permit-required time period of 20 h per week during peak business hours.

New York City takes a different approach. Under current New York regulations, "No establishment shall make facilities available for the purpose of sexual activities where anal intercourse, vaginal intercourse or fellatio take place." [19]. In practice, no sex is allowed in public spaces within the CSV, but despite the regulations, sexual activity does take place in private spaces, even though it is illegal, and clubs continue to operate. In practice, therefore, nearly all responsibility for reducing transmission falls to the individual.

One notable difference that may influence the varying approaches in the three cities is the ownership of the venues. In Los Angeles and San Francisco, the venues are mostly owned by gay men, who have many ties to local civic and community organizations, and whose own lives were affected significantly by the HIV epidemic. These men were typically much more willing to collaborate with community-based HIV prevention organizations and local health departments. In contrast, in New York, CSVs are typically owned by individuals with fewer ties to the gay community, and whom health departments have often found harder to reach.

There are no conclusive data as to the impact of these different strategies. Venues have been reluctant to participate in such comparative studies. When public health departments attempted to conduct such studies, venues resisted; health departments then ended their attempts to carry out the research. One significant step towards determining the impact was a study published in 2003 [20]. This study looked at reports of unprotected sex by men who reported attending bathhouses in four different cities—San Francisco, New York, Chicago, and Los Angeles. It found that men in all four cities reported similar levels of unprotected sex. What differed, however, was that men in San Francisco reported having fewer unprotected exposures inside the commercial venues. The prohibition of unprotected anal sex most likely drove it outside the venues. Thus, while the policy failed at reducing risk in the community as a whole, it may have effectively reduced unprotected sex inside venues. Did the policy fail, as some have suggested, because it did not reduce risk behavior throughout the community? Or did it succeed because it moved it away from venues?

Is Epidemiology Missing the Mark?

This question highlights one of the key epidemiologic challenges facing public health interventions regarding sexual risk. If one asks whether the policy succeeded in reducing risk behavior, one could reasonably conclude that the policy failed. If, however, one looks at whether it affected where risk behavior took place, one may reasonably reach another conclusion.

Advocates for and against regulating CSVs rely on conflicting epidemiologic constructs to support their efforts. These epidemiologic frames—one, individual and the other, structural—both reflect and support belief systems which in turn suggest different programmatic interventions.

In an individualist framework, epidemiologists focus on individual's risk. Multiple studies have looked at the reported risk of individual patrons. In the 1980s and 1990s, two studies in different locations on the west coast reported that approximately 10 % of CSV patrons report unprotected sex [21, 22]. However, the impact of this percentage will vary considerably depending on the number of partners that those 10 % report [23].

As a later survey, conducted in 1996, of a west-coast bathhouse which found that only a small minority of men reported unprotected anal sex, this might be enough to sustain an HIV epidemic [22].

However, mapping these networks is extremely difficult. No network maps have ever been drawn of a bathhouse patron's partnership selection and it is unlikely that we will have one for the foreseeable future. One study did attempt to measure some of the network factors in venues, but excluded the most frequent patrons [24].

In turn, risk is usually attributed to psychological factors such as lack of information, low self-esteem, and low self-efficacy. Multiple theories, including the Health Belief Model [25], Theory of Reasoned Action [26], or the AIDS Risk Reduction Model [27], despite some differences, suggest that information, self-efficacy, and access to the means of protection (for example, condoms) are key to reducing individual risk.

Thus, in CSVs, this frame is exemplified by the statement often repeated in debates about the role of venues: "it's not where you do it, but what you do" [28].

The interventions that are suggested by this paradigm typically include social marketing outreach, and counseling. HIV and STD testing are also promoted. Risk is assumed to be at the individual level, and to the individual. Individuals are also assumed to be completely empowered, able to act in their own best interest, and given complete freedom to take whatever level of risk they wish. When they do not act in their own best interest, it is assumed to be due to factors which may be addressed by behavioral interventions which are effective enough to reduce their risk behavior.

Adherents to this framework, furthermore, believe that venues are the best place to reach high-risk individuals [24, 29]. Evidence, however, suggests that in practice, these interventions reach few individuals. Data from the National HIV Behavioral Surveillance (NHBS) System reveal that fewer than 3 % of bar, bathhouse, and club patrons participated in educational interventions—and only a quarter of the men took free condoms [30].

In contrast, structuralists believe that these venues are some of the riskiest places to be for uninfected lower risk individuals. In addition to being concerned with reducing unprotected sex, they are also concerned with the risk that an individual's partners may confer depending on *their* partners' risk. If a partner rarely takes risks, then they pose less risk to an individual; if a partner frequently takes risk, they pose more. Venues are relevant to transmission, therefore, because they can affect how sexual mixing can take place between individuals who take a great deal of risk and those who do not.

In this paradigm, in addition to psychosocial factors, the environment emerges as an important factor that can increase the risk of HIV transmission. Specifically, in the case of CSVs, two of the most important environmental variables which can affect mixing between those men at highest risk and those who take less risk are the absence or presence of regulations forbidding high-risk (unprotected anal) sex, and the absence or presence of private rooms which can make it easier or more difficult to enforce those regulations.

Venues may affect sexual networks even if sex does not take place in them, but serve to bring individuals together. For example, a bar in western Canada was found to be where individuals met new sexual partners, and attendance at the bar was associated with being exposed to gonorrhea [31].

This difference in paradigms—individual or structural—is not without consequences. Evidence regarding secondhand smoke was an important factor in developing policies which regulated smoking in public [32]. The existence of secondhand risk of sexual transmission through networks is well accepted as part of the epidemiology of STDs. However, it has been difficult to operationalize this concept beyond partner notification.

The data surrounding environmental variables and sexual networks do not add up to a level of causation regarding the role of venues in affecting transmission that health policy makers are likely to feel confident relying upon when considering what, if any, regulatory action they should take. Causation is less clear than in other areas of public health, such as the link between tobacco smoking and cancer.

However, practitioners would do well to remember that even greater certainty in determining the role of venues may not necessarily lead to greater action on the part of public health. There can still be considerable opposition from the industry and from individuals. For example, in tobacco control, the industry has frequently questioned the science behind studies, and supported their arguments by attributing all responsibility to smokers themselves. As a result, businesses will enjoy fewer costs, and an important group of patrons will enjoy certain benefits.

The Core Group's Power: Not Sought, But Acquired Nonetheless

When it comes to STDs one group of individuals has acquired a significant amount of power—even though it has not formed itself as a constituency.

In the case of STD and HIV transmission, the core group—a small number of individuals who have high levels of risk both in terms of number of partners and lack of consistent use of condoms—is a long-established concept, although some definitional issues persist [33]. But public health has not examined its relationship to issues of individual freedoms and policy.

Without any active efforts or lobbying on their own, a core group's members are the de facto beneficiaries of the lack of regulation in many cities. In part, this is because they can count on the support of advocates who are not at high risk or who do not even attend venues, but who, out of a belief that individual freedom is paramount, particularly when threatened by a majority, will support individuals' rights to sexual expression in public venues.

Some have hypothesized that if a majority of club patrons are safe, there is enough of a market that will support regulated venues which forbid unsafe behavior (Bense, personal communication). However, this assertion fails to take into account one important feature of bathhouse attendance.

Data from the NHBS conducted in 2003/04 revealed that in San Francisco, the frequency of bathhouse attendance is highly skewed (Fisher Raymond, personal communication). An analysis of bathhouse patrons residing in San Francisco who in 2004 reported at least one potentially discordant relationship in the previous six months revealed that a majority attended less than once each month. 22 % of bathhouse patrons who reported at least one potentially discordant relationship attended less than once a month; 10 % monthly; 4 % weekly; and 3 % daily.

These data reveal that the most frequent users are also amongst the riskiest.

Of daily and weekly users, 74 % were HIV positive. Fully 98 % had more than one potentially discordant partnership (meaning that they may not have known their partner's status) in the past six months. Of these, 36 % reported unprotected insertive anal intercourse and 19 % had unprotected receptive anal intercourse. A quarter of these men reported having an STD in the previous year. Not only are these patrons at high risk to themselves, but they also represent a significant risk to their partners.

Given the number of total visits to venues and partnerships they represent over a year's time, the likelihood of high levels of mixing taking place between them and men who only occasionally take risks is high. This mixing is unlikely to be addressed solely by behavioral interventions, which, as we have seen, reach few individuals and have limited effectiveness.

The benefit accruing to those at highest risk may have parallels in other areas of public health. In a national survey, frequent alcohol bingers were found to make up only 6 % of the population, but consume 50 % of the alcohol (National Household Survey, 1999). Thus, their importance to the alcohol marketplace, the policies that protect the marketplace, and their cost to society are disproportionate to their numbers. Heavy drinkers, by their numbers, have the most to gain individually from having lower taxes on alcohol, and the most to lose if they are raised.

Thus, there are risks and costs to society when individual rights are held paramount. The highest risk individuals end up acquiring the most freedom and, without seeking it, they may reap the most benefit from the lack of regulation.

In the case of CSVs, public health regulation may pose a potential risk to individual freedoms. However, adopting a purely behavioral or educational public health approach in such venues may result in risk to the community's health. Judging from past findings, individually oriented interventions are likely to be ineffective at reducing HIV and STD transmission, leaving businesses and the core, high-risk group to benefit, and the rest of the population to bear the increased risk and personal and health care costs of disease.

The Adult Film Industry

The adult film industry provides another important example of how public health has grappled with conflicts between individuals and the public: in this case, the right of individuals to be protected from harm and the public's right not to bear costs which are externalized by the industry.

Most debates about the effect of the adult film industry and its impact have focused on their impact on the viewer and not on the health risks to the performers. In 1988 the California Supreme Court, in *People v. Freeman*, found adult film production to be protected free speech under the first amendment. In this case, Freeman, the producer, was found not to be engaged in pandering and such films were not considered obscene based on the prevailing community standard. The US Supreme Court refused to hear and let stand the decision of the California Supreme Court [34]. Thus, the adult film industry was legalized in California through case law, not by statute, and has for the most part escaped governmental oversight. In 2005, the US adult entertainment industry was estimated to generate over $12 billion in revenue with Los Angeles County, the largest center for adult film production worldwide.

Data regarding the impact of pornography on viewers' risk is inconclusive. One study found that gay men who preferred unprotected sex also watched films which showed unprotected sex. However, it is impossible to conclude that the films caused the viewers to have unprotected sex, since it is also possible that the viewers simply preferred seeing behaviors that they engaged in.

However, one study did show that many young MSM, who receive very little education about reducing risk in same-sex relationships from their teachers or parents, frequently do name pornography as an important source of information [35]. This suggests that more consideration be given to the content and its effect on viewers' behaviors.

Typically the industry has fought regulation, citing infringement of free speech and relying on copyright laws to prevent duplication and unauthorized distribution of their product [36]. Producers have organized themselves into a "Free Speech Coalition," (http://www.freespeechcoalition.org), to combat government efforts to censor or otherwise regulate the adult film industry.

The industry also has a significant impact on the performers. In this section, we describe how occupational health policies have been utilized to protect performers' health.

Although the total population of performers at any one time may appear small, they have a very large sexual network and serve as a bridge population for STD transmission to and from the general population. Until 2000, surveillance for HIV and STDs in the industry had been limited. Sporadic case reports of HIV among performers were reported in the media throughout the 1990s. In 1998 one HIV-positive male performer infected five female performers. An outbreak of HIV followed in April of 2004 when a male performer who had tested regularly and believed he was negative infected three of thirteen female sexual partners exposing a total of 61 primary and secondary sexual contacts in a 23-day period [37]. Since that time the Los Angeles County Department of Public Health has tracked gonorrhea and chlamydia infections, reporting over 3,200 cases between 2004 and 2008 among approximately 1,800 performers with reinfection rates within a 1-year period as high as 26.1 % [38].

Although the Occupational Health and Safety Act (OSHA) was passed in 1970, and required employers to provide a safe and healthful workplace for employees, working conditions have not changed nor have any regulations been promulgated or enforcement occurred that would protect workers in the adult film industry. Regulation of the industry in the United States has been limited to prevention and prosecution of child pornography, and prohibits performers under age 18 (Title 18, Section 2257 of the United States Code of Regulations). This federal law requires producers to document and maintain records that all performers engaged in sexual contact are over age 18 [39].

In the occupational setting, the employer has an obligation to ensure a safe and healthful work environment and must provide personal protective equipment (PPE) to protect a worker from any "residual" hazard which cannot be eliminated through the use of engineering controls. Further, the employer is required to pay into a workmen compensation fund should an employee become injured despite the best efforts of the employer to protect that worker.

Individual employees do not have the option of not using any required PPE, nor may an employer or an employee dismantle any engineering controls from operating as designed. Thus, a guard cannot be removed from a saw or a high-speed drill, and an employee cannot work without safety glasses, steel toed shoes, or hard hats. If an employee refuses to utilize all required PPE or follow safety procedures, he or she may be removed from the work environment.

While some performers are aware of occupational hazards of STDs, in general they lack an understanding of their risks or their rights to a workplace free from such hazards or their employer's responsibility to protect their health and provide a safe and healthy workplace. Workers may also be reluctant to file a complaint, fearing they may lose their job.

Furthermore, the industry has tended to avoid contact with any public governmental entity. Since the industry has often been prosecuted or perceived to be illegal, there is little incentive for adult film industry producers to comply with regulations.

After the 2004 HIV outbreak in the industry, to improve performer awareness of the health risks and the production companies' responsibilities to their workers, Cal/OSHA developed an online resource that outlined the workplace requirements and key elements of a model exposure control plan [40]. Cal/OSHA had determined that California's Bloodborne Pathogen Standard applied to this industry and required the employer to have an exposure control plan, an injury and illness prevention plan, and a worker training plan.

There is a precedent for regulation in similar industries. The state of Nevada has demonstrated the feasibility of lowering STD rates among sex workers through strict regulations for its legal brothel industry. The mandatory use of condoms in brothels was instituted in 1988, and HIV testing became mandatory for brothel prostitutes in the state in 1986. The sex workers in brothels are tested for chlamydia and gonorrhea on a weekly basis and for syphilis and HIV on at least a monthly basis. Since the implementation of these regulations, not a single individual has tested positive for HIV while working in the brothel [41]. Of more than 7,000 STD tests conducted between 1982 and 1989 among brothel workers, only 20 positive STD cases were diagnosed, all of which occurred before implementation of the mandatory condom law [42].

Because of the Nevada regulations, commercial sex workers have become virtually free of STDs, and the few that do contract them do so primarily before entering the industry or from boyfriends and husbands when on leave from the brothel. Regulation of the Nevada brothel system is a feasible model for the adult film industry. Sex workers in both industries typically stay in the business for only a brief time, and they carry out similar types of work. The average career of an adult film performer is estimated at just 18 months, signifying that thousands of performers enter and exit this industry over the years [43].

One of the main barriers to enforcing OSHA regulations in the adult film industry has been that OSHA only applies to employees, not temporary hires or contract workers. When OSHA has levied fines against companies, these companies have appealed decisions in the courts on the grounds that the performers are not considered employees, and therefore OSHA regulations do not apply. This will likely remain an unresolved matter until settled through legislation or until specific regulations are written for this industry.

Implications for Interventions

Unintended Consequences: A Biased Concern?

Public health practitioners have different perspectives on which set of interventions to implement. As discussed above, individualists tend to favor behavioral interventions while structuralists prefer more regulatory approaches.

Structural interventions often include regulation or taxation, and as such, some limitation on absolute individual freedom. They are often criticized for not taking into account the potential for unintended consequences.

With respect to CSVs, a criticism that has often been levied opposing any further regulation or against shutting down bathhouses is that they would only push the same high-risk behaviors into other venues, such as public parks [12]. This was particularly common before the advent of the Internet as a major avenue for finding new partners.

While some reports indicate that some men did go to more public settings following increased CSV regulation, significant arguments weigh against this notion. One hypothetical explanation is that for many, the costs outweigh the benefits. While the monetary costs associated with finding a new partner in a park or other noncommercial sites may be less than in a CSV, it is likely to have other costs, including the potential for being arrested, or subject to harassment. It may also be a much less efficient way to find a new partner.

Regarding the adult film industry, critics of regulation have charged that greater regulation will only drive the industry to other states or countries. While to some extent this is true, there is also a cost/benefit argument that would argue to the contrary. The industry benefits from its geographic proximity to mainstream film production, also located in Los Angeles. This proximity allows for individuals, in particular technicians, to work both in adult and mainstream film production.

In contrast to these criticisms against structural interventions, public health has not examined whether behavioral interventions themselves might also have unintended consequences. To the extent that behavioral interventions do not address the environment itself, since they require change only from the individual, they may leave untouched many of the features of the environments which may increase risk, such as the absence of enforceable policies regarding individual behavior. This may threaten to undermine any benefits that behavioral interventions have. Furthermore, they may also result in the venues or producers gaining political support from other stakeholders from having collaborated with public health, for example, by allowing outreach and testing to take place onsite. This political support can be useful when appealing to policymakers who may be considering more regulatory approaches.

Sexual Health Practitioners' Unique Relationship with the Private Sector

Public health efforts frequently have to take into account the role of business in either preventing or promoting the risk for disease. Where cooperation is possible, public health has sought it, and many examples of partnerships exist. This is true in nutrition, injury prevention, and alcohol prevention, for example.

In other situations, public health has had to take a more confrontational approach. Many states sued tobacco companies in order to recuperate costs associated with smoking. To a great extent, the history of public health has been closely related to the history and philosophy of progressive movements [44], which includes regulating businesses so that they do not harm individuals or communities.

Frequently, those on both sides of debates over the role of regulation also have contrasting viewpoints regarding who holds primary responsibility for health. Antiregulatory conservatives often believe that individuals are the masters of their own destiny, and that if they are sick, they are often responsible and should bear the consequences for their personal behavioral choices. In this paradigm, if individuals choose to smoke, choose to drink soda, and eat junk food, they deserve the consequences of their choices.

Pro-regulation progressives are more likely to believe that businesses and other larger social factors are responsible for individuals' health. In this paradigm, companies are responsible for aggressively marketing tobacco and soda and alcohol, and ought not to leave the public sector to absorb the costs of prevention and treatment of cancer, obesity, alcoholism, and STDs and HIV.

In most areas of public health, assigning responsibility, together with determining who profits in the private sector, helps determine who should pay for the costs associated with prevention. Thus, states have successfully sued cigarette companies to recuperate the social costs associated with the risks of smoking. They have also taxed consumers. This was, in part, in order to reduce consumption, which they have succeeded in accomplishing [45]. Second, they have done so in order to finance prevention efforts [46].

In much of the dialogue around HIV and STD prevention, these paradigms often get turned inside-out and the alliances between progressives and those in favor of regulation get fractured. Questioning of businesses' motives will often be drowned out by the combination of high demand

for these businesses' services, as well as by calls for protecting individual freedoms.

Rather than collaborate or confront businesses who may be profiting from encouraging risk, producing pornography, or facilitating individuals meeting partners in settings that may facilitate transmission, much of public health as well as community-based advocates have often chosen to ignore these businesses. With little or no community constituency to press for change from businesses, neither governmental nor nongovernmental, community-based public health institutions are likely to assert any authority or press for change. Rather, they often go further, embracing these businesses as partners and accepting their terms of engagement regarding who can conduct educational efforts or research. Advocates and researchers who take this route consider bathhouses, for example, to be a valuable community institution and partner, and an ally to their efforts to promote health [47, 48]. In general, HIV and STD prevention practitioners have shied away from critically examining these partnerships and looking at who bears the costs, or who profits.

Examples of Constituency Building to Advance Sexual Health

In both the case of CSVs and the adult film industry, it is important to recognize that there is a range of business responses to collaboration with public health. Similar to other business sectors [49–51], some venue owners and adult film producers have taken extraordinary steps in terms of prohibiting unprotected sex. As we have seen, some clubs prohibit unprotected sex and are able to enforce it by eliminating all private spaces [52]. Some adult film producers have also refused to film any unprotected sex, and will not hire individual performers who have had unprotected sex during a film shoot [53]. Yet these are the minority, and they have often taken these actions independently of being asked to do so by public health.

Public health's challenge of gaining collaboration from businesses is made more difficult if there is substantial demand for those businesses' services and products. Furthermore, without a constituency, taking an assertive stance is even more challenging. Early advocates pointed out as early as 1984 that gay and bisexual men continued to support venues even though they made not even a minimal effort to encourage safe behavior, and that producers of adult films already were uncertain about the development of videos featuring protected sex [54]. Several notable attempts have been made to engage other businesses within each of these sectors. With regard to commercial sex venues, as mentioned above, Los Angeles succeeded in gaining some collaboration from the owners. Similarly, in San Francisco, owners pay for staffing to inform patrons of the rules, and to enforce them. This was largely done as a result of a coalition of community-based organizations coming together with sex club owners. Only after these requirements were adopted informally did the coalition disband and enforcement of similar rules begin to be carried out by the local health department.

Efforts to regulate the adult film industry have also included strategies to force the industry to assume a greater responsibility in protecting workers' health. In December 2009, a community-based HIV medical provider, AIDS Healthcare Foundation, sought to amend the Bloodborne Pathogen Standard to clarify requirements for worker protection in the adult film industry. They advocated for the standard to specifically address health hazards in the adult film industry [55]. An excerpt from the petition follows:

> Although workers in adult films should enjoy protections under the current phrasing of the regulation, as well as the Board's [CalOSHA] determination that adult film workers are employees, the adult film industry has steadfastly refused to take any steps to protect its workers from diseases spread by bloodborne pathogens, resulting in thousands of employees becoming infected with sexually transmitted diseases. Clarification and enhanced enforcement of the rules are called for.

In response to the petition and after a hearing of the CalOSHA Standards Board in March of 2010, a series of public statewide meetings were initiated to discuss whether the regulations should be amended to specifically address the adult film industry. It remains to be seen what, if any, action will be taken to regulate the industry.

Advocates have also sought to mobilize national organizations to support their efforts. Both the American Public Health Association [56] and the National Coalition of STD Directors [57] have called for mandatory labeling at the beginning of each adult film that states that the adult film was produced pursuant to OSHA workplace requirements and prohibiting the distribution and sales of adult films produced in violation of OSHA requirements to hotels, cable television content providers, and others in commercial settings when condoms were not used by performers.

While films featuring unprotected sex have gained more and more acceptance in the gay community, it has been largely believed that these films featured HIV-positive performers. Community-based health organizations largely stayed silent on the issue, given that there was no risk of additional HIV transmission taking place on the set, and they were not concerned about transmission of any other STDs. Interestingly, there has been virtually no questioning of the role of promoting unprotected sex to viewers. While the data, as described above, are far from conclusive, this silence is in marked contrast to the considerable advocacy efforts by these same agencies to encourage promotion of safe sex images.

Only when a company began promoting films featuring unprotected sex between HIV-positive and HIV-negative individuals did any community-based organizations begin to question gay producers' responsibility. Their efforts have included both calling attention to their activities in the press and asking for the cooperation of the producer; to date, no changes have been announced [58].

Implications for Surveillance

Measuring only individual risk behaviors can often result in being unable to detect key features of communicable diseases. Asking individuals about their own behavior may yield useful information about risk, but it is not sufficient and cannot account for why some groups get infected much faster than others even when their risk behavior is similar, or when the disparities in risk behavior are much smaller than the disparities in infection rates.

If the mission of public health is to assure conditions in which people can be healthy, then it stands to reason that surveillance must focus not only on disease, or risk, or individuals' health—but on the conditions, sexual networks, and circumstances that affect an individual's health.

Focusing epidemiology on individual risk and disease rates may also have another unintended consequence of reinforcing the notion that risk is at the individual level, and as such, remains something inherently private. By rendering the interconnectedness of nonmonogamous sexual partners nearly invisible, notions of secondhand risk—similar to that created by smokers—also remain invisible, and sexual behavior remains an issue of individuals and their sexual partners. This then reinforces the idea that neither the private sector nor the public sector has any responsibility to change the conditions, and more specifically, the environments in which this risk occurs.

Because of the relative ease of measuring individual risk behaviors, it should be no surprise that a large proportion of those interventions considered to be effective, and therefore replicable, are focused at the individual level [59, 60]. These interventions rely heavily on individual will and self-efficacy, often supporting the intent to change through creating social norms favoring healthy behavior. Notably, none of these pose any limitations on individual rights or the rights of businesses.

There are no easy solutions, despite advances in network science [61–64]. Being able to map sexual networks remains challenging, whether in sexual venues, on the Internet, or in the adult film industry.

There are, nonetheless, other community-level indicators that may yield useful information for studying and preventing the transmission of HIV and other STDs. In the same way that a community's social economic status can affect health of

individuals, it may be true that a number of community-level factors, both proximally and distally related to individual-level behavior, may also contribute to STD transmission in a community. This would include the number of CSVs, the number of patrons, and the frequency of their visits, as well as total revenues generated.

With regard to the adult film industry, one indicator some researchers have already examined is the level of unprotected sex in films. An analysis of condom use by Grudzen et al. found that condoms are used only 3 % of the time for penile–vaginal intercourse in the heterosexual industry [65].

Important indicators also include the number of adult film performers and production companies in an area; the number of permits issued to adult film producers in an area; and sales and rental data on adult films made with and without condoms.

Gathering data on the number of major producers and attempting to estimate the percentage of adult film content viewed which is produced by major producers, US-based producers, or by individuals making less expensive video and broadcasting it through the Internet may also be useful to better understand industry practices. Additionally, being able to track how much revenue in hotels comes from viewing adult film content may be useful when developing collaborations with a potentially important partner—the hotel industry itself. Film rentals have accounted for significant revenues for hotels, although the in-room viewing of adult film may be shifting from the hotel as the source to travelers' laptop computers [66].

While many of the private companies' revenues are difficult to ascertain if not publicly traded, some data may be available through looking at the number of employees estimated to be in each company.

Both surveillance and epidemiology in this arena need to remain vigilant to the different phases of HIV and STD epidemics [67]. Strategies that may have had a significant impact in one phase may have less of an impact in later phases. For example, while shutting down bathhouses early in the HIV epidemic may have had a significant impact, it would arguably have less of an impact in later phases of the epidemic [68]. This may be due to a combination of factors, including the relative impact of the core group on transmission, decreasing infectivity due to greater access to treatment, as well as the advent of new venues for meeting partners such as the Internet.

Conclusion

The history of attempting to balance individual, business, and public health interests in the sexual health arena is one that should give public health practitioners both pause and some hope for optimism.

The unintentional coalescing of forces of advocates for absolute individual freedom for sexual expression, and a strong business sector which can count on the demand for its services, can provide formidable challenges to reducing HIV and STD transmission. Surveillance efforts and prevention practitioners have alternately reflected on the effect of these forces on their efforts; at other times, grappled with them; and still at other times, contributed to them.

Ultimately, public health acting alone has few tools to change those individuals who want to have unprotected sex, or to change the community cultural norms often promoted by businesses. It is not reasonable to expect that behavioral and low-scale structural interventions can bring down disease incidence without bringing the private sector into greater alignment with their interests [69, 70].

While CSVs have much less impact on the epidemic than they used to have, due in part to the advent of the Internet as well as the widespread access to treatments which reduce infectivity, they still pose important questions that public health will need to grapple with in the future. This will be necessary for reducing all STDs, including HIV. Public health will need to develop more forthright strategies to better understand how venues can affect transmission not just at the individual but also at the network and population level. It will need to better grapple with diversity not just of demographics such as age, race, and ethnicity but also of risk level as well.

Only by doing so can it reduce the potential impact of these venues on the transmission of STDs.

Public health has useful tools at its disposal to deal with reducing STD transmission among adult film industry performers. However, it will require ongoing collaboration with occupational health, and grappling with a powerful set of industry interests. Again, the effect of the Internet on decentralizing production will also be important to consider.

Efforts to promote sexual health will also require stronger efforts at coalition building. In addition to building stronger ties with other groups specifically interested in similar missions, it will require bringing to the table stakeholders who bring diverse strengths, assets, and constituencies to the table. Some of these stakeholders will come from the industries themselves, particularly those venue owners and adult film industry producers who have already shown themselves willing to invest in their customers and workers' health. Other public health efforts have shown themselves able to do so, and that should be encouraging to sexual health promotion advocates and practitioners as well.

The story of reducing individual and community levels of risk associated with attending sex venues or working in the adult film industry began with good epidemiology: detecting outbreaks. It is important to take a lesson from what followed. Public health epidemiologists, researchers, and interventionists must not focus on individual risk alone, but must carefully examine the relationships between individuals and the contexts in which those relationships flourish. In these two cases, the contexts are both physical and economic. Public health must carefully consider the interests of all the affected constituencies, including business owners, their employees, and their customers, as well as the communities in which they operate and which may suffer unintended consequences. This will require careful assessment and analysis, and a good deal of listening. It will also require leadership and forthright decision-making along with a commitment to fulfilling society's interest in creating conditions in which people can be healthy.

References

1. Institute of Medicine (U.S.). Committee for the Study of the Future of Public Health. The future of public health. Washington, DC: National Academy Press; 1988.
2. Centers for Disease Control and Prevention. Establishing a holistic framework to reduce inequities in HIV, viral hepatitis, STDs, and tuberculosis in the United States. Atlanta: U.S. Department of Health and Human Services, Centers for Disease Control and Prevention; 2010.
3. Armstrong EA. Forging gay identities: organizing sexuality in San Francisco, 1950–1994. Chicago: University of Chicago Press; 2002.
4. Lorch P. Gay men dying: shifting gears, part I. San Francisco: Bay Area Reporter; 1983. p. 6.
5. Shilts R. The mayor of Castro street: the life and times of Harvey Milk. 1st ed. New York: St. Martin's Press; 1982.
6. Winkelstein W, Wiley JA, Padian NS, et al. The San Francisco Men's Health study: continued decline in HIV seroconversion rates among homosexual/bisexual men. Am J Public Health. 1988;78(11):1472–4.
7. Auerbach DM, Darrow WW, Jaffe HW, Curran JW. Cluster of cases of the acquired immune deficiency syndrome. Patients linked by sexual contact. Am J Med. 1984;76(3):487–92.
8. Thiede H, Jenkins RA, Carey JW, et al. Determinants of recent HIV infection among seattle-area men who have sex with men. Am J Public Health. 2009;99 Suppl 1:S157–64.
9. Brewer DD, Golden MR, Handsfield HH. Unsafe sexual behavior and correlates of risk in a probability sample of men who have sex with men in the era of highly active antiretroviral therapy. Sex Transm Dis. 2006;33(4):250–5.
10. Bayer R. Private acts, social consequences: AIDS and the politics of public health. New York: The Free Press; 1989.
11. Shilts R. And the band played on: politics, people, and the AIDS epidemic. New York: St. Martin's Press; 1987.
12. Berube A. The history of gay bathhouses. 1984. J Homosex. 2003;44(3–4):33–53.
13. Huberman R, Jones C, Kraus B. Three gay figures join the AIDS debate. San Francisco: Bay Area Reporter; 1983. p. 4.
14. Wohlfeiler D, Teret S, Woodruff AJ, Marcus J. The venues project: reducing human immunodeficiency virus (HIV) and sexually transmitted infections in bathhouses, sex clubs, internet sites, and circuit parties. Paper presented at National HIV Prevention Conference, Atlanta, GA, December 3, 2007.
15. Rotello G. Sexual ecology: AIDS and the destiny of gay men. New York: Dutton; 1997.
16. Savage D. Regulating bathhouses. 2006. http://slog.thestranger.com/2006/01/regulating_bath. Accessed 5 May 2011.
17. Kramer L. The tragedy of today's gays. New York: Penguin; 2005.
18. Garthwaite TJ, Fielding J. Memo to Los Angeles board of supervisors. 21 June 2004.
19. New York State Sanitary Code 24-2.2.
20. Woods WJ, Binson D, Pollack LM, Wohlfeiler D, Stall RD, Catania JA. Public policy regulating private and public space in gay bathhouses. J Acquir Immune Defic Syndr. 2003;32(4):417–23.
21. Richwald G, Kyle G. Sexual activities in bathhouses in Los Angeles county: implications for AIDS prevention education. J Sex Res. 1988;25:169–80.
22. Van Beneden CA, O'Brien K, Modesitt S, Yusem S, Rose A, Fleming D. Sexual behaviors in an urban bathhouse 15 years into the HIV epidemic. J Acquir Immune Defic Syndr. 2002;30(5):522–6.
23. Wohlfeiler D, Potterat JJ. Using gay men's sexual networks to reduce sexually transmitted disease (STD)/human immunodeficiency virus (HIV) transmission. Sex Transm Dis. 2005;32(10 Suppl):S48–52.
24. Woods WJ, Binson D, Blair J, Han L, Spielberg F, Pollack LM. Probability sample estimates of bathhouse sexual risk behavior. J Acquir Immune Defic Syndr. 2007;45(2):231–8.
25. Rosenstock IM, Strecher VJ, Becker MH. Social learning theory and the Health Belief Model. Health Educ Q. 1988;15(2):175–83.
26. Ajzen I, Fishbein M. Understanding attitudes and predicting social behavior. Englewood Cliffs, NJ: Prentice-Hall; 1980.
27. Catania JA, Kegeles SM, Coates TJ. Towards an understanding of risk behavior: an AIDS risk reduction model (ARRM). Health Educ Q. 1990;17(1):53–72.
28. Woods WJ, Binson D. Public health policy and gay bathhouses. J Homosex. 2003;44(3–4):1–21.
29. Binson D, Woods WJ, Pollack L, Paul J, Stall R, Catania JA. Differential HIV risk in bathhouses and public cruising areas. Am J Public Health. 2001;91(9):1482–6.
30. Sanchez T, Finlayson T, Drake A, et al. Human immunodeficiency virus (HIV) risk, prevention, and testing behaviors–United States, National HIV Behavioral Surveillance System: men who have sex with men, November 2003–April 2005. MMWR Surveill Summ. 2006;55(6):1–16.
31. De P, Singh AE, Wong T, Yacoub W, Jolly AM. Sexual network analysis of a gonorrhoea outbreak. Sex Transm Infect. 2004;80(4):280–5.
32. United States. Public Health Service. Office of the Surgeon General. The health consequences of involuntary smoking: a report of the surgeon general. Washington, DC: United States. Public Health Service. Office on Smoking and Health; 1986.
33. Thomas JC, Tucker MJ. The development and use of the concept of a sexually transmitted disease core. J Infect Dis. 1996;174 Suppl 2:S134–43.
34. California v. Freeman (1989) 488 U.S. 1311.
35. Kubicek K, Carpineto J, McDavitt B, et al. Integrating professional and folk models of HIV risk: YMSM's perceptions of high-risk sex. AIDS Educ Prev. 2008;20(3):220–38.

36. Bartow A. Pornography, coercion, and copyright law 2.0. Vand J Ent Tech Law. 2008;10:799–840.

37. Taylor MM, Rotblatt H, Brooks JT, et al. Epidemiologic investigation of a cluster of workplace HIV infections in the adult film industry: Los Angeles, California, 2004. Clin Infect Dis. 2007;44(2):301–5.

38. Goldstein BY, Steinberg JK, Aynalem G, Kerndt PR. High Chlamydia and Gonorrhea incidence and reinfection among performers in the adult film industry. Sex Transm Dis. 2011;38(7):644–8.

39. Record keeping requirements. 18USC §2257. Available at http://codes.lp.findlaw.com/uscode/18/I/110/2257; http://uscode.house.gov/download/pls/18C110.txt.

40. Division of Occupational Safety and Health. Vital information for workers and employers in the adult film industry. Available at http://www.dir.ca.gov/DOSH/AdultFilmIndustry.html#PPE. Accessed 1 Nov 2010.

41. Reade R, Richwald G, Williams NT. The Nevada legal brothel system as a model for AIDS prevention among female sex industry workers. Abstract SC 715. Paper presented at International Conference of AIDS; 1990. Accessed 2 Feb 2010.

42. Nevada State Health Division Office of Health Statistics and Surveillance. Overview of STD/HIV prevention in the brothels; 2010 (Unpublished data).

43. Huffstutter PJ. See no evil. Los Angeles Times Magazine. 2003.

44. Krieger N, Birn AE. A vision of social justice as the foundation of public health: commemorating 150 years of the spirit of 1848. Am J Public Health. 1998;88(11):1603–6.

45. Zaza S, Briss PA, Harris KW, Task Force on Community Preventive Services (U.S.). The guide to community preventive services: what works to promote health? New York: Oxford University; 2005.

46. Chaloupka FJ. Tobacco pricing and price manipulation: one economist's perspective. Presentation at California Tobacco Control Program Regional Forum, Los Angeles, CA, January 20, 2011.

47. Woods WJ, Erwin K, Lazarus M, Serice H, Grinstead O, Binson D. Building stakeholder partnerships for an on-site HIV testing programme. Cult Health Sex. 2008;10(3):249–62.

48. Hu TW, Sung HY, Keeler TE. Reducing cigarette consumption in California: tobacco taxes vs an anti-smoking media campaign. Am J Public Health. 1995;85(9):1218–22.

49. Simon PA, Fielding JE. Public health and business: a partnership that makes cents. Health Aff (Millwood). 2006;25(4):1029–39.

50. Grant M, Leverton M. Working together to reduce harmful drinking. New York, NY: Brunner-Routledge; 2009.

51. Easton A. Public-private partnerships and public health practice in the 21st century: looking back at the experience of the Steps Program. Prev Chronic Dis. 2009;6(2):A38.

52. Bense B. Step through the buzzer door: safer sex and public sex. Focus. 2002;17(10):5–6.

53. Cam BD, Creg H, Mills B, Keith W. Titan media public policy statement – "bareback" or high risk behavior. http://static.titanmedia.com/unlocked/images/promotions/public/NEWS/pages/barebacking.pdf. 2004.

54. Helquist M, Osmon R. Beyond the baths: the other sex businesses. 1984. J Homosex. 2003;44(3–4):177–201.

55. Occupational Safety and Health Standards Board. Petition File No. 513: bloodborne pathogens. http://www.dir.ca.gov/oshsb/petition513.html. Accessed 12 Jan 2011.

56. American Public Health Association. Policy statement, prevention and control of sexually transmitted infections and HIV among performers in the adult film industry. 9 Nov 2010.

57. National Coalition of STD Directors. Policy statement on worker health and safety in the adult film industry. 6 Oct 2010.

58. Hemmelgarn S. Porn company's 'role models' draw concerns of AIDS advocates. Bay Area Reporter. 2 Dec 2010.

59. Mullen PD, Ramirez G, Strouse D, Hedges LV, Sogolow E. Meta-analysis of the effects of behavioral HIV prevention interventions on the sexual risk behavior of sexually experienced adolescents in controlled studies in the United States. J Acquir Immune Defic Syndr. 2002;30 Suppl 1:S94–105.

60. Centers for Disease Control and Prevention. Compendium of HIV prevention interventions with evidence of effectiveness. Atlanta: U.S. Department of Health and Human Services; 1999 (revised).

61. Aral SO. Sexual network patterns as determinants of STD rates: paradigm shift in the behavioral epidemiology of STDs made visible. Sex Transm Dis. 1999;26(5):262–4.

62. Morris M. Sexual networks and HIV. AIDS. 1997;11(Suppl A):S209–16.

63. Rothenberg RB, Potterat JJ, Woodhouse DE. Personal risk taking and the spread of disease: beyond core groups. J Infect Dis. 1996;174 Suppl 2:S144–49.

64. Potterat JJ, Muth SQ, Rothenberg RB, et al. Sexual network structure as an indicator of epidemic phase. Sex Transm Infect. 2002;78 Suppl 1:i152–58.

65. Grudzen CR, Elliott MN, Kerndt PR, Schuster MA, Brook RH, Gelberg L. Condom use and high-risk sexual acts in adult films: a comparison of heterosexual and homosexual films. Am J Public Health. 2009;99 Suppl 1:S152–56.

66. Marriott pulls plug on in-room adult movies. The Independent. 22 Jan 2011. http://www.independent.co.uk/travel/news-and-advice/marriott-pulls-plug-on-inroom-adult-movies-2191452.html. Accessed 9 May 2011.

67. Wasserheit JN, Aral SO. The dynamic topology of sexually transmitted disease epidemics: implications for prevention strategies. J Infect Dis. 1996;174 Suppl 2:201–13.

68. Reidy WJ, Goodreau SM. The role of commercial sex venues in the HIV epidemic among men who have sex with men. Epidemiology. 2010;21(3):349–59.

69. Institute of Medicine. No time to lose: getting more from HIV prevention. Washington, DC: National Academy Press; 2001.

70. Wohlfeiler D, Ellen J. The limits of behavioral interventions for HIV prevention. In: Cohen L, Chávez V, Chehimi S, editors. Prevention is primary: strategies for community well-being. 2nd ed. San Francisco, CA: Jossey-Bass; 2010. p. 352–70.

Part II

Critical Factors in Approaches to Prevention

Distribution of Prevention Resources and Impact on Sexual Health in the USA

7

Harrell W. Chesson, Steven D. Pinkerton, and David R. Holtgrave

The hypothesis that reductions in sexually transmitted disease (STD) prevention resources can lead to subsequent increases in STD rates is known in the STD field as "Brown's Law." This aphorism is named for Dr. William Brown, the former leader of what is now the Division of STD Prevention within the Centers for Disease Control and Prevention (CDC), who warned against premature reductions in STD prevention budgets [1, 2]. "As the point of eradication is approached," he said, "it is more often the program that is eradicated than the disease." [2].

As a corollary to Brown's Law, the level of funding allocated for STD and HIV prevention would be expected to be an important determinant of STD and HIV incidence rates. Federal funding for STD and HIV prevention typically amounts to about $1 billion per year in the USA. Although substantial, public investment in STD

H.W. Chesson (✉)
Division of STD Prevention, Centers for Disease Control and Prevention, 1600 Clifton Road, NE, MS E-80, Atlanta, GA 30333, USA
e-mail: hbc7@cdc.gov

S.D. Pinkerton
Center for AIDS Intervention Research (CAIR), Department of Psychiatry and Behavioral Medicine, Medical College of Wisconsin, 2071 North Summit Avenue, Milwaukee, WI 53202, USA

D.R. Holtgrave
Bloomberg School of Public Health, Johns Hopkins University, 624 N Broadway, Baltimore, MD 21205, USA

prevention is quite small compared to the economic burden of STDs (including HIV) in the USA, which has been estimated at $13.0 billion to $21.6 billion in 2008 US dollars [3–6].

Several studies have provided evidence that the level of funding allocated for STD and HIV prevention does indeed impact the incidence of STD and HIV (or STD/HIV-related behaviors), providing direct support for Brown's Law [7–11]. For example, decreases in prevention funding were associated with increases in STD incidence rates, and vice-versa [7]. Model-based studies have also suggested that the funding levels are an important determinant of STD and HIV incidence rates [12–17]. These studies, when combined with the vast literature documenting the impact and cost-effectiveness of specific STD and HIV prevention interventions [18–29], offer strong evidence that funding STD and HIV prevention programs is not an example of merely "throwing money at the problem." Instead, STD and HIV prevention expenditures are generally a cost-effective use of public health resources and have a substantial impact on sexual health.

The magnitude of the impact of prevention funding on sexual health depends on three key issues: How much, to whom, and for what? The first issue (how much?) refers to the amount of money allocated for STD and HIV prevention. The second issue (to whom?) refers to the recipients of STD and HIV prevention funding, and involves such questions as how federal prevention resources should be distributed across states.

S.O. Aral, K.A. Fenton, and J.A. Lipshutz (eds.), *The New Public Health and STD/HIV Prevention: Personal, Public and Health Systems Approaches*, DOI 10.1007/978-1-4614-4526-5_7,
© Springer Science+Business Media New York 2013

The third issue (for what?) refers to how prevention resources are allocated, generally within states (e.g., which interventions to deliver, which risk groups to target).

This chapter is organized as follows. Section "STD and HIV Prevention Funding Levels" focuses on STD and HIV prevention funding levels. In this section, we report how much money is allocated for STD and HIV prevention by federal and state governments, and we show how federal allocations have changed over time. We also describe the distribution of federal funds to state and local health departments (and other entities, such as community-based organizations) and examine how the distribution of prevention resources compares to the distribution of the burden of disease.

Section "Studies of the Impact of Prevention Funding" focuses on published studies of the impact of STD and HIV prevention funding levels on sexual health. In this section, we review published studies of the association between prevention funding and STD and HIV incidence (and other related health outcomes), and review model-based estimates of what STD and HIV rates might have been in the absence of prevention funding or in the presence of increased prevention resources.

Section "Resource Allocation for STD and HIV Prevention" focuses on resource allocation methods. Our discussion of resource allocation primarily is limited to a description of resource allocation models available for decision makers and a discussion of cost-effectiveness league tables. Many key issues relevant to resource allocation decisions are addressed in other chapters of this book and elsewhere [30–43]. These issues include choosing the mix of interventions, targeting populations at risk, and evaluating interventions.

STD and HIV Prevention Funding Levels

Although some STD and HIV prevention activities are funded through private sources, the large majority of prevention funding in the USA is allocated by governmental agencies at the federal, state, and local level [6]. This section begins with a review of past and present federal allocations for STD and HIV prevention. When comparing past and present funding allocations, we include inflation-adjusted estimates to account for the declining purchasing power of these prevention resources over time. We also present estimates of the contribution of state governments to STD and HIV prevention, drawn from recent reports by the American Social Health Association (ASHA), Kaiser Family Foundation (KFF), and the National Alliance of State and Territorial AIDS Directors (NASTAD) [44, 45]. Before these reports were published, little information was available regarding the levels of STD and HIV prevention funding available from state and local governments.

Federal Prevention Funding

The bulk of federal funding for STD and HIV prevention is allocated to CDC. In a typical year, more than 85% of federal HIV prevention funding is directed to CDC [46]. Similarly, CDC's Division of STD Prevention is the lead federal agency for STD prevention, although the exact percentage of overall federal STD prevention funding that is allocated to CDC is difficult to estimate with precision [6].

In recent years, CDC's annual domestic HIV and STD prevention budgets have been about $750 million and $150 million, respectively [9, 47, 48]. Most of the federal funding allocated to CDC for STD and HIV prevention is distributed to state and local agencies, particularly state and local health departments. Roughly 80% of CDC's HIV prevention funding is distributed to external partners [49]. Similarly, 74% of CDC's STD prevention funding is distributed to state and local health departments, and another 8% is allocated to prevention training centers, and for research and program grants [50].

As shown in Fig. 7.1, CDC's HIV prevention budget increased sharply in the early 1980s in response to the rapid growth of the US AIDS epidemic [9, 47]. HIV prevention funding continued to increase (although not steadily) through 2002. From 2002 to 2008, however, HIV prevention funding decreased by 7%, unadjusted for inflation. When adjusted for overall inflation, the

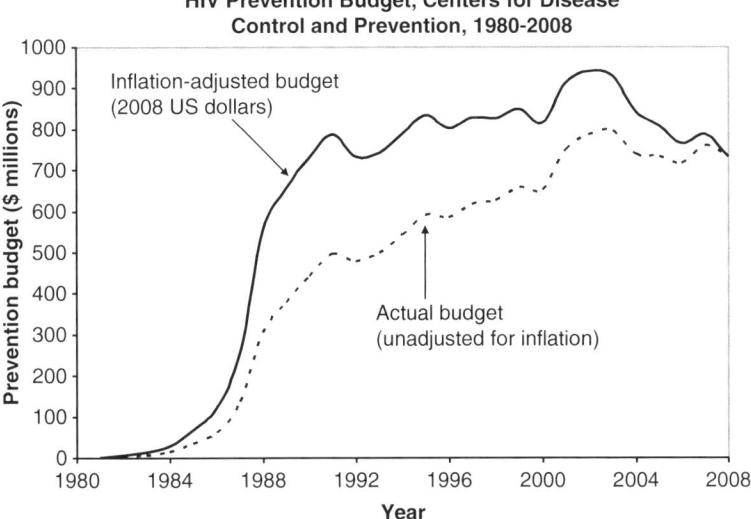

Fig. 7.1 HIV prevention funding was obtained from Holtgrave and Kates for years up to 1999 and from CDC appropriation records for years 2000 and beyond [9, 47]. These figures include funding for all domestic HIV pre- vention across CDC. Updates for inflation were calculated using the "all items" component of the consumer price index for all urban consumers (US Bureau of Labor Statistics, http://www.bls.gov/cpi/)

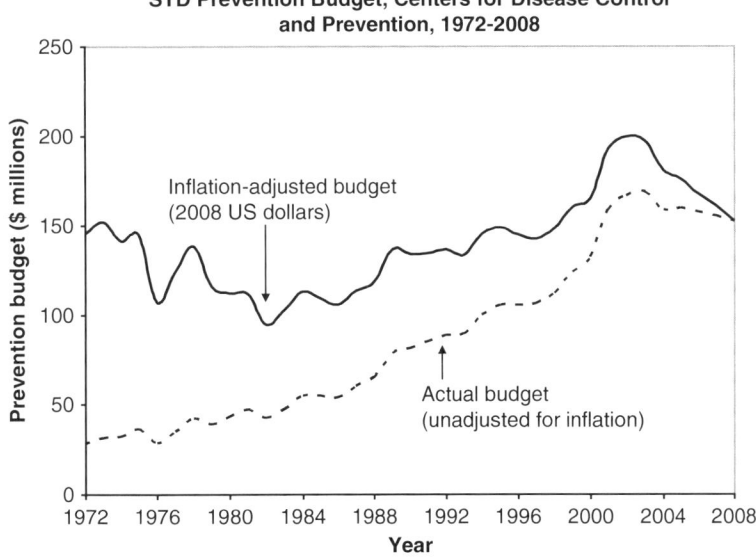

Fig. 7.2 STD prevention funding includes appropriations to the Division of STD Prevention, CDC and was obtained from unpublished CDC records [48]. Updates for inflation were calculated using the "all items" component of the consumer price index for all urban consumers (US Bureau of Labor Statistics, http://www.bls.gov/cpi/)

decrease in HIV prevention funding over this period was 22%.

CDC's STD prevention budget (Fig. 7.2) increased from 1972 to 2002, with a subsequent decline and leveling-off of funding from 2003 to 2008 [48]. From 2002 to 2008, inflation-adjusted STD prevention funding decreased by 24%. On average, over the entire 1972–2008 period, STD funding just kept pace with inflation. That is, inflation-adjusted STD

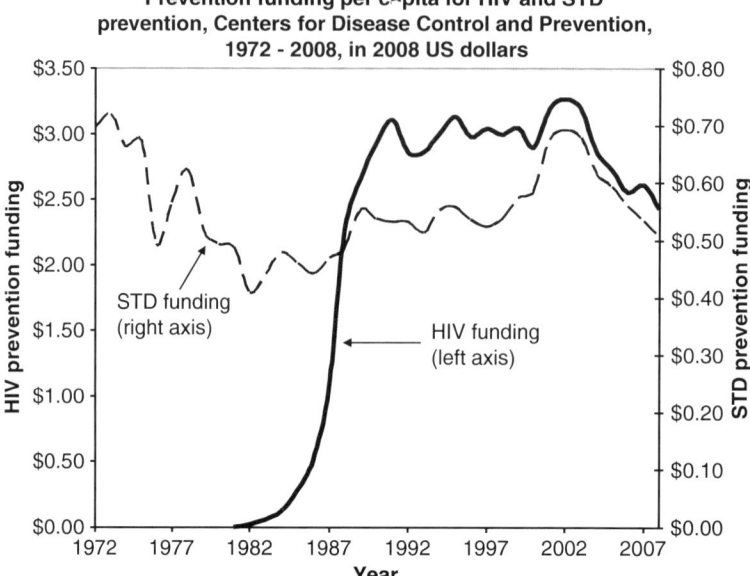

Fig. 7.3 Per-capita funding estimates were calculated using national population estimates maintained by CDC as described in annual surveillance reports [54]. Sources for funding data are as described in Figs. 7.1 and 7.2 [9, 47, 48]. Updates for inflation were calculated using the "all items" component of the consumer price index for all urban consumers (US Bureau of Labor Statistics, http://www.bls.gov/cpi/)

prevention funding in 2008 was quite similar to that of 1972.

These inflation-adjusted funding allocations provide a more accurate illustration of trends in the purchasing power of prevention funding than do the unadjusted (actual) funding allocations. Furthermore, when comparing trends in prevention funding over time it is important to consider the impact of population growth as well. All else equal, as the size of the population increases, per-capita prevention funding decreases. Trends in inflation-adjusted STD and HIV prevention funding per capita are shown in Fig. 7.3. From 2002 to 2008, the decrease in inflation-adjusted per capita prevention funding was 26% for HIV and 27% for STD. In fact, the funding for HIV in 2008 ($2.43 per capita) was the lowest since 1988 ($2.27 per capita). Similarly, the funding for STD in 2008 was the lowest since 1988. At $0.51 per capita in 2008, STD prevention funding was near the lowest point ($0.41 per capita in 1982) observed over the 1972–2008 period.

Table 7.1 presents the CDC budget for fiscal year 2007 for STD and HIV prevention and other selected public health purposes. In total, the CDC budget was about $9.1 billion, or about $30 per capita. Slightly more than one-third of this budget went toward immunization (including the Vaccines for Children program), and another $4.84 per person was spent on terrorism preparedness and emergency response. Funding for HIV/AIDS prevention ($2.49) and STD prevention ($0.51) totaled $3 per capita in fiscal year 2007, and accounted for about 11% of the overall CDC budget. To put these per-capita budget amounts in context, estimates suggest that each year Americans spend an average of about $29 per person on candy, $53 per person on bottled water, and $184 per person on lotteries in states that have lotteries (Table 7.1).

State and Local Prevention Funding

A recent collaborative report from NASTAD and KFF provides detailed information regarding the contribution of state funding to overall HIV prevention funding [45]. This report on state

Table 7.1   Centers for Disease Control and Prevention budget, by selected categories, fiscal year 2007, and estimated annual spending by Americans on Candy, Bottled Water, and Lotteries

Budget category[a]	Budget (dollars in billions)	Funding per capita (dollars per person)
Total	$9.1	$29.98
Immunization, including Vaccines for Children	$3.3	$10.92
Terrorism preparedness & emergency response	$1.5	$4.84
Health promotion	$0.9	$3.11
HIV/AIDS	$0.8	$2.49
Sexually transmitted diseases	$0.2	$0.51
Spending category[b]	Spending (dollars in billions)	Spending per capita (dollars per person)
Candy	$8.8	$28.94
Bottled water	$16	$52.62
Lotteries (in states that have lotteries)	n/a	$184.25

[a]CDC budget estimates adapted from CDC's *FY 2009 Budget Submission* (http://www.cdc.gov/fmo/topic/Budget%20 Information/appropriations_budget_form_pdf/FY07-09_Functional_Table.pdf) and *FY 2010 Justification of Estimates for Appropriation Committees* (http://www.cdc.gov/fmo/topic/Budget%20Information/appropriations_budget_form_ pdf/FY2010_CDC_CJ_Final.pdf), obtained from the internet on January 11, 2010. "Health promotion" includes activities such as the prevention of chronic disease and birth defects
[b]Spending estimates for candy (http://www.businessweek.com/globalbiz/content/jun2009/gb20090624_590587.htm), bottled water (http://articles.moneycentral.msn.com/Investing/Extra/BottledWaterARiverOfMoney.aspx), and lotteries (http://www.taxfoundation.org/publications/show/1302.html) were obtained from the internet on January 11, 2010. Average spending per capita on lotteries includes video lottery games and applies to states which have lotteries

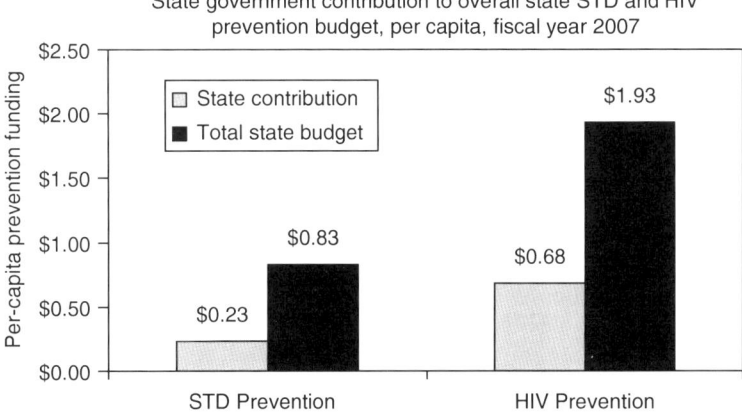

Fig. 7.4   STD data were obtained from ASHA report and HIV data were obtained from NASTAD/KFF report [44, 45]. The total state STD prevention budget was calculated based on the average state contribution ($0.23 per capita) and reported federal contribution ($0.60 per capita) [44]. The $0.60 per capita estimated federal contribution for STD prevention is higher than suggested in Fig. 7.3 because Fig. 7.3 includes only appropriations to CDC's Division of STD Prevention

investment in HIV prevention provides state-specific estimates of such factors as per-capita HIV prevention funding from state and federal sources. In fiscal year 2007, state contributions toward HIV prevention totaled just over $200 million nationwide. The average state contribution to HIV prevention was $0.68 per capita (Fig. 7.4), representing about 35% of the $1.93 per-capita funding available to the state from all public sources. The relative importance of state funds varied markedly across states, with estimates of the state contribution to overall HIV prevention funding ranging from 0 to over 70%.

Table 7.2 Distribution of CDC STD and HIV prevention funds by state quintile, 2006: average (range)

	STD prevention funding per capita	HIV prevention funding per capita
All states	$0.43 ($0.19–$1.50)	$1.40 ($0.49–$3.79)
Lowest fifth	$0.24 ($0.19–$0.29)	$0.62 ($0.49–$0.75)
Second fifth	$0.32 ($0.29–$0.35)	$0.87 ($0.79–$0.95)
Middle fifth	$0.39 ($0.35–$0.42)	$1.18 ($0.95–$1.41)
Fourth fifth	$0.49 ($0.44–$0.53)	$1.69 ($1.42–$2.08)
Highest fifth	$0.70 ($0.54–$1.50)	$2.61 ($2.12–$3.79)

Source: National Center for HIV/AIDS, Viral Hepatitis, STD, and TB prevention
State health profiles (http://www.cdc.gov/nchhstp/stateprofiles/usmap.htm)

The 2009 NASTAD/KFF estimates are consistent with a 2000 report by NASTAD in which state contributions for HIV prevention totaled about 27% of the amount allocated to states by CDC for HIV prevention [13]. Further, these results are generally consistent with unpublished reports provided to CDC from 40 states in 2000, in which state and local funding accounts for about 40% of the combined local, state, and federal HIV prevention funding [7].

Just as the NASTAD/KFF report provides information on state contributions for HIV prevention, a recent report from ASHA provides detailed information regarding the state contributions for STD prevention funding [44]. On average, state-contributed funding accounted for about one-fourth of each state's overall STD prevention budget. The average state contribution was $0.23 per capita (Fig. 7.4), representing only 0.61% of the average $43.14 per capita of state funding for public health. The median state contribution ($0.14 per capita) was notably lower than the mean.

The estimated state contributions to STD prevention in the recent ASHA report as a percentage of overall STD prevention funding are notably lower than estimates from the mid-1990s during which state and local contributions were estimated at 58% of the total public STD prevention funding [6]. These differences may reflect changes over time in the state and federal contributions to STD prevention efforts. It is also possible that these differences can be attributable, at least in part, to the inclusion of contributions of local governments or to changes over time in how STD program funding is categorized in state budgets [6].

Geographic Distribution of CDC Funding for STD and HIV Prevention

Overall CDC funding for STD and HIV prevention is reviewed above. Here, we focus on the distribution of CDC funds across states. The average state allocation of CDC prevention funding in 2006 was $0.43 per capita for STD prevention and $1.40 per capita for HIV prevention (Table 7.2) [51]. Per-capita funding across states ranged from $0.19 to $1.50 for STD prevention and from $0.49 to $3.79 for HIV prevention. Per-capita funding in the highest quintile of states was $0.70 for STD prevention and $2.61 for HIV prevention, about three to four times higher than the per-capita funding in the lowest quintile of states. CDC allocations to states for STD prevention were highly correlated with allocations for HIV prevention. That is, states with below-average funding for STD prevention tended to be the same states with below-average funding for HIV prevention.

The distribution of federal STD and HIV prevention funds by CDC to the states can be illustrated with Lorenz curves and Gini coefficients [52]. To plot the Lorenz curve for distribution of CDC prevention resources, we first ranked the states in ascending order of per-capita CDC STD prevention funding (e.g., states with the lowest per-capita funding were ranked first). We then plotted the cumulative proportion of CDC STD prevention funding accounted for by a cumulative proportion of the population (Fig. 7.5). The Lorenz curve for HIV prevention funding was drawn in an analogous manner. The Gini coefficient can range from 0 (no inequality) to 1 (complete inequality), and is measured as twice

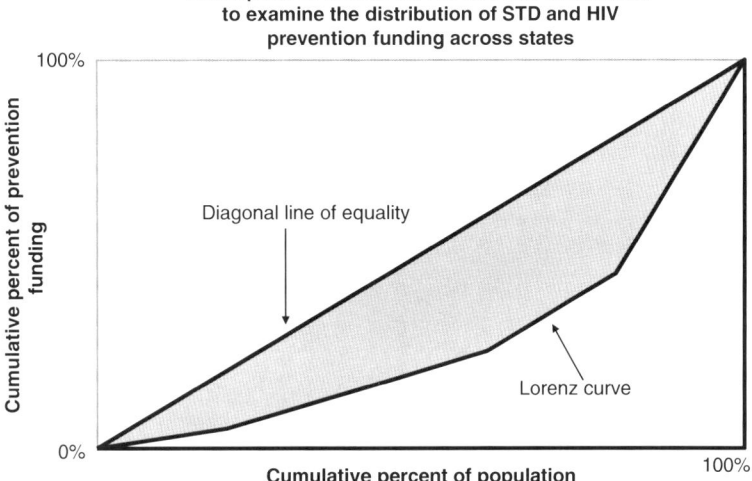

Description of Lorenz curves and Gini coefficients to examine the distribution of STD and HIV prevention funding across states

Fig. 7.5 To plot the Lorenz curve for distribution of CDC prevention resources, we first ranked the states in ascending order of per-capita CDC STD prevention funding (e.g., states with the lowest per-capita funding were ranked first). We then plotted the cumulative proportion of CDC STD prevention funding accounted for by a cumulative proportion of the population. The Lorenz curve for HIV prevention funding was drawn in an analogous manner. The Gini coefficient can range from 0 (no inequality) to 1 (complete inequality), and is measured as twice the area between the diagonal line of equality and the Lorenz curve (the shaded area in the hypothetical example above)

the area between the diagonal line of equality and the Lorenz curve (the shaded area in the hypothetical example in Fig. 7.5) [52].

Federal STD prevention funds are distributed slightly more evenly across states than are HIV prevention funds, as illustrated in Fig. 7.6. One possible explanation for this finding is that STDs like chlamydia are more evenly distributed across states than are HIV cases, which are more concentrated geographically. As shown in Fig. 7.6, the distribution across states of STD prevention funding is similar to that of STD cases, and the distribution across states of HIV prevention funding is similar to that of cumulative AIDS cases. We note Fig. 7.6 shows cumulative AIDS cases (rather than current HIV incidence) by state, owing to a lack of HIV incidence data for all states.

The similarity between the distribution of prevention funding and the distribution of cases of disease is not surprising, as prevention funding is allocated to state and local health departments based in part on the number of cases of disease [30, 45, 53]. The phrase "proportional allocation" is used to describe the allocation of prevention resources in which the prevention funding is distributed in the same proportion as the burden of disease. There are several justifications for using a proportional allocation scheme, including the desirability of targeting prevention resources to geographical areas with greatest need, fairness of allocation across geographical areas (in terms of dollars per AIDS case or per STD case), and ease of use (as no complex resource allocation models are required). A main argument against proportional allocation is that such an allocation rewards the reporting of new cases, not the prevention of new cases, and does not necessarily maximize the number of averted cases [30, 53]. Further, the completeness of reporting may vary across states owing to differences in surveillance systems and policies [54]. Issues regarding the allocation of prevention resources are discussed in a later section of this chapter.

Section Summary

The CDC's budget for STD and HIV prevention declined by about 25% from 2002 to 2008 when

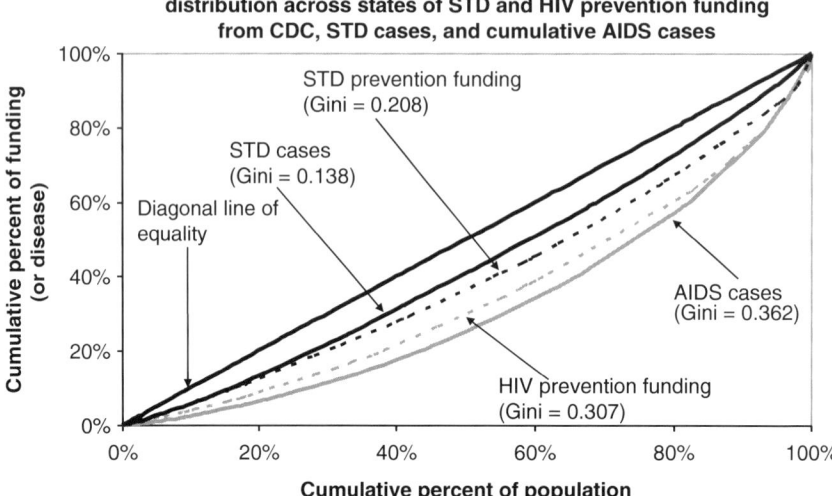

Fig. 7.6 As inequality in the distribution across states increases, the Lorenz curve moves further from the line of equality and the Gini coefficient increases. AIDS cases are cumulative cases through 2005 and prevention funding for STD and HIV is from 2006 [51]. STD cases are the combined gonorrhea and chlamydia cases reported in 2006 [54]

adjusted for inflation and population growth. In 2008, the CDC's budget for STD and HIV prevention was about $0.9 billion (or $3 per capita), most of which was distributed to state and local partners. The distribution of CDC's STD and HIV prevention funding across states is similar to the distribution of the burden of disease across states. The average state contribution was $0.68 per capita for HIV prevention and $0.23 per capita for STD prevention.

Studies of the Impact of Prevention Funding

Although numerous studies have documented the impact and cost-effectiveness of various STD and HIV prevention activities [18–29], only a handful of studies have examined the question, "Does funding for STD and HIV prevention matter?" In this section, we review empirical studies that have examined the relationship between prevention expenditures and incidence rates (or other STD/HIV-related health outcomes). We also review modeling studies that have examined the

potential consequences of changes in prevention funding allocations.

Empirical Studies of the Impact of STD/HIV Prevention Funding

Cutler and Arnold noted that substantial cuts in federal appropriations for venereal disease control in the early 1950s were followed by increases in syphilis rates in the late 1950s, and attributed this increase at least in part to the decreased prevention funding [55]. More recently, Chaulk and Zenilman plotted national-level STD rates against STD prevention funding and reported that decreases in federal STD prevention funding were followed by increases in syphilis and gonorrhea rates [1]. For example, decreases in STD funding in the 1950s were followed by increases in gonorrhea rates in the 1960s. Based on plots of national-level HIV incidence rates and HIV prevention funding, Holtgrave and Pinkerton presented evidence suggesting that increases in HIV prevention funding in the mid to late 1980s corresponded with notable decreases in new HIV

Table 7.3 Summary of studies examining impact of STD/HIV prevention funding on STD/HIV-related health outcomes

Study	Data examined	Main findings
Chesson et al. [7]	State-level CDC funding allocations for STD and HIV prevention and state-level gonorrhea rates, 1981–1998	Greater amounts of prevention funding in a given year were associated with lower gonorrhea rates in subsequent years
Linas et al. [8]	State-level CDC HIV prevention funding (1996–2003) and HIV testing data from the Behavioral Risk Factor Surveillance System (2003)	The odds of having been tested for HIV were higher in states with greater amounts of HIV prevention funding. Prevention funding was also positively associated with increased knowledge of methods to prevent mother-to-child HIV transmission
Holtgrave and Kates [9]	National-level HIV prevention allocations and national-level HIV incidence estimates, 1978–2006	After the mid-1980s, national investment in HIV prevention in a given year was inversely correlated with HIV incidence in the subsequent year
Sansom et al. [10]	Surveillance data (proportion of HIV-infected women prescribed perinatal prophylaxis and perinatal HIV transmission rate) from 1999 and 2001 in six CDC-funded areas and five unfunded areas	In the funded areas, the proportion of women prescribed prophylaxis increased from 1999 to 2001 and the perinatal HIV transmission rate decreased from 1999 to 2001
Chesson and Owusu-Edusei [11]	State-level syphilis rates and state-level CDC allocation for syphilis elimination activities 1997–2005	Greater levels of syphilis elimination funding in a given year were associated with lower syphilis rates in subsequent years

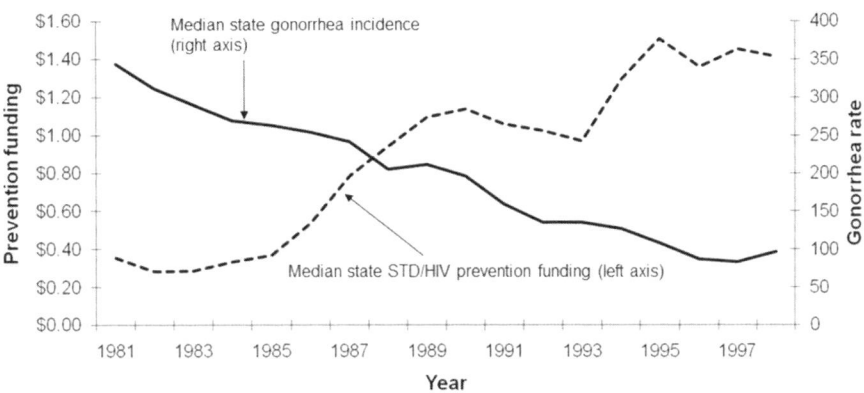

Median state gonorrhea incidence rate (new reported cases per 100,000) and CDC STD/HIV prevention funding per capita (2008 US dollars), 1981-1998

Fig. 7.7 Source: Chesson et al. [7]. Updates for inflation were calculated using the "all items" component of the consumer price index for all urban consumers (US Bureau of Labor Statistics, http://www.bls.gov/cpi/)

cases [56]. This analysis did not, however, examine this relationship statistically.

The idea behind Brown's Law—that STD prevention resources are an important determinant of STDs rates—is certainly plausible, as illustrated by the examples above. Until recently, however, the relationship between STD/HIV prevention resources and STD/HIV-related health outcomes had not been examined rigorously.

Empirical studies of the impact of prevention expenditures on incidence rates and other health outcomes are described below and summarized in Table 7.3.

Chesson and colleagues examined the relationship between gonorrhea rates and combined CDC STD and HIV prevention funding at the state level from 1981 to 1998 (Fig. 7.7). In this study, larger prevention funding allocations in a

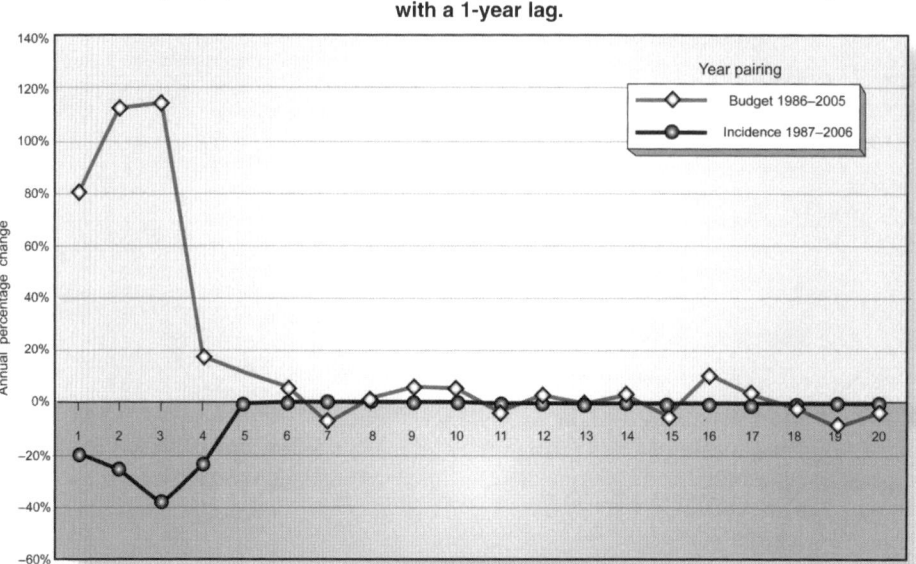

Percent change in HIV incidence (1987–2006) and CDC's HIV prevention budget (adjusted for inflation and expressed in 1983 dollars; 1986–2005), with a 1-year lag.

Fig. 7.8 Source: Holtgrave and Kates [9]. © 2007 American Journal of Preventive Medicine

given year were associated with reductions in reported gonorrhea incidence rates in subsequent years [7]. Each one dollar of prevention funding (per capita, adjusted to 2008 dollars) for a given state in a given year was associated with reductions in gonorrhea rates of about 2–20%, depending on the regression model used, in the subsequent 1–3 years. Although this study examined combined STD and HIV prevention funding, a subsequent (unpublished) analysis by the lead author found that the results of the combined study were generally consistent when focusing only on STD prevention funding or only on HIV prevention funding.

Linas and colleagues examined the relationship between state-level CDC HIV prevention funding and HIV testing using data from the Behavioral Risk Factor Surveillance System (BRFSS) [8]. In their analysis, increased HIV prevention funding was associated with an increased probability of HIV testing and an increased awareness of methods to prevent mother-to-child transmission of HIV [8]. The authors estimated that about 13 million more people were tested for HIV between 1998 and

2003 than would have been tested in an alternative scenario of reduced funding for HIV prevention.

Holtgrave and Kates correlated national-level HIV incidence estimates and CDC HIV prevention funding from 1978 to 2006 and found that, after the mid-1980s, prevention expenditures in a given year were inversely associated with HIV incidence in the subsequent year (Fig. 7.8) [9]. Owing to factors such as the limited sample size ($n=29$ years of national-level data), the authors described their study as "exploratory." Nonetheless, theirs was the first study (and to our knowledge the only study to date) to document a statistically significant association between federal HIV prevention expenditures and reductions in HIV incidence at the population level.

Sansom and colleagues examined the impact of federally funded activities to prevent perinatal HIV transmission [10]. Two outcomes (the proportion of HIV-infected women prescribed perinatal prophylaxis and the proportion of HIV-infected women whose infants were HIV infected) were assessed in six CDC-funded areas and in five unfunded areas from 1999 to 2001.

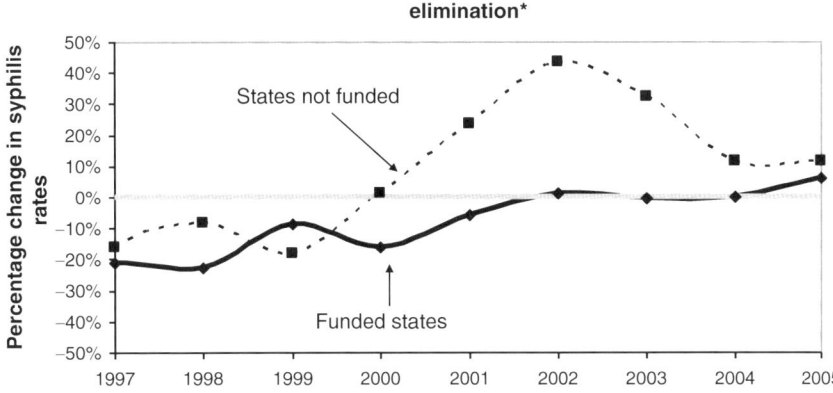

Fig. 7.9 A state was considered an initially funded state if that state (or a city within that state) received CDC funding for syphilis elimination 1998 or 1999. Washington, DC, was included as an initially funded "state." Source: Chesson and Owusu-Edusei [11]

The proportion of women prescribed prophylaxis increased in the funded areas and decreased in the unfunded areas, and this difference in trends between the funded areas and the unfunded areas was statistically significant. The decline in the rate of perinatal HIV transmission was more pronounced in the funded areas than in the unfunded areas, but this difference was not statistically significant.

Chesson and Owusu-Edusei examined the impact of CDC funding for syphilis elimination on syphilis rates at the state level from 1997 to 2005 [11]. Although primary and secondary (P&S) and early latent syphilis rates increased from 2002 to 2005, these increases were much more pronounced in states that did not receive CDC funding for syphilis elimination compared to funded states (Fig. 7.9). Regression analyses of state-level syphilis rates and syphilis elimination funding over time were used to examine whether these findings were attributable to syphilis elimination efforts. Controlling for differences in race, poverty, crime, and other factors across states, these analyses suggested a significant inverse correlation between state-level funding in a given year and state-level syphilis rates in subsequent years. Every dime of prevention funding (per capita) was associated with reductions in syphilis rates of about 33% over the next 1–3 years.

Model-Based Estimates of the Impact of Prevention Funding

The studies described above examined associations between prevention funding and STD/HIV-related health outcomes over time. In addition to these empirical studies of the impact of prevention funding, several model-based studies have been conducted to estimate the impact of STD and HIV prevention expenditures on STD and HIV incidence rates in the USA. Often, models are the best available option for estimating what the STD and HIV incidence might have been in the absence of prevention efforts [57–59].

Holtgrave and colleagues conducted scenario analyses in which they compared the HIV epidemic observed in the USA against hypothetical scenarios in which no HIV prevention programs were in place (Fig. 7.10) [12, 13]. HIV incidence in these hypothetical scenarios of no HIV prevention was based on the expected natural dynamics of HIV in the absence of prevention interventions.

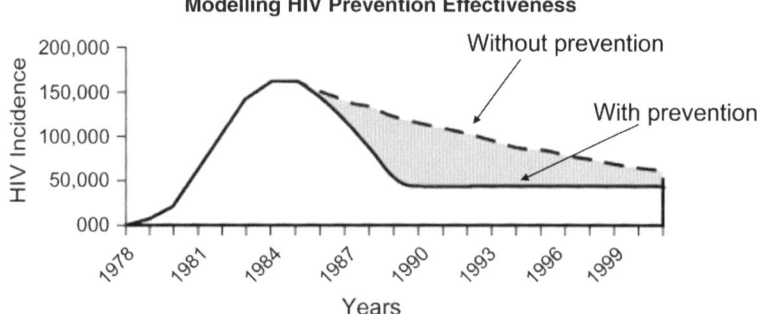

Fig. 7.10 Source: Holtgrave [13]. © 2002 AIDS

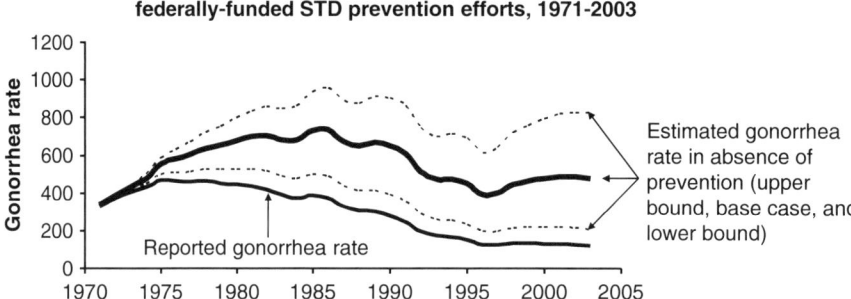

Fig. 7.11 Source: Chesson [16]

In these hypothetical scenarios, HIV incidence was expected to increase over time until it reached a peak, after which incidence would remain stable or would decrease. Owing to the uncertainty in estimating what HIV incidence rates in the USA might have been without prevention efforts, the authors conservatively assumed that the peak HIV incidence rate in the absence of prevention would not have exceeded the peak HIV incidence rate actually observed in the USA.

In one such application of this approach, it was estimated that HIV prevention activities averted an estimated 204,000–1,585,000 HIV infections in the USA from the onset of the AIDS epidemic through 2000 [13]. Another study suggested that an additional $93 million in HIV prevention funding in 2007 targeted toward HIV counseling and testing in high-risk communities would avert 1,223–2,537 HIV infections [12]. In another application, Holtgrave and colleagues estimated that CDC's HIV prevention budget in fiscal year 2007 would have to be about $1.3 billion to address unmet prevention needs [14, 15]. Holtgrave testified before Congress in 2008 that a reduction in HIV incidence of 50% in 5 years should be possible with such a level of additional funding [60].

Model-based estimates of the impact of prevention funding are not as common for STDs other than HIV. Chesson developed a simple model in which the change in the gonorrhea rate from year to year depended in part on the amount of federal funding for gonorrhea prevention [16], as suggested by an earlier study of the association between prevention funding and gonorrhea rates [7]. This modeling approach suggested that 32 million gonorrhea cases were averted over the 33-year period from 1971 to 2003 as a result of federally funded STD prevention efforts. It was estimated that in the absence of prevention, gonorrhea rates in 2003 would be roughly four times higher than the observed rate (Fig. 7.11).

A model by White and colleagues noted that two equilibrium levels of STD rates were possible for the same set of model parameter values, depending on starting conditions [17]. In one potential outcome (the "virtuous circle"), adequate provision of STD services keeps the demand for STD services low. In the other potential outcome (the "vicious circle"), inadequate provision of STD services leads to a high demand for STD services, and the resulting unmet prevention needs serve to maintain high STD incidence. Although this model was not used to assess the impact of prevention funding, the authors noted the possibility that a short-term increase in STD prevention funding could succeed in shifting from a vicious circle with high STD incidence and high unmet prevention needs to a virtuous circle with lower STD rates and adequate STD prevention services. The short-term increase in prevention funding could easily be offset by the medical costs averted by achieving the "virtuous circle" with its lower rates of STD incidence.

Section Summary

Several studies have documented an association between increases in expenditures for STD and HIV prevention and decreases in STD and HIV incidence rates (or STD/HIV risk behaviors). Model-based studies have also suggested that funding levels are an important determinant of STD and HIV incidence rates. These empirical and model-based studies offer strong evidence of the impact of federally funded STD and HIV prevention efforts, especially when considered alongside the numerous studies documenting the impact and cost-effectiveness of various STD and HIV prevention interventions.

Resource Allocation for STD and HIV Prevention

Resource allocation models seek to maximize the benefit (in terms of reduction in disease incidence and burden of disease) of a given level of prevention resources. Detailed descriptions and discussions of resource allocation for STD and HIV

prevention are available elsewhere [30–43]. Our discussion of resource allocation is limited primarily to a description of selected resource allocation models for STD and HIV prevention in the USA. We also discuss the use of league tables to facilitate the incorporation of cost-effectiveness information into resource allocation decisions.

The allocation of federal prevention resources includes the distribution of resources across states and the within-state allocation of these prevention resources across different prevention strategies or different target populations. A recent modeling study by Zaric and Brandeau examined the importance of these two steps: a higher-level allocation of funds (such as the decision at the federal level of how to allocate federal prevention funds to the states) and a lower-level allocation of funds (such as a state's decision of how to allocate its federal funding across different interventions) [61]. At each level, two allocations were compared: a proportional allocation in which funding was based on the burden of HIV and the most efficient allocation (as suggested by the model) in terms of preventing the most new cases of HIV. The modeling results suggested that efficient allocations (as compared to proportional allocations) were more important at the lower level than the higher level.

STD and HIV Resource Allocation Models for the USA

The Institute of Medicine Report, "*No Time To Lose: Getting More From HIV Prevention*," released in 2000, called for an efficient allocation of prevention resources geared to maximize the number of HIV infections averted [30]. The resource allocation model presented in the IOM report was based on four key inputs: (1) the annual incidence of HIV in three main risk groups (injection drug users, men who have sex with men [MSM], and high-risk heterosexuals), (2) the reductions in the annual risk of HIV that could be achieved by various HIV prevention programs, (3) the number of people that could be reached by each intervention, and (4) the cost of the interventions [30]. In the model's base case scenario,

$412 million in HIV prevention would avert 3,000 cases if allocated across MSM, IDU, and high-risk heterosexuals in proportion to HIV incidence in these groups and would avert 3,900 cases if allocated most efficiently according to the resource allocation model [30, 53].

Since the IOM report calling for more focus on resource allocation decisions, several resource allocation models have been made available to guide decision-makers toward a more efficient allocation of prevention resources. A selection of such models applicable to the USA is described briefly below. Resource allocation models are also available for resource-poor settings [39, 62, 63], but are not described in this review.

The HIV Prevention Funding Allocation Model (HPFAM) is a spreadsheet-based resource allocation model designed to optimize the impact of HIV prevention activities [41]. This tool takes into account efficiency and equity tradeoffs, and facilitates the incorporation of input from community planning groups regarding priority populations. In the example provided for a state health department, the optimal allocation without equity constraints prevented roughly twice as many new HIV infections as the allocation in which all risk groups received an equal amount of funding.

"Maximizing the Benefit" is a spreadsheet-based resource allocation model that can be used to rank more than 20 interventions based on cost-effectiveness and other factors such as acceptability [37, 64, 65]. A Bernoullian model of HIV acquisition is used to estimate the potential impact of most interventions. In an application of the model at the national level, the authors estimated that a re-allocation of CDC HIV prevention funds could avert 20,000 HIV cases per year instead of the 7,300 averted by focusing on the four interventions recommended by CDC at the time [37]. The model is available at http://www.rand.org/health/surveys_tools/maximizing_benefit/index.html.

Resource allocation models have been developed by the Division of HIV/AIDS Prevention (DHAP) at CDC for internal use to help guide DHAP on allocation strategies that might improve the overall effectiveness of HIV prevention efforts. A resource allocation model presented at the 2009 National HIV Prevention Conference combined a dynamic compartmental model of HIV transmission with an optimization model to determine the allocation scenario that minimizes HIV incidence over a 5-year horizon [66]. The intervention types considered by the model were HIV screening interventions, with or without partner referral services, and programs to reduce risk behaviors. These interventions were targeted to population subgroups defined by transmission risk category (high-risk heterosexuals, men who have sex with men and injection drug users), gender, race, and HIV status. The number of new infections in each population subgroup under the optimal allocation scenario is compared to that under the current funding scenario to estimate the number of infections averted and the cost per infection averted.

Models are also available to guide (non-HIV) STD prevention resource allocation. One example is the Screening Optimally for Chlamydia: Resource Allocation, Testing and Evaluation Software (SOCRATES) model, which helps resource allocation decision makers determine which chlamydia screening strategies to adopt in order to maximize the associated health benefits [67]. Though the default SOCRATES model inputs are dated, users can manually update the model parameters by changing the input values, such as those regarding the costs and performance of the various diagnostic options.

Results from a resource allocation model by Tao and colleagues [68] can also help in determining optimal screening strategies for chlamydia, such as which age groups to screen and which diagnostic tests and treatments to use. For any fixed budget, the model can determine the chlamydia screening strategy that maximizes the number of women with chlamydia who are treated or the chlamydia screening strategy that maximizes costs saved (averted medical costs minus program costs), depending on the goals of the user.

Finally, STIC (Sexually Transmitted Infection Costs Saved) FIGURE is a spreadsheet tool available for STD and HIV prevention programs to estimate the costs averted through various prevention activities [69]. These activities include HIV testing and counseling and the treatment of persons with chlamydia, gonorrhea, and syphilis. The tool is based primarily on previously published estimates of the impact of these prevention activities and the direct and indirect costs of STDs including HIV [70]. Though not a resource allocation model, the tool can help in assessing the cost-effectiveness of STD and HIV prevention activities.

League Tables

Decision-makers can use cost-effectiveness studies to help them choose their mix of interventions and target population(s) without having to apply a dedicated resource allocation model. "League tables" have been developed to facilitate this process for HIV prevention and other health-related resource allocation decisions. In the league table approach, interventions for different at-risk populations (e.g., MSM, high-risk heterosexual men, high-risk women, IDUs) are listed in individual tables. Each league table lists potential interventions for the target group in order of increasing cost per client. The tables also specify the impact of the interventions (e.g., HIV infections averted or quality-adjusted life-years saved) and their incremental cost-effectiveness ratios (e.g., additional cost per additional infection averted) compared to the next less expensive intervention. These tables help decision makers to determine whether they should fund the least expensive intervention for a particular group or whether it would be economically sound to fund the next most expensive intervention, the third most expensive intervention, and so on.

Resource allocations across multiple groups (e.g., MSM, high-risk women, etc.) can be optimized by considering not only the incremental cost-effectiveness ratios within each group, but also how these ratios compare across groups [71]. At each step of the resource allocation algorithm, the available intervention with the smallest incremental cost-effectiveness ratio (ICER) is selected for funding.

A 3-group example focusing on HIV prevention is presented in Table 7.4 (panels A and B).

This example assumes that there are 1,000 people in each group (X, Y, and Z) and that there are three candidate interventions for Group X (X1, X2, and X3), three candidate interventions for Group Y (Y1, Y2, and Y3), but only two candidate interventions for Group Z (Z1 and Z2). This example also assumes that a person can participate in at most one intervention, although it is possible to offer different interventions within a given group (e.g., some members of Group X can be offered intervention X1 while others in Group X are offered intervention X2, as explained in more detail below). The cost of the intervention is calculated by multiplying the intervention cost per person by the number of people participating in the intervention. Similarly, the impact of the intervention (number of cases of HIV averted) is calculated by multiplying the intervention impact per person by the number of people participating in the intervention. The number of persons provided a given intervention can range from 0 to 1,000 (the entire risk group).

Table 7.4 (panel A) presents the intervention data (the "league tables") used in the analysis. From this information, optimal resource allocations can be determined for a range of prevention budgets. The first intervention selected for funding is X1 because, among the least expensive interventions in the three groups (X1, Y1, and Z1), it has the smallest ICER. However, because intervention X2 also has a smaller ICER than interventions Y1 and Z1, if the prevention budget is sufficiently large, intervention X2 should be funded, rather than X1, if the goal is to maximize the number of HIV infections averted. Interventions Y1 and Z1 (which have the smallest ICERs among remaining interventions) would be funded next. If there is enough money remaining, intervention X3 would then replace X2, then Z2 would replace Z1, and so on.

Table 7.4 (panel B) shows the optimal mix of interventions for fixed budgets ranging from $0 to $440,000. Because X1 is the first intervention selected for funding, X1 will be provided to as many clients in group X as possible (at a cost of $40 per client) when the budget is less than or equal to $40,000. Because X2 is the second

Table 7.4 Example of league table-based resource allocation

Panel A: costs, effectiveness, and incremental cost-effectiveness ratios of hypothetical prevention interventions for three risk groups (X, Y, Z)

Intervention	Intervention cost per person	Intervention effect (HIV cases averted per person)	Incremental cost-effectiveness ratio (cost per case of HIV averted)
Group X			
None	$0	0	–
X1	$40	0.004	$10,000
X2	$80	0.006	$20,000
X3	$130	0.007	$50,000
Group Y			
None	$0	0	–
Y1	$60	0.002	$30,000
Y2	$130	0.003	$70,000
Y3	$210	0.004	$80,000
Group Z			
None	$0	0	–
Z1	$40	0.001	$40,000
Z2	$100	0.002	$60,000

Panel B: intervention provided to clients in Groups X, Y, and Z under optimal resource allocation algorithm, assuming a fixed prevention budget

Prevention budget	Group X	Group Y	Group Z
$0	None	None	None
>$0 to <$40,000	None or X1	None	None
$40,000	X1	None	None
>$40,000 to <$80,000	X1 or X2	None	None
$80,000	X2	None	None
>$80,000 to <$140,000	X2	None or Y1	None
$140,000	X2	Y1	None
>$140,000 to <$180,000	X2	Y1	None or Z1
$180,000	X2	Y1	Z1
>$180,000 to <$230,000	X2 or X3	Y1	Z1
$230,000	X3	Y1	Z1
>$230,000 to <$290,000	X3	Y1	Z1 or Z2
$290,000	X3	Y1	Z2
>$290,000 to <$360,000	X3	Y1 or Y2	Z2
$360,000	X3	Y2	Z2
>$360,000 to <$440,000	X3	Y2 or Y3	Z2
$440,000	X3	Y3	Z2

This example illustrates how leagues tables can be used to achieve optimal resource allocation across three distinct groups at risk for HIV/STI acquisition (e.g., MSM, at-risk women, and heterosexual men). The example assumes that there are 1,000 people in each group (X, Y, Z) and that there are three candidate interventions for Group X (X1, X2, and X3) and Group Y (Y1, Y2, and Y3), but only two for Group Z (Z1 and Z2). Each person can participate in at most one intervention. *Panel A* of the table presents the intervention data (the "league tables") used in the analysis; *Panel B* identifies the optimal allocation of resources to fund interventions for the three groups assuming a fixed overall prevention budget. At each step of the resource allocation algorithm, the intervention with the smallest incremental cost-effectiveness ratio (ICER) is selected for funding intervention selected for funding, X2 will be offered to as many clients in Group X as possible (in place of the intervention X1) when the budget is between $40,000 and $80,000. For budgets at or above $80,000 up to $140,000, X2 will be offered to all clients in Group X and Y1 will be offered to as many clients as possible of Group Y. Only after the budget exceeds $140,000 will Z1 be offered to clients in Group Z. For greater budgets, more expensive (but more effective) interventions will be offered. At a budget of $440,000, for example, it is possible to provide all clients with the most expensive, most effective intervention: X3 for clients in Group X; Y3 for clients in Group Y, and Z2 for clients in Group Z.

Although this resource allocation algorithm ensures that the maximum number of HIV infections is prevented for a given budget, it does not necessarily guarantee that an intervention will be provided to each group. For example, the optimal allocation of a $140,000 budget would include intervention X2 for all members of Group X and intervention Y1 for all members of Group Y, but no intervention for Group Z (see Table 7.4, panel B). It is simple enough to modify the algorithm to ensure equity across groups (e.g., divide the available funds between the groups equally). However, the resulting resource allocation does not necessarily maximize the number of cases of HIV prevented for the given budget.

In a 2001 article, Pinkerton and colleagues provided league tables that ranked HIV prevention interventions for three target populations (MSM, at-risk men, and at-risk women) by the cost per HIV infection averted by the interventions [19]. For at-risk women, for example, the cost per infection averted ranged from < $50,000 for several interventions (such as condom distribution, basic outreach, and a single-session video intervention) to over $50 million (for post-exposure prophylaxis following receptive vaginal intercourse).

In another example, Hornberger and colleagues ranked 106 interventions (62 focusing on averting new HIV infections, and 44 dealing with managing persons with HIV) by cost–utility ratio [18]. Specifically, interventions were ranked by their cost per quality-adjusted life year

(QALY), which takes into account both gains in life expectancy and in quality of life. In their review, interventions ranged from "cost-saving" (such as HIV screening for pregnant women with HIV prevalence of 1% or greater) to costing over $100,000 per QALY gained (such as post-exposure prophylaxis for heterosexual men after insertive anal sex).

Although league tables can help to inform resource allocation decisions, the use of league tables is not without potential pitfalls [31, 72, 73]. Most notably, results listed in league tables might come from studies with important disparities, such as in the values applied (e.g., values for the discount rate, program costs, and health costs), the scope of the analysis (such as what costs and benefits are included), or the comparison strategy to which cost-effectiveness ratios were calculated [31, 72, 73]. These potential pitfalls are not limited to league tables, however. Resource allocation models often incorporate results from a range of cost-effectiveness studies, and could therefore be subject to many of these potential limitations as well.

Section Summary

Resource allocation models seek to maximize the benefit (in terms of reduction in disease incidence and burden of disease) of a given level of prevention resources. Several resource allocation models have been made available to guide decision-makers toward a more efficient allocation of STD and HIV prevention resources in the USA. "League tables" can also help decision-makers to use cost-effectiveness studies in choosing their mix of interventions and target population(s).

Summary and Conclusion

Our review of studies of the distribution of prevention resources and consequent impact on sexual health revealed three important themes. First, the amount of funding for prevention is an important determinant of STD and HIV incidence rates. In support of Brown's Law, both empirical and model-based studies provide evidence that incidence and prevalence would likely be notably higher in the absence of prevention efforts. Second, for any level of prevention resources, the magnitude of the impact of those resources will depend upon how those resources are allocated. The resource allocation models we reviewed suggest that substantial increases in the impact of prevention resources can be achieved by allocating prevention resources more efficiently. Third, the distribution of federal prevention funds across states is generally proportional to the distribution of the burden of disease across states. While a proportional distribution may be desirable in some aspects, such as to address equity concerns, such a distribution likely does not maximize the reduction in the burden of STDs and HIV [53].

Other Considerations

Maximizing the impact of STD and HIV prevention programs is not the sole consideration of resource allocation decision makers. Often, issues regarding social justice, equity, and intangible benefits of prevention programs are important concerns that can influence the allocation or prevention resources [30, 74]. There is no standard for the weight that cost-effectiveness should have in the resource allocation decision relative to other important concerns [75]. Further, differences of opinion regarding the optimal allocation of STD and HIV prevention resources would still exist even if cost-effectiveness were the sole concern of all those involved in the allocation of STD and HIV prevention resources. As Valdiserri and colleagues noted, "…there is no universally-agreed to, optimal configuration for HIV-prevention interventions, at either the federal or local level." [75].

Barriers to the Use of Economic Studies

There are many important barriers to the use of cost-effectiveness information and resource-allocation tools to guide STD and HIV policy decisions [74, 76–79]. Weinstein and Melchreit identified numerous such barriers, including lack of relevant, useful cost-effectiveness studies; lack

of available expertise in economic analysis and program evaluation; resistance to controversial interventions (such as needle exchange programs); and conflicts of interest, such as support for a particular intervention or for interventions targeted to a particular population that exceeds the level of support that can be justified based on the cost and effectiveness of the interventions [78]. Similarly, Kahn and colleagues noted that advocacy groups often have more influence on resource allocation decisions for HIV/AIDS prevention than for other areas of prevention [80].

Addressing Barriers to the Use of Economic Studies

The barriers to the use of economic studies as described by Weinstein and Melchreit in 1998 were echoed in 2008 by Neumann and colleagues who lamented "the disconnect between health economists and public health practitioners." [74]. Noting that little seemed to have changed from the Weinstein and Melchreit report in 1998 to the Neumann and colleagues report in 2008, Holtgrave warned that actions must be taken now to prevent a similar report in 2018 [77]. Specific strategies that have been suggested to incorporate health economic studies in the field of STD and HIV prevention include: routine collection of cost data to facilitate economic evaluations of STD and HIV prevention interventions, establishment of on-going partnerships between analysts and STD and HIV prevention practitioners, improvement of methods to measure the value of STD and HIV prevention interventions, and increased communication of the value of STD and HIV prevention to elected officials and the general public [74, 77].

This chapter has presented examples of several strategies to facilitate the use of health economic studies. For example, the recent studies documenting a direct link between increases in STD and HIV prevention funding and decreases in the incidence of STD and HIV (and STD/HIV-associated behaviors) represent new developments in methods to measure the value of STD and HIV prevention activities. Prior to these recent studies (Table 7.3), there was remarkably little empirical evidence to support the assertion that federally funded STD/HIV prevention activities can reduce STD/HIV incidence rates at the population level. The resource allocation models and league tables described in this chapter are examples of ways to link analysts with STD and HIV prevention practitioners. These tools can facilitate the incorporation of STD and HIV cost-effectiveness studies into public health practice.

Conclusion

In conclusion, studies reviewed in this chapter offer strong evidence that funding for STD and HIV prevention does indeed bring about important public health benefits in a cost-effective manner. Economic evaluations and resource allocation models are available to help guide decisions about how to spend STD and HIV prevention dollars more efficiently. Although these tools are not without limitations, and cost-effectiveness is but one of the important factors that decision makers must consider, the use of cost-effectiveness studies and resource allocation models can help to maximize the impact of public investment in STD and HIV prevention. Further steps should be taken to facilitate the use of health economics in the field of STD and HIV prevention.

References

1. Chaulk CP, Zenilman J. Sexually transmitted disease control in the era of managed care: "magic bullet" or "shadow on the land"? J Public Health Manag Pract. 1997;3:61–70.
2. Etheridge EW. Sentinel for health: a history of the Centers for Disease Control. Berkeley and Los Angeles, CA: University of California Press; 1992.
3. Siegel JE. Estimates of the economic burden of STDs: review of the literature with updates. In: Eng TR, Butler WT, editors. The hidden epidemic: confronting sexually transmitted diseases. Washington, DC: National Academy Press; 1997. p. 330–56.
4. Alexander LL, Cates JR, Herndon N, Ratcliffe JF, American Social Health Association. Sexually transmitted diseases in America how many cases and at what cost? Menlo Park, CA: Kaiser Family Foundation; 1998.
5. Chesson HW, Blandford JM, Gift TL, Tao G, Irwin KL. The estimated direct medical cost of sexually transmitted diseases among American youth, 2000. Perspect Sex Reprod Health. 2004;36:11–9.
6. Institute of Medicine (Committee on Prevention and Control of Sexually Transmitted Diseases). The hidden epidemic: confronting sexually transmitted diseases. Washington, DC: National Academy Press; 1997.
7. Chesson HW, Harrison P, Scotton CR, Varghese B. Does funding for HIV and sexually transmitted disease prevention matter? Evidence from panel data. Eval Rev. 2005;29:3–23.
8. Linas BP, Zheng H, Losina E, Walensky RP, Freedberg KA. Assessing the impact of federal HIV prevention spending on HIV testing and awareness. Am J Public Health. 2006;96:1038–43.
9. Holtgrave DR, Kates J. HIV incidence and CDC's HIV prevention budget: an exploratory correlational analysis. Am J Prev Med. 2007;32:63–7.
10. Sansom SL, Harris NS, Sadek R, Lampe MA, Ruffo NM, Fowler MG. Toward elimination of perinatal human immunodeficiency virus transmission in the United States: effectiveness of funded prevention programs, 1999–2001. Am J Obstet Gynecol. 2007;197: S90–5.
11. Chesson H, Owusu-Edusei Jr K. Examining the impact of federally-funded syphilis elimination activities in the USA. Soc Sci Med. 2008;67:2059–62.
12. Holtgrave DR. The president's fiscal year 2007 initiative for human immunodeficiency virus counseling and testing expansion in the United States: a scenario analysis of its coverage, impact, and cost-effectiveness. J Public Health Manag Pract. 2007;13:239–43.
13. Holtgrave DR. Estimating the effectiveness and efficiency of US HIV prevention efforts using scenario and cost-effectiveness analysis. AIDS. 2002;16:2347–9.
14. Holtgrave DR. When "heightened" means "lessened": the case of HIV prevention resources in the United States. J Urban Health. 2007;84:648–52.
15. Holtgrave DR, Pinkerton SD, Merson M. Estimating the cost of unmet HIV-prevention needs in the United States. Am J Prev Med. 2002;23:7–12.
16. Chesson HW. Estimated effectiveness and cost-effectiveness of federally funded prevention efforts on gonorrhea rates in the United States, 1971–2003, under various assumptions about the impact of prevention funding. Sex Transm Dis. 2006;33:S140–4.
17. White PJ, Ward H, Cassell JA, Mercer CH, Garnett GP. Vicious and virtuous circles in the dynamics of infectious disease and the provision of health care: gonorrhea in Britain as an example. J Infect Dis. 2005;192:824–36.
18. Hornberger J, Holodniy M, Robertus K, Winnike M, Gibson E, Verhulst E. A systematic review of cost-utility analyses in HIV/AIDS: Implications for public policy. Medical Decision Making. 2007;27:789–821.
19. Pinkerton SD, Johnson-Masotti AP, Holtgrave DR, Farnham PG. Using cost-effectiveness league tables

to compare interventions to prevent sexual transmission of HIV. AIDS. 2001;15:917–28.

20. Holtgrave DR, Qualls NL, Curran JW, Valdiserri RO, Guinan ME, Parra WC. An overview of the effectiveness and efficiency of HIV prevention programs. Public Health Rep. 1995;110:134–46.

21. Oakley A, Fullerton D, Holland J. Behavioural interventions for HIV/AIDS prevention. AIDS. 1995;9: 479–86.

22. Stephenson JM, Imrie J, Sutton SR. Rigorous trials of sexual behaviour interventions in STD/HIV prevention: what can we learn from them? AIDS. 2000;14 Suppl 3:S115–124.

23. Mullen PD, Ramirez G, Strouse D, Hedges LV, Sogolow E. Meta-analysis of the effects of behavioral HIV prevention interventions on the sexual risk behavior of sexually experienced adolescents in controlled studies in the United States. J Acquir Immune Defic Syndr. 2002;30 Suppl 1:S94–105.

24. Johnson WD, Hedges LV, Ramirez G, et al. HIV prevention research for men who have sex with men: a systematic review and meta-analysis. J Acquir Immune Defic Syndr. 2002;30 Suppl 1: S118–129.

25. Semaan S, Des Jarlais DC, Sogolow E, et al. A meta-analysis of the effect of HIV prevention interventions on the sex behaviors of drug users in the United States. J Acquir Immune Defic Syndr. 2002;30 Suppl 1:S73–93.

26. Neumann MS, Johnson WD, Semaan S, et al. Review and meta-analysis of HIV prevention intervention research for heterosexual adult populations in the United States. J Acquir Immune Defic Syndr. 2002;30 Suppl 1:S106–117.

27. Semaan S, Kay L, Strouse D, et al. A profile of U.S.-based trials of behavioral and social interventions for HIV risk reduction. J Acquir Immune Defic Syndr. 2002;30 Suppl 1:S30–50.

28. Honey E, Augood C, Templeton A, et al. Cost effectiveness of screening for Chlamydia trachomatis: a review of published studies. Sex Transm Infect. 2002;78:406–12.

29. Lyles CM, Kay LS, Crepaz N, et al. Best-evidence interventions: findings from a systematic review of HIV behavioral interventions for US populations at high risk, 2000–2004. Am J Public Health. 2007;97:133–43.

30. Institute of Medicine (Committee on HIV prevention strategies in the United States). No time to lose: getting more from HIV prevention. Washington, DC: National Academy Press; 2000.

31. Paltiel AD, Stinnett AA. Resource allocation and the funding of HIV prevention. In: Holtgrave DR, editor. Handbook of economic evaluation of HIV prevention programs. New York: Plenum; 1998. p. 135–52.

32. Brandeau ML. Difficult choices, urgent needs: optimal investment in HIV prevention programs. In: Kaplan EH, Brookmeyer R, editors. Quantitative evaluation of HIV prevention programs. New Haven: Yale University Press; 2002. p. 97–117.

33. Kaplan EH, Pollack H. Allocating HIV prevention resources. Socioecon Plann Sci. 1998;32:257–63.

34. Kahn JG. The cost-effectiveness of HIV prevention targeting: how much more bang for the buck? Am J Public Health. 1996;86:1709–12.

35. Bautista-Arredondo S, Gadsden P, Harris JE, Bertozzi SM. Optimizing resource allocation for HIV/AIDS prevention programmes: an analytical framework. AIDS. 2008;22 Suppl 1:S67–74.

36. Brandeau ML, Zaric GS, de Angelis V. Improved allocation of HIV prevention resources: using information about prevention program production functions. Health Care Manag Sci. 2005;8:19–28.

37. Cohen DA, Wu SY, Farley TA. Cost-effective allocation of government funds to prevent HIV infection. Health Aff (Millwood). 2005;24:915–26.

38. Earnshaw SR, Hicks K, Richter A, Honeycutt A. A linear programming model for allocating HIV prevention funds with state agencies: a pilot study. Health Care Manag Sci. 2007;10:239–52.

39. Lasry A, Carter MW, Zaric GS. S4HARA: System for HIV/AIDS resource allocation. Cost Eff Resour Alloc. 2008;6:7.

40. Richter A, Brandeau ML, Owens DK. An analysis of optimal resource allocation for prevention of infection with human immunodeficiency virus (HIV) in injection drug users and non-users. Med Decis Making. 1999;19:167–79.

41. Richter A, Hicks KA, Earnshaw SR, Honeycutt AA. Allocating HIV prevention resources: a tool for state and local decision making. Health Policy. 2008;87: 342–9.

42. Pinkerton SD, Abramson PR. Model-based allocation of HIV-prevention resources. AIDS Public Policy J. 1996;11:153–5.

43. Bibus DP. A model for distributing HIV-prevention resources. AIDS Public Policy J. 1994;9:197–207.

44. American Social Health Association. Show me the money: state investment in STD prevention, FY2007. 2008.

45. Kates J, Penner M, Kern D, Carbaugh A, Ginsberg B, Jorstad C. The national HIV prevention inventory: the state of HIV prevention across the U.S. A report by NASTAD and the Kaiser Family Foundation. Menlo Park, CA: National Alliance of State and Territorial AIDS Directors; 2009.

46. Summers T, Alagiri P, Kates J. Federal HIV/AIDS spending. A budget chartbook: fiscal year 2002. Kaiser Family Foundation; 2003.

47. Department of Health and Human Services. Justification of estimates for appropriation committees: Centers for Disease Control and Prevention. Fiscal year 2010; 2009.

48. Division of STD Prevention, CDC. CDC history of STD funding. 2009.

49. Centers for Disease Control and Prevention. CDC's HIV/AIDS prevention activities. 2002.

50. Douglas Jr JM. Sexually transmitted infections in young women. Congressional Briefing, 24 April 2008. 2008.

51. National Center for HIV/AIDS, Viral Hepatitis STD and TB Prevention. NCHHSTP state profiles. 2009.

52. Colander DC. Economics. 5th ed. New York: McGraw-Hill; 2004.

53. Kaplan EH, Merson MH. Allocating HIV-prevention resources: balancing efficiency and equity. Am J Public Health. 2002;92:1905–7.

54. Centers for Disease Control and Prevention. Sexually transmitted disease surveillance, 2007. Atlanta: US Department of Health and Human Services, Centers for Disease Control and Prevention; 2008.

55. Cutler JC, Arnold RC. Venereal disease control by health departments in the past: lessons for the present. Am J Public Health. 1988;78:372–6.

56. Holtgrave DR, Pinkerton SD. Implications of economic evaluation for national HIV prevention policy makers. In: Kaplan EH, Brookmeyer R, editors. Quantitative evaluation of HIV prevention programs. New Haven: Yale University Press; 2002. p. 32–52.

57. Hallett TB, White PJ, Garnett GP. Appropriate evaluation of HIV prevention interventions: from experiment to full-scale implementation. Sex Transm Infect. 2007;83 Suppl 1:i55–60.

58. Walker PT, Hallett TB, White PJ, Garnett GP. Interpreting declines in HIV prevalence: impact of spatial aggregation and migration on expected declines in prevalence. Sex Transm Infect. 2008;84 Suppl 2:ii42–48.

59. Heaton LM, Komatsu R, Low-Beer D, Fowler TB, Way PO. Estimating the number of HIV infections averted: an approach and its issues. Sex Transm Infect. 2008;84 Suppl 1:i92–96.

60. U.S. House of Representatives, Committee on Oversight and Government Reform. The domestic epidemic is worse than we thought: a wake-up call for HIV prevention. Committee on Oversight and Government Reform; 2008.

61. Zaric GS, Brandeau ML. A little planning goes a long way: multilevel allocation of HIV prevention resources. Med Decis Making. 2007;27:71–81.

62. The Futures Group International. Resource allocation for HIV/AIDS programs: using the goals model to relate expenditures to program goals. The Futures Group International; 2001.

63. World Bank. Optimizing the allocation of resources for HIV prevention: the allocation by cost-effectiveness (ABC) model. Guidelines. Washington, DC: World Bank; 2002.

64. Cohen DA, Farley T, Wu S. Maximizing the benefit: HIV prevention planning based on cost-effectiveness. A practical tool for community planning groups and health departments. RAND; 2004.

65. Cohen DA, Wu SY, Farley TA. Comparing the cost-effectiveness of HIV prevention interventions. J Acquir Immune Defic Syndr. 2004;37:1404–14.

66. Lasry A, Sansom SL, Hicks KA, Uzunangelov V. Modeling the impact of HIV prevention strategies in the United States. 2009 National HIV Prevention Conference; 2009.

67. Division of STD Prevention. SOCRATES: Screening optimally for chlamydia: resource allocation, testing and evaluation software. Atlanta: Centers for Disease Control and Prevention; 2003.

68. Tao G, Gift TL, Walsh CM, Irwin KL, Kassler WJ. Optimal resource allocation for curing Chlamydia trachomatis infection among asymptomatic women at clinics operating on a fixed budget. Sex Transm Dis. 2002;29:703–9.

69. Chesson H, Collins D, Koski K. STIC Figure. Sexually Transmitted Infection Costs saved. Instruction manual. Atlanta: Division of STD Prevention, Centers for Disease Control and Prevention; 2008.

70. Chesson HW, Collins D, Koski K. Formulas for estimating the costs averted by sexually transmitted infection (STI) prevention programs in the United States. Cost Eff Resour Alloc. 2008;6:10.

71. Karlsson G, Johannesson M. The decision rules of cost-effectiveness analysis. Pharmacoeconomics. 1996;9:113–20.

72. Drummond M, Torrance G, Mason J. Cost-effectiveness league tables: more harm than good? Soc Sci Med. 1993;37:33–40.

73. Mason J, Drummond M, Torrance G. Some guidelines on the use of cost effectiveness league tables. BMJ. 1993;306:570–2.

74. Neumann PJ, Jacobson PD, Palmer JA. Measuring the value of public health systems: the disconnect between health economists and public health practitioners. Am J Public Health. 2008;98:2173–80.

75. Valdiserri RO, Robinson C, Lin LS, West GR, Holtgrave DR. Determining allocations for HIV-prevention interventions: assessing a change in federal funding policy. AIDS Public Policy J. 1997;12: 138–48.

76. Holtgrave DR, Curran JW. What works, and what remains to be done, in HIV prevention in the United States. Annu Rev Public Health. 2006;27:261–75.

77. Holtgrave DR. Measuring the value of public health systems. Am J Public Health. 2009;99:775–6.

78. Weinstein B, Melcchreit RL. Economic evaluation and HIV prevention decision making. In: Holtgrave DR, editor. Handbook of economic evaluation of HIV prevention programs. New York: Plenum; 1998. p. 153–62.

79. Lasry A, Richter A, Lutscher F. Recommendations for increasing the use of HIV/AIDS resource allocation models. BMC Public Health. 2009;9 Suppl 1:S8.

80. Kahn JG, Brandeau ML, Dunn-Mortimer J. OR modeling and AIDS policy: from theory to practice. Interfaces. 1998;28:3–22.

Scaling Up, Coverage, and Targeting

8

David H. Peters, Gita Sinha, and Robert C. Bollinger

In this chapter, we examine the current state of knowledge and practice concerned with scaling up and achieving universal coverage of HIV and sexually transmitted diseases (STD) health services, and targeting interventions to specific populations. Recognizing that routes of disease transmission and the consequences of disease cross international borders, the processes of scaling up HIV and STD prevention programs are inherently global issues. Nonetheless, understanding specific local and national contexts is essential to effectively scale up health programs. As illustrated by the emerging research initiatives and resources for program implementation, there is also a push in the USA to build the theory and evidence to improve program performance and scale up programs that contribute to HIV and STD prevention, both nationally and globally. These issues are of importance not only for HIV and STD prevention programs, but they also raise significant political, economic, social, and technical concerns beyond these programs, for many stakeholders at local and national

levels. These issues have a prominent place on the global health agenda, and particularly for low and middle-income countries and under-served populations, where HIV and STD prevention have the greatest potential to address the largest burden of disease.

The concepts of scaling up, coverage, and targeting in the health sector are related to each other. Although there is no consensus on a precise definition of scaling up, there is an assumption that scaling up in the health sector can be considered "an ambition or process of expanding the coverage of health interventions" [1]. There are more formal definitions of coverage, which can be measured as the extent to which the services rendered cover the potential need for those services in a population in a given time period [2]. This definition of coverage of health services differs from a common but more specific reference to the coverage of health insurance in the USA. Universal coverage of a health service means that everyone who needed a service would receive it. But coverage levels of health services are rarely universal and tend to vary across populations, while the needs for services also differ. In situations where health risks, conditions, or services are not identical for everyone in a population, then targeting strategies are often pursued, usually for those most at risk, or those least able to obtain a health service. There is no standardized definition of targeting in public health, but it can be considered the process of designing and implementing an intervention, program, or policy

D.H. Peters (✉)
Bloomberg School of Public Health, Johns Hopkins University, 615 N. Wolfe St, E8-132, Baltimore, MD 21205, USA
e-mail: dpeters@jhsph.edu

G. Sinha • R.C. Bollinger
Center for Clinical Global Health Education, Johns Hopkins University School of Medicine, 600 N. Wolfe Street, Phipps 521, Baltimore, MD 21287, USA

S.O. Aral, K.A. Fenton, and J.A. Lipshutz (eds.), *The New Public Health and STD/HIV Prevention: Personal, Public and Health Systems Approaches*, DOI 10.1007/978-1-4614-4526-5_8,
© Springer Science+Business Media New York 2013

for a specified and identifiable group of recipients in a broader population or region [3]. In this chapter, we discuss how concepts of scaling up need to go deeper than the simple notions of quantitative coverage of health services, by learning from theories of change about how the processes of scaling up can lead to sustainable effects. In this context, targeting approaches are assessed as ways to improve the effectiveness, equity, and efficiency of health service delivery.

Scaling Up

Scaling up health services has long been an important organizing principle in global health. STD and HIV prevention programs have the potential to address gaps and barriers that have long been recognized in the history of scaling up disease-specific and more general health services. The Declaration of Alma Ata of 1978, with its slogan of "Health for All by the Year 2000," rallied people around the desire to have universal access to primary health care [4]. Many countries have embedded this perspective in their policies and laws, in many cases defining universal access to health services as a human right [5, 6]. Yet the ability to scale up health services to achieve universal coverage has been far from successful. Neither the comprehensive "Health for All" initiative nor the sometimes competing selective primary care approaches, such as the campaign to achieve "Universal Childhood Immunization by 1990," a key initiative of the so-called Child Survival Revolution, were able to achieve their ambitious goals. In the case of the Universal Childhood Immunization campaign, the campaign was not able to sustain high national immunization coverage rates, or in many cases to reach vulnerable populations within countries, despite its successes in obtaining resources, political commitment, and rapidly implementing standardized approaches that initially did achieve high levels of coverage in many countries [7].

Since 2000, when the United Nations General Assembly adopted the Millennium Development Goals (MDGs), the interest in scaling up high impact health services, particularly in low-income countries, has again taken center stage [1]. The MDGs set ambitious targets for reducing child and maternal mortality, combating HIV/AIDS and malaria, and set targets for countries to achieve high levels of coverage for basic health services. The international response to the HIV/AIDS pandemic has also aggressively promoted universal access to antiretroviral therapy around the world. A number of new global health initiatives (e.g., the Global Fund to Fight AIDS, Tuberculosis, and Malaria (GFATM), the World Bank Multi-Country HIV/AID Program (MAP), the US President's Emergency Fund for AIDS Relief (PEFFAR), the GAVI Alliance, the Roll Back Malaria Partnership, and the Stop TB Partnership have each taken up the mantle to promote universal access to specific health services around the world, and have been accompanied by substantial new financial resources [8]. These initiatives have raised expectations to deliver health programs at large scale, including HIV and STD prevention programs. Unfortunately, many countries are not on track to achieve the MDG health goals by 2015 [9], and between one quarter and one half of developing countries are unlikely to achieve the various health service coverage targets [10]. Given the trajectory of countries toward achieving the MDGs, and the large gap between expectations and achievement of the global health initiatives, further investigation into the reasons for shortcomings is needed. This should include an appraisal of the assumptions behind scaling up and a better understanding of what scaling up should mean in practice, and particularly to understand the logic models or theories of change that can guide practice and research that has been notably absent in the discussions around how to scale up to reach MDG targets [11].

Most of the literature concerning scaling up by global health initiatives has implicit assumptions about common pathways to scaling up health interventions to reach common targets. For the most part, scaling up is understood as the replication of specific health interventions that had been shown to be effective in research settings or on a small scale in any developing country, but are subsequently delivered through a better resourced and enlarged public health delivery system. In this regard, HIV/AIDS plans for scaling up are different, since most HIV/AIDS

Table 8.1 Conceptual frameworks for scaling up health services

Name of framework	Author (reference)	Year of publication
A Learning Process Approach	Korten [24]	1980
Alternative Strategies for Scaling Up NGOs	Uvin [25]	1995
Diffusion of Innovations	Rogers [26]	1995
SEED-Scale	Taylor-Ide and Taylor [27]	2002
Scaling Up Management Framework-SUM	Kohl and Cooley [28]	2003
Expandnet Framework	Simmons, Fajan, and Ghiron [11]	2008

programs actively include large numbers of non-governmental organizations (NGOs) for advocacy and service delivery. Nonetheless, for large scale global health initiatives like GFTAM, GAVI, and PEPFAR, scaling up has meant increasing coverage of services through swift disbursement of funds, increasing access to services through more points of service delivery, and expanding partnerships, ensuring sustainable funding and promoting participatory ownership [12–14]. The underlying model of replication is exemplified through a number of articles that estimate the costs of scaling up specific health interventions in these programs. The approach involves multiplying the unit costs of an effective public service delivery system in small area by the number of areas in a country and then around the world, with some adjustments made for economies of scale, but not the interacting effects that different programs have on each other [15]. Similar methods have also been used to estimate human resource requirements for scaling up health services [16]. In the specific case of costing of anti-retroviral therapy (ART) for HIV infection, recent models have tried to take account of the fact that people must take medicines for the rest of their life, and therefore the projected costs must also address the effects of ART on longevity, the likelihood of requiring second line drugs and need for treatment for opportunistic infections [17]. In South Africa, financing the cost of scaling up ART in the context of a scheme for universal coverage of health services would require substantial increases in resources in public health, nearly doubling the proportion of GDP spent on publicly funded health care over 10 years [18].

There have also been a number of recent analyses that look beyond the more straightforward considerations of resource constraints and cost-effective interventions that need to be scaled up. A recent review of the literature identified a number of common constraining factors that need to be tackled in order to scale up in international health, including the lack of absorptive capacity, weak health systems, human resource constraints, and high costs [1, 19]. In analyses that examine success stories, strong leadership and management, realistic financing, and technical innovation were shown to be common characteristics of successful large scale health programs [20, 21]. In a case study comparing the scale-up of three antiretroviral programs in South Africa, Schneider and colleagues found that despite having common models for care, factors related to managerial and political leadership, along with local implementation and monitoring processes, were more important determinants of success than financing or human resource capacity issues [22].

Recognizing that scaling up is not a new concept in the health sector, there is also much that can be learned from previous experience and analysis about how to manage organizational and social change that is clearly a critical component needed to implement and sustain HIV and STD prevention programs on a large scale. In Table 8.1, we present six conceptual models based on experience with scaling up health programs based on a review by Subramanian and colleagues [23]. The six models emerged out of two backgrounds: the concern with how to scale up pilot projects, and the experience with scaling up innovations. None of these models have been applied by the recent global health initiatives. In contrast to the global health initiatives, these analyses are more concerned with the process of scaling up, the adaptability of the innovation or service that is being scaled up, and the capacity of the organizations or communities that are implementing the expansion, which are summarized below.

Models for Scaling Up

Korten defines successful scaling up in three stages: (1) Adequate resources are provided along with technical input, capacity building, and understanding of community culture to demonstrate effectiveness; (2) Inputs per output are minimized along with assuring a good fit between the program requirements and the realistic capabilities of the organizations involved to demonstrate efficiency; (3) Expansion through innovation and increasing organizational capacity to respond to large-scale requirements [24]. The Scaling up Management (SUM) framework developed by Kohl and Cooley builds on Korten's analysis by identifying successful replication when other organizations increase their uptake and use of the innovation [28]. Successful collaboration occurs when formal and informal partnerships and networks are developed.

Uvin's framework identifies NGO expansion in four dimensions: (1) Quantitative — an organization increases size (including increasing human resources, financial resources, and inputs) and coverage of people who are served; (2) Functional — an organization adds new activities or services to its existing work; (3) Political — an organization adds activities involving advocacy, empowerment, and making changes in policies; and (4) Organizational — an organization strengthens and adds variety to its financial sources and mechanisms and its organizational structures and functions [25]. The Expandnet framework defines success when there is an increase in the impact of health service innovations that have been successfully tested in pilot and experimental projects to foster policy and program development on a lasting basis [11].

Rogers described his theories on the diffusion of innovation as focusing on the transfer of knowledge as the basis for successful scaling up of an innovation, with examples involving health behaviors or services [26]. The Taylors' SEED-Scale framework defines successful scaling up in terms of community involvement, where successful community projects are developed and promoted, and transformed into learning centers for other organizations seeking to learn how to implement the innovation, so that the projects are then systematically extended throughout different regions with other groups [27].

Absorptive capacity is recognized as important to the process of scaling up, which has been described in both financial and more operational terms. The current global health initiatives have largely considered absorptive capacity as the ability to spend donor funds on activities related to the MDGs [29], or in relation to the macroeconomic implications of high volume of aid inflows [30, 31]. In contrast, Uvin focuses on overcoming human resource inadequacies, developing efficient systems and policies for the smooth channeling of funds, and providing adequate incentives for efficient and effective use of resources to ensure that organizations have the adequate capacity to absorb and utilize funds for scaling up [25]. Absorptive capacity within the implementing organization has also been described as dependent upon the implementation capacity of the organization (adequate human resources, logistics and supplies, sound management, strong leadership, policy and legal framework set in place, supportive environment, and adequate physical facilities) and the harmonization between the resource and user organization to ensure a smooth process of scaling up [11].

Diffusion of innovations theory stresses that the receptive context/climate of an organization is important to incorporate innovations and increase its absorptive capacity for new knowledge. Characteristics of a receptive context include presence of strong leadership; a clear strategic vision, both for the organization and for scaling up; good management relations; "champions" in critical positions; a climate that is conducive to experimentation and risk-taking; and effective monitoring systems to capture and use important data [32].

There is a similarity in the models for scaling up in their emphasis on process and learning, the adaptability of the innovation or service that is being scaled up, and the capacity of the organizations or communities that are implementing the expansion. Although there does not seem to be a clear advantage of adapting one model over another, they each challenge the utility of any "one size fits all" strategy, and the assumption that strategies can simply be adapted to local conditions. Rather, they indicate that specific strategies need to be developed in ways that are appropriate to individual countries and areas within a country, so that they can better involve and build local institutions and address local contexts. It is also clear that the current focus of global health initiatives on achieving quantitative coverage targets provides little insight for the actions needed for further growth or sustainability. Rather, lessons from the past suggest the need for attention to political, organizational, and functional dimensions of scaling up, as well as the nurturing of local organizations.

Coverage

Up to this point, we have discussed access and coverage of health services in very general terms. Historically, much of the rhetoric has centered on improving access to health services, though there are many different ways of interpreting what this means. Most researchers recognize that "access" is related to the timely use of health services according to need [33]. Although some researchers distinguish between the supply and opportunity for use of services and the actual utilization of health services [34], most view access to health services as including realized need [35]. It is relatively straightforward to define and measure coverage of a health service where a universal need can be assumed. Examples include immunization coverage rates among children aged 12–23 months, or safe deliveries for all women with a delivery in the last year. It is more challenging to measure coverage for conditions that are not easily recognized or do not affect entire populations, such as the proportion of HIV-infected people who

receive anti-retroviral therapy in a given year. Assessing effective coverage is even more challenging. This is defined as the proportion of health gain actually delivered by a health system compared to the maximum health gain that a person with a health need could obtain from the health system, a description that combines the concepts of the coverage of health interventions, the demand for care, and access to quality health care [36]. Methods have been developed to estimate people's health needs and potential gains in health life expectancy [36, 37], but formal measurements of effective coverage are not in widespread use, and rely on the availability of considerable data and contestable assumptions about disability and the maximum effectiveness of interventions. In the case of HIV, estimating effective coverage would require knowing who in the population actually needs specific HIV preventive and treatment services and estimating the amount of healthy life they have gained through the specific HIV services, compared with an estimate of how much healthy life could be gained at maximum coverage and quality of care for those needing them.

In this chapter, we use a framework that builds on longstanding descriptions of access to health services that includes coverage or the actual use of services, but outline the determining factors most commonly considered as constraints to access to health care (Fig. 8.1) [38]. In this framework, the four main dimensions of access each have a supply and demand element, and include

1. Geographic Accessibility—the physical distance or travel time from service delivery point to the user.

2. Availability—having the right type of care available to those who need it, such as hours of operation and waiting times that meet demands of those who would use care, as well as having the appropriate type of service providers and materials.

3. Financial Accessibility—the relationship between the price of services (in part affected by their costs) and the willingness and ability of users to pay for those services, as well as be protected from the economic consequences of health costs.

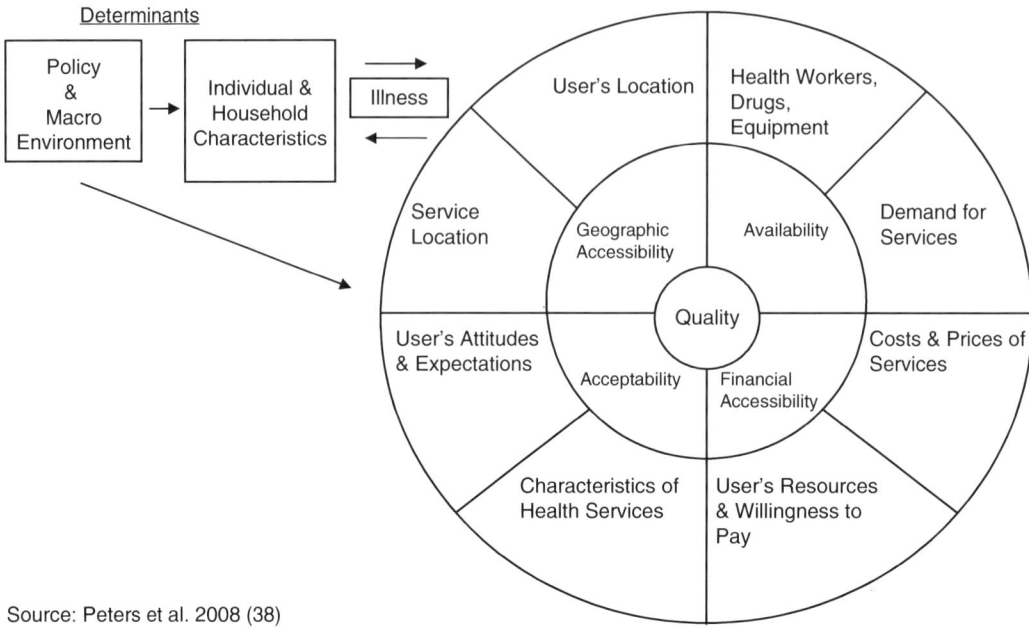

Source: Peters et al. 2008 (38)

Fig. 8.1 Framework for understanding access to health services adapted from: Peters et al. [38]

4. Acceptability—the match between how responsive health services providers are to the social and cultural expectations of individual users and communities.

Quality of care is at the center of the circle of all four dimensions of access to health services, since it is an important component of each dimension, and is ultimately related to the technical ability of health services to make an impact on people's health. To the left of the circle are sets of more distal determinants of health service access, shown at the policy or macro-environmental level, as well as the individual and household levels. Poverty can be examined as a determinant of illness or health needs, as well as by looking at disparities within the different dimensions of health-care access.

One consistent finding in the literature on access to health services is that people in poor countries have less access to health services than those in better off countries, and within a country, the poor tend to have less access to health services [38]. The lack of financial resources and less access to information creates barriers for the poor, though it is important to note the causal relationship between access to health services and poverty also runs in the other direction. The deprivation of poverty leads to ill health, and when health care is needed yet delayed or not obtained, people's health worsens, which in turn leads to lost income and higher health-care costs, both of which contribute to poverty [39, 40]. The relationship between poverty and access to health care is often characterized as a vicious cycle, where poverty leads to ill health, and ill health maintains poverty [41]. As is the case with primary care more generally, STD and HIV prevention programs face similar challenges in overcoming disparities in access to services.

In practice, few national governments have been able to assure that health policies that benefit the poor are successful. Benefit–incidence studies in low- and middle-income countries have shown that in the large majority of countries, public spending on health disproportionately benefits wealthier citizens [42–44]. Among the poorest countries of the world, few have proposed strategies to improve health services or financing to the poor [45].

Within LMICs, there are also large differences between the poor and better off that vary widely between the type of service and the region. Within countries, the poor and other deprived groups tend to have the lowest access to health services, despite their greater need. Gwatkin demonstrated that tertiary and secondary hospital services were more likely to favor the better off than primary care and preventive services [46]. In an analysis of 56 low and middle-income countries, Gwatkin and colleagues further reinforced this point [47]. Medically attended deliveries were shown to have the greatest disparity the poorest and wealthiest quintile within countries, whereas cheaper and more widely available oral rehydration therapy (ORT) and antenatal care showed the smallest disparities among the services they were able to examine. Victora et al. examined co-coverage of maternal and child health interventions across countries and also found large differences between those who received comprehensive health services and those who did not [48]. For example, the percentage of children in Cambodia who did not receive BCG, DPT or measles vaccines, vitamin A supplementation, or safe water was 0.3%, but only 0.8% of children received all of the interventions. In the poorest wealth quintile, 31% of Cambodian children received no interventions and 17% only one intervention. These findings suggest that even greater effort is needed to address the challenge of bringing health services to poor and disadvantaged populations around the world. Of relevance to HIV and STD prevention is that many specific prevention programs need to be integrated into existing healthcare programs. From a policy perspective, a well-functioning health delivery system is considered important for the success of HIV and STD prevention [49].

Targeting

Targeted approaches are intended to address situations where the risks or burdens of a disease or intervention are not shared equally within a population. Ensuring that health programs are targeted to the poorest or most vulnerable populations is a common public policy goal, but one that has challenged governments, funders and implementing organizations for many years. In STD and HIV prevention, targeted approaches, as compared to universal approaches, have gained higher policy and program priority [49].

Targeting in HIV and STD prevention can occur in multiple ways, including the following:

- At the disease/clinical level, researchers, community stakeholders, and/or service providers identify specific clinical, behavioral, and/or social vulnerabilities for acquiring HIV and/or STDs.
- At the program level, newly designed pilot initiatives target specific individuals and/or groups to demonstrate efficacy for HIV/STD prevention outcomes.
- At the policy level, agencies prioritize and allocate resources for program dissemination to implementers serving desired target recipient groups.

Targeting: Importance

In HIV and STD prevention, epidemiology has specified individual- and population-level disease risks and contexts, leading prevention programs and policies to support targeting methods. Targeting is a potentially resource-efficient and logistically feasible method for program efficacy as well as effectiveness. Targeting promotes efficacy by defining the specific characteristics of a new program's recipients, both as warranted in the development phase, and as actually observed during pilot program evaluation(s). Targeting processes can be used as part of a pilot program's further dissemination or scale-up strategy. Consequently, targeting promotes effectiveness by informing how to disseminate impactful programs to recipients in additional, "real world" settings. Effective targeting has the potential to ultimately promote prevention program sustainability in vulnerable populations and settings. Preventing HIV and/or STDs in the targeted population(s) is thought to efficiently and sustainably benefit the wider public health against the broader repercussions of these diseases [48].

Targeting: Approaches

Sources

Most of the time, the relative strength or weakness of a targeting approach is presumed to be linked to the program's end result or outcome, such as the efficacy of the program in a controlled study environment, or the cost-effectiveness of the intervention from a program or policy-related evaluation. There are virtually no published studies or reviews directly comparing "targeted" versus "universal" interventions for HIV or STD prevention; such comparisons are difficult to design and implement. The expanding field of implementation science aims to address some of these major gaps in the science of HIV and STD prevention.

Lessons about targeting are therefore best sought from a wide variety of sources, including primary agency reports, the published literature, and, as increasingly called for, new implementation research efforts. The US Centers for Disease Control has compiled a synthesis of evidence-based HIV and STD prevention interventions that have been evaluated for their implementation and dissemination potential and efficacy, known as the DEBI (Dissemination of Evidence-Based Interventions) project [3]. Additional sources include program reports from major implementing agencies such as the Population Council, Family Health International, state/local health departments, and other policy-defining organizations such as the World Health Organization.

Indicators for Targeting

Targeting is all about defining "who" receives the intervention. In developed country settings, public health surveillance, including methods such as clinical case reporting, contact tracing, and community-based screening, have helped to define specific risk groups who are commonly diagnosed with HIV and STDs, and thus considered the highest priority for prevention interventions. These groups may be defined on the basis of several types of indicators, including the following:
- Geographic location(s)
- Specific risk behaviors
- Access to existing services or "capture points" such as clinics

- Means or capacity to participate in the intervention(s)

In addition to clinical case identification, community- and clinic-based reviews and primary descriptive research studies have helped to define the clinical, behavioral, and social contexts of these highly affected individuals, as indicators of their disease vulnerability. These in turn have led to a number of potential indicators for targeting. Examples include the following:
- Geographic/Environmental/Residential
  - Prisoners
  - Highly disease-prevalent cities/districts/neighborhoods
- Social
  - Age (e.g., adolescents)
  - Gender
  - Ethnicity
  - Socio-economic status
- Behavioral
  - Sexual practices (e.g., men who have sex with men, transactional sex)
  - Drug Abuse
  - Alcohol Abuse
  - Domestic Violence
- Clinical
  - Co-incident diagnoses
  - Culprit symptoms
  - Utilization of STD/HIV testing services
  - Hospital/Emergency Room presentation

Targeting Methods

Practically speaking, in many cases, targeting occurs by circumstance, according to whom an agency or implementer already serves. For example, an intervention is newly designed for a known subgroup or community with which an implementer has a pre-existing relationship [50]. Alternatively, efficacious pilot interventions are disseminated from one target population to a similar target population in a different setting, or, in other cases, adapted to new target populations [50]. DEBI provides a framework for identifying and implementing or adapting an intervention for a target population group. Specific steps include
1. Identifying the target population and its subgroups. Understanding the heterogeneity within a target group is important, from the intervention planning stage.

2. Identifying the specific factors that influence the intervention design and implementation, including clinical and behavioral risk factors.
3. Assessing recent trends in the population, including factors such as demographic changes, mobility, disease, or resource access.
4. Choosing the specific factors/determinants to target with the intervention.
5. Identifying where, when, and how to reach the target audience. The intervention's content is related in great part to the specific behaviors or risk factors that influence the acquisition of disease, but must also account for how readily these risk factors can be identified, accurately, in order to be addressed.

Assessing an implementing agency's capacity is an important factor in the potential to successfully reach an intended targeted population. DEBI guides intervention planners to ask the following questions when assessing target populations:

1. What is the agency history and/or capacity in working with the specified community?
2. What are the behaviors that place the target population at risk for acquisition or transmission of disease?
3. What factors influence the above behaviors?
4. Which one or two factors can be prioritized by and addressed by the agency?
5. What data support the above information? How representative are these data for the target population?

Ultimately, there is no blueprint for effective targeting. Targeting approaches derive from the earliest assessment and planning stages, and continue to evolve as programs are evaluated and further expanded.

Targeting Versus "Universal" Approaches

Researchers, program implementers, and policymakers have yet to resolve the debate of whether targeted versus universal approaches to HIV and STD prevention are more effective. Targeted versus universal prevention strategies have traditionally been framed by characterizing the underlying epidemic as "concentrated" or "generalized." In a concentrated epidemic, the assumption is that disease acquisition and transmission affects

specific, identifiable subpopulation(s), leading to targeted strategies aimed at the group(s) considered most at risk. Historically, a generalized epidemic, defined as affecting over 1% of the general population, has led to prevention strategies aimed at all groups, regardless of classified risk. However, these so-called universal approaches have inevitably faced limited resources for implementation and sustainability, and failure to achieve desired outcomes, such as reduced disease incidence.

Using more sophisticated methods such as multi-level analyses, mathematical modeling, and mixed-methods analyses, recent HIV epidemiology has characterized sexual transmission dynamics and socio-cultural contexts that redefine epidemics as "mixed" rather than simply concentrated versus generalized [51]. Thus, even within traditionally defined generalized epidemics, targeted approaches have been identified. These include prevention strategies for those engaged in high-risk concurrent sexual partnerships, bridge populations between high and low-prevalent geographical settings, and community-based "hotspots" of high-risk sexual behavior such as sex work [51, 52]. "Test and treat" is another evolving strategy, targeting high risk groups to promote 100% HIV testing coverage and early antiretroviral treatment.

Advantages of Targeting

Targeting confers specific advantages over more generalized approaches to HIV and STD prevention. The most cited advantage is that it can enhance the "efficiency" by which the intervention reaches the most vulnerable or "in-need" groups [49]. Additionally, targeted approaches, at their best, enable a deeper understanding of the cultural, social, and other factors for the recipients, making the intervention more relevant, and therefore more utilized and adopted. Targeted programs, when incorporated within and by the community of interest, can support a sense of ownership by the recipients, and directly support the program's effectiveness and sustainability over time.

In contrast, universal prevention strategies may be considered too broad to be effective and the specific messages too diluted to make an impact on specific at-risk groups. The costs associated with reaching all individuals in a population can be considerable. Demonstrating the evidence for efficacy and effectiveness of universal approaches is both challenged methodologically and constrained by prevailing time and available resources.

Disadvantages of Targeting

Targeting has considerable methodological and other disadvantages, particularly in HIV and STD prevention. These include ensuring that the processes of identifying and engaging individuals of interest are feasible, ethical, and accurate. Typically HIV- and STD-vulnerable populations are significantly marginalized from mainstream society, making it difficult to find them, as well as to engage and sustain their program participation. Even agencies or implementers with prior experience with a target group will face the challenge of engaging them with new materials or programs. It is important that the targeting process as well as intervention participation does not stigmatize the participant from the target group itself, or further from the general population.

There are also trade-offs between the methods of targeting and the effectiveness of providing services to everyone who could potentially need a service in a population, and thereby achieve full coverage. For example, interventions delivered in STD clinics are going to reach a select sub-population, which may exclude the at-risk, non-health-care-seeking groups. In contrast, non-targeted approaches are intended for everyone in the population, and have the potential to reach all, including non-identified people or those groups defined as at risk for HIV or STDs.

Despite allocating significant resources to specified groups, targeted interventions face the additional risk of inadvertently "leaking" such resources to unintended recipients: this risk demands continuous and, compared to universal approaches, more intensive process evaluation to ensure that the program is reaching its intended targets.

Effective targeting for vulnerable groups also requires, from the outset, the "buy-in" from

stakeholders and individuals within the identified communities, as well as administrative and policy stakeholders who may oversee priorities in the general population. Rationalizing a targeted approach is intrinsically linked to showing how the program's more limited participation will ultimately benefit the wider population.

The Efficacy and Effectiveness of Targeting: How Do You Know It Worked?

The "reach" of an intervention is one indicator of effective targeting: both for increasing access and utilization of an intervention, and for the content to be relevant to the intended population, as discussed in the RE-AIM framework [53]. Other process measures to demonstrate effective targeting include attitudes toward the intervention, including willingness to share or utilize, or to share knowledge of the intervention with others. Additionally, it is important for the evaluation sample to demonstrate representation of the target population in general. More traditional outcome measures for the intervention, such as population-level disease incidence, and their changes over time, are ultimate, though indirect, indicators of targeting effectiveness. It is important, from the earliest planning stages, that an intervention is designed to measure its ability to effectively target the intended group, and to demonstrate that the impact on the targeted group is of benefit to both that group and the general public health outcomes.

Implementation Matters

It is clear from the above discussion that processes of scaling up and the ability to target health services are very much dependent on how an organization is able to implement health programs in a given context. A recent book synthesized the literature on addressing the challenge of implementation of health services in developing countries [54]. Using a series of systematic reviews, quantitative and qualitative analyses of existing data, and mixed-methods country case studies, the research examined questions of what evidence exists on what strategies work to strengthen health services, as well as how they are implemented in real situations. The good news is that there are many ways that have been shown to improve service delivery. However, there is not a clearly defined intervention or strategy that can be reliably shown to improve implementation of health services, not the least of which is because many interventions have the same label are actually implemented in very different ways in different settings, and are not very replicable in detail. Rather than finding specific interventions or programs that can be well implemented, there are some generalizable lessons on how to improve implementation. It is important to recognize that how a strategy is implemented matters a great deal: the initial and continuous adaptation to local context is associated with more complete strategy implementation, though such adaptation tends to be easier in small-scale interventions. Carefully consulting and involving community stakeholders, particularly those involved with oversight, implementation, and beneficiaries themselves, has been shown to improve outcomes, and is particularly important for being able to utilize local resources and ensure the accountability that is usually needed for sustained and effective implementation. The type of "learning and doing" practices that underlie successful health delivery strategies involves engaging key stakeholders, asking difficult questions about performance and who is benefiting, and using data intelligently to guide decisions, inform stakeholders, and manage incentives to promote good outcomes. Not surprisingly, strategies to improve services for vulnerable populations are more effective when there are explicit plans for benefits to reach the disadvantaged, when there is regular measurement of impact on the disadvantaged, and where there is oversight to ensure that such populations benefit from services.

Although there are examples where careful implementation of an HIV program can strengthen implementation of other services [55, 56], there is insufficient evidence to claim that HIV or other disease-specific programs are an effective way to strengthen health services beyond their specific area of concern. On the other hand, strategies to strengthen implementation of disease-specific programs in one area of a country can be successfully scaled up nationally [54]. Careful process documentation and evaluation, including the definition of any targeting methods, are essential to taking an HIV or STD prevention program from one locale to a larger region or national setting.

Although no specific health program or strategy was identified as one that repeatedly fails to be implemented well, the analysis by Peters and colleagues did identify conditions where strategies to strengthen implementation were more likely to fail [54]. The absence of consistent and strong leadership usually contributes to failure. What appears important is the ability to communicate a clear mandate for implementation from top management that is backed up by clear authorities, resources, and accountabilities throughout an organization. Overly simplistic strategies, such as the ad hoc training of health workers, or introducing simplistic policy changes like the introduction of clinical guidelines by themselves, tend to have little success. Focusing on the institutional support, such as supervision and accountability systems, offers more promise. On the other hand, overly complex strategies that outstrip the management capacity of an organization to provide services also lead to failure. Interestingly, multiple-component strategies to strengthen organizations tended to have higher rates of failure, but also higher average effects when they succeed. This suggests that an important task for planning is to diagnose when a strategy is exceeding the capacity of the service delivery organization, and adjusting efforts accordingly.

Conclusions

Universal coverage of health services, including HIV and STD prevention services, is a central political and public health issue in the USA and around the world. In this chapter, we reviewed some of the historical and current thinking around how to scale up programs to increase access and utilization of health services. Unfortunately, many of the global health initiatives have taken a rather simplistic approach that views scaling up as largely a question of providing more resources to increase coverage of health interventions, and have done little to learn from the past about how to achieve and sustain health programs. History teaches us that understanding context is critical to success, along with the engagement of key stakeholders in the design and implementation of programs, the creation of appropriate incentives and account-abilities, and the use of data for continued prob-lem-solving. We reviewed six perspectives that have much to teach HIV and STD prevention pro-grams on how to scale up and sustain programs.

We also proposed a systematic way to exam-ine questions of access to health services of appropriate quality that also included an exami-nation of both supply and demand side factors affecting geographic access, availability of ser-vices, financial access, cultural and social accept-ability. This provides a framework for problem-solving in a way that recognizes that one size of prevention program cannot fit all cir-cumstances. Recognizing that targeting of health programs is an important strategy for reaching public policy goals, we identified many different ways to target HIV and STD prevention services that should be designed and implemented through a structured process and subject to frequent revi-sion. Such "learning by doing" strategies that use information to empower communities and imple-menting agencies, while holding key stakehold-ers accountable, are important keys to the successful expansion and sustainability of HIV and STD prevention programs.

References

1. Mangham LJ, Hanson K. Scaling up in international health: what are the key issues? Health Policy Plan. 2010;25:85–96.
2. Last J, editor. A dictionary of epidemiology. 2nd ed. New York: Oxford University Press; 1988.
3. Collins C. et al. The Diffusion of Effective Behavioral Interventions Project: Development, Implementation, and Lessons Learned. *Aids Education and Prevention*. 2006.;18(Suppl A):5-20.
4. World Health Organization. Declaration of Alma-Ata; 1978. http://www.who.int/hpr/NPH/docs/declaration_almaata.pdf. Accessed December 14, 2010.
5. Braveman P, Gruskin S. Poverty, equity, human rights and health. Bull World Health Organ. 2003;81(7): 539–45.
6. Hunt P. The human right to the highest attainable stan-dard of health: new opportunities and challenges. Trans R Soc Trop Med Hyg. 2006;100:603–7.
7. Black M. The children and the nations: the story of UNICEF. Sydney, Australia: UNICEF; 1986.
8. Ravishankar N, Gubbins P, Cooley RJ, Leach-Kemon K, Michaud MC, Jamison TD, Murray JLC. Financing of global health: tracking development assistance for health from 1990 to 2007. Lancet. 2009;373:2113–24.
9. United Nations. *The Millennium Development Goals Report 2008*. New York: The United Nations. 2008.
10. Matsubayashi T, Peters DH, Rahman MH. Analysis of cross-country changes in health services. In: El-Saharty S, Siadat B, Janovsky K, Vujicic M, Peters DH, editors. Improving health service delivery in developing countries. Washington, DC: World Bank; 2009. p. 173–202.
11. Simmons R, Fajans P, Ghiron L, editors. Scaling up health service delivery: from pilot innovations to poli-cies and programmes. Geneva, Switzerland: World Health Organization; 2008.
12. PEPFAR. US five-year global HIV/AIDS strategy. Washington, D.C: PEPFAR; 2004.
13. The Global Fund. The Global Fund Annual Report 2007. Geneva, Switzerland: The Global Fund; 2007.
14. GAVI. GAVI alliance handbook: country proposal and monitoring processes. Geneva, Switzerland: GAVI; 2008.
15. Johns B, Tan Torres T. Costs of scaling up health interventions: a systematic review. Health Policy Plan. 2005;20:1–3.
16. World Health Organization. World health report 2006: working together for health. Geneva, Switzerland: World Health Organization; 2006.
17. Leisegang R, Maartens G, Hislop M, Regensberg L, Cleary S. Improving the evidence base of Markov models used to estimate the costs of scaling up antiret-roviral programmes in resource-limited settings. BMC Health Serv Res. 2010;10 Suppl 1:S3.
18. Cleary S, McIntyre D. Financing equitable access to antiretroviral treatment in South Africa. BMC Health Serv Res. 2010;10 Suppl 1:S2.
19. Hanson K, Cleary S, Schneider H, Tantivess S, Gilson L. Scaling up health policies and services in low-and middle-income settings. BMC Health Serv Res. 2010;10 Suppl 1:S1.
20. What Works Working Group, Levine R, Kinder M. Millions saved: proven successes in global health. Washington, DC: Center for Global Development; 2004.
21. Medlin CA, Chowdhury M, Jamison DT, Measham AR. Improving the health of populations: lessons of experience. In: Jamison DT, Berman JG, Measham RA, Alleyne G, Claeson M, Evans BD, Musgrove P, editors. Disease control priorities in developing coun-tries. 2nd ed. Washington, D.C: World Bank; 2006. p. 181–94.

22. Schneider H, Coetzee D, Van Rensburg D, Gilson L. Differences in antiretroviral scale up in three South African provinces: the role of implementation management. BMC Health Serv Res. 2010;10 Suppl 1:S4.

23. Subramanian S, Naimoli J, Peters D H. Scaling Up and the Millenium Development Goals. 2010; *Manuscript under review.*

24. Korten CD. Community organization and rural development: a learning process approach. Public Adm Rev. 1980;40(5):480–511.

25. Uvin P. Fighting hunger at the grassroots: paths to scaling up. World Dev. 1995;23(6):927–39.

26. Rogers ME. Diffusion of innovations. 4th ed. New York: The Free Press; 1995.

27. Taylor-Ide D, Taylor EC. Just and lasting change: when communities Own their futures. Baltimore, MD: The Johns Hopkins University Press; 2002.

28. Kohl R, Cooley L. Scaling Up-a conceptual and operational framework. Washington, DC: Management Systems International; 2003.

29. De Renzio P. Scaling up versus absorptive capacity: challenges and opportunities for reaching the MDGs in Africa. ODI Briefing Paper. London: Overseas Development Institute; 2005.

30. Department for International Development. *The Macroeconomic Effects of Aid.* London: Department for International Development. 2002

31. International Monetary Fund. *Fiscal Policy Response to Scaled-up Aid.* Washington, DC: International Monetary Fund. 2007.

32. Greenhalgh T, Robert G, Macfarlane F, Bate P, Kyriakidou O. Diffusion of innovations in service organizations: systematic review and recommendations. Milbank Q. 2004;82(4):581–629.

33. Campbell SM, et al. Defining quality of care. Soc Sci Med. 2000;11:1611–25.

34. Mooney G, et al. Utilisation as a measure of equity: weighing heat? J Health Econ. 1991;4:475–80.

35. Culyer AJ, van Doorslaer E, Wagstaff A. Access, utilisation and equity: a further comment. J Health Econ. 1992;11:207–10.

36. Shengelia B, Tandon A, Adams O, Murray CJL. Access, utilization, quality, and effective coverage: an integrated conceptual framework and measurement strategy. Soc Sci Med. 2005;61(1):97–109.

37. Lozano R, Soliz P, et al. Benchmarking of performance of Mexican states with effective coverage. Lancet. 2006;368(9548):1729–41.

38. Peters DH, Garg A, Bloom G, Walker DG, Brieger WR, Rahman MH. Poverty and access to health care in developing countries. Ann NY Acad Sci. 2008;1136:161–71.

39. Narayan D, et al. Voices of the poor: Can anyone hear us? New York: Oxford University Press; 2000.

40. Smith J. Healthy bodies and thick wallets: the dual relation between health and socioeconomic status. J Econ Perspect. 1999;13:145–66.

41. Wagstaff A. Poverty and health sector inequalities. Bull World Health Organ. 2002;80:97–105.

42. Castro-Leal F, et al. Public spending on health care in Africa: Do the poor benefit? Bull World Health Organ. 2000;78:66–74.

43. Makinen M, et al. Inequalities in health care use and expenditures: empirical data from eight developing countries and countries in transition. Bull World Health Organ. 2000;78:55–65.

44. Gwatkin DR, et al. Reaching the poor with health, nutrition and population services-what works, what doesn't, and why. In: Gwatkin DR et al., editors. Why were the reaching the poor studies undertaken? Washington: The World Bank; 2005.

45. Laterveer L, et al. Pro-poor health policies in poverty reduction strategies. Health Policy Plan. 2003;2: 138–45.

46. Gwatkin DR. Are Free Government Health Services the Best Way to Reach the Poor? *World Bank, HNP Discussion Paper.* 2004:1–8.

47. Gwatkin DR, et al. Socio-economic differences in health, nutrition, and population: overview. Washington: The World Bank; 2007.

48. Victora CG, et al. Co-coverage of preventive interventions and implications for child-survival strategies: Evidence from national surveys. Lancet. 2005;9495: 1460–6.

49. World Health Organization. Towards Universal Access: Scaling up priority HIV/AIDS interventions in the health sector. *Progress Report 2010.* 2010. http://whqlibdoc.who.int/publications/2010/9789241500395_eng.pdf. Accessed December 14, 2010.

50. McKleroy VS, Galbraith JS, Cummings B, Jones P, Harshbarger C, Collins C, Gelaude D, Carey JW, ADAPT Team. Adapting evidence-based behavioral interventions for new settings and target populations. AIDS Educ Prev. 2006;18(Suppl A):59–73.

51. Wilson D, Fraser N. Mixed HIV epidemic dynamics: Epidemiology and program implications. Presentation at *HIV Prevention in Mixed Epidemics,* Accra, Ghana, February 8, 2011. http://www.aidstar-one.com/sites/default/files/David%20Wilson.pdf. Accessed 15 Apr 2011.

52. Tanser F, Bärnighausen T, Newell M-L. Identification of Localized Clusters of High HIV Incidence in a Widely Disseminated Rural South African Epidemic: A Case for Targeted Intervention Strategies. Presentation at *Conferences on Retroviruses and Opportunistic Infection,* Boston, USA, March 2, 2011. http://www.retroconference.org/2011/Abstracts/41395.htm. Accessed 15 Apr, 2011.

53. Glasgow RE, McKay HG, Piette JD, Reynolds KD. The RE AIM framework for evaluating interventions: what can it tell us about approaches to chronic disease management? Patient Educ Couns. 2001;44(2): 119–27.

54. Peters DH, El-Saharty S, Siadat B, Janovsky K, Vujicic M. Improving health service delivery in developing countries. Washington D.C: World Bank; 2009.

55. Matsubayashi T, Manabe YC, Etonu A, Kyegombe Y, Muganzi A, Coutinho A, Peters DH. The effects of an HIV project on HIV and non-HIV services at local government clinics in urban Kampala. BMC Int Health Hum Rights. 2011;11(Suppl):S9.

56. Walton DA, Farmer PE, Lambert W, Léandre F, Koenig SP, Mukherjee JS. Integrated HIV prevention and care strengthens primary health care: lessons from rural Haiti. J Public Health Policy. 2004;25(2): 137–58.

Cornelis A. Rietmeijer and Mary McFarlane

Introduction

The past 15 years have seen an incredible growth in the number of people worldwide who have access to the Internet whether through fixed or mobile devices. By the end of the first decade of the new millennium, the large majority of Americans were online in one way or another while the number of people living in developing countries are increasingly gaining access as well, mostly through the use of mobile telephones. The digital divide, meaning the discrepancy in access to the Internet and mobile telephony across social, demographic, and geographic strata, still exists but is rapidly closing. In a 2010 survey among adults in the USA, the Pew Research Center found that 80% of white, non-Hispanic adults used the Internet compared to 69% of blacks and 66% of Hispanics [1]. Conversely, Hispanics are leading whites in the use of mobile phone

C.A. Rietmeijer, M.D., Ph.D., M.S.P.H. (✉)
Rietmeijer Consulting LLC
533 Marion Street, Denver, CO 80218, USA
e-mail: kccs@rietmeijer.us

M. McFarlane, Ph.D.
Division of STD Prevention, Centers for Disease Control and Prevention, 1600 Clifton Rd., NE, MS E-02, Atlanta, GA 30333, USA

technology. In 2011, more than 87% of English-speaking US Hispanics owned a cell phone, vs. 80% of non-Hispanic whites. Another Pew study found that, compared to the general American population, Hispanics use their cell phones more often, and they use more features on their phones [2]. In developing countries the use of the Internet and mobile telephones is also rapidly increasing. In 2010, approximately 11% of African adults used the Internet. While considerably lower than the US, there has been a 25-fold increase of Internet use in Africa between 2000 (4.5 million users) and 2010 (111 million users), by far the fastest growth in the world [3].

Simultaneously, another shift has taken place. Originally the Internet was mostly a large repository of information that could be tapped in increasingly clever ways, but the transfer of information was mostly unidirectional, i.e., from the World Wide Web to the end user. In the past 10 years, though, the Internet has become a two-way street, where the uploading of (personal) information has become at least as important as the downloading of data. This has set the stage for the formation of online social networks on websites like MySpace, Facebook, Twitter, YouTube, as well as professional networking sites like LinkedIn, and closer to the STI field, STD Prevention Online (www.stdpreventiononline. org). The efficient way provided by the Internet to allow people to reach other people for a virtually endless range of purposes, may have

S.O. Aral, K.A. Fenton, and J.A. Lipshutz (eds.), *The New Public Health and STD/HIV Prevention:*
Personal, Public and Health Systems Approaches, DOI 10.1007/978-1-4614-4526-5_9,
© Springer Science+Business Media New York 2013

both negative and positive implications for public health. Thus, worries about the Internet facilitating sexual relationships and propagating sexually transmitted infections (STI), including HIV transmission, as well as the contrasting enthusiasm to use the new media as a highly efficient tool for STI/HIV prevention and care could have been anticipated from the beginning.

The purpose of this chapter is four-fold: (1) to provide an updated overview of the scientific literature that has covered the Internet as an environment for STI/HIV risk, prevention and care; (2) to place the major findings from this literature in an explanatory context; (3) to propose avenues for future research and development of innovation at the interface between electronic media and the prevention and care of STI/HIV; and (4) to suggest the role of new technologies in shaping a new approach to public health.

Risk

The use of the Internet for sexual purposes has been well established. While statistics have been difficult to verify, some estimate that the Internet accounts for US$ 2.5 billion in pornography sales annually and is an increasingly important component of the overall pornography industry [4]. Globally, there are an estimated four million pornographic Websites (about 12% of all Internet sites) and over 25% of Internet searches are for pornographic material. More than 25% of US men and over 10% of women admit to using *work* computers to view pornography on the Internet [5]. Of course, viewing sexual explicit material whether online or offline does not cause transmission of STIs and since watching porn predominantly leads to masturbation, it could even be considered "safe sex." Perhaps this is why, published despite its extensive use, there has not been much in terms of scientific exploration of pornography in relation to STI risk or prevention.

However, pornographic sites or social networking sites can also be used to find sex partners and the use of the Internet for this specific purpose has been the topic of intense research interest ever since a string of syphilis infections was linked to

an online sexual network and published in a major medical journal [6]. Since then, numerous studies have been published about online sex seeking and associated risks for STI and HIV transmission, particularly among men who have sex with men (MSM) [7–11]. The general conclusion from these studies appears to be that the Internet may act as a risk-enhancing environment for two reasons: first, people who have Internet partners are more likely to engage in high risk sex acts and second, the efficiency of finding sex partners online increases the absolute number and potential concurrency of sex partners. In terms of the Anderson–May equation [12] both the "β" and "c" factors are increased with consequent effects on R_0. Moreover, even if sex with Internet partners would be equally protected as sex with offline partners (i.e., β stays the same), the absolute number of sex acts and thus the number of unprotected sex acts would increase, and with that the increased risk for STI/HIV transmission.

However, there have been considerable limitations to the early studies. Importantly, some of the studies showing higher risks among MSM who had online partners had as comparison groups MSM who did not have such partners. Thus, to the extent that lower-risk MSM were over-represented in the latter group, having online partners may have simply been a marker for high-risk behaviors and not necessarily a cause [13, 14]. Subsequent studies that examined online versus offline risk behaviors among MSM who had both types of partners, painted a more nuanced picture. A study from the UK, for example showed that HIV positive men who met other positive men online were more likely to engage in unprotected anal intercourse than HIV positive men who met other positive men offline (see discussion on serosorting below). However, regardless of HIV serostatus, MSM were just as likely to have unprotected anal intercourse with partners met online or offline if these partners were serodiscordant or of unknown HIV status [15]. Similarly, a more recent study from the USA showed no association between unprotected anal intercourse and source of partner recruitment, offline or online, among MSM recruited in bars and other gay venues as part of the National HIV Behavioral Surveillance System. While MSM reported slightly higher levels of unprotected anal intercourse with online partners, this association disappeared after controlling for multiple (online and offline) partnerships. Furthermore, men reported higher levels of risk with serodiscordant partners met offline than with partners met online, but this finding was limited to men who reported both online and offline partners [16].

Most of the studies on the relationship of Internet sex seeking and STI/HIV risk have investigated (self-reported) risk behaviors but not actual STIs, and most of them have focused on MSM. While some studies have found a relationship between history of STIs and online risk behaviors [17, 18], there is only one published study to date that has assessed the prevalence of gonorrhea or chlamydia in relation to both recent and longer term histories of online partnering among visitors of an urban STI clinic—and did not find any association for MSM. Interestingly, while internet sex partnering was far less common among heterosexual men and women in this study, there was actually a lower risk for prevalent STIs among heterosexual men and women who reported online sexual partnerships [19]. Explanations for this preventive effect include the possibility that the formation of online partnerships may include more or less intensive communications including risk negotiations before an offline, in-person contact is made. Conversely, typical offline venues such as bars, parties, and bath houses may not be conducive to such negotiations [20]. That these types of negotiations do not invariably result in higher levels of protected sex is illustrated by a special case of sexual behavior negotiation: (HIV) serosorting. Serosorting can be defined as making decisions about protected or unprotected sex based on the (perceived) concordant HIV serostatus of the sex partner. Studies indicate that the Internet may facilitate serosorting, and Internet sex partnering may be particularly common about HIV-infected persons who are looking for seroconcordant partners [21, 22]. Serosorting among HIV-negative persons may be problematic because seronegativity among prospective sex partners cannot be taken for granted, as it depends on when the last negative HIV test occurred and on the veracity of self-reported status. Among HIV seropositive persons, these factors may be less of an issue and serosorting in this group may more likely result in "true" seroconcordant relationships. Foregoing protection in such relationships may be defended on the basis that no further HIV transmission occurs and serosorting as an effective public health prevention strategy is currently under debate [23–25]. Still, there is concern that serosorting among HIV positive persons may result in superinfection with other (potentially resistant) HIV strains and also in transmission of other STIs [25]. In fact, the current epidemic of syphilis among MSM may in part be the result of HIV serosorting.

While the use of the Internet as a communication tool has predominantly taken off among older adults, the use of text messaging is the medium of choice among adolescents and young adults. According to a recent survey by the Pew Research Center's Internet and American Life Project, 75% of 12–17-year-olds in the USA own cell phones and 72% of all adolescents (88% of cell phone users) use text messaging regularly. Texting is by far the most common form of communication among teens: 54% contact friends daily via text messaging compared to 38% who call on a cell phone, 33% who talk face-to-face, and 11% who send an e-mail. A typical teen in this study sends about 50 texts a day. After texting, the sharing of photos is the most popular feature of cell phone contacts. However, teens also experience negative effects of texting, including being bullied or harassed (26% of respondents). A small proportion (4%) of respondents admitted to "sexting," i.e., sending sexually explicit texts or photos; however, 15% reported to have received "sexts" [26]. As with sex seeking on the Internet, there is considerable concern about sexting and some have even considered legislation against it [27]. However, there are no studies to date that link sexting to sexual risk behaviors and STI transmission. Indeed, in a recent study among young Hispanic women, Ferguson found no evidence that sexting behaviors (reported by 20% of the sample) were associated with other high-risk sexual behaviors [28].

So, what is one to conclude? Does the Internet enhance risk behaviors, is it equivocal to risk behaviors, or might it indeed reduce risks, at least for some? One way out of this conundrum may be to see online sex seeking and sex partnering as a complex behavior with both potential risk increasing and risk reducing consequences. The problem is that the studies to date do not provide the level of detail needed to help us better understand online sex partnering. To the extent that online partnering is becoming increasingly common, not only among adolescents and young adults, but increasingly so among older adults, especially those recently divorced or widowed, more research is clearly needed to inform not only potential risks, but also the potential benefits of online partnering and ways that interventions may be developed to lower the former and boost the latter.

Prevention

With the recognition of the Internet as a potential risk environment for HIV/STI risk behaviors came the realization that this emerging risk "venue" could also be used to target prevention messages to those engaging in risky behaviors online. Over the past decade, numerous interventions have been deployed that can be broadly divided in two categories: (1) creation of prevention-oriented Websites that draw potentially at-risk people into education and other prevention activities; and (2) outreach into Websites where online partnering is occurring, e.g., chat rooms of sex-oriented Websites. Generally, the challenge of the former approach is to entice and engage high-risk individuals into meaningful risk reduction activities on Websites that many and perhaps the most at-risk individuals have little incentive to visit. The challenge of the second approach is to negotiate the fine line between gaining access to sex-seeking Websites in a sufficiently unobtrusive way that such presence will be tolerated by site patrons and owners while still offering sufficiently effective interventions to have an impact on risk-taking behaviors.

In their simplest form, prevention Websites, whether stand-alone or in conjunction with other services (e.g., STI clinic or family planning Websites) offer information on HIV and STIs and ways to prevent these infections such as safer sex and regular testing. There are numerous Websites that could serve as examples, including the public Websites of the Centers for Disease Control and Prevention (www.cdc.gov/nchstp) and the American Social Health Association (www.ashastd.org). These sites are generally well-maintained, regularly updated and relatively easy to navigate. However, the information stream is one-directional, there is little or no targeting of information to the individual requesting the information, and the focus of the sites is generally on the provision of information rather than individual-level prevention. Yet, the development of the Internet in recent years, especially its potential for interactivity, has promised the possibility of developing online interventions using the unique characteristics of the Internet, including its ability to quickly process a large amount of data and to execute complex algorithms resulting in a virtually endless array of possible outcomes. For example, to the extent that offline research, including Project RESPECT, had shown that individualized prevention plans based on a person's unique sexual history result in reductions in risk behavior lowering the incidence of subsequent STIs [29], the development of an online version of such an intervention that would create highly individual intervention plans based on computer algorithms driven by an online self-administered questionnaire was technically possible. The fact that this process could be entirely automated with costs largely limited to up-front development coupled with the virtually unlimited reach of the Internet, added to the appeal to develop such interventions. Moreover, a number of computer-based (but not online) interventions had demonstrated technical feasibility as well as efficacy in terms of behavioral modification, including condom use following the intervention [30].

However, there have been relatively few randomized studies of interactive online prevention interventions and the results have been mixed [31]. For example, preliminary results from a study among MSM in the Netherlands, showed efficacy in changing self-reported behaviors among men who were exposed to tailored messages based on computer algorithms when compared to control conditions [32]. An early US-based study also showed some efficacy, but the retention of study subjects in the study was too low to allow the authors to arrive at meaningful conclusions [33]. Retention of samples recruited online has been a challenge in other studies as well and is one of the major impediments in online research. However, retention was good in a more recently published US-based randomized intervention study among 650 MSM, demonstrating a modest, borderline statistically significant reduction in unprotected anal intercourse among men exposed to the highly interactive online intervention after 3 months, but no lasting intervention effect after 12 months [34]. Another, smaller study among MSM demonstrated risk reduction in both intervention and control conditions, however, greater risk reduction with high-risk partners in the online intervention group [35]. An online randomized controlled trial among youth showed very slight increases in social norms supporting condom use behaviors among an online recruited sample but not in a clinic-recruited sample. However, no behavior change in terms of actual increased condom use was observed in this study [36]. HIV testing behaviors among MSM were enhanced in yet another online intervention trial [37], and an intervention among MSM by Bowen et al. demonstrated the short-term efficacy on behavioral predictors, including knowledge, self-efficacy and outcome expectations immediately after the online risk reduction intervention and 1 week later. Finally, a randomized controlled online intervention among MSM in Hong Kong did not show any efficacy [38].

While to date, we are not aware of any of the above-described interventions that have been sustained beyond the study phase, outreach interventions in chat rooms and other sex-seeking environments have been implemented and are ongoing in a number of places (including the popular gay Websites ManHunt and Adam-for-Adam) despite the fact that the efficacy of such interventions has not been studied. The genesis of these interventions, however, is different in that they have mostly originated from health departments extending their HIV/STI partner notification efforts online rather than an academic interest into the development and evaluation of innovative behavioral interventions on the Internet. The foray of health departments' partner notification efforts onto the Internet was prompted by the resurgence of syphilis and other STIs among MSM in the mid-1990s when risk behaviors increased as the perceived threats associated with HIV infection decreased—an unintended side effect of the HAART revolution. As described earlier, the syphilis resurgence was also linked to finding sex partners online and since these partners were mostly anonymous except for their chat room pseudonym (also known as "handler"), outreach into chat rooms was initiated to trace these "pseudonymous" partners [39]. Chat room outreach may go beyond simple partner notification and could include engaging visitors to chat rooms into one-on-one discussions of HIV risks and safer sex. However, as briefly alluded to above, chat room outreach is a delicate enterprise as workers engaged in such interventions must constantly be aware not to overstep their boundaries and jeopardize their presence on the site. To assist the online outreach worker in negotiating the many pitfalls of working in this environment, the National Coalition of STD Directors (NCSD) has issued a set of useful Internet STD/HIV prevention guidelines [40]. Nonetheless, a number of studies suggest that Internet outreach is effective for partner notification [41–44] and anecdotal information suggests there may be benefits for behavioral prevention as well. For example, a recently published study from New York demonstrated that Internet partner notification led to an 8% increase in the overall number of syphilis patients with at least one treated sex partner, 26% more sex partners being medically examined and treated if necessary, and 83% more sex partners notified of their STD exposure [39]. Furthermore, this type of "field work" may be particularly efficient since a single worker can serve a number of Websites simultaneously without having to leave the office. Indeed, as suggested elsewhere, there are no technical limitations to centralizing these services and offering them across state lines, thus further enhancing the efficiency of this approach [45].

An innovative approach to online partner notification has been the stand-alone, fully user-driven inSPOT Website (www.inspot.org). Initially developed in response to the resurgence of syphilis among MSM, the site later expanded to include other STIs and risk populations beyond MSM. This program allows persons diagnosed with or suspected to have an STI to contact their partners by sending them an "e-card" (electronic post cards) specifying the STI they may have been exposed to, with or without the sender's identifying information. E-card recipients are then encouraged to attend STD clinics or other health-care providers for evaluation, diagnosis, and treatment. When promoted in the media, the Website has been shown to draw considerable attention and motivate the sending of e-cards [46]. However, recently published data from two STD clinics, one a randomized controlled trial [47], the other a survey-based study [48], have raised doubt about the program's effectiveness in these settings.

Short messaging service (SMS), a.k.a text messaging on mobile phones is increasingly used for the purposes of STI/HIV prevention. Examples include communication between providers and patients, partner notification, and sexual health promotion and education. While many programs appear to have used SMS/text messaging effectively, few of them have been rigorously evaluated [49, 50]. Still, some studies have shown the effectiveness of text messaging as a reminder system for anti-retroviral therapy [51, 52] and human papillomavirus immunization [53], but not for contraception adherence [52, 54]. SMS reminders were also shown to increase HIV/STI re-testing among HIV-negative MSM [55]. Finally, a recently published randomized study from Australia demonstrated efficacy of an SMS-based intervention to enhance STI knowledge and testing, but no effect was seen on condom use [56].

Care/Services

Online Testing

The introduction of nucleic acid amplification testing (NAAT) for chlamydia and gonorrhea infections in the mid-1990s heralded a revolution in STI control. Where, in the past, specialized clinics were needed to conduct invasive and unpleasant procedures to obtain specimens from the cervix or urethra for chlamydia and gonorrhea culture, NAAT allowed for the testing of urine and self-obtained vaginal or penile specimens that were much less invasive and could be conducted in a variety settings, including the privacy of one's own home. Over the past 15 years, the new testing technologies have allowed for the testing of many more people for chlamydia and gonorrhea and detect many more infections. Indeed, the continued increase in reported chlamydia infections in the US and Europe is probably still due to the increased use of NAAT in settings where chlamydia screening has only recently been introduced rather than a true increase in incidence [57].

The exponential use of the Internet for a virtually unlimited variety of services has led to the development of online STI testing programs. Researchers at Johns Hopkins University should be credited for pioneering in this area with the "I Want The Kit" program (www.iwantthekit.org). This program allows interested individuals to go online and order self-testing kits. After submitting the specimens via mail to the laboratory, they receive chlamydia, gonorrhea, and trichomonas test results within a week and are referred to local clinics for treatment, should any of the tests be positive [58]. A program similar to "I Want the Kit" is the "I Know" campaign targeting young women in the Los Angeles area (www.dontthink-know.org) since 2007 [59]. A large-scale online chlamydia testing program was also recently conducted in the Netherlands, involving over 10,000 men and women [60].

These and other online testing programs have clearly demonstrated a proof of concept: people respond to these campaigns, they order kits, most receive results, and the majority of them will get treated if they are found to be positive. Moreover, these people are not just the "worried well"—the chlamydia positivity rate found in these programs is actually quite high and comparable to the rates found among asymptomatic patients in STD clinics. For example, the "I Want the Kit" program reports 13% chlamydia positivity rates among men [61] and 10.3% among women [58]. A somewhat lower rate (8%) was found among women participating in the "I Know" campaign [59].

However, despite the innovative nature of these programs and considerable expenses incurred in program development and marketing, the overall yield in terms of absolute number of tests submitted and number of chlamydia cases diagnosed is still limited. For example, the "I Know" campaign reported 1,286 tests and 108 chlamydia cases diagnoses during 9 months of the campaign, or approximately 144 positive tests on an annual basis, which represents less than 1% of the 55,000 cases reported for the entire Los Angeles jurisdiction. These limited results occur against the backdrop of substantial expenses for campaign development and implementation and despite great enthusiasm of project staff. A cost-effectiveness analysis of the "I Know" campaign estimated a cost of over $600,000 per quality adjusted life year (QALY) saved, considerably more than the $50,000/QALY that is generally considered cost-effective [59].

To be fair, it could be argued that once the websites are built and the logistics of sending and receiving kits and test results are in place, the marginal cost of each additional test will be falling. However, we also know that the "build it and they will come" slogan does not necessarily hold for online testing; without ongoing and costly marketing and advertising, demand will quickly reduce to a trickle (Denver Public Health, unpublished observation). Yet, there are a number of potential advantages to the concept of online testing that may yet prove to assist with cost-effective scale-up of the intervention. First, since a single Web-based program can be accessed everywhere, there is, at least in theory, no reason why these programs need to be replicated in each STI prevention jurisdiction. A single national

Website could function as well as, and probably better than, a large array of similar programs at the state level. Similarly, there is no need to involve a multitude of laboratories in an online testing program. Once a specimen is in the mail, for the purposes of sample integrity or programmatic logistics, it does not matter much whether the sample is shipped locally or across state boundaries. So, only involving one or few labs is theoretically possible and would substantially increase efficiency since a large volume of specimens would allow for economies of scale, and the training of only a few people dedicated to the program would enhance program quality as well. Finally, marketing and advertising could be centralized and easily included with existing national STI awareness campaigns, like the "Get Yourself Tested" campaign that is launched annually in the US as part of the April STD Awareness Month. In summary, there is proof of concept for online testing programs, but the tipping point for arriving at the status of a viable national STI prevention strategy may only be reached if inherent characteristics of the intervention are fully exploited [62].

Technological Advances in the Clinical Setting

While the real-world feasibility and effectiveness of many innovative online STI prevention programs have yet to be established, closer to home, the use of Internet technologies in the clinical environment, especially the development and implementation of browser-based and Internet-connected electronic medical records (EMR) is rapidly demonstrating its practical applicability. It is true that electronic medical record systems are not always very user-friendly and often involve a steep learning curve, especially for staff not used to working with computers or the Internet. Also, off-the-shelve EMR products are often built with billing in mind and may not meet the specific demands of a public health clinical environment. Yet, there are many advantages to a browser/Web-based system, a number of which will be reviewed below. Foremost, a real-time electronic clinical management system through internal error checks and algorithm-based prompts can greatly enhance the quality of data collection and thus the quality of care delivered. This would include the basics of appropriate clinical examination, diagnosis and treatment, but systems can also be revised to accommodate the inclusion of new clinical protocols that traditionally take considerable time to be fully implemented due to slow clinician uptake. For example, at the Denver Metro Health Clinic (DMHC), prompts were included in the EMR recently to support the implementation of expedited partner therapy (EPT) resulting in a rapid increase in providers offering EPT to eligible partners [63].

Interfacing the EMR with the Internet allows for a number of additional benefits, including real-time connections to other online systems, such as laboratory services and automated transmission of reportable STIs from the clinic to the reporting jurisdiction, not only significantly shortening the reporting time lapse but also avoiding transcription errors and saving considerable clerical time. At DMHC an interface was built to provide STI test results online, currently used by approximately 50% of clients and saving additional clerical time [64]. Finally, a high-quality EMR facilitates program monitoring and evaluation and also allows for effectiveness research. For example, the Safe in the City study, involving over 38,000 patient records across the three participating study sites [65], could not have been conducted at the Denver site without the EMR. Similarly, the Denver STD clinic EMR, in place since 2005, was instrumental in establishing the effectiveness of EPT in reducing chlamydia and gonorrhea re-infections [66].

Closing Comments

The purpose of this book is to examine an integrated view of personal and public health aspects of, and approaches to, STI/HIV prevention in developed country settings, incorporating systems issues that include the use of technologies discussed in this chapter. One of the corollaries of this view is a shift in the STI/HIV prevention research paradigm from one that focuses on efficacy of interventions in a specialized environment, to one that emphasizes the applicability of interventions in the real world setting of compounding public health problems and public health needs. In the context of effectiveness, an intervention's feasibility, efficiency and reach (scale) are key characteristics. The Internet and the increasing use of mobile media offer great promises for all three and it is somewhat frustrating that we have not made greater strides in online prevention offerings beyond their proof of concept. In the closing paragraphs of this chapter, we therefore examine some of the underlying reasons for our seemingly slow progress and offer some suggestions for future interventions and research using the Internet and other electronic media.

First, STI/HIV prevention interventions, however nicely packaged, are not likely to attract much attention from those visitors on the Internet who are not concerned about their risk for STIs. Also, STI risk perception and subsequent behavior change is dependent on cues, for example the development of genital symptoms or having a partner with an STI. In this context it is important to consider that behavioral interventions that have been shown to be effective in reducing STI incidence, such as Project RESPECT [29] and Safe in the City [65], have been conducted in the STI clinical setting. Not only do persons recruited from STI clinics have higher STI risks (and thus an intervention effect may be easier to measure), but also they are acutely aware of their risk, thus creating a "teachable moment"; in terms of the Transtheoretical Model [67], they are "ready for action" to reduce risk behaviors. However, once the crisis subsides, so will the readiness to take action. Thus we cannot assume that once we build our online interventions that everybody will flock to our Websites and will engage in STI risk reduction activities. Rather, we should start to think to bring the interventions to places where at-risk individuals might go to find information. For example, to the extent that it is likely that they would land at information sites developed by CDC or the American Social Health Association, these sites could be expanded to include online intervention programs. Videos form an attractive media that can be produced at relatively low cost (given their reach), have been shown to be effective in high-risk settings [65, 68, 69], and are very popular among teens and young adults. Moreover, in an online environment, they may be selected from a video repository based on automated interactive, risk-based algorithms [36].

As it has proven difficult to develop a large reach for primary STD/HIV prevention interventions online, it is appealing to use large-scale online programs that reach adolescents and young adults, especially on popular social networking sites like Facebook, Twitter, and YouTube. Parenthetically, as this is a rapidly changing field, new networking sites may gain in popularity where others are fading. Consequently, future characteristics and reach of these sites will undoubtedly dictate developments of future online public health interventions. Nonetheless, many STI/HIV prevention programs and organizations have a presence on the most popular sites, yet their effectiveness remains to be determined. Specific risk-reduction interventions have also been developed in these environments and are currently undergoing evaluation (SS Bull, — personal communication). We may also find partners who have an established presence in these environments. Consider for example, Kicesie's Sex Ed [70] a YouTube site posting "vlogs" (video logs) on a variety of sexual health topics. According to YouTube site statistics, these vlogs have been viewed an astounding 298 million times. Collaborations between such sites and STI prevention programs might provide the reach and scale the former has and the latter needs [71]. In this context, it is important to note that the popularity of this Website is in part due to the focus of its contents on sex-positive messages, rather than sexual diseases. Currently, in the STI and HIV prevention field, there is an ongoing discourse on shifting the emphasis from reduction of sexual risk (individual behavior focus) to the promotion of sexual health (population norm focus) [72, 73]. This important offline discourse may prove to have major implications for online STI prevention. In a broader sense, this discourse lives in the context of an ever-evolving and increasingly domineering electronic technological environment that redefines how people learn and think about STIs as well as how public health addresses them.

Acknowledgments The Internet and STD Center for Excellence is supported by the Association for Prevention Teaching and Research (APTR) and the Centers for Disease Control and Prevention (CDC) — APTR/CDC COOPERATIVE AGREEMENT Grant TS-1400.

References

1. Internet and American Life Project 2011 http://www.pewinternet.org/Static-Pages/Trend-Data/Whos-Online.aspx. Accessed 31 May, 2011.
2. Hispanics lead U.S. embrace of mobile technology 2011 http://www.pewinternet.org/Media-Mentions/2011/Hispanics-lead-US-embrace-of-mobile-technology.aspx. Accessed 31 May 2011.
3. Internet World Stats 2011 http://www.internetworldstats.com/stats.htm. Accessed 31 May 2011
4. Internet Pornography Statistics 2006 http://internet-filter-review.toptenreviews.com/internet-pornography-statistics.html. Accessed 30 May 2011
5. The tangled web of porn in the the the office. In: Newsweek; 2008.
6. Klausner JD, Wolf W, Fischer-Ponce L, Zolt I, Katz MH. Tracing a syphilis outbreak through cyberspace. JAMA. 2000;284:447–9.
7. Bull SS, McFarlane M. Soliciting sex on the Internet: what are the risks for sexually transmitted diseases and HIV? Sex Transm Dis. 2000;27:545–50.
8. McFarlane M, Bull SS, Rietmeijer CA. The Internet as a newly emerging risk environment for sexually transmitted diseases. JAMA. 2000;284:443–6.
9. Liau A, Millett G, Marks G. Meta-analytic examination of online sex-seeking and sexual risk behavior among men who have sex with men. Sex Transm Dis. 2006;33:576–84.
10. McFarlane M, Bull SS, Rietmeijer CA. Young adults on the Internet: risk behaviors for sexually transmitted diseases and HIV(1). J Adolesc Health. 2002;31:11–6.
11. McFarlane M, Kachur R, Bull S, Rietmeijer C. Women, the Internet, and sexually transmitted infections. J Womens Health (Larchmt). 2004;13:689–94.
12. May R, Anderson R. Transmission dynamics of HIV infection. Nature. 1987;326:137–42.
13. Rietmeijer CA, Bull SS, McFarlane M. Sex and the internet. AIDS. 2001;15:1433–4.
14. Rietmeijer CA, Bull SS, McFarlane M, Patnaik JL, Douglas Jr JM. Risks and benefits of the internet for populations at risk for sexually transmitted infections (STIs): results of an STI clinic survey. Sex Transm Dis. 2003;30:15–9.
15. Bolding G, Davis M, Hart G, Sherr L, Elford J. Gay men who look for sex on the Internet: is there more HIV/STI risk with online partners? AIDS. 2005;19:961–8.

16. Jenness SM, Neaigus A, Hagan H, Wendel T, Gelpi-Acosta C, Murrill CS. Reconsidering the internet as an HIV/STD risk for men who have sex with men. AIDS Behav. 2010;14:1353–61.
17. Daneback K, Mansson SA, Ross MW. Using the Internet to find offline sex partners. Cyberpsychol Behav. 2007;10:100–7.
18. Elford J, Bolding G, Sherr L. Seeking sex on the Internet and sexual risk behaviour among gay men using London gyms. AIDS. 2001;15:1409–15.
19. Al-Tayyib AA, McFarlane M, Kachur R, Rietmeijer CA. Finding sex partners on the internet: what is the risk for sexually transmitted infections? Sex Transm Infect. 2009;85:216–20.
20. Rietmeijer CA, Lloyd LV, McLean C. Discussing HIV serostatus with prospective sex partners: a potential HIV prevention strategy among high-risk men who have sex with men. Sex Transm Dis. 2007;34: 215–9.
21. Grov C, DeBusk JA, Bimbi DS, Golub SA, Nanin JE, Parsons JT. Barebacking, the Internet, and harm reduction: an intercept survey with gay and bisexual men in Los Angeles and New York City. AIDS Behav. 2007;11:527–36.
22. Berry M, Raymond HF, Kellogg T, McFarland W. The Internet, HIV serosorting and transmission risk among men who have sex with men, San Francisco. AIDS. 2008;22:787–9.
23. Snowden JM, Raymond HF, McFarland W. Seroadaptive behaviours among men who have sex with men in San Francisco: the situation in 2008. Sex Transm Infect. 2011;87:162–4.
24. Eaton LA, Kalichman SC, O'Connell DA, Karchner WD. A strategy for selecting sexual partners believed to pose little/no risks for HIV: serosorting and its implications for HIV transmission. AIDS Care. 2009;21:1279–88.
25. Meeting Summary: "Consultation on Serosorting Practices among Men who Have Sex with Men" 2009 http://www.cdc.gov/hiv/topics/research/resources/other/serosorting.htm. Accessed 30 May 2011
26. The New Centrality of Mobile Phones:How adolescents text & talk with friends and how that compares with other forms of interpersonal communication. 2011. http://www.pewinternet.org/Presentations/2011/Mar/~/media/Files/Presentations/2011/Mar/SRCD_Teens_Texting_talking_w_Friends_033111_pdfLenhart.pdf. Accessed 31 May 2011.
27. Illinois lawmakers send sexting bill to governor. 2010. http://articles.chicagotribune.com/2010-04-27/news/ct-met-sexting-bill-0428-20100427_1_sexting-lieutenant-governor-quinn-spokesman-bob-reed. Accessed 31 May 2011.
28. Ferguson CJ. Sexting Behaviors Among Young Hispanic Women: Incidence and Association with Other High-risk Sexual Behaviors. The Psychiatric quarterly 2010.
29. Kamb ML, Fishbein M, Douglas Jr JM. et al. Efficacy of risk-reduction counseling to prevent human immunodeficiency virus and sexually transmitted diseases: a randomized controlled trial. Project RESPECT Study Group. JAMA. 1998;280:1161–7.
30. Noar SM, Black HG, Pierce LB. Efficacy of computer technology-based HIV prevention interventions: a meta-analysis. AIDS. 2009;23:107–15.
31. Chiasson MA, Hirshfield S, Rietmeijer C. HIV prevention and care in the digital age. J Acquir Immune Defic Syndr. 2010;55 Suppl 2:S94–7.
32. Davidovich U, De Wit J, Stroebe W. Using the Internet to reduce risk of HIV infection in steady relationships. A randomized controlled trial of a tailored intervention for gay men. Amsterdam: Roel & Uitgeefprojecten; 2006.
33. Bull SS, Lloyd L, Rietmeijer C, McFarlane M. Recruitment and retention of an online sample for an HIV prevention intervention targeting men who have sex with men: the Smart Sex Quest Project. AIDS Care. 2004;16:931–43.
34. Rosser BR, Oakes JM, Konstan J, et al. Reducing HIV risk behavior of men who have sex with men through persuasive computing: results of the Men's INTernet Study-II. AIDS. 2010;24:2099–107.
35. Carpenter KM, Stoner SA, Mikko AN, Dhanak LP, Parsons JT. Efficacy of a web-based intervention to reduce sexual risk in men who have sex with men. AIDS Behav. 2010;14:549–57.
36. Bull S, Pratte K, Whitesell N, Rietmeijer C, McFarlane M. Effects of an Internet-based intervention for HIV prevention: the Youthnet trials. AIDS Behav. 2009;13:474–87.
37. Blas MM, Alva IE, Carcamo CP, et al. Effect of an online video-based intervention to increase HIV testing in men who have sex with men in Peru. PLoS One. 2010;5:e10448.
38. Lau JT, Lau M, Cheung A, Tsui HY. A randomized controlled study to evaluate the efficacy of an Internet-based intervention in reducing HIV risk behaviors among men who have sex with men in Hong Kong. AIDS Care. 2008;20:820–8.
39. Ehlman DC, Jackson M, Saenz G, et al. Evaluation of an innovative internet-based partner notification program for early syphilis case management, Washington, DC, January 2007-June 2008. Sex Transm Dis. 2010;37:478–85.
40. National Guidelines for Internet-based STD and HIV Prevention 2008. http://www.stdpreventiononline.org/index.php/resources/detail/277. Accessed 30 May 2011.
41. CDC. Internet use and early syphilis infection among men who have sex with men. MWR Morb Mortal Wkly Rep 2003;52:1229–32.
42. CDC. Using the Internet for partner notification of sexually transmitted diseases--Los Angeles County, California, 2003. MMWR Morb Mortal Wkly Rep 2004;53:129-31.
43. Mimiaga MJ, Fair AD, Tetu AM, et al. Acceptability of an internet-based partner notification system for sexually transmitted infection exposure among men who have sex with men. Am J Public Health. 2008;98:1009–11.

44. Hogben M, Kachur R. Internet partner notification: another arrow in the quiver. Sex Transm Dis. 2008;35:117–8.

45. Rietmeijer CA, McFarlane M. STI prevention services online: moving beyond the proof of concept. Sex Transm Dis. 2008;35:770–1.

46. Levine D, Woodruff AJ, Mocello AR, Lebrija J, Klausner JD. inSPOT: the first online STD partner notification system using electronic postcards. PLoS Med. 2008;5:e213.

47. Kerani RP, Fleming M, Deyoung B, Golden MR. A Randomized, Controlled Trial of inSPOT and Patient-Delivered Partner Therapy for Gonorrhea and Chlamydial Infection Among Men Who Have Sex With Men. Sex Transm Dis. 2011;38:941–6.

48. Rietmeijer CA, Westergaard B, Mickiewicz TA, et al. Evaluation of an Online Partner Notification Program. Sex Transm Dis. 2011;38(5):359–64.

49. Lim MS, Hocking JS, Hellard ME, Aitken CK. SMS STI: a review of the uses of mobile phone text messaging in sexual health. Int J STD AIDS. 2008;19:287–90.

50. Swendeman D, Rotheram-Borus MJ. Innovation in sexually transmitted disease and HIV prevention: internet and mobile phone delivery vehicles for global diffusion. Curr Opin Psychiatry. 2010;23:139–44.

51. Kelly JD, Giordano TP. Mobile phone technologies improve adherence to antiretroviral treatment in a resource-limited setting: a randomized controlled trial of text message reminders. AIDS. 2011;25:1137.

52. Pop-Eleches C, Thirumurthy H, Habyarimana J, et al. Mobile phone technologies improve adherence to antiretroviral treatment in a resource-limited setting: a randomized controlled trial of text message reminders. AIDS. 2011;25:825–34.

53. Kharbanda E, Stockwell M, Fox H, Andres R, Lara M, Rickert V. Text message reminders to promote human papillomavirus vaccination. Vaccine. 2011;29:2537–41.

54. Hou M, Hurwitz S, Kavanagh E, Fortin J, Goldberg A. Using daily text-message reminders to improve adherence with oral contraceptives: a randomized controlled trial. Obstet Gynecol. 2010;116(3):633–40.

55. Bourne C, Knight V, Guy R, Wand H, Lu H, McNulty A. Short message service reminder intervention doubles sexually transmitted infection/HIV re-testing rates among men who have sex with men. Sex Transm Infect. 2011;87:229–31.

56. Lim MS, Hocking JS, Aitken CK, et al. Impact of text and email messaging on the sexual health of young people: a randomised controlled trial. J Epidemiol Community Health. 2012;66(1):69–74.

57. Prevention CfDCa. Sexually Transmitted Disease Surveillance 2009. Atlanta: Department of Health and Human Service; 2010.

58. Gaydos CA, Dwyer K, Barnes M, et al. Internet-based screening for Chlamydia trachomatis to reach non-clinic populations with mailed self-administered vaginal swabs. Sex Transm Dis. 2006;33:451–7.

59. Kerndt P, Rotblatt H, Papp J, Gift TL. "I Know:" Combining Home Testing Technology, Social Marketing, & Lessons From E-Commerce to Fight Chlamydia & Gonorrhea Disparities Among Young Women In: 2010 STD Prevention Conference. Atlanta; 2010.

60. Greenland KE, Op de Coul EL, van Bergen JE, et al. Acceptability of the Internet-Based Chlamydia Screening Implementation in the Netherlands and Insights Into Nonresponse. Sex Transm Dis. 2011;38(6):467–74.

61. Chai SJ, Aumakhan B, Barnes M, et al. Internet-based screening for sexually transmitted infections to reach nonclinic populations in the community: risk factors for infection in men. Sex Transm Dis. 2010;37:756–63.

62. Online STI Testing—Moving Beyond the Proof of Concept. 2011. http://www.stdpreventiononline.org/index.php/blog/edit/817.)

63. Mickiewicz TA, Al-Tayyib AA, Mettenbrink C, Rietmeijer CA. Implemetation of an Expedited Partner Therapy (EPT) Program in an Inner-City STD Clinic in Denver, CO. In: 19th Meeting of the Interational Society for STD Research. Quebec City, Canada; 2011.

64. Ling SB, Richardson DB, Mettenbrink CJ, et al. Evaluating a Web-Based Test Results System at an Urban STI Clinic. Sex Transm Dis. 2010;37(4):259–63.

65. Warner L, Klausner JD, Rietmeijer CA, et al. Effect of a brief video intervention on incident infection among patients attending sexually transmitted disease clinics. PLoS Med. 2008;5:e135.

66. Mickiewicz TA, Al-Tayyib AA, Mettenbrink C, Rietmeijer CA. Use and Effectiveness of Expedited Partner Therapy in an Inner-City STD Clinic In: 19th Meeting of the International Society for STD Research. Quebec City, Canada; 2011.

67. Norcross J, Krebs P, Prochaska J. Stages of change. J Clin Psychol. 2011;67:143–54.

68. O'Donnell LN, Doval AS, Duran R, O'Donnell C. Video-based sexually transmitted disease patient education: its impact on condom acquisition. Am J Public Health. 1995;85:817–22.

69. O'Donnell L, San Doval A, Duran R, O'Donnell CR. The effectiveness of video-based interventions in promoting condom acquisition among STD clinic patients. Sex Transm Dis. 1995;22:97–103.

70. Kicesie's Sex Ed. 2011. http://www.youtube.com/user/kicesie?blend=1&ob=5. Accessed 1 June 2011.

71. Blogging and You-Tube: Homegrown Internet Education 2010. http://cdc.confex.com/cdc/std2010/webprogram/Paper21656.html.

72. Swartzendruber A, Zenilman J. A national strategy to improve sexual health. JAMA. 2010;304:1006.

73. Sexual Health. 2011. http://www.cdc.gov/sexual-health/. Accessed 20 October 2011

Twenty-First Century Leadership for Public Health and HIV/STI Prevention

10

Kevin A. Fenton

Introduction

As we enter the second decade of the twenty-first century, the epidemic spread of HIV and other sexually transmitted infections (STI) presents severe and pervasive challenges for public health [1]. With more than 33 million people infected with HIV globally, and more than 45 million acquiring new STIs annually, the resultant morbidity and mortality associated with undiagnosed or untreated disease are major public health concerns in developed and developing country settings [2]. Accompanying this growing and substantial disease burden are concerns about the ability and capacity of existing public health systems to meet current and future needs. Among the many challenges facing HIV and STI prevention programs is the complex and evolving nature of the available interventions which need to be selected, targeted, combined, and implemented by a range of community, clinical, programmatic,

Disclaimer
The findings and conclusions in this chapter are those of the author and do not necessarily represent the views of the Centers for Disease Control and Prevention or the Agency for Toxic Substances and Disease Registry.

K.A. Fenton, M.D., Ph.D. (✉)
National Center for HIV/AIDS, Viral Hepatitis, STD, and TB Prevention; Centers for Disease Control and Prevention, 1600 Clifton Road, NE, Mailstop E07, Atlanta, GA 30333, USA
e-mail: kfenton@cdc.gov

and policy participants [3]. Unlike the clinical workforce that is well defined with clear accreditation systems, the boundaries of the HIV/STI prevention workforce are not always well defined. This absence of uniformity affects the strategic positioning and accountability of HIV/STI prevention programs at the national and local levels, as well as the coordination, consistency, and quality of HIV/STI prevention services [4].

From a broader systems perspective, another challenge facing HIV/STI prevention is the diffuse locus of control for effecting change, monitoring progress, and ensuring quality and accountability. The overall leadership and governance of prevention and public health programs remain a complex but critical component of the health system. Successful implementation and scale-up of prevention programs often necessitate overseeing and guiding the whole health system—including private, public, and community sectors—and require both political action and technical solutions. It also involves reconciling competing demands for limited resources, in changing circumstances, with rising performance expectations [5]. While it is often the responsibility of public health leaders and governments to oversee effective national and local HIV/STI prevention responses, this does not mean that all leadership and governance functions can or should be carried out by central ministries or departments of health [6, 8].

Effective public health leadership, including leadership for HIV/STI prevention and sexual health programs, encompasses mastery of a

S.O. Aral, K.A. Fenton, and J.A. Lipshutz (eds.), *The New Public Health and STD/HIV Prevention: Personal, Public and Health Systems Approaches*, DOI 10.1007/978-1-4614-4526-5_10, © Springer Science+Business Media New York 2013 range of competencies including policy making, management, coalition building, regulation, systems thinking and design, accountability, and communication. Grabowski [7] argues that leadership in the public health setting is a challenging, highly visible activity that requires individuals to innovate ideas, to execute agency objectives, to motivate and guide personnel, to plan and allocate agency resources, to sense and respond to changes in an agency's environment, and to relate their actions to the needs of the general population. Yet, despite these challenging demands, there is currently no standardized blueprint for effective public health leadership and governance of sexual health or HIV/STI prevention programs, and there has been little attention to systematically defining factors that influence the development and maintenance of strong leadership within these fields [8]. Given the opportunities for improving care, treatment, prevention, and research, and the need to balance demands for limited resources, effective leadership that fosters collaboration is urgently needed to advance change in complex and under-resourced health systems.

This chapter examines leadership and governance as essential building blocks of effective health systems, robust public health responses, and ultimately, effective HIV/STI prevention and sexual health programs in western industrialized settings. It begins by examining some of the challenges facing the public health workforce and critically examines the evolving definitions of leadership within the context of public health, HIV/STI prevention, and sexual health programs. Case studies of innovative ways in which leadership development for the new public health is being conceptualized, packaged, and integrated into training programs for public health and sexual health workers are explored. The chapter ends by identifying key domains for strengthening leadership for HIV/STI prevention and the new public health.

The Public Health Workforce Challenges

Public health workers may be defined as all persons responsible for providing the essential services of public health regardless of the organization in which they work [9]. The public health workforce is a complex mix of health, social service, and other professionals from many disciplines inside and outside the health and social service sectors. While the core of the public health workforce is easier to identify, the rest of the workforce merges with many other groups who have overlapping or congruent missions [10].

For example, in the USA, the term "public health workforce" is frequently used to define individuals employed by State and local health-related agencies who design and implement programs, policies, and allied activities aimed at improving the community's health. The public health workforce may also be considered to include other professionals—for example, those working in academia who educate students, train practitioners, or perform research—whose actions influence, inform, or contribute to the public's health [10]. Additionally, as private sector health care delivery organizations provide more community-based public health services, their employees could also be considered part of the public health workforce [10]. Finally, given our current understanding of the social determinants of health [11, 12], individuals from many sectors of a community (e.g., education and economic development) influence health and well-being [13].

Impact of the Global Economic Downturn

Whichever definition is used, there are a number of threats that require urgent responses facing the public health workforce in economically advanced industrialized countries. These challenges are likely to have tremendous impacts on our ability to effectively address HIV/STI prevention and other public health needs during the next decade. Chief among these challenges is the recent global economic downturn [14, 15], which threatens, or is resulting in, unprecedented restrictions in the size, scope, funding, support, and performance of public health programs. Many countries are now grappling with record budget deficits and have responded by restricting public spending, eliminating duplication and waste, and fundamentally rethinking the role of government in providing safety net and support services. Health system transformation and reorganization is the order of the day in many developed countries as governments look for ways to reduce health care spending and increase value for money, while driving towards increased health impact.

The impact of the global recession is tangible, and has been devastating to local public health. In the USA, the National Alliance of State and Territorial AIDS Directors (NASTAD) found that 54% of state health departments experienced a budget reduction in federal Fiscal Year 2009 and 71% anticipated reductions in Fiscal Year 2010—greatly impacting HIV prevention staff capacity, through staff furloughs, hiring freezes, elimination of positions, and early retirement [16]. Similar challenges to the public sector workforce are being experienced in the United Kingdom; these challenges force the remaining public health workers to try to do more for more people with fewer resources. The global financial crisis, however, is one of a number of challenges to public health programs and the workforce [17]. Others include workforce ageing, diversity, technological and programmatic reforms, and migration.

Workforce Ageing

In the USA, public health leaders, and indeed the entire public health workforce, are ageing [18]. The average health department-based public health worker is 47 years old—7 years older than the rest of the US workforce. Soon, a large portion of the national public health workforce, including the leadership cadre, will be retiring. Current estimates suggest that 23% of the current workforce—almost 110,000 workers—will be eligible to retire by 2012 [18]. The public health workforce is diminishing over time (there were 50,000 fewer public health workers in 2000 than in 1980); a trend accelerated by the global economic downturn, which has resulted in unprecedented reductions in staff cadre and a consequential shrinking, in the USA, of HIV/STI prevention capacity. The Association of Schools of Public Health (ASPH) estimates that 250,000 more public health workers will be needed by 2020 [19], and that to replenish the workforce and avert a crisis, schools of public health will have to train three times the current number of graduates over the next 11 years. The ageing workforce has major implications for sexual health programs since this loss translates into dissolution of critical expertise and leadership at a time when programs are facing tremendous fiscal challenges; when longstanding and robust professional relationships and partnerships are critical for the survival of programs; and when there is an urgent need to mentor, train, and support the next generation of sexual health workers, both in the community and government sectors.

Workforce Diversity

In addition to the overall worker shortage, the lack of diversity in some public health professions raises special concern [20]. These concerns are heightened for those working in sexual health in western industrialized settings, given the increasing concentration of adverse sexual health outcomes among the poor, racial/ethnic and sexual minorities—the socioeconomically disadvantaged who have limited access to curative services without subsidies and others who have high prevalence of risk behaviors [21, 22]. A more diverse public health workforce is needed to help ensure that health services and decisions made about health care reflect the values and beliefs of the entire population, and are provided with cultural sensitivity by people with whom the public identifies [23]. In the USA, underrepresented ethnic/racial groups comprise 25% of the population but only 10% of health professionals—a percentage that is growing very modestly. For example, Hispanics account for 12% of the US population, but only 2% of nurses and 3.5% of physicians. Less than 1 in 20 African Americans are doctors or dentists, even though 1 in 8 persons in the USA are African American [20]. By increasing the number of underrepresented groups in the health professions, many existing health disparities may more likely be reduced because of a higher sensitivity to the needs, values, and cultures of minority and underserved populations. Although the diversity of the public health workforce has improved over the last 30 years, there remains a need to continue recruitment efforts to sustain past gains by attracting students and new professionals to the public health fields.

Succession Planning

Economic challenges and a workforce that is both ageing and lacking in needed diversity requires that the field of public health plan for, develop, and train a new, and more diverse, generation of leaders at local, state, and federal levels. The largest barrier to the adequate staffing of governmental public health agencies is a shrinking or constant budget [20]. Budget constraints result in both limited numbers of positions and staff receiving noncompetitive salaries for high levels of responsibility and heavy workloads. These factors often push workers to the private sector, which often offers higher salaries and benefits, and less overall responsibility. Succession planning—the continuous process and critical strategy an organization employs to ensure effective leadership despite staff turnover, including identifying how executive positions will be filled—is critical [18, 24]. Succession plans may include preparing talent from within an organization, or planning recruitment activities for external candidates, and are especially important in an economic environment and job market in which agencies will be increasingly competing for experienced leaders. These plans are also important to ensure that public health agencies minimize risk to the populations they serve and maintain a reliably strong response system in the case of emergencies [18].

Using Technology to Improve Communication and Information Management

Inadequate knowledge exists about the competencies and related training and education resources the public health and sexual health workforce will need to meet future challenges. Increasingly complex and matrix-managed health systems demand the emergence of new ways to build constituencies, to develop interoperable electronic health systems, and to grow relevant public health leadership. Similarly, knowledge and understanding of telecommunications and information technology will need to be quickly and appropriately harnessed [25]. This includes understanding which information-based technologies can best support public health goals, and which communications technologies are the most appropriate for a specific cause (e.g., intervention, and prevention). The Internet, World Wide Web, and corporate and private intranets offer great potential for the lifelong training and education of public health workers [26]. These same technologies also provide an infrastructure for integrating national efforts with local community needs and concerns [26].

Migration of Health Leaders

A more general challenge facing the global public health workforce is the migration of highly educated and trained health personnel away from countries with health systems in crisis. While the international migration of health personnel can bring mutual benefits to both source and destination countries, the balance of gains and losses of health personnel migration should have a net positive impact on the health systems of developing countries [27]. Globally, the debate on international health worker recruitment and its impact on health systems has been intense in recent years [28–30]. In resolution WHA57.19, the World Health Assembly (WHA) noted with concern that, "highly trained and skilled health personnel from the developing countries continue to emigrate at an increasing rate to certain countries," thereby weakening health systems in the countries of origin [31]. In May 2006, the WHA adopted Resolution WHA59.23 [32] urging Member States to affirm their commitment to the education and training of more health workers. This Resolution gave the World Health Organization (WHO) a mandate to: (1) provide technical support to Member States, as needed, in their efforts to revitalize health education and training institutions, and rapidly increase the health workforce; (2) encourage global health partners to support education and training institutions; (3) encourage Member States to engage in partnerships intended to improve the capacity and quality of health-professional education in developing countries; and (4) encourage and support Member States in the development of health-workforce planning teams and the use of innovative approaches to teaching, including the use of information and communications technology.

Ultimately, the mobilization and strengthening of human resources for health is central to combating health crises in both developed and developing country settings and is crucial for building sustainable health systems. Nearly all countries are challenged by worker shortage, skill-mix imbalance, weak knowledge base, inadequate investment, and migration. Within the context of the new public health, workforce planning, capacity building, and leadership development are shared problems requiring shared responsibility and strategic action.

What Is Leadership?

Public health scholars have long recognized that effective leadership is a necessary requirement for the effective translation of existing knowledge about the prevention and control of disease into policies that lead to longer and healthier lives [33]. Rowitz [34] defines leadership as creativity in action, and the ability to see the present in terms of the future while maintaining respect for the past. He goes on to say that, "leading is in part a visionary endeavor, but it requires the fortitude and flexibility needed to put vision into action and the ability to work with others and to follow when someone else is the better leader." Leadership and governance is 1 of the 6 WHO building blocks of a health system described in its Framework for Action, *Strengthening Health Systems to Improve Health Outcomes* [35]. Public health leadership includes a commitment to the community and the values for which it stands [36]. Such a community perspective requires a

systems thinking orientation. It also requires a commitment to social justice that is as strong as our commitment to a well-designed public health agenda.

Dimensions of Leadership

Leaders are especially important as they establish organizational values and purpose and the shared norms that act as a contract with their staff and colleagues, which may, in turn, foster positive performance [37]. In general, leaders need to be good managers or have good managers around them, although leadership itself is more about vision (ends) and management more about mission (means) [34]. The management and leadership continuum gives some guidance to understanding the differences between managers and leaders, although skill sets do overlap [38]. Leaders in organizations and programs should remember that strong leadership with weak management is no better, and is sometimes actually worse, than the reverse. The real challenge is to combine strong leadership and strong management and use each to balance the other [39]. In examining strategic management in government, Moore [40] summarized the three most important aspects of every public manager's job as including: (1) Establishing the value of their purpose and vision; (2) Managing upwards, towards the interface with politics, to invest their purpose with legitimacy and support; and (3) Managing downwards, towards their staff, to improve the organization's capabilities to achieve the desired purpose. Ultimately, leadership is about managing and coping with change—leaders and organizations need to work with the external environment to create change [41]. This is especially pertinent given the tremendous social, cultural, and economic changes in which public health is practiced today. More change demands more leadership. In addition, Rowitz [38] argues that the effective public health leader understands the importance of vision and modifying organizational structures, within a dynamic and complex environment, to improve the capacity of the organization and deliver high-quality programs and services.

Table 10.1 Dimensions of leadership

Management in agencies skills	Organizational leadership skills	Transactional leadership skills	Strategic leadership skills	Transformational leadership skills
Planning	Developing others	Relationship building	Systems thinking	Paradigm busting
Organizing	Coaching	Collaboration	Strategic planning	Policy innovation
Staff management	Mission/vision	Communication	Stakeholder analysis	Change orientation
Controlling	Matrix structures	Sharing power and influence	Negotiation	Complexity thinkers
Budgets	Portfolio management	Developing collaborative structures	Policy analysis	Systems transformation
Conflict management	Team building		Futures orientation	
	Problem solving		Analytic	
	Decision making			

Adapted from Rowitz [38]

Building teams inside the organization becomes critical to the sharing of power as well as the recognition that all employees have experiences and skills to offer. Working collaboratively with others means that organizational leaders often need to manage the program portfolios of those inside and outside the organization working together on some programmatic priority [38].

Rowitz further characterizes other dimensions of leadership as including: transactional, strategic, and transformational leadership skills (Table 10.1) [38]. In transactional leadership, the key skills of collaboration are critical since organizations and their leaders need to increasingly look outwards, working with a variety of partners to achieve health outcomes. Leading other leaders (meta-leadership) is critical for building relationships, maximizing communication, and exploring ways to share power and influence.

Strategic leadership is about justifying and planning for change, and requires competence in systems thinking approaches to make policies and programs work better. Strategic leaders use analytic skills to extract useful information from data applying that knowledge to solve big problems faced by the whole organization. The tools of community assessment, stakeholder analysis, community-building approaches, performance measurement, accreditation, and other tools often guide and aid the strategic leader in decision making.

Transformational leadership requires complex thinking and practical skills in how to select the right partners to be involved in policy and programmatic change. The ultimate outcome is population health improvement enabled by systems transformation driven by leadership, with less focus on structure and process, and more focus on policy, and programmatic outcomes [38].

Leadership in Sexual Health

Leadership in sexual health combines the general characteristics of public health leadership with special skills required to lead the unique partnerships, issues, and contexts that face sexual health in any given setting. These special skills may include leading programs that address highly stigmatizing issues, involve socially marginalized constituencies, and that need to address particularly sensitive or proscribed behaviors, attitudes or practices. Although there are no definitive descriptions of the competencies required for leadership in sexual health, UNAIDS [42] has identified ten essential roles and responsibilities for HIV prevention leadership (Table 10.2) which are illustrative of the wider leadership functions and priorities for promoting sexual health, as a strong component of HIV/STI prevention efforts in modern public health practice. This section reflects on key aspects of these responsibilities, and their relevance to the intersection between public health and sexual health.

Table 10.2 Possible roles and responsibilities of the National AIDS Authority for HIV prevention leadership (UNAIDS) [42]

- Provide overall leadership and advocacy for HIV prevention
- Coordinate various actions on HIV prevention and integrate with treatment, care, and support elements of the national AIDS strategy
- Create platforms for policy debate on HIV prevention
- Build a vocal constituency for HIV prevention
- Monitor and evaluate HIV prevention programs within the overall AIDS response
- Support resource mobilization and capacity building of the National AIDS Authority to scale up HIV prevention
- Coordinate inputs around HIV prevention for national AIDS and development planning
- Assess response capacity within each ministry and civil society sector and identify measures to strengthen capacity
- Analyze human resource, legal, and social protection needs and identify measures to build human resources and scale up legal and social protection services
- Analyze the extent to which each sector contributes to reducing HIV vulnerability and identify measures of vulnerability reduction

Leadership and Advocacy

Leadership and advocacy for HIV/STI prevention and sexual health remain critical, especially in an environment challenged by both a devastated economy and inadequate workforce. This requires the development of health sector policies and frameworks that fit within broader national development policies and resource frameworks that are underpinned by commitments to human rights, equity, and gender equality. A critical component of this work is articulating the distinct roles of governments in promoting and maintaining sexual health. Multiple examples of transformative leadership have been exercised by national governments in responding to HIV/STI prevention and sexual health through the publication of national strategic plans [43, 44, 49]; advancing policies which facilitate and promote sexual health [45, 46]; funding core infrastructure, training, and capacity building [47]; and investing in research [48]. Strong leadership by governments can facilitate the development of robust responses at subnational levels including regional, state, or local responses.

Coordination and Integration

Today's leaders in sexual health should be adept in coordinating sexual health activities across programs, settings, and organizations to integrate

prevention, treatment, care, and support elements at national, regional, and local levels. This networked functioning is critical to leverage and make more efficient use of resources, promote greater harmonization, and limit missed opportunities for prevention. In the USA, improved coordination and integration has been identified as a core strategic pillar of the National HIV/AIDS Strategy [49], and the US Centers for Disease Control and Prevention (CDC) has launched and funded its Program Collaboration and Service Integration (PCSI) strategic priority to enhance integration across HIV, hepatitis, STD, and TB prevention programs [50]. Key leadership priorities for PCSI include investing in workforce training and capacity building; removing administrative barriers and burdensome reporting requirements; integrating surveillance; and promoting more holistic approaches to prevention. National leadership has also been evidenced by global [46], regional [51], and national [43, 45, 52] approaches to strategic leadership on sexual health. These approaches promote more holistic and coordinated, health- and wellness-based efforts to enhance traditional vertical HIV/STI prevention, treatment, and care programs.

Encouraging Policy as Intervention

Leaders must create forums for policy debate on HIV/STI prevention and sexual health, especially given the highly sensitive nature of the issues' associated stigma and discrimination, and the inconsistency with which elected officials and other policymakers will often engage on these issues [42]. Critical policy priorities in public health and sexual health include: policy guidance actions and formulating sector strategies and specific technical policies; defining goals, directions, and spending priorities across sexual health services; and identifying the roles of public, private, and voluntary actors as well as civil society. Today's challenges require leaders who have the competence to facilitate, negotiate, and collaborate in an increasingly competitive and contentious political environment. A critical and allied role in this area is the ability to generate and interpret intelligence and research on policy options. In the USA, public health policy leadership has been a critical part of the response to the AIDS epidemic [53], and more recently, has resulted in shepherding changes in approaches to HIV testing; federal funding for syringe services programs; removal of the ban on entry of HIV-positive individuals into the country; and the development of a national strategy [54].

Building a Well-Informed Constituency for HIV Prevention

Effective leadership in HIV/STI prevention and sexual health requires the ability to collaborate across organizational boundaries and build coalitions across government ministries, with the private sector and with communities. To achieve successful coalitions, leaders must understand how to act on key determinants of health; protect workers' health; ensure the health needs of the most vulnerable are properly addressed; and anticipate and address the health impact of public and commercial investments [42]. Collaboration and coalition building have been key strategies in a number of western industrialized countries. For example, the US National Chlamydia Coalition [55] was convened in 2008 to address the continued high burden of chlamydia infection, especially among women aged 25 and younger. The Act Against AIDS Leadership Initiative was launched by the CDC as part of its Act Against AIDS communication campaign in 2009 [56]. The initiative initially brought together some of the nation's foremost African-American organizations to intensify HIV prevention efforts in African-American communities. These coalitions—which include partners across sectors in government and actors outside government, including civil society—aim to influence action on key determinants of health and access to health services; to generate support for public policies; and to keep the different parts connected.

Research, Monitoring, and Evaluation

HIV/STI prevention and sexual health leaders must leverage their ability to select and apply the appropriate tools to monitor and evaluate programs to improve effectiveness, impact, and quality. This focus on evaluation is critical at both the start-up and scale-up phases of program implementation, and leaders must ensure that real-time adjustments to programs are made as experience is gained. Robust program monitoring and evaluation data also provide the necessary intelligence to reassure funders and elected officials to expand and maintain prevention programs [42]. In the USA, evaluation frameworks have been developed for classifying behavioral interventions with evidence of effectiveness in reducing sex and drug injection risk behaviors. These recommendations were published in 1999 (and updated in 2001) in a document entitled *Compendium of HIV Prevention Interventions with Evidence of Effectiveness* [57]. The *Tiers of Evidence Framework* [58] is a conceptual framework that provides a multi-tiered system for classifying all HIV behavioral interventions based on the type and level of evidence for reducing HIV risk. For program implementation, the CDC has also developed the *Evaluation Guidance Handbook: Strategies for Implementing the Evaluation Guidance for CDC-Funded HIV Prevention Programs* [59]. This manual describes various strategies that can be used by health departments to collect, analyze, report, and use program data.

Tackling Vulnerability and Inequity

Finally, leaders in public health and sexual health must continue to analyze the extent to which their programs contribute to reducing HIV vulnerability and identify measures of vulnerability reduction [42]. This accountability must be supported in several ways: through the organization's work on monitoring health system performance as set out in the building block on information; by ensuring that all health system actors are held publicly accountable; and through identification of champions at senior levels of the organization who address health equity and social determinants of health (SDH). They can lead others in the organization to understand why social determinants and health equity should be addressed and how to incorporate social determinants in day-to-day work. Finally, leaders can promote the adoption of policies that address SDH in the organization, including identifying priorities, assessing progress toward meeting objectives derived from those priorities, and reporting the progress on a regular basis (e.g., in annual reports).

Leadership recommendations for addressing sexual health inequalities have been published by the CDC [60] and provide a framework for changing organizational culture and engagement to address health disparities. The European Center for Disease Prevention and Control (ECDC) has also identified issues related to migration and HIV in the European Region as a major area of strategic focus to enhance European surveillance, screening, and care programs, and to ensure greater regional awareness and focus on health inequity related to migrants [61, 62].

Case Studies: Leadership Development for the Twenty-First Century

As economically advanced industrialized countries struggle with the challenges of identifying the most effective and efficient ways to improve the health of their societies, the public health workforce is concomitantly challenged by capacity, turnover, and the need for up-to-date knowledge and skills to deliver quality essential public health services [63]. To meet the training and continuing education needs of an evolving workforce, a clearer understanding is required concerning the functions and composition of the public health workforce, both now and in the future. This information needs to be communicated clearly to legislators and other government leaders so that policy can be based on an understanding of the current demand for public health services and the supply of trained professionals required to meet that demand. Furthermore, because this workforce is geographically dispersed and demographically diverse, new strategies for presenting efficient and effective training must be developed. Having an adequate and accessible public health workforce is fundamental to an integrated health system and for the provision of essential health services in developed and developing countries [64].

In this section, models for addressing and integrating public health leadership training to build long-term health system capacity in global and developed country contexts are explored. The following examples demonstrate how different countries are prioritizing leadership development and training for their public health workforce generally, and their sexual health workforce in particular, and how they ensure appropriate strategic planning and integration in this training. While not meant to be exhaustive, these case studies provide a sense of what opportunities might and can exist in this arena.

Leadership Development for the Sexual Health Workforce: In-Service Training for GUM Registrars in the United Kingdom

In the United Kingdom, Genitourinary Medicine (GUM) is the specialty that informs the prevention and management of STIs, including HIV. The core elements of the specialty are the clinical management of STIs and HIV/AIDS; surveillance and reporting; and the prevention of morbidity and mortality due to STIs and HIV through

Table 10.3 Integrated epidemiology, public health, leadership, and management competencies in UK GUM Registrar training programs

- *Epidemiology and Public Health*: Progressively develop the ability to understand and use epidemiological and public health data relating to service users and the wider community in order to participate in leading the planning of clinical services aimed at improved health and reduced health inequality for the population
- *Personal Qualities*: To demonstrate the personal qualities required to plan, deliver, and develop GUM services. The trainee will be required to draw upon their own values, strengths, and abilities to deliver high standards of care
- *Working with others*: To show leadership by working with others in teams and networks to deliver and improve GUM services
- *Managing services*: To acquire the knowledge, skills, and attitudes to manage services effectively and therefore, ensure the success of the organizations in which the trainees work
- *Improving services*: To be able to deliver safe and effective GUM services by maintaining quality and improving services
- *Setting Direction*: To acquire the knowledge, skills, and attitudes necessary for effective participation in an organization by setting direction and contributing to its vision and aspirations

initiation of treatment, partner notification, and behavioral change. GUM physicians are required to have specialist skills for the delivery of HIV and GUM services in a cross-section of disciplines to address all these elements. The specialty of GUM has a strong multidisciplinary team ethos and requires excellent communication skills [65].

The GUM training curriculum is trainee-centered and outcome-based. A spiral approach has been adopted, which provides a learning experience that revisits topics and themes, each time expanding the levels of sophistication about knowledge, attitudes, and decision-making regarding that topic. This approach aids reinforcement of principles, the integration of topics, and the achievement of higher levels of competency. The Medical Leadership Competency Framework [66], developed by the Academy of Medical Royal Colleges and the NHS Institute for Innovation and Improvement, has informed the inclusion of leadership competencies in this curriculum (Table 10.3).

The GUM training program illustrates the critical importance of integrating leadership and management as well as epidemiology and public health in the training of future sexual health professionals. This integration is a critical component of many specialist training programs in other western industrialized countries and recognizes the importance of the public health and leadership component of specialty training, such as sexual health, in building workforce capacity.

Leadership Development for the Public Health Workforce: The US Centers for Disease Control and Prevention's I LEAD Program

The US Centers for Disease Control and Prevention is committed to building better public health leaders for the agency and its mission. CDC recognizes that it must remain at the forefront of public health leadership to accomplish its mission of improving people's health and safety. The Initiative for Leadership Enhancement and Development (I LEAD) is a competency-based framework for the CDC's leadership building efforts. I LEAD offers a structured pathway through the leadership curriculum called a Leadership Development Map (LDM).

The LDM provides a pathway that reflects the individual's current involvement in leadership in four levels: Getting Ready for Leadership; Leading and Managing People and Teams; Leading and Managing People and Programs; and Leading Organizations. Developed through extensive research inside and outside the CDC, the I LEAD curriculum combines courses and experiential learning activities to help current and future leaders build the skills and competencies they need to be effective in leadership and management roles and addresses organizational leadership challenges. All staff are required to incorporate these leadership training opportunities into their annual "Individual Development Plans (IDP)" and to use dedicated learning resources (Individual Learning Accounts [ILAs]) to support their development.

The I LEAD Program is explicit in identifying key, functional competencies that cross multiple occupations and job series. These are derived from competencies developed by the US Department of Health and Human Services, the Office Personnel Management, and practitioners in leadership development. The target level of expertise (proficiency) is designated based upon the employee's involvement in leadership for each competency. Finally, with each competency, the agency is explicit about its definition and key behaviors to be mastered. A range of courses offered as part of the I LEAD program are associated with each competency so that employees are able to select the training which best meets their strategic leadership development needs.

The I LEAD program provides an example of ongoing leadership development for those who are currently working in the development, delivery, and support of public health (including sexual health) programs. By adopting a strategic, transparent, and competency-based approach to leadership development for all employees, the I LEAD program clearly demonstrates the agency's prioritization of leadership development through access to state of the art training.

Leadership Development for Public Health Professionals: The National Public Health Leadership Institute

The National Public Health Leadership Institute (NPHLI) is a leadership development program in the USA sponsored by the CDC. The Institute's mission is to strengthen the leadership competencies of senior public health leaders and to build a network of senior leaders who can work together and share knowledge on how to address public health challenges. The CDC founded NPHLI in 1991 and supported its development, implementation and evaluation through cooperative agreement funding and technical assistance until 2011.

The NPHLI is a 1-year public health development program for public health leaders. It is designed for selected senior public health leaders who are committed not only to leading their own organizations and communities but also to leading public health system change with a diverse range of partners across sectors, borders, and the country. The NPHLI convenes new leaders and new public health partners who will confront the new challenges in public health together. The NPHLI is designed to attract new partners from across the public health system: legislative leaders, media leaders, business leaders, and leaders in and out of the government sector.

The design of the NPHLI curriculum centers around two key priorities: leading people and leading system change. For leading people, the NPHLI believes that effective leaders inspire trust and confidence. In public health, that means not only leading people within organizations but also leading community improvement with diverse partners across sectors, across borders, and across the country. For leading system change, the NPHLI teaches that leadership is ultimately measured by outcomes. The set of new challenges for public health leaders is diverse. The course design responds to this diversity by helping leaders investigate their roles and responsibilities in creating positive change that resonates from the local level to the national level. Topics covered include individual assessment, coaching, team leadership, collaboration, authentic leadership, effective networks, and expansion of the leadership pipeline.

Multiple evaluations of the NPHLI demonstrated its impact and benefit to leadership development and practice in the public health domain. A recent evaluation [67] by the Center for Health Leadership and Practice, Public Health Institute, and the University of North Carolina team headed by Dr. Karl Umble confirmed that the NPHLI has made a major difference in the lives of public health leaders across the nation. Specifically, the program was successful in several areas: ensuring professionals learned valuable concepts and put them into practice; providing a better understanding of the roles they could play locally and nationally in improving public health systems; strengthening professional networks; improving leadership confidence and competence; and encouraging meta-leadership within and outside of traditional public health settings.

The NHPLI continues to evolve: In September 2011, the CDC selected the Center for Health Leadership and Practice (CHLP) at the Public Health Institute (PHI) to run a new national program focused on improving community health by developing collaborative, multi-sectoral leadership teams across the country. CHLP entered into a 3-year cooperative agreement with the CDC under which the CHLP will assemble, train and provide technical assistance to at least 20 local teams from around the nation working on community health improvement projects. Similar to the NHPLI, the team members will be drawn from multiple sectors—including government, nonprofit and community-based organizations, and health care—and will be trained in applied, team-based and collaborative leadership development.

Leadership Development for Global Public Health Professionals: The Field Epidemiology Training Program

The CDC's Field Epidemiology Training Program (FETP) was developed in order to support countries throughout the world to have effective and equitable public health systems which protect communities and enable people to live healthy and productive lives. The FETP works with Ministries of Health and public health partners to strengthen public health systems and develop the workforce to build sustainable capacity. Built on the best science, innovative programs, and a commitment to meet our partners' national priorities, the FETP works with partners to strengthen the global public health workforce, strengthen public health systems, and strive for program sustainability through key strategies that emphasize applying public health science and practice, and demonstrating measurable public health results.

The FETP partners with Ministries of Health and other public health institutions to strengthen their countries' epidemiologic workforce through a residency-based program in applied epidemiology. A combination of classroom-based instruction and mentored practical work allows trainees to receive hands-on, multi-disciplinary training in public health surveillance, outbreak investigation, laboratory management, program evaluation, and other aspects of epidemiology research and methods.

The FETP also works with partner Ministries of Health to strengthen their public health surveillance and response systems for priority disease conditions. FETP trainees learn detection, confirmation, reporting, and analysis of disease data and implementation of effective public health responses in a participatory approach and receive regular feedback during the process. As graduates, they apply these skills in their work for the Ministry to operate and further strengthen the surveillance and response systems. In turn, the information is used for more effective disease detection, control, and prevention.

FETP helps countries develop sustainable public health capacity to deliver effective leadership and management development programs through the Sustainable Management Development Program (SMDP) [68]. Through strategic partnerships with public health training institutions, faculty development, and technical program assistance, FETP develops leadership and management programs for public health professionals. The program combines experiential training and supervised applied management improvement projects to help public health professionals acquire the knowledge and skills needed to improve organizational performance, shape the public health agenda, and strengthen public health practice in their countries.

FETP is a 2-year, full-time training program with approximately 25% of the time spent in classroom instruction and 75% spent in field assignments. The training is competency-based with close supervision. The trainees provide epidemiologic services to the Ministry of Health during their training, including surveillance system assessments and outbreak investigations. Graduates receive a certificate or, in some programs, a degree. FETP trainees take courses in epidemiology, communications, and economics and management. They also learn about quantitative and behavior-based strategies. In addition, FETP trainees work in the field, where they conduct epidemiologic investigations and field surveys; evaluate surveillance systems; perform

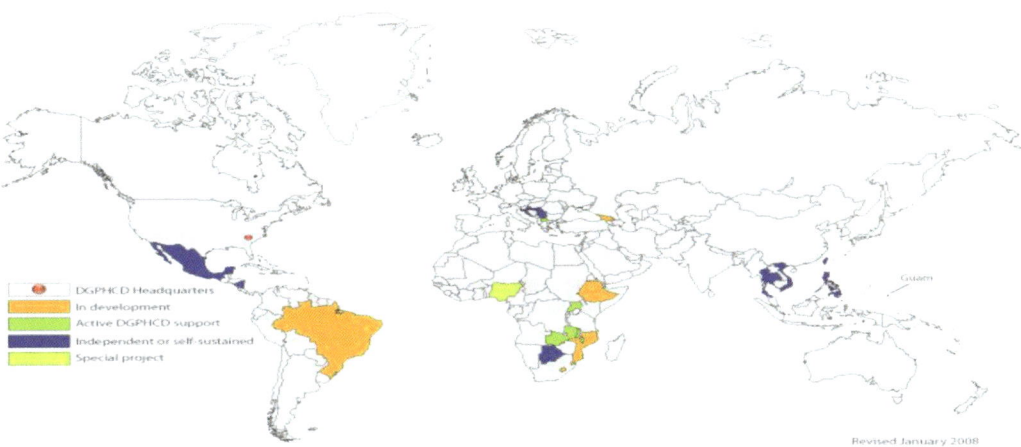

Division of Global Public Health Capacity Development (DGPHCD)
Sustainable Management Development Programs by Development Stage

disease control and prevention measures; report their findings to decision and policy makers; and train other health workers.

FETPs are developed as Ministry programs, not CDC programs. The program is located in the Ministry of Health and is tailored to the country's needs and priorities. In order for an FETP to be successful, the Ministry of Health must be actively engaged and supportive. To attract the best trainees to the program, the Ministry must provide support for the trainees during the program and develop an attractive career ladder for them after graduation. In order for the program to move toward sustainability, the Ministry must provide a Ministry of Health employee to serve as the counterpart to the resident advisor.

Leadership and the New Public Health

To more effectively address the challenges that lay ahead in sexual health and public health, we need new types of leaders working at every level of the health system. Although the specific work commitments and associated performance measures may differ from one setting to another, the key responsibilities of effective leadership for the new public health remain the same. Key among these attributes are the ability to clearly articulate vision and values, build effective teams, understand and organize for performance and scale, improve measurement and accountability, learning to live with complexity, and understanding and dismantling cultural barriers.

Clearly Articulate Vision and Values

Effective leaders must be clear about what they want to achieve, within what time frame, and at what cost. If leaders do not drive the process of program development, implementation, and scale-up with a clear vision, then programs are likely to fail. If our public health institutions and sexual health programs do not embody a clear set of values that empower managers and staff to continuously challenge themselves to perform more effectively and harmoniously, the programs will be inefficient and unsustainable. Similarly, if individuals within institutions are not offered the incentives to push themselves and others to scale up successful interventions, then the current pattern of pervasive "short-termism" and fragmentation of effort will continue to characterize national policies and programs as well as policies and approaches of donors.

Building Effective Teams

The new public health will be increasingly networked, requiring new, robust, and effective partnerships with traditional and nontraditional partners. Effective program performance requires effective teamwork, and new public health leaders must be trained and skilled in thinking about the nature, shape, and form of partnerships required for effective program functioning and impact. Individual practitioners tend to have limited control over the fate of clients and systems, therefore, teamwork across disciplines is generally required if value and outcomes are to improve. New public health leaders must integrate the focus on outcomes and impact with the effective use of performance measurement as a motivating tool to organize their colleagues and drive improvement.

Organize for Performance and Scale

The new public health focus on scale, coverage, and impact is occurring at a time characterized by diminishing resources, a drive towards better value for money, and increasing the efficiency and impact of our public health investments. For the new public health leader, this means incorporating a renewed focus on performance and scale. In general, ideas about what will work and visions of scale emanate from people in and around the public health workforce [69], and the presence of a "champion" of these ideas is generally necessary for scaling up efforts. A champion believes in the potential of an idea, model, or intervention, is committed to promote its scaling up, sticks with the agenda, and can convince others to follow her or his lead. A common feature of effective champions is that they are persistent, well connected, have coalition-building skills, articulate a clear vision amidst complexity, and have credibility that facilitates the mobilization of resources [69]. It is also desirable for them to know how to generate commitment by appealing to social values, to identify the critical challenges in their environments, and to have the relevant technical competence, management skills, and capacity to motivate and train others [70].

Learning to Live with Complexity

The nature of the activities required to effectively manage and improve sexual health-related issues in any setting are increasingly complex, involving numerous diverse and independent processes, activities, partnerships, and relationships [71]. These complex, adaptive systems consist of a number of heterogeneous agents, each of which makes decisions about how to behave and which may evolve over time. These agents interact with each other leading to an emergence of a "whole" that is more than the sum of its parts. Therefore, one cannot understand the whole system by simply looking at its individual parts. This makes the job of leaders in prevention increasingly difficult as it becomes more challenging to predict what will happen with budgets, staffing, programs, or the interactions between various parts of a program. The same starting conditions may yield different results and, in a complex and changing environment, actions may yield unintended consequences. In addition, rare events can be more significant than average ones, and may occur more often than planned for. Today's leaders must be able to navigate complexity, often by making changes to the way(s) in which they approach key tasks, engage partners, and prioritize actions [72]. For example, new skills, including forecasting, risk assessment and mitigation, prioritization, and managing tradeoffs, will become increasingly important for the new public health leader, and in turn, help these policy makers, planners, implementers, and researchers to explore different and innovative approaches for reaching populations in need with effective, equitable, and efficient health services [72] (Table 10.4).

Dismantling Cultural Barriers

Cultural barriers challenge the ability to collaborate and develop partnerships—essential skills for dealing with complex or chaotic environments. Such environments are characterized by

Table 10.4 Leading in complex contexts

Characteristics of complex systems:
- Involves large number of interacting elements
- The interactions are nonlinear and minor changes can produce disproportionately major consequences
- The system is dynamic, the whole is great than the sum of its parts
- The system has a history, the past is integrated with the present, and evolution is irreversible
- Hindsight does not lead to foresight as the external conditions and systems constantly change
- Since the agents and systems constrain each other, one cannot predict or forecast what will happen

Leadership strategies in complex systems:
- *Open up the discussion.* Complex contexts require more interactive communication than other domains
- *Set barriers to limit or delineate behavior.* Once present, barriers allow the system to self-regulate within those boundaries
- *Stimulate attractors.* Phenomena that arise when small stimuli or probes resonate with people who provide structure and coherence
- *Encourage dissent and diversity.* Dissent and debate encourage the emergence of well-forged patterns and ideas
- *Manage starting conditions and monitor for emergence.* Since outcomes are unpredictable, leaders need to focus on creating environments from which good things can emerge, rather than trying to bring about predetermined results

Adapted from Snowden and Boone [73]

flux and unpredictability, no right answers, multiple competing priorities and ideas, and the need for creative and innovative solutions. In these environments, leaders will be increasingly tasked to more rapidly probe, sense, and respond; create environments that allow patterns to emerge; increase their level of interaction and communication; and encourage dissent and diversity to generate ideas. The twenty-first century leader must be comfortable with a range of strategies that both address cultural barriers and create work environments in which cultural differences are valued. Cultivating such an environment will require leaders who are trained and competent to openly discuss cultural backgrounds and values. They must be able to identify and eliminate forms of dominance (by hierarchy, function, race, gender, etc.) that inhibit team members' full contributions while also acknowledging and swiftly resolving the inevitable tensions that arise when

employees from different backgrounds share ideas and emotions [74]. Other strategies for managing multi-cultural teams include adaptation (acknowledging cultural gaps openly and working around them), structural interventions (changing the shape, structure, or functioning of the team), managerial interventions (management directed resetting of productive group norms and culture), and exit interventions (removing team members when other options have failed) [75]. For the future improvement of our prevention programs, structural and operational changes including performance measurement, process improvement, and teamwork must become the norm.

Conclusions

Public health's bottom line ultimately equates to our effectiveness at promoting and protecting the health of a diverse public, and is usually measured in health outcomes. The global spread of HIV and other STIs, along with our prevention responses, are complicated by complex social, cultural, and political environments that are constantly evolving; health systems that are fragmented; and a public health workforce that is seriously challenged. Achieving real and sustained improvements to these challenges requires new types of leaders at every level. As we increasingly shift towards a more value-oriented, performance-driven health care, we will require leaders working in sexual health and public health that can similarly evolve, adapt, and reject previously enshrined ways of working. Today and in the future, sexual health leaders must increasingly organize and work in teams effectively, measure their performance by the health outcomes and impact of their activities, apply financial and behavioral incentives, improve processes, and address ineffective practices that impede health impact.

An increasing range of instruments and institutions exist to carry out the array of functions required for effective leadership and governance [5]. However, the added challenge for governments is to provide vision and direction for the whole health system, and oversee implementation of agreed-upon health policies through systems that are faced with critical governance and stewardship challenges. Whether in developed or resource-poor settings, many challenges remain consistent and include: reconciling competing demands for resources; working across government to promote health outcomes; managing growing private sector provision; tackling corruption; responding to decentralization; engaging with an increasingly vocal civil society; and a growing array of international health agencies [5].

Ultimately, a fundamental problem with leadership and values in public health and sexual health is that they will not last unless carefully nurtured. Without such nurturing, the values and incentives that move prevention programs to operate both effectively and efficiently may quickly turn into bureaucratic paralysis. Finding ways to perpetuate good leadership and institutional values dedicated to development, implementation, scaling up, evaluation, and quality improvement are some of the main challenges and opportunities for leadership in the twenty-first century.

References

1. World Health Organization. Global prevalence and incidence of curable STIS. Geneva, 2001 (WHO/CDS/CDR/EDC/2001.10).
2. Fenton KA. Sexually Transmitted Infections: why are they important? Chapter in ABC of sexually transmitted infections. 6th ed. Oxford: Blackwell Publishing; 2011.
3. Merson M, Padian N, Coates TJ, Gupta GR, Bertozzi SM, Piot P, Mane P, Bartos M. Lancet HIV Prevention Series Authors. Combination HIV prevention. Lancet. 2008;372(9652):1805–6.
4. Kelley RT, Johnson K. Capacity-building assistance and structural challenges in HIV prevention services. Am J Public Health. 2010;100(5):773–4.
5. World Health Organization. Strengthening health systems to improve health outcomes. Who's framework for action. http://www.who.int/healthsystems/strategy/everybodys_business.pdf. (2011) Accessed 16 Aug 2011.
6. Szekeres G, Coates TJ, Ehrhardt AA. Leadership development and HIV/AIDS. AIDS. 2008;22 Suppl 2:S19–26.
7. Grabowski JG. An ecological perspective of public health leadership. APHA 135th Annual Meeting. November 3-7, 2007. Abstract #159126. 3411.0: Monday, November 05, 2007—Table 3. http://apha.confex.com/apha/135am/techprogram/paper_159126.htm (2011). Accessed 16 Aug 2011.
8. Szekeres G. The next 5 years of global HIV/AIDS policy: critical gaps andstrategies for effective responses. AIDS. 2008;22 Suppl 2:S9–17.
9. DHHS, Public Health Service, The Public Health Workforce: An Agenda for the Twenty-first Century (Washington: U.S. Government Printing Office, 1994), 4
10. Gebbie K, Merrill J, Tilson HH. The Public Health Workforce. Health Aff. 2002;21(6):57–67.
11. World Health Organization. Closing the gap in a generation: Health equity through action on the social determinants of health. Report from the Commission on Social Determinants of Health. 2008. http://www.who.int/social_determinants/thecommission/finalreport/en/index.html.
12. Dean HD, Fenton KA. Addressing social determinants of health in the prevention and control of HIV/AIDS, viral hepatitis, sexually transmitted infections, and tuberculosis. Public Health Rep. 2010;125 Suppl 4:1–5.
13. Health Resources and Services Administration. Public health workforce study. [Internet]. Washington, D.C: US Department of Health and Human Services; 2005 Jan [cited 2009 Sept 24]. 29 p. http://bhpr.hrsa.gov/healthworkforce/reports/publichealth/default.htm
14. Voelker R. One casualty of global economic crisis: uncertain finances for HIV/AIDS programs. JAMA. 2010;304(3):259–61.
15. Gray RT, Heymer KJ, Hoare A, Kwon JA, Thein HH, Lote N, Siba P, Saramony S, Saphonn V, Worth H, Kaldor JM, Wilson DP. What impact might the economic crisis have on HIV epidemics in Southeast Asia? Curr HIV Res. 2009;7(6):656–65.
16. Summary results. (2009) Impact of State General Revenue Cuts in HIV/AIDS and Viral Hepatitis Programs. http://www.nastad.org/Docs/highlight/2009426_State%20Budget%20Cuts%20-%20Summary%20Results%20-%20Final.pdf. Accessed June 2009
17. Institute of Medicine, Committee for the Study of the Future of Public Health. The Future of Public Health. Washington: National Academy Press; 1988.
18. Heishman H. Public Health's Aging Workforce, Aging Leaders. Northwest Public Health. Fall/Winter 2007. 2011 http://www.nwpublichealth.org/webspecials/aging-leaders. Accessed 16 Aug 2011.
19. ASPH. Policy Brief. Confronting the Public Health Workforce Crisis. December 2008.http://www.asph.org/document.cfm?page=1038. Accessed 16 Aug 2011.
20. APHA issue brief. The Public Health Workforce Shortage: Left Unchecked, Will We Be Protected? September 2006. http://www.apha.org/NR/rdonlyres/8B9EBDF5-8BE8-482D-A779-7F637456A7C3/0/workforcebrief.pdf

21. Aral SO, Adimora AA, Fenton KA. Understanding and responding to disparities in HIV and other sexually transmitted infections in African Americans. Lancet. 2008;372(9635):337–40.

22. Aral SO, Fenton KA, Holmes KK. Sexually transmitted diseases in the USA: temporal trends. Sex Transm Infect. 2007;83(4):257–66.

23. Gilson L. Acceptability, Trust and Equity. In: Mooney G, McIntyre D, editors. The economics of health equity. Cambridge: Cambridge University Press; 2007.

24. NASTAD. Workforce recruitment and retention challenges and responses. Leadership development Issue Brief. No. 3. September 2009. http://www.nastad.org/Files/042600_NASTADBrief3. FINAL.pdf. Accessed 16 Aug 2011.

25. Walter H. Curioso, New Technologies and Public Health in Developing Countries: The Cell PREVEN Project. http://faculty.washington.edu/wcurioso/libro_cell.htm. Accessed 16 Aug 2011.

26. U.S. Department of Health and Human Services Public Health Service. The Public Health Workforce: An Agenda for the 21st Century. http://www.health.gov/phfunctions/pubhlth.pdf

27. Chen L, Evans T, Anand S, Boufford JI, Brown H, Chowdhury M, Cueto M, Dare L, Dussault G, Elzinga G, Fee E, Habte D, Hanvoravongchai P, Jacobs M, Kurowski C, Michael S, Pablos-Mendez A, Sewankambo N, Solimano G, Stilwell B, de Waal A, Wibulpolprasert S. Human resources for health: overcoming the crisis. Lancet. 2004;364(9449):1984–90.

28. Health Workforce Advocacy Initiative. Addressing the Health Workforce Crisis. http://www.healthworkforce.info/advocacy/HWAI_advocacy_toolkit.pdf. Accessed 16 Aug 2011.

29. World Health Organization, World Health Report 2006 (2006), at xix. http://www.who.int/whr/2006/en/index.html.

30. Narasimhan V, Brown H, Pablos-Mendez A, et al. Responding to the global human resources crisis. Lancet. 2004;363:1469–72.

31. Imhan, H Brown and A Pablos-Mendez et al. Responding to the global human resources crisis, *Lancet* 363:(2004) 1469–72. //www.who.int/mediacentre/news/releases/2004/wha4/en/http://www.who.int/mediacentre/news/releases/2004/wha4/en/. Accessed 26 Dec 2007

32. Resolution WHA59.23. Rapid scaling up of health workforce production. In: Fifty-ninth World Health Assembly, Geneva, 22-27 May 2006. Geneva: World Health Organization; 2006.

33. Coye JM, Foege WH, Rober WL. Leadership in Public Health. Milbank Memorial Fund. 1994 http://www.milbank.org/mrlead.html#intro. Accessed 16 Aug 2011.

34. Rowitz L Public Health Leadership. Putting Principles into Practice. 2nd Ed. Jones and Bartlett Publishers LLC. 2009. LLC.

35. World Health Organization. Everybody business: strengthening health systems to improve health outcomes : WHO's framework for action. 2007. http://www.who.int/healthsystems/strategy/everybodys_business.pdf ISBN 978 92 4 159607 7

36. Beaglehole R, Dal Poz MR. Public health workforce: challenges and policy issues. Hum Resource Health. 2003;1(1):4.

37. Gilson L. What sort of stewardship and health system management is needed to tackle health inequity, and how can it be developed and sustained? http://www.wits.ac.za/files/res6698635c22a-043b6ab501602421b6ffb.pdf Accessed 16 Aug 2011.

38. Rowitz L. Management and Leadership. J Public Health Manage Pract [1078-4659] 2010;16(2): 174–6

39. Kotter JP. What leaders really do. Harv Bus Rev. 1990;68(3):103–11.

40. Moore M. Creating Public Value: Strategic management in government. Cambridge: Harvard University Press; 1995.

41. Alvord, S.H., Brown, D., Letts, C.W. (2003). Social entrepreneurship. Leadership that facilitates societal transformation—an explanatory study. Working Papers. In: Centre for Public Leadership (Ed.).

42. UNAIDS. Possible roles and responsibilities of the National AIDS Authority for HIV Prevention Leadership. http://hivpreventiontoolkit.unaids.org/support_pages/faq_effective_leadership.aspx. Accessed 16 Aug 2011.

43. Department of Health. The national strategy for sexual health and HIV. London: Department of Health; 2001.

44. National HIV/AIDS strategy. Revitalising Australia's Response 2005-2008. http://www.health.vic.gov.au/hivaids/5th_hiv_strategy.pdf. Accessed 16 August 2011.

45. U.S. Public Health Service. The Surgeon General Call to Action to Promote Sexual Health and Responsible Sexual Behaviors. Washington, DC, 2001. http://www.surgeongeneral.gov/library/sexualhealth/call.htm.

46. World Health Organization. Defining sexual health: Report of a technical consultation on sexual health 28–31 January 2002, Geneva. Geneva, Switzerland; 2006. http://www.who.int/reproductivehealth/topics/gender_rights/defining_sexual_health.pdf

47. Sutton MY, Jones RL, Wolitski RJ, Cleveland JC, Dean HD, Fenton KA. A review of the Centers for Disease Control and Prevention's response to the HIV/AIDS crisis among Blacks in the United States, 1981-2009. Am J Public Health. 2009;99 Suppl 2:S351–9.

48. NIH Office of AIDS Research. FY2012 National Institutes of Health Trans-NIH AIDS research by-pass budget estimate and Trans-NIH plan for HIV-related research. http://www.oar.nih.gov/strategicplan/fy2012/index.asp. Accessed 16 Aug 2011.

49. The White House. National HIV/AIDS strategy for the United States. http://www.whitehouse.gov/sites/default/files/uploads/NHAS.pdf. Accessed 16 Aug 2011.

50. CDC. Program collaboration and service integration: Enhancing the prevention and control of HIV/AIDS, Viral Hepatitis, STD, and TB in the United States. An NCHHSTP Green paper. July 2007. http://www.cdc. gov/nchhstp/programintegration/attachments/ I-NCHHSTP-PCSIGreenPaper_508.pdf. Accessed 25 Sep 2009.

51. Pan American Health Organization. Sexual Health and Development of Adolescents and Youth in the Americas: Program and Policy Implications. 2003. http://www.paho.org/English/HPP/HPF/ADOL/SRH. pdf. Accessed 16 Aug 16 2011.

52. National HIV/AIDS Strategy. Revitalising Australia's Response 2005–2008. http://www.health.vic.gov.au/ hivaids/5th_hiv_strategy.pdf.

53. De Cock KM, Jaffe HW, Curran JW. Reflections on 30 years of AIDS. Emerg Infect Dis. 2011;17(6): 1044–8.

54. Millett GA, Crowley JS, Koh H, Valdiserri RO, Frieden T, Dieffenbach CW, Fenton KA, Benjamin R, Whitescarver J, Mermin J, Parham-Hopson D, Fauci AS. A way forward: the National HIV/AIDS Strategy and reducing HIV incidence in the United States. J Acquir Immune Defic Syndr. 2010;55 Suppl 2:S144–7.

55. National Chlamydia Coalition. Information. http:// ncc.prevent.org/. Accessed 16 Aug 2011.

56. CDC. Act Against AIDS Leadership Initiative. Harnessing the Strength of National Organizations to Reach the Communities Hardest Hit by HIV. http:// www.cdc.gov/hiv/aaa/leadership_initiative.htm. Accessed 16 Aug 2011.

57. CDC. Compendium of HIV Prevention Interventions with Evidence of Effectiveness. http://www.cdc.gov/ hiv/topics/research/prs/compendium-evidence-based-interventions.htm. Accessed 16 Aug 2011.

58. CDC. Tiers of Evidence: A Framework for Classifying HIV Behavioral Interventions. http://www.cdc.gov/ hiv/topics/research/prs/tiers-of-evidence.htm. Accessed 16 Aug 2011.

59. CDC. Evaluation Guidance Handbook: Strategies for Implementing the Evaluation Guidance for CDC-Funded HIV Prevention Programs. http://www.cdc. gov/hiv/topics/evaluation/health_depts/guidance/ strat-handbook/index.htm. Accessed 16 Aug 2011.

60. CDC. Establishing a Holistic Framework to Reduce Inequities in HIV, Viral Hepatitis, STDs, and Tuberculosis in the United States. Atlanta (GA): U.S. Department of Health and Human Services, Centers for Disease Control and Prevention; October 2010. www. cdc.gov/socialdeterminants. Accessed 16 Aug 2011

61. European Centre for Disease Prevention and Control. Migrant health: HIV testing and counselling in migrant populations and ethnic minorities in EU/EEA/EFTA Member States. Stockholm: ECDC; 2011.

62. European Centre for Disease Prevention and Control (2009). Migrant health: Access to HIV prevention, treatment and care for migrant populations in EU/ EEA countries. Technical report. http://ecdc.europa. eu/en/publications/Publications/0907_TER_ Migrant_health_HIV_Access_to_treatment.pdf. Accessed 16 Aug 2011.

63. U.S. Department of Health and Human Services. The Public Health Workforce: An Agenda for the 21st Century. A Report of the Public Health Functions Project. http://www.health.gov/phfunctions/pubhlth. pdf. Accessed 16 Aug 2011.

64. World Health Assembly. International recruitment of health personnel: draft global code of practice A63/8. 15 April 2010. http://apps.who.int/gb/ebwha/pdf_files/ WHA63/A63_8-en.pdf. Accessed 16 Aug 2011.

65. Joint Royal Colleges of Physicians Training Board. Specialty training curriculum for Genitourinary Medicine. August 2010. http://www.gmc-uk.org/ Genito_urinary_medicine_curriculum_2010. pdf_32485349.pdf. Accessed 31 Jul 2011.

66. NHS Institute for Innovation and Improvement and the Academy of Medical Royal Colleges. Medical Leadership Competency Framework. Enhancing Engagement in Medical Leadership. Third Edition, July 2010. http://www.institute.nhs.uk/images/docu-ments/Medical%20Leadership%20Competency%20 Framework%203rd%20ed.pdf. Accessed 16 Aug 2011.

67. Umble K, Diehl S, Gunn A, and Haws S. Developing Leaders, Building Networks: An Evaluation of the National Public Health Leadership Institute—1991-2006 National Public Health Leadership Institute Final Evaluation Report. http:// www.phli.org/evalreports/ExecSummary.pdf. Accessed 31 Jul 2011

68. CDC. Global Health. Sustainable Management Development Program (SDMP). http://www.cdc.gov/ globalhealth/smdp/. Accessed 16 Aug 2011.

69. Hartmann A. and Linn JF. Scaling up. A framework and lessons for development effectiveness from litera-ture and practice. CALING UP.

70. Simmons R, Shiffman J. Scaling up health service innovations: a framework for action. In: Simmons R, Fajans P, Ghiron L, editors. Scaling up health services delivery: from pilot innovations to policies and programmes. Geneva: WorldHealth Organisation; 2006.

71. Sherr L, Fishbein M, Spire B, Paul Moatti J, Shishana O, Prince B, Catalan J, Hedge B, van den Boom F. Contexts and complexity—special considerations in HIV and socialscience. AIDS Care. 2008;20(5): 507–8.

72. Paina L. Peters DH. Health Policy Plan: Understanding pathways for scaling up health services through the lens of complex adaptive systems; 2011.

73. Snowden DJ and Boone ME. A Leader's framework for decision making. Harvard Business Review. November 2007. Reprint R0711C. www.hbrreprints. org. Accessed 16 Aug 2011.

74. Thomas DA and Ely RJ. Making differences matter: A new paradigm for managing diversity. Harvard Business Review. September 1996. Product no. 96510

75. Brett J, Behar K, and Kern MC. Managing multicul-tural teams. Harvard Business Review. November 2006. Reprint R0611D. www.hbrreprints.org. Accessed 16 Aug 2011.

Part III

Critical Reviews: New Public Health Focus for Populations at Risk for STI/HIV

Enhancing Women's Sexual Health: Prevention Measures in Diverse Populations of Women

11

Jeanne M. Marrazzo

Introduction

The landscape of interventions to prevent transmission of sexually transmitted infections (STI), including human immunodeficiency virus (HIV), has changed considerably in the last decade. Of particular relevance to women are the licensure and uptake of highly effective immunization against genital human papillomavirus (HPV) and associated prevention against associated consequences, including cervical cancer; encouragement about the use of topical antiretroviral agents as pre-exposure prophylaxis to reduce risk of HIV and genital herpes acquisition; enhanced emphasis on expedited partner management and rescreening for persons infected with *C. trachomatis* and *N. gonorrhoeae*; and the availability of a modified female condom. While these advances are encouraging, effective prevention of HIV and the other STI remains a high priority, both internationally and domestically, and most urgently among women. UNAIDS reported in 2010 that while the rate of new HIV infections

has fallen in several countries, these favorable trends are at least partially offset by increases in new infections in others; moreover, the proportion of infections in women is increasing in several countries, and young people ages 15–24 account for 41% of new HIV infections in sub-Saharan Africa [1]. In 2008, the CDC revised its estimates of the annual incidence of new HIV infections in the USA by 40% (an increase from an estimated 40,000 new infections annually to approximately 56,000) [2]. Moreover, a large proportion of new HIV infections continue to be diagnosed in late stages of the disease, and women are not exempt from these trends [3, 4]. As discussed below, rates of reportable non-HIV STI either have not declined or have actually increased in women. This chapter will review the current state of prevention interventions for HIV/STI in diverse populations of women.

It is worth noting from the outset that the complexities that underlie women's vulnerability to many of the infections discussed here serve to highlight that structural interventions with the potential to effect system change are needed. Globally, women's socioeconomic and educational status is by far below that of men, and power dynamics often place women at the lower end of hierarchies within relationships and families, and in the workplace. For many prevention interventions to have a meaningful impact, these inequities will need to be addressed, or at least acknowledged.

J.M. Marrazzo, M.D., M.P.H. (✉)
Division of Allergy and Infectious Diseases,
Department of Medicine, University of Washington,
Seattle, WA, USA

Division of Infectious Diseases, Harborview Medical Center, 325 Ninth Avenue, Mailbox #359932, Seattle, WA 98104, USA
e-mail: jmm2@uw.edu

S.O. Aral, K.A. Fenton, and J.A. Lipshutz (eds.), *The New Public Health and STD/HIV Prevention: Personal, Public and Health Systems Approaches*, DOI 10.1007/978-1-4614-4526-5_11,
© Springer Science+Business Media New York 2013

Epidemiologic Trends for High-Impact Infections in Women, with Emphasis on Adverse Impacts on Sexual/Reproductive Health

Chlamydia trachomatis is the most commonly reported infectious disease in the USA, and typically infects the cervix with occasional infection of the urethra in some women. In 2009, >1.2 million diagnoses of *C. trachomatis* were reported to CDC, but approximately 3 million new cases are estimated to occur annually [5]. Most chlamydial infections cause neither signs nor symptoms and thus are able to ascend without notice to the upper reproductive tract. There, chronic infection can elicit immunopathogenesis with consequent scarring of the fallopian tubes, ovaries, endometrial lining, and occasionally, the adjacent peritoneum [6]. Thus, genital chlamydial infection is the leading cause of preventable infertility and ectopic pregnancy [7]. Selective screening of appropriate women is necessary to control this infection and its sequelae, and most experts agree that it has effected widespread declines in reproductive tract sequelae; whether it has effected declines in prevalent infection is a question of debate [8]. The U.S. Preventive Services Task Force and the CDC recommend that all sexually active women age 25 years or younger be screened annually for *C. trachomatis*, with screening of older women based on behavioral risk criteria [9]. Despite this, rates of appropriate screening in young women remain suboptimal, and interventions to enhance screening in target populations are needed [10].

In 2009, the number of reported cases of gonorrhea in the USA remained stable, with the highest attack rates occuring in 15- to 24-year-old women and men; however, after adjustment for sexual experience, the highest rates are seen in sexually active 15- to 19-year-old women [11]. According to the population-based National Health and Nutrition Examination Survey (NHANES), in 1999–2002, the prevalence was higher among non-Hispanic black persons relative to white (1.2%; CI, 0.7–1.9%), and 46% of those infected with gonorrhea also had *C. trachomatis* detected [12]. The Ad Health study of young adults showed similar results in 2001–2002.

Among 12,548 persons aged 18–26 years, the prevalence of gonorrhea was 0.43% (95% CI, 0.29–0.63%), and strikingly higher in blacks than whites (2.13%; 95% CI 1.46–3.10%) [13]. Overall, more cases of gonorrhea are reported in men than women, which probably reflects both a greater ease of diagnosis in men and a substantially higher rate of infection in men who have sex with men (MSM) than in heterosexual men and women. The rate of gonorrhea in African American populations in the USA is almost 25 times higher than that in whites or persons of Asian ancestry; Latino populations and Native Americans experience intermediate rates. Only a small portion of these differences can be explained by greater attendance of nonwhite populations at public clinics, where case reporting is more complete than in private health facilities. Race and ethnicity are demographic markers of increased risk, not factors that directly denote a high risk for gonorrhea or other STDs. Differing incidence rates between population subgroups are related less to variations in numbers of sex partners than to complex and poorly understood differences in sex partner networks, as well as access to health care and related societal factors. A detailed analysis of rising gonorrhea incidence in California from 2003 to 2005 raised the importance of contact with a recently incarcerated partner as a major risk, and highlighted the relatively understudied contribution of this infection in corrections settings, especially for women [14].

The major current concern with gonorrhea is advancing antimicrobial resistance. Overall, prevalence of fluoroquinolone-resistant strains, which was <1% during 1990–2001, increased to 4.1% in 2003, and 13.8% in 2006. [15] Such increases prompted CDC to recommend in 2007 that fluoroquinolones no longer be used to treat gonorrhea in the USA [16]. Highlighting this relentless trend, the CDC reported the first case of a clinical isolate of *N. gonorrhoeae* with high-level resistance to azithromycin from a woman evaluated in Hawaii in early 2011 [17]. Of note, the CDC's Gonococcal Isolate Surveillance Project (GISP), the sole national system designed to monitor emergence of antimicrobial resistance in this pathogen, tests isolates only from men with symptoms of urethritis who are seeking care at selected Sexually Transmitted Disease (STD) Clinics. These data may approximate antimicrobial resistance patterns in women, but the implications of potential differences in the spectrum of gonorrhea in women are worth noting: antibiotic regimens for pelvic inflammatory disease (PID) should retain excellent activity against gonorrhea, and options in the current landscape are quite limited. Infertility resulting from fallopian tube obstruction is the most common serious consequence of PID and occurs in 15–20% of women after a single episode and 50–80% of those who experience three or more episodes [18]. Infertility may be more common after chlamydial than gonococcal PID, perhaps because the more acute inflammatory signs associated with gonorrhea bring women to diagnosis and treatment sooner. Moreover, *N. gonorrhoeae* is a nefarious player in PID. The PID Evaluation and Clinical Health (PEACH) study enrolled over 800 women aged 14–37 with symptomatic PID [19]. Despite clinical cure and apparent microbiologic eradication of gonorrhea, as evidenced by lower tract cultures, infertility rates were 13% for women with *N. gonorrhoeae* identified, 19% for those with *C. trachomatis*, and 22% for those with anaerobic bacteria over 35 median months of follow-up [20]. Rates of chronic pelvic pain were 27% among women with gonococcal infection [21].

The resurgence of syphilis in the USA, and in many other industrialized countries, has largely involved men who have sex with men (MSM) [5]. In 2009, cases of primary and secondary syphilis comprised the highest number of cases reported since 1995, and the majority of these occurred in men [5]. However, some data suggest that an epidemiologic shift of the syphilis resurgence into heterosexual networks may be underway [22]. Congenital syphilis continues to occur in the U.S., largely in situations where prenatal screening was not obtained. For example, high rates of congenital syphilis in Maricopa County, Arizona (U.S.) prompted an analysis of syphilis case report data from state and county health departments [23]. This showed that among 970 women reported to have syphilis, 49% were Hispanic, of whom 49% were non-US citizens. Of the latter group, the majority (64%) reported having a male sex partner who reported drug use or anonymous sex. These data indicate the complex interplay of limitations in successful access to care and sexual networks that are likely needed to sustain outbreaks of this devastating neonatal disease, and the interventions needed to prevent them [24].

Sexually transmitted herpes simplex virus (HSV) infections now cause most genital ulcer disease throughout the world and an increasing proportion of cases of genital herpes in developing countries with generalized HIV epidemics, where the positive feedback loop between HSV and HIV transmission is a growing, intractable problem. Despite this consistent link, randomized trials evaluating the efficacy of suppressive antiviral therapy to suppress HSV in both HIV-uninfected and HIV-infected persons have not demonstrated a protective effect against acquisition or transmission of HIV [25, 26]. In the USA, the prevalence of antibody to HSV-2 began to fall in the late 1990s, especially among adolescents and young adults; the decline is presumably due to delayed sexual debut, increased condom use, and lower rates of multiple (≥ 4) sex partners, as is well documented in the U.S. Youth Risk Behavior Surveillance System (YRBSS) [27].

Genital human papillomavirus (HPV) remains the most common sexually transmitted pathogen in this country, infecting 60% of a cohort of initially HPV-negative, sexually active Washington state college women within 5 years in a study conducted from 1990 to 2000 [28]. The scale-up of HPV vaccine coverage among young women—discussed in detail in text that follows—promises to lower the incidence of infection with the HPV types included in the vaccines. The available vaccines target the major oncogenic HPV types (16/18), responsible for the majority of cervical cancers; the quadrivalent vaccine targets the two HPV types that cause genital warts (6/11) as well. Uptake of the vaccines has generally been good, with the majority of US pediatricians offering it to older adolescents; however, barriers remain, most significantly, high cost [29]. A great deal of activity in designing post-immunization surveillance programs to monitor genital HPV infection and related consequences is now underway [30].

Finally, vaginal infections are an under-recognized cause of morbidity in women, and in the case of trichomoniasis and bacterial vaginosis (BV), increase the risk of acquisition of other STI, including HIV [31]. Up to 50% of women of reproductive age in developing countries have bacterial vaginosis (arguably acquired sexually), and trichomoniasis remains a sexually transmitted cause of vaginitis worldwide. Although few nationally representative surveys have been performed, trichomoniasis prevalence measured by culture of vaginal fluid was reported for women in the National Health and Nutrition Survey (NHANES), which uses a complex, stratified, multistage probability sample design with unequal probabilities of selection to obtain a nationally representative sample of the U.S. civilian noninstitutionalized population. Of over 3,754 women in the 2001–2004 NHANES who supplied a self-collected swab of vaginal secretions for *T. vaginalis* PCR assay, prevalence was 3.1% (95% CI, 0.7–2.3%) [32]. Prevalence was 1.3% among non-Hispanic white women, 1.8% among Mexican American women, and 13.3% among non-Hispanic Black women. Independent risks for infection included non-Hispanic black race/ethnicity, being born in the U.S., higher number of lifetime sex partners, increasing age, lower educational level, poverty, and douching. Only 15.2% with trichomoniasis reported vaginal symptoms. Of significant interest is that 49.8% of women with trichomoniasis also had bacterial vaginosis. Using PCR assay applied to 12,449 participants in the National Longitudinal Study of Adolescent Health, overall prevalence was 2.3% (95% CI, 1.8–2.7%), and higher in women (2.8%), especially Black women (10.5%) [33]. In a study of trichomoniasis in over 13,000 women in the second trimester of pregnancy, the prevalence by culture was 13%. Infection by *T. vaginalis* was associated with Black race, being unmarried, a history of gonorrhea, and having multiple sexual partners during pregnancy. The high prevalence of this sexually transmitted pathogen in pregnant women is of concern because data suggest that trichomoniasis is linked with an increased risk of low birth weight. However, treatment of symptomatic trichomoniasis has not been shown to reduce preterm birth [34].

Demographic Trends in Sexual Risk Behaviors

Specific Practices and Associated Risk

Vaginal, Oral, Anal Sex
Several recent reviews have described patterns of sexual behavior across various age groups and populations [35]. Of great interest for populations most susceptible to bacterial STI are surveys of adolescents. The 2009 Youth Risk Behavior Surveillance System (YRBSS) was conducted among students in grades 9–12. Among high school students nationwide, 34.2% were currently sexually active, 38.9% of currently sexually active students had not used a condom during their last sexual intercourse, and 2.1% of students had ever injected an illegal drug [36].

Same- and Opposite-Sex Behavior
According to the 2006–2008 National Survey of Family Growth, 13% of women aged 15–44 and 5.2% of men reported same sex behavior in their lifetime [37]. Women who have sex with women (WSW) represent diverse communities of women who may exclusively have sex with women, or historically (or currently) engage in sexual partnerships with both men and women. Despite the fact that same sex behavior is not infrequent among women in the USA and despite the widespread prevalence of chlamydia, little data at the clinic, community, or population levels are available that describe its prevalence among these sexual minority communities. Numerous studies support that greater than 90% of women who self-identify as lesbian report a sexual history with men [38]. Moreover, recent studies indicate that some communities of WSW, particularly adolescents and young women might be at increased risk for STDs and HIV as a result of certain reported risk behaviors [39–41], including

sex with high risk men. Same-sex sexual behavior is likely underreported to care providers [42]. Moreover, tremendous gaps of knowledge exist in understanding what specific sexual behaviors among WSW place them at risk for STI. Sexual practices involving digital-vaginal or digital-anal contact and those including penetrative sex objects represent plausible means for transmission of cervicovaginal secretions.

Genital Hygiene Measures

Vaginal douching does not protect against acquisition of STD/HIV, and increases the risk of certain vaginal infections, notably BV. Among HIV-uninfected Kenyan female sex workers, increased frequency of vaginal washing was associated with a higher likelihood of BV, as were vaginal lubrication with petroleum jelly (OR 2.8, 95% CI=1.4–5.6), lubrication with saliva (OR=2.3, 95% CI=1.1–4.8), and bathing less than the median for the cohort (14 times/week; OR=4.6, 95% CI=1.2–17.5). The authors concluded that modification of intravaginal and general hygiene practices should be evaluated as potential strategies for reducing the risk of BV [43].

Genital hygiene methods for washing after sexual exposure, including vaginal washing and douching, are ineffective in protecting against HIV and STD and may increase the risk of bacterial vaginosis, some STD, and HIV [44].

Hormonal Contraception

While exogenous hormones may modulate mucosal immunity to STD/HIV, data remain insufficient to recommend that women modify their hormonal contraceptive practices to reduce their risk of STD/HIV acquisition. Hormonal contraceptives do not provide protection against STD/HIV acquisition, and need to be used in conjunction with barrier methods of protection (condoms) in women at risk. A systematic review of data from 1966 through early 2005 concluded that studies of combined oral contraceptive and depot medroxyprogesterone use generally reported positive associations with cervical chlamydial infection, although not all associations were statistically significant. For other STI, the

findings suggested no association between hormonal contraceptive use and STI acquisition, or the results were too limited to draw any conclusions. Evidence was generally limited in both amount and quality, including inadequate adjustment for confounding, lack of appropriate control groups and small sample sizes. Thus, observed positive associations may be due to a true association or to bias, such as differential exposure to STI by contraceptive use or increased likelihood of STI detection among hormonal contraceptive users [45].

The relationship between hormonal contraception and HIV acquisition was recently examined in two well done observational studies. The largest and most sophisticated cohort investigation prospectively followed 6109 HIV-uninfected women from family planning clinics in Uganda and Zimbabwe to assess risk of HIV acquisition over 15–24 months [46]. Neither combined oral contraceptives (HR, 0.99; 95% CI, 0.69–1.42) nor DMPA (HR, 1.25; 95% CI, 0.89–1.78) was associated with risk of HIV acquisition overall, including among participants with cervical or vaginal infections. However, hormonal contraceptive users who were HSV-2 seronegative had an increased risk of HIV acquisition (for combined oral contraceptive use, HR, 2.85; 95% CI, 1.39–5.82; for DMPA, HR, 3.97; 95% CI, 1.98–8.00).

A second study accounted for HSV-2 serostatus in a prospective cohort study of 1206 HIV seronegative sex workers from Mombasa, Kenya who were followed monthly. 233 women acquired HIV (8.7/100 person-years). HSV-2 prevalence (81%) and incidence (25.4/100 person-years) were high. In multivariate analysis, including adjustment for HSV-2, HIV acquisition was associated with use of oral contraceptive pills (adjusted HR, 1.46; 95% CI, 1.00–2.13) and depot medroxyprogesterone acetate (adjusted HR, 1.73; 95% CI, 1.28–2.34). The effect of contraception on HIV susceptibility did not differ significantly between HSV-2 seronegative and seropositive women. HSV-2 infection was associated with elevated HIV risk (adjusted HR, 3.58; 95% CI, 1.64–7.82). These authors concluded that in this group of high-risk African women, hormonal contraception and HSV-2 infection were both associated with increased risk for HIV acquisition. HIV risk associated with hormonal contraceptive use was not related to HSV-2 serostatus [47].

A retrospective cohort study at a U.S. university clinic assessed STI incidence among 304 HIV-infected women, 82 of whom received DMPA and 222 who did not. No significant differences in trichomoniasis, chlamydial infection, and gonorrhea occurred between the women receiving or not receiving DMPA [48].

Groups with Specific Concerns

Adolescents

Adolescent females have the highest rates of chlamydia and gonorrhea in the USA. Risk is elevated in this group relative to other age groups likely due to a combination of biological predisposition (cervical ectopy, which exposes more vulnerable columnar epithelium to these pathogens), behavior (participation in sexual networks with high levels of infection) and access to care (inability to independently pay for health care and concerns for confidentiality). In 2009, rates of chlamydia increased in 15–19 year-old women 1.8% from the prior year, to 3,329.3 cases per 100,000 population [5]. While women in this age group continue to have the highest gonorrhea rates (568.8 cases per 100,000 population), this number actually represented a decline of 10.5% from 2008.

Data support the need for adolescents to receive comprehensive, current, and accessible information on prevention of STD/HIV and pregnancy, including condoms. Data from the 1994 to 2002 National Longitudinal Study of Adolescent Health (Add Health) compared subsequent sexual behaviors and risk of STI among adolescents who did and did not use a condom at their sexual debut [49]. Adolescents who reported condom use at sexual debut were more likely to report condom use at most recent intercourse (on average, 6.8 years after sexual debut), and were half as likely to test positive for chlamydia or gonorrhea (adjusted OR 0.50; 95% CI, 0.26–0.95).

Reported number of lifetime sexual partners did not differ between the two groups. A separate analysis of Add Health data included teens enrolled in 2001 who were followed 1 and 3 years later; those teens who took a virginity pledge reported a longer time until sexual debut than teens who did not take similar pledges [50]. However, overall sexual behaviors subsequent to pledging, including patterns of condom use, did not differ between these groups. A more recent analysis demonstrated that teens who took the pledge and who did have sex were less likely to use condoms at sexual debut [51].

Pregnant Women

Surprisingly few data are available on STI/HIV incidence in pregnancy, but data suggest that this period is a time of enhanced vulnerability for acquisition of these infections, particularly HIV. Moreover, women who acquire HIV during pregnancy are more likely to transmit the virus to their infants in utero, probably due to a combination of the high plasma HIV viral loads associated with the primary infection period and cell-mediated immunomodulation during pregnancy. Of course, non-HIV STI transmission to the neonate can have devastating consequences as well; the majority of congenital syphilis cases likely result in spontaneous abortion, for example, and both *C. trachomatis* and *N. gonorrhoeae* cause serious ophthalmic and (in the case of chlamydia) respiratory problems.

Sexual Minorities

Prior studies indicate that women who practice same sex behavior, including exclusively same sex behavior, are at risk for STIs, including genital types of human papillomavirus (HPV), HIV, genital herpes, and trichomoniasis [52–58]. Moreover, bacterial vaginosis (BV) occurs commonly among women who report sex with women, and there is a high degree of concordance among monogamous same sex couples, suggesting a potential role for sexual transmission in this group [59]. These observations emphasize the need for healthcare providers and public health advocates to address the sexual and reproductive health care needs of this group of women in a comprehensive and informed manner. Beyond exploring the sex and number of sex partners of their WSW patients, providers should elicit history of past and current sex with men, history of preventive health examinations (including Papanicolaou smears and STI screens), detailed sexual practices (oral sex, anal sex, penetrative sex with toys/objects, etc.), use of safer sex methods (dental dams, condoms, etc.) and associated drug use.

In the first analysis of its kind, investigators found that women aged 15–24 years attending family planning clinics in the U.S. Pacific Northwest 1997 through 2005 and who also reported same sex behavior had higher positivity of *C. trachomatis* than women who reported exclusively heterosexual behavior [60]. Factors associated with chlamydial infection among WSW in this study included use of nucleic acid amplification tests (NAAT) for diagnosis, testing at a non-"routine visit," report of genitourinary symptoms and report of a sex partner with chlamydial infection. Over the study period, WSW who reported sexual behavioral risks also had the highest chlamydia positivity compared to women reporting sex only with or women who reported sex with men and women who reported similar risks. Interestingly, a greater proportion of women reporting sex with men and women reported sexual risk behaviors compared with both heterosexual women and those reporting sex only with women; despite this, *C. trachomatis* positivity was not highest in this group. Of note, there was relatively high chlamydia positivity among American Indian/Alaska Native WSW, a finding that is consistent with racial/ethnic disparities previously described from the Region X IPP data [61]. The finding of higher chlamydia positivity among WSW relative to women reporting sex exclusively with men was unexpected. Possible explanations for this observation relate to differences in these two groups' use of reproductive health care services (including chlamydia screening), biological susceptibility to lower genital tract infection, infrequent use of barrier methods to prevent STI transmission with female partners, trends towards higher risk behaviors, and differential characteristics of their respective sexual networks.

Several investigators have reported that WSW are less likely to undergo routine Papanicolaou smear screening—and generally, preventive gynecologic care, often sought in the context of obtaining birth control—relative to their exclusively heterosexual counterparts [62, 63]. This would logically reduce the number of health care encounters at which chlamydia testing would likely be performed. Moreover, most women who report same sex behavior often do not believe that they are at risk of acquiring STI from their female partners [64]. This may lead to less frequent use of some preventive measures (for example, washing sex toys between partners) or infrequent use of barrier methods (including gloves, condoms, dental dams) for STI prevention [65]. Further, health care providers do not always obtain a complete sexual history and may thus fail to elicit reports from WSW of higher risk behaviors that would prompt *C. trachomatis* screening and related prevention counseling [66].

Another potential explanation for finding of some STI, including chlamydia, among WSW relates to selection of sex partners. Some women who report same sex behavior may be more likely to select higher risk sex partners and participate in higher risk behaviors, including unprotected vaginal and anal sex with homosexual or bisexual men [38, 67]. One large cross-sectional survey across health care sites in the USA found that women who identified as lesbians reported more male sex partners and higher numbers of male sex partners who reported sex with other men in the past year than either heterosexual or bisexual women [41]. In a Seattle-based study of women reporting sex with at least one woman in the past year, concurrency (overlap between partnerships reported by participant) was common, especially among bisexual women [68]. Bisexual women frequently reported inconsistent condom use with either vaginal or anal intercourse with men. Many of these women (16%) believed their male partner had sex with another man at some point in time. Additional studies have demonstrated other high-risk behaviors among some WSW, including use of injection drugs and crack cocaine, and exchange of sex for drugs or money [38, 69–72].

Taken together, the data cited above emphasize that WSW should undergo routine age-based annual screening for *C. trachomatis* as recommended by current guidelines. No data are available to inform screening for *N. gonorrhoeae* in this group.

In the USA, the National Health and Nutrition Examination Surveys (NHANES) have provided the principal window into population-based trends in HSV seroprevalence in adults since the survey first reported on this outcome in 1989 [73]. Using audio computer assisted self-interview (A-CASI) obtained from women ages 18–59 years who participated in NHANES 2001–2006, Xu and colleagues assessed participants' report of recent and life time same-sex behavior [74]. In addition, a subset of these women, ages 18–49 years, had type-specific serologic testing for HSV that, as they point out, can serve as a valuable surrogate marker for cumulative lifetime sexual risk. The percentage of participants who reported ever having had sex with another woman translates to 5.7 million (95% CI, 4.9–6.6), a number that will serve as a useful denominator for future analyses and that emphasizes the normative aspects of this behavior. Moreover, more than half of all respondents who reported having sex with another woman in their lifetime identified themselves as heterosexual, including 25% who reported having had sex with another woman in the prior year. These findings are very good reminders that equating sexual behavior to sexual identity—a tendency still evident in many clinical interactions and some guidelines—is neither reliable nor advisable, and is essentially scientifically irresponsible.

In the NHANES group, 7.1% of women reported ever having had sex with a woman (95% CI, 6.1–8.2), significantly lower than the 11.2% reported in the 2002 National Survey of Family Growth (another large, U.S. population-based survey) [75], but higher than the 4.9% reported in the U.K.'s National Survey of Sexual Attitudes and Lifestyles (NATSAL 2000, 1999–2001) [63]. It is unlikely that the true prevalence differs greatly between the USA and the U.K., but several factors may have contributed to these discrepancies: interviewing methodology,

phrasing of survey questions and the changing sociopolitical climate. Using CASI has been shown to increase the frequency of reporting of potentially stigmatized behaviors; paradoxically, CASI was not used in the NSFG study, but was employed in both NHANES and NATSAL. The phrasing of questions regarding sexual practices differed: the NSFG study asked participants about "a sexual experience," the definition of which could conceivably be open to interpretation, while NHANES and NATSAL asked more specifically about sexual practice. And lastly, timing is everything—particularly in reference to generational attitudinal shifts. Report of any lifetime same-sex behavior in NHANES was considerably higher in younger women, peaking at 9.4% in ages 18–29 years, and in fact, was negatively correlated with increasing age. The higher overall prevalence of lifetime same-sex behavior in this age group has been suggested by other data, and may truly reflect that times really are changing: more open attitudes and evident tolerance for homosexuality has likely created a freer climate for young women to pursue and to report sexual relationships with other women.

Xu and colleagues found strikingly high seroprevalence of HSV-2 in certain subgroups of women who reported ever having had sex with a woman, and identified some intriguing risks as well. The most intriguing finding was that HSV-2 seroprevalence was significantly higher among the groups of women reporting same-sex behavior. The HSV-2 seroprevalence of women who identified as heterosexual and reported no lifetime same-sex behavior was 23.8%, compared to 45.6% of women who identified as heterosexual with some lifetime same-sex behavior, or 35.9% of women who identified as bisexual—although the bisexual group reported a higher number of lifetime male sex partners than the former (median, 17.6 vs. 10.8). HSV-2 seroprevalence was 30.3% for those sexually active with women in the past year and 36.2% for those ever active with women. Interestingly, the seroprevalence of HSV-2 among women who self-identified as "homosexual" (8.2%) was nearly identical to that in a much smaller, clinic-based sample done in Seattle nearly a decade ago [56]. It is worth noting, though, that even among (the admittedly small number of) self-identified homosexual or lesbian participants in NHANES, most (84%) had had at least one male sex partner, so the authors could not estimate HSV-2 seroprevalence among women who reported no lifetime sex with men. Report of same-sex behavior—whether during the lifetime or more recently—was also associated with earlier sexual debut and higher numbers of total lifetime sex partners; however, self-identification (as homosexual, bisexual, or heterosexual) significantly impacted this association. Again, even these relatively straightforward data collected at the population level emphasize the complex interplay between sexual behavior, identity, and orientation.

Prevention Interventions in Women, with Emphasis on Relevance to and Access for Key Vulnerable Populations

Barrier Methods

Male Condoms

When used consistently and correctly, male latex condoms are effective in preventing sexual transmission of HIV and other STDs, including chlamydia, gonorrhea, syphilis, genital HPV, and trichomoniasis. By limiting lower genital tract infections, male condoms might also reduce the risk of women developing pelvic inflammatory disease (PID) [76]. In heterosexual serodiscordant relationships in which condoms were consistently used, HIV-negative partners were 80% less likely to become HIV-infected compared with persons in similar relationships in which condoms were not used [77]. Condom use may also reduce the risk for transmission of herpes simplex virus-2 (HSV-2), although data for this effect are more limited [78, 79]. Finally, condom use reduces the risk of HPV [80, 81] and HPV-associated diseases (e.g., genital warts and cervical cancer) [82]. Use of condoms has been associated with regression of cervical intraepithelial neoplasia (CIN) [83] and clearance of HPV infection in women, and with regression of HPV-associated penile lesions in men [84].

A prospective study among newly sexually active college women demonstrated that consistent condom use was associated with a 70% reduction in risk for genital HPV transmission. Investigators followed 82 female university students who reported their first intercourse with a male partner either during the study period of within 2 weeks before enrollment [81]. Cervical and vulvovaginal samples for HPV DNA testing and Pap smears were collected every 4 months. Incidence of genital HPV infection was 37.8 per 100 patient-years at risk among women whose partners used condoms for all instances of intercourse during the 8 months before testing, compared with 89.3 per 100 patient-years at risk in women whose partners used condoms less than 5% of the time (adjusted hazard ratio (HR) 0.3, 95% CI, 0.1–0.6). In women reporting 100% condom use by their partners, no cervical squamous intraepithelial lesions (SIL) were detected in 32 patient-years at risk, whereas 14 incident lesions were detected during 97 patient-years at risk among women whose partners did not use condoms or used them less consistently.

In an analysis that pooled data from all published studies that prospectively assessed condom use and HSV-2 incidence, persons who always used condoms had a 30% decreased risk of acquiring HSV-2 compared with those who reported no condom use ($P=0.01$) [85]. Moreover, risk of acquiring HSV-2 decreased by 7% for every additional 25% increment in the time that condoms were used ($P=0.01$). Conversely, HSV-2 acquisition rose steadily with report of increasing frequency of unprotected sex acts. These effects were consistent for men and women.

Two general categories of nonlatex condoms exist. The first type is made of polyurethane or other synthetic material and provides protection against STD/HIV and pregnancy equal to that of latex condoms. These condoms provide an acceptable alternative for persons unable to use latex condoms. A Cochrane review concluded that while one nonlatex condom (eZon) did not protect against pregnancy as well as its latex comparison condom, no differences were found in the typical use efficacy between the Avanti and the Standard Tactylon and their latex counterparts. The nonlatex condoms had higher rates of clinical breakage than latex comparators (OR for clinical breakage, 2.64 (95% CI, 1.63–4.28) to 4.95 (95% CI, 3.63–6.75)). Contraceptive efficacy of nonlatex condoms could not be estimated, and will require more research [86]. The FDA has published draft guidelines modifying the labeling on male latex condoms to reflect these findings [87].

Female Condoms

Laboratory studies indicated that the original version of the female condom (Reality™) is an effective mechanical barrier to viruses and semen. If used consistently and correctly, the female condom might substantially reduce the risk for STI. Female condoms are safe to use repeatedly if proper care procedures are followed. Two systematic reviews support the potential effectiveness of female condoms. The first reviewed 137 articles and abstracts on various aspects of the female condom and five randomized controlled trials on its effectiveness [88]. The review concluded that while the evidence is limited, "the female condom is effective in increasing protected sex and decreasing STI incidence among women." A second systematic review concluded that "randomised controlled trials provide evidence that female condoms confer as much protection from STIs as male condoms." [89].

The comparative effectiveness of the male condom and female condom was assessed in a randomized controlled trial that assigned women to sequential use of ten male latex condoms, then ten female polyurethane condoms [90]. The association between frequency and types of self-reported mechanical failure and semen exposure were measured by prostate-specific antigen. Moderate to high postcoital prostate-specific antigen (PSA) levels were detected in 3.5% of male condom uses and 4.5% of female condom users (difference 1.4; 95% CI, 1.6–3.7). PSA levels were more frequent with mechanical problems and less frequent with other problems or correct use with no problems. Although mechanical problems were more common with the female condom, the risk of semen exposure was probably similar.

The FDA held an advisory meeting in December 2008 to review evidence in support of a new version of the female condom [91]. The new version has a slightly modified shape, no seam, and is made from nitrile (as opposed to polyurethane, the material of the first version). Modifications to the manufacturing process as a result of this shift have resulted in considerable cost reductions to the product. The advisory panel voted to support FDA approval of the new female condom, and it became available in 2009. The new female condom is already in use in many countries outside of the USA and has been endorsed by the World Health Organization (WHO) after a similar review process. This new design should theoretically afford protection similar to the polyurethane female condom and allows for lower manufacturing cost.

Diaphragms

Observational studies demonstrate that diaphragm use protects against cervical gonorrhea, chlamydia, and trichomoniasis [89]. The MIRA trial examined the effect of a diaphragm plus polycarbophil (Replens) lubricant on HIV acquisition in women in Zimbabwe and South Africa. The authors found no additional protective effect of latex diaphragm, lubricant gel, and condoms on HIV acquisition compared to condoms alone [92]. A subsequent analysis of data from this study evaluated outcomes of chlamydia and gonorrhea [93]. Median follow-up time was 21 months, and the retention rate was over 93%. Four hundred seventy-one first chlamydia infections occurred, 247 in the intervention arm and 224 in the control arm with an overall incidence of 6.2/100 woman-years (relative hazard (RH) 1.11, 95% CI: 0.93–1.33) and 192 first gonococcal infections, 95 in the intervention arm and 97 in the control arm with an overall incidence of 2.4/100 women-years (RH 0.98, 95% CI: 0.74–1.30). Results indicated that when diaphragm adherence was defined as "always use" since the last visit, a significant reduction in gonorrhea incidence occurred among women randomized to the intervention (RH 0.61, 95% CI: 0.41–0.91). The authors concluded that while no difference by study arm was found in the rate of acquisition of chlamydia or gonorrhea, per-protocol results suggested that consistent use of the diaphragm may reduce acquisition of gonorrhea.

Another analysis from the MIRA trial estimated the diaphragm's effect on HPV incidence and clearance in women in Zimbabwe [94]. No overall difference in HPV incidence occurred at the first post-enrollment visit and at 12 months, or in HPV clearance at 12 months among women HPV-positive at enrollment. However, clearance of HPV type 18 was lower in the diaphragm group at exit visit (RR 0.55; 05% CI: 0.33–0.89) but not at 12 months. Women reporting diaphragm/gel use at 100% of prior sex acts had a lower likelihood of having one or more new HPV types detected at 12 months (RR 0.75; 95% CI: 0.58–0.96). The authors concluded that diaphragms did not reduce HPV incidence or increase clearance.

Diaphragms should not be relied on as the sole source of protection against STI or HIV infection. Diaphragms used with nonoxynol-9 (N-9) spermicides have been associated with an increased risk for bacterial urinary tract infections in women.

Other Methods

Microbicides

In general, results of topical microbicides with nonspecific antimicrobial activity for the prevention of HIV and STD have been disappointing [95, 96]. Although a randomized controlled trial comparing vaginal application of 0.5% PRO 2000 (a synthetic polyanionic polymer that blocks attachment of HIV to the host cell) to BufferGel (a vaginal buffering agent), placebo gel, and condom use only found that PRO 2000 was associated with a 30% reduction in risk of HIV acquisition relative to no gel use (adjusted HR 0.70 (95% CI, 0.46–1.08; $P=0.10$)) or to placebo gel use (adjusted HR 0.67 (05% CI, 0.44–1.02; $P=0.06$)), and that women randomized to the PRO2000 arm who had high adherence to gel and used condoms infrequently experienced a 78% reduction in risk [97], a considerably larger study (the MDP301 trial, conducted in four sub-Saharan African countries) assessing 0.5%

PRO2000 relative to placebo gel found no protective effect [98]. Taken together, these studies do not support further testing of polyanion-type compounds with nonspecific activity against STD and HIV.

Other microbicide products have not fared well either. A randomized controlled trial compared coitally dependent use of Carraguard (a carrageenan derivative with in vitro activity against HIV) to methylcellulose gel placebo among South African women at high risk for HIV infection. After 2 years follow-up, HIV incidence in the Carraguard group ($N=3,011$) was 3.3 per 100 woman-years, and 3.8 per 100 woman-years in the placebo group ($N=2,994$) (adjusted HR 0.87 (95% CI: 0.69–1.09)). Applicator dye testing—one means of measuring actual vaginal insertion of the product—indicated that adherence to product was low (42% of sex acts overall). Self-reported product use was substantially higher than the estimate obtained from applicator testing, and some investigators have reported low accuracy for applicator dye testing [99, 100].

Two randomized controlled trials compared daily 6% cellulose sulfate (an HIV entry inhibitor) vaginal gel to corresponding placebo. A multicountry trial enrolled 1398 African women at high risk for HIV. Twenty-five newly acquired HIV infections occurred in the cellulose sulfate group and 16 in the placebo group, with an estimated hazard ratio of infection for the cellulose sulfate group of 1.61 ($P=0.13$). This result, which is not significant, is in contrast to the interim finding that led to the trial being stopped prematurely (hazard ratio, 2.23; $P=0.02$) and the suggestive result of a preplanned secondary (adherence-based) analysis (hazard ratio, 2.02; $P=0.05$). No significant effect of cellulose sulfate as compared with placebo was found on the risk of gonorrhea (HR, 1.10; 95% confidence interval [CI], 0.74–1.62) or chlamydia (hazard ratio, 0.71; 95% CI, 0.47–1.08). The authors concluded that cellulose sulfate did not prevent and may have increased risk of HIV acquisition [101]. A second randomized, placebo-controlled trial of cellulose sulfate in Nigeria was stopped prematurely after the data safety monitoring board of the multicountry trial concluded that cellulose sulfate might be increasing the risk of HIV [101, 102].

With the limited data available, cellulose sulfate gel appeared not to prevent transmission of HIV, gonorrhea, or chlamydial infection.

Two trials of the effectiveness of 1.0% C31G (Savvy; a surfactant) in preventing HIV acquisition were similarly disappointing. In the first, more women in the SAVVY group reported reproductive tract adverse events than placebo [103]. In the second, 33 seroconversions (21 in the SAVVY group and 12 in the placebo group) occurred in the 2,153 participants. The cumulative probability of HIV seroconversion was 2.8% in the SAVVY group and 1.5% in the placebo group ($P=0.121$) with a hazard ratio of 1.7 for SAVVY versus placebo (95% CI: 0.9, 3.5) [104]. The trials indicated that SAVVY did not reduce the incidence of HIV infection, and may have been associated with increased risks.

Pre-exposure Prophylaxis for HIV and STD
In the last 2 years, the field of pre-exposure prophylaxis (PrEP) has been galvanized by the results from clinical trials of antiretroviral medications (ART) to impact transmission and acquisition of HIV. In HIV-infected persons, ART reduces viral load and presumably reduces infectiousness. A recent trial, HPTN 052, provided more optimism about the use of ARVs for prevention [105]. Focusing on the HIV infected partner of discordant couples, HPTN 052 was a randomized, multicenter, clinical trial to evaluate the effectiveness of ARV in preventing sexual transmission. To be eligible, the HIV-infected partner needed to have a CD4 cell count of 350–550 cells/mm^3, above the level of current WHO recommendations to initiate therapy. Couples were randomized to one of two study arms: (1) immediate initiation of ARVs in the index case upon enrollment, or (2) delayed initiation of ARVs until two consecutive CD4 cell counts were below 250 cells/mm^3 or with an AIDS defining illness. The HPTN 052 results were striking, and validated findings from seven previous observational studies [106]. Participants in the immediate ARV initiation arm had a 96% lower risk of acquiring HIV than those in the delayed arm. Moreover, the HIV-infected partner in the immediate arm also suffered fewer HIV-related complications than those in the delayed arm.

In HIV-uninfected persons, ART reduces susceptibility to infection, a concept supported by animal studies and by a study of safety and acceptability in West African women. Most recently the results of the CAPRISA 004 and the iPrEX studies have provided proof of concept for both topical and oral PrEP [107–109]. CAPRISA 004 randomized 889 women in South Africa to coitally dependent use (up to 12 h before and within 2 h after intercourse, not to exceed two administrations in 1 day) of 1% tenofovir gel inserted vaginally, or to corresponding placebo gel, for a median of 30 months. Women randomized to the tenofovir gel group had a significantly reduced rate of HIV acquisition: 5.6 per 100 women-years, compared to 9.1 per 100 women-years (incidence rate ratio 0.61; 95% CI=6–60). The risk of HSV-2 acquisition was also reduced in the tenofovir group (by 51%; $P=0.003$).

In the first clinical trial reporting on the efficacy of oral PrEP (iPrEx), nearly 3,000 men at high risk for HIV acquisition through sex with other men were randomized to daily oral tenofovir-emtricitabine (TDF-FTC) or placebo and followed for a median of 1.2 years [110]. Men in the TDF-FTC arm experienced a 42% reduction in incidence of HIV (95% CI=18–60) [111]. A nested case-control analysis compared drug levels in men randomized to the TDF-FTC group. Among men with detectable drug level, as compared with those without a detectable level, the odds of HIV infection were lower by nearly 13-fold (O.R. 12.9; 95% CI, 1.7–99.3), corresponding to a relative reduction in HIV acquisition risk of 92% (95% CI, 40–99). Of note, adherence among men randomized to the active study product as estimated by TDF or FTC levels in peripheral blood mononuclear cells (PBMC) was approximately 50%. More recently, the iPrEx investigators reported that daily oral TDF-FTC use for 2 years in HIV-uninfected men was associated with small but significant loss of bone mineral density at the femoral neck (net effect, −1.1% (95% CI, −0.4 to −1.9)) [112]. The encouraging findings from the iPrEx study prompted CDC to publish interim guidance on the use of TDF-FTC for PrEP in MSM [113]. Planning is underway to issue full guidelines, expected sometime in 2011.

While the results of iPrEx and CAPRISA 004 are extremely encouraging, a Phase III, double-blind, randomized, placebo-controlled trial of daily oral TDF-FTC among African women at high risk for HIV acquisition was stopped early when its Independent Data and Monitoring Committee concluded that the study would be unable to determine if oral Truvada is effective in preventing HIV infection in high-risk women [114]. An equal number of HIV infections ($n = 28$) were observed in each arm among the 1,951 women enrolled to that point. The study had planned to enroll 3,900 women and follow them for 1 year. Complete analysis of the final data set must occur before a plausible explanation for this disappointing result can be offered, and is anticipated in the next several months. In the interim, other randomized controlled trials of PrEP are underway which examine different dosing strategies (daily vaginal use of 1% tenofovir gel in the VOICE study (MTN 003)) [115], risk behavior (heterosexual acquisition in reproductive age women in the VOICE study and in HIV serodiscordant couples in the Partners in Prevention Study), and geographic locale. Information on these studies is available at http://www.avac.org.

Two studies examined suppression of HSV as a means of reducing acquisition or transmission of HIV. Infection with herpes simplex virus type-2 (HSV-2) is a significant risk for acquisition and transmission of HIV [116]. A meta-analysis of 19 prospective observational studies reported that infection with HSV-2 increased risk of HIV acquisition 2.7-fold in men and 4.4-fold in women [117]. However, two studies of daily suppressive acyclovir therapy in HIV-uninfected adults in Africa did not show a reduction in risk of HIV acquisition, despite high rates of reported adherence and excellent retention in one [25, 118]. A similar study among HIV-infected persons showed that although acyclovir treatment reduced the frequency of genital ulcers by 73% and HIV plasma viral load by 40% ($0.25 \log_{10}$ copies/ml) compared to placebo, it did not effect a reduction in risk of HIV acquisition [26, 119]. Notably, participants treated with acyclovir had a small but significant reduction in risk of progression to HIV-related disease including decline of CD4 cells to <200 cells/mm^3, initiation of antiretroviral medication, or death.

Regarding PrEP for other STD prevention, as described earlier, an unexpected finding from the CAPRISA 004 trial was the protective effect of 1% tenofovir gel on HSV-2 acquisition [120]. Earlier work had shown that oral tenofovir did not produce drug levels in the vagina necessary to reach the EC50 against herpes. However, topical tenofovir allows local drug concentrations nearly 1,000 times higher than oral dosing. In CAPRISA 004, the higher level of tenofovir in cervicovaginal fluid was associated with significantly reduced rates of HSV-2 acquisition. The relationship between vaginal tenofovir gel use and HSV-2 acquisition will also be assessed in heterosexual women participating in the ongoing VOICE study, with results expected in early 2013.

Another randomized trial of STI pre-exposure prophylaxis evaluated other vaginal infections. It assessed the effect of directly observed oral treatment with 2 g of metronidazole plus 150 mg of fluconazole compared with metronidazole placebo plus fluconazole placebo administered monthly in reducing vaginal infections among Kenyan women at risk for HIV-1 acquisition. Of 310 HIV-1-seronegative female sex workers enrolled (155 per arm), 303 were included in the primary end points analysis. Compared with control subjects, women receiving the intervention had fewer episodes of BV (HR, 0.55; 95% CI, 0.49–0.63) and more frequent vaginal colonization with any *Lactobacillus* species (HR, 1.47; 95% CI, 1.19–1.80) and hydrogen peroxide-producing *Lactobacillus* species (HR, 1.63; 95% CI, 1.16–2.27). The incidences of vaginal candidiasis (HR, 0.84; 95% CI, 0.67–1.04) and trichomoniasis (HR, 0.55; 95% CI, 0.27–1.12) among treated women were less than those among control subjects, but the differences were not statistically significant. The authors concluded that periodic presumptive treatment reduced the incidence of BV and promoted colonization with normal vaginal flora [121]. Another trial randomized women with asymptomatic BV to observation or treatment and prophylaxis with twice weekly intravaginal metronidazole gel. Women in the metronidazole gel arm had fewer chlamydial infections over the subsequent 6 months [122].

Postexposure Prophylaxis for STI/HIV, and Unintended Pregnancy

In the USA, an emergency contraception (EC) pill with the brand name Plan B is available over the counter to women aged 17 years and older and by prescription to younger women. Plan B contains two tablets of 0.75 mg levonorgestrel, which may be taken 12 h apart as labeled or together as a single dose. If Plan B is not readily accessible, oral EC also may be provided using many commonly available brands of oral contraceptive pills by instructing the woman to take a specified number of tablets at once. Emergency insertion of an IUD up to 7 days after sex can reduce pregnancy risk by more than 99%. However, this method is not advisable for a woman who may have untreated cervical gonorrhea or chlamydia, who is already pregnant, or who has other contraindications to IUD use. All oral EC regimens are most efficacious when initiated as soon as possible after unprotected sex but have some efficacy as long as 5 days later. EC is ineffective (but is also not harmful) if the woman is already pregnant [123]. More information about EC is available in the 19th edition of *Contraceptive Technology* [124], or at http://www.arhp.org/healthcareproviders/resources/contraceptionresources.

A Cochrane review summarized the efficacy, safety, and convenience of various methods of emergency contraception. The review concluded that mifepristone middle dose (25–50 mg) was superior to other hormonal regimens. Mifepristone low dose (<25 mg) could be more effective than levonorgestrel 0.75 mg (two doses) but this was not conclusive. Levonorgestrel proved more effective than the Yuzpe regimen. The copper IUD was another effective emergency contraceptive that can provide ongoing contraception [123].

CDC guidelines for the use of postexposure prophylaxis with antiretroviral therapy aimed at preventing HIV acquisition as a result of sexual exposure are available [125], as are recommendations for STI prophylaxis after sexual assault.

Immunization

Preexposure vaccination is one of the most effective methods for preventing transmission of two main STDs: HPV and hepatitis B. In March 2007, the Advisory Committee on Immunization Practices (ACIP) issued guidelines for administration of the quadrivalent HPV vaccine to females aged 25 years and younger [126]. Specific details are available at http://www.cdc.gov/std/hpv. This vaccine confers protection against HPV types 6/11 (responsible for 90% of genital warts) and 16/18 (responsible for 70% of cervical cancers). In published clinical trials, the quadrivalent HPV vaccine has demonstrated efficacy for prevention of vaccine HPV type-related cervical, vaginal, and vulvar cancer precursor and dysplastic lesions, and external genital warts [127]. Universal vaccination of females aged 11–12 years is recommended, as is catch-up vaccination for females aged 13–26 years. The vaccine is also efficacious in preventing infection in women aged 24–45 years not already infected with the relevant HPV types [128]. Data on the efficacy of the quadrivalent HPV vaccines in protecting young men from vaccine-type HPV acquisition indicates similarly high levels of protection [129, 130], and the ACIP issued permissive guidance for immunization to prevent genital warts in young men in 2010. Both men and women are also likely to benefit from protection against anal intraepithelial neoplasia afforded by the quadrivalent vaccine. A bivalent vaccine that is effective in preventing cervical neoplasia associated with HPV types 16/18 has also been approved for use in the USA, and is recommended by ACIP [131, 132].

Immunization against hepatitis B has been routinely recommended for infants since 1991 and was subsequently recommended for adolescents. While this has been temporally associated with marked declines in HBV incidence in the USA [133], sexual transmission still accounts for the majority of new infections, which are especially common among unvaccinated MSM. Consequently, hepatitis B vaccination is recommended for all adults who are at risk for sexual infection, including sex partners of hepatitis B surface antigen (HBsAg)-positive persons, sexually active persons who are not in a long-term, mutually monogamous relationship, persons seeking evaluation or treatment for a STD, and

MSM [134]. Moreover, all HIV-infected persons should be immunized against hepatitis B, as the natural history of hepatitis B is accelerated in the setting of HIV, and coinfection imposes specific considerations in selection of antiretroviral agents. Hepatitis A vaccine is licensed and is recommended for MSM and illicit drug users (both injecting and noninjecting) [135]. Specific details are available at http://www.cdc.gov/hepatitis.

Prospects for an effective HIV vaccine remain on the distant horizon. Recent disappointing results from human trials have stimulated a renewed focus on the basic biology of HIV pathogenesis. Two phase III trials of a vaccine aimed at eliciting neutralizing antibodies against the envelope glycoprotein 120 did not find protection against HIV infection [136, 137]. A phase IIB trial of the first T-cell vaccine (Merck's MRKAd5 HIV-1 gag/pol/nef trivalent product, using a replication-defective adenovirus type-5 vector with three HIV genes) was stopped in September 2007. Interim analysis revealed no protective effect against HIV acquisition, and no reduction in initial viral loads among participants infected with HIV [138, 139]. Further analysis showed that pre-existing immunity to adenovirus type-5 was directly associated with a significantly higher risk of acquiring HIV, and that this untoward effect was further augmented among uncircumcised men. A community-based, randomized, double-blind, placebo-controlled trial performed in over 16,000 Thai adults evaluated four priming injections of a recombinant canary pox vector vaccine (ALVAC-HIV) plus two booster injections of a recombinant glycoprotein 120 subunit vaccine (AIDSVAX B/E) [140]. There was a trend toward HIV prevention in the intention-to-treat analysis (vaccine efficacy 26.4% (95% CI -4.0 – 4.79)), but not in the per protocol analysis (vaccine efficacy 26.2% (95% CI -13.3 – 51.9)). Vaccination did not affect HIV viral load or CD4 count in participants who acquired HIV during the trial.

Circumcision in Male Sex Partners

Three randomized controlled trials performed in healthy African men showed that male circumcision was effective in preventing HIV acquisition.

In studies performed in Uganda, South Africa, and Kenya, men were randomized to be offered immediate or delayed (24 months) circumcision, and followed over 2 years for acquisition of HIV and other STDs [141–144]. The summary rate ratio for reduction of HIV acquisition in the men who underwent immediate circumcision for the three trials was 0.42 (95% CI 0.31, 0.57), identical to that obtained from observational studies, which translates into a protective effect of male circumcision of 58% [142]. On the basis of these findings, a WHO and UNAIDS consultation in March 2007 recommended that circumcision be recognized as an effective intervention for HIV prevention of heterosexual HIV acquisition in men [145]. WHO and UNAIDS also recommended that male circumcision be offered to HIV-negative men in addition, but not as a substitute, to other HIV risk-reduction strategies.

Circumcision also affords a similar level of protection against acquisition of other STI, particularly nonulcerative pathogens, including high-risk genital HPV and genital herpes [146–148]. In South Africa, after 21 months of follow-up, circumcision protected against high-risk HPV (OR 0.57; 95% CI, 0.43–0.75), but not gonorrhea [146]. The association between trichomoniasis and male circumcision remained borderline when controlling for age, ethnic group, number of lifetime partners, marital status, condom use and HIV status (adjusted OR, 0.48, $p=0.069$). In the as-treated analysis, this association became significant (OR, 0.49, $p=0.030$ and adjusted OR, 0.41, $p=0.03$). The authors concluded that male circumcision reduces incident trichomoniasis among men. Men in Uganda were also followed for acquisition of STD for 2 years. At 24 months, the cumulative probability of HSV-2 seroconversion was 7.8% in men randomized to circumcision (1,684 men who were initially HSV2-seronegative) and 10.3% in the control group (1,709 men initially HSV2-seronegative) (adjusted HR 0.72 (95% CI, 0.56–0.92; $P=0.008$)) [148]. The prevalence of high-risk HPV genotypes was 18.0% in the intervention group and 27.9% in the control group (adjusted risk ratio, 0.65; 95% CI, 0.46–0.90; $P=0.009$). However, no significant difference between the two study groups was observed in the incidence of syphilis (adjusted HR, 1.10; 95% CI, 0.75–1.65; $P=0.44$). Among men enrolled in the Kenya study, circumcision afforded no protection against incident gonorrhea, chlamydia, or trichomoniasis [149].

No randomized controlled trials of circumcision have been performed among men in the USA. However, a cross-sectional analysis reported that among 394 heterosexual African-American men attending a Baltimore STD clinic who reported known HIV exposure, circumcision was significantly associated with lower HIV prevalence (10.2% vs. 22.0%); adjusted prevalence rate ratio (PRR) 0.49 (95% CI, 0.26–0.93). No such association was seen for men with unknown HIV exposure [150]. The benefits of circumcision to MSM are unproven. A meta-analysis of studies reported that overall, circumcised MSM had lower odds of being infected with HIV (OR, 0.86; 95% CI, 0.65–1.10), an association that did not reach statistical significance and that was similar among men who reported primarily engaging in insertive anal sex [151].

Unfortunately, the benefits of male circumcision in reducing HIV acquisition in men do not extend to women; however, other benefits may occur. Female sex partners of men who participated in the Uganda circumcision trial were followed to assess effects on their genital symptoms and vaginal infections [152]. Among women with normal vaginal flora scores at enrollment, rates of BV at follow-up were significantly lower in wives of men who had been circumcised compared to men who had not (prevalence risk ratio (PRR) 0.80; 95% CI, 0.65–0.97). In women with BV at enrollment, persistent BV at 1 year was significantly lower in the intervention arm than control arm women (PRR 0.83; 95% CI, 0.72–0.96). The adjusted prevalence risk ratio of GUD among wives of circumcised men compared with uncircumcised men was 0.78 (95% CI, 0.61–0.99), consistent with circumcision efficacy of 22%. The adjusted prevalence risk ratio for trichomoniasis in intervention arm wives relative to controls was 0.55 (95% CI, 0.34–0.89; efficacy 45%). The authors concluded that male circumcision may have direct benefits for prevention of genital ulceration, trichomoniasis, and BV in female partners and that this should be considered when planning scale-up of male circumcision programs for HIV prevention.

Implementation of male circumcision as a HIV prevention strategy remains to be fully defined. Concerns include possible disinhibitory effects on sexual risk behaviors, complications from unsafe or inexperienced providers, and acceptability by substantial numbers of men at highest risk for HIV [96]. Male circumcision is a compliment to, not a substitute for, other HIV risk-reduction strategies. WHO and UNAIDS recommend that countries with hyperendemic and generalized HIV epidemics and low prevalence of male circumcision expand access to safe male circumcision services within the context of ensuring universal access to comprehensive HIV prevention, treatment, care, and support.

Interactive Counseling Strategies

New data continue to support the use of individual client-centered counseling to reduce recipients' risk of acquiring HIV/STD. The U.S. Preventive Services Task Force (USPSTF) recently reviewed the evidence base on this topic [153, 154], and concluded with the following summary statement:

> The USPSTF recommends high-intensity behavioral counseling to prevent sexually transmitted infections (STIs) for all sexually active adolescents and for adults at increased risk for STIs. This is a grade B recommendation. The USPSTF concludes that the current evidence is insufficient to assess the balance of benefits and harms of behavioral counseling to prevent STIs in non-sexually active adolescents and in adults not at increased risk for STIs [153].

Training modules are available to help providers develop skills in this area; one consolidated resource is at http://www.stdhivpreventiontraining.org. Patient-centered counseling can have a beneficial impact on the likelihood of patients' assuming new or enhancing current risk-reduction practices. All providers should routinely obtain a sexual history from their patients, and address management of risk reduction as indicated [155, 156]. This is particularly important for routine care of HIV-infected persons, and for adults and adolescents at risk for acquisition of STI.

Systems-Based Approaches for Improving Women's Sexual Health: Priorities

Because women—and their infants—are uniquely vulnerable to the consequences of the infections discussed above, structural interventions that can effect wide-scale system change have the most potential to promote positive change. Examples include the adoption of chlamydia screening as a standard of care that is linked to provider (or health plan) performance and the provision of antimicrobial therapy for sex partners without requiring that they be examined (expedited partner management).

Optimization of selective screening for chlamydial infection remains a cornerstone of the interventions available to promote and protect women's health [157]. Randomized controlled trials have evaluated the effect of rescreening for chlamydia or gonorrhea in preventing repeat infection, and have uniformly provided support. The largest study randomly assigned women and heterosexual men with gonorrhea or chlamydial infection to have their partners receive expedited treatment or standard referral. The expedited-treatment group was offered medication to give to their partners, or if they preferred, study staff contacted partners and provided them with medication without examination. Persons assigned to standard partner referral were advised to refer partners for treatment and offered assistance notifying partners. Persistent or recurrent gonorrhea or chlamydia occurred in 13% assigned to standard partner referral and 10% assigned to expedited treatment of sexual partners (relative risk, 0.76; 95% CI, 0.59–0.98). Expedited treatment was more effective than standard referral of partners in reducing persistent or recurrent infection among patients with gonorrhea (3% vs. 11%, $P=0.01$) than in those with chlamydia (11% vs. 13%, $P=0.17$) ($P=0.05$ for comparison of treatment effects) and remained independently

associated with a reduced risk of persistent or recurrent infection after adjustment for other predictors of infection at follow-up (relative risk, 0.75; 95% CI, 0.57–0.97). Patients assigned to expedited treatment of sexual partners were significantly more likely than those assigned to standard referral of partners to report that all of their partners were treated and significantly less likely to report having sex with an untreated partner [158].

Additional observational studies support that this strategy should continue to be emphasized. Among 897 female adolescents attending school-based health centers, 236 had one or more subsequent positive tests for a cumulative incidence of reinfection in one year of 26.3% (95% CI, 23.4–29.2) [159]. Project RESPECT data were used to determine the incidence of new infections during the year after a visit to a STD clinic. Among 1,236 women, 25.8% had one or more new infections (11.9% acquired *C. trachomatis*, 6.3% *N. gonorrhoeae*, and 12.8% *T. vaginalis*); among 1,183 men, 14.7% had 1 or more new infections (9.4% acquired *C. trachomatis*, and 7.1% *N. gonorrhoeae*). The authors concluded that individuals who receive diagnoses of any of these STI should return in 3 months for rescreening [160]. This approach has also been used successfully for trichomoniasis [161]. Rescreening several months after a diagnosis of chlamydia, gonorrhea, or trichomoniasis detects substantial numbers of new infections, and can be recommended as a population-level prevention method. Community-level behavioral interventions since these have been extensively reviewed elsewhere [162].

Conclusion

A range of preventive interventions is needed to reduce the risks of acquiring STI and HIV among sexually active people. A flexible approach targeted to specific populations should integrate combinations of biomedical, behavioral, and structural interventions. These would ideally involve an array of prevention contexts, including (1) communications and practices among sexual partners, (2) transactions between individual clients and their health care providers and (3) comprehensive population-level strategies for prioritizing prevention research, ensuring accurate outcome assessment, and formulating health policy.

References

1. UNAIDS report on the global HIV/AIDS epidemic 2010. 2010.
2. Hall HI, Song R, Rhodes P, et al. Estimation of HIV incidence in the United States. JAMA. 2008;300:520–9.
3. Hall HI, Geduld J, Boulos D, et al. Epidemiology of HIV in the United States and Canada: current status and ongoing challenges. J Acquir Immune Defic Syndr. 2009;51 Suppl 1:S13–20.
4. Brooks JT, Kaplan JE, Holmes KK, Benson C, Pau A, Masur H. HIV-associated opportunistic infections – going, going, but not gone: the continued need for prevention and treatment guidelines. Clin Infect Dis. 2009;48:609–11.
5. Centers for Disease Control and Prevention. Sexually transmitted disease surveillance, 2009. Atlanta, GA: U.S. Department of Health and Human Services; 2010.
6. Gottlieb SL, Brunham RC, Byrne GI, Martin DH, Xu F, Berman SM. Introduction: the natural history and immunobiology of Chlamydia trachomatis genital infection and implications for chlamydia control. J Infect Dis. 2010;201 Suppl 2:S85–7.
7. Haggerty CL, Gottlieb SL, Taylor BD, Low N, Xu F, Ness RB. Risk of sequelae after Chlamydia trachomatis genital infection in women. J Infect Dis 2010;201 Suppl 2:S134–55.
8. Gottlieb SL, Berman SM, Low N. Screening and treatment to prevent sequelae in women with Chlamydia trachomatis genital infection: how much do we know? J Infect Dis. 2010;201 Suppl 2: S156–67.
9. Meyers DS, Halvorson H, Luckhaupt S. Screening for chlamydial infection: an evidence update for the U.S. Preventive Services Task Force. Ann Intern Med. 2007;147:135–42.
10. Chlamydia screening among sexually active young female enrollees of health plans – United States, 2000–2007. MMWR Morb Mortal Wkly Rep. 2009;58:362–5.
11. Centers for Disease Control and Prevention. Sexually transmitted disease surveillance, 2006. Atlanta, GA: U.S. Department of Health and Human Services; 2007.
12. Datta SD, Sternberg M, Johnson RE, et al. Gonorrhea and chlamydia in the United States among persons 14 to 39 years of age, 1999 to 2002. Ann Intern Med. 2007;147:89–96.
13. Miller WC, Ford CA, Morris M, et al. Prevalence of chlamydial and gonococcal infections among young adults in the United States. JAMA. 2004;291: 2229–36.
14. Barry PM, Kent CK, Klausner JD. Risk factors for gonorrhea among heterosexuals – San Francisco, 2006. Sex Transm Dis. 2008.
15. Centers for Disease Control and Prevention. Sexually transmitted disease surveillance 2006 supplement, Gonococcal Isolate Surveillance Project (GISP) annual report 2006. Atlanta, GA: U.S. Department of Health and Human Services, Centers for Disease Control and Prevention; 2008.
16. Update to CDC's sexually transmitted diseases treatment guidelines, 2006: fluoroquinolones no longer recommended for treatment of gonococcal infections. MMWR Morb Mortal Wkly Rep. 2007;56:332–6.
17. Neisseria gonorrhoeae with reduced susceptibility to azithromycin – San Diego County, California, 2009. MMWR Morb Mortal Wkly Rep. 2011;60:579–81.
18. Westrom L, Joesoef R, Reynolds G, Hagdu A, Thompson SE. Pelvic inflammatory disease and fertility. A cohort study of 1,844 women with laparoscopically verified disease and 657 control women with normal laparoscopic results. Sex Transm Dis. 1992;19:185–92.
19. Ness RB, Soper DE, Peipert J, et al. Design of the PID Evaluation and Clinical Health (PEACH) study. Control Clin Trials. 1998;19:499–514.
20. Ness RB, Soper DE, Holley RL, et al. Effectiveness of inpatient and outpatient treatment strategies for women with pelvic inflammatory disease: results from the Pelvic Inflammatory Disease Evaluation and Clinical Health (PEACH) randomized trial. Am J Obstet Gynecol. 2002;186:929–37.
21. Haggerty CL, Schulz R, Ness RB. Lower quality of life among women with chronic pelvic pain after pelvic inflammatory disease. Obstet Gynecol. 2003;102:934–9.
22. Primary and secondary syphilis – Jefferson county, Alabama, 2002–2007. MMWR Morb Mortal Wkly Rep. 2009;58:463–7.
23. Kirkcaldy RD, Su JR, Taylor MM, et al. Epidemiology of syphilis among hispanic women and associations with congenital syphilis, Maricopa county, Arizona. Sex Transm Dis. 2011;38(7):598–602.
24. Bhutta ZA, Yakoob MY, Lawn JE, et al. Stillbirths: what difference can we make and at what cost? Lancet. 2011;377:1523–38.
25. Celum C, Wald A, Hughes J, et al. Effect of aciclovir on HIV-1 acquisition in herpes simplex virus 2 seropositive women and men who have sex with men: a randomised, double-blind, placebo-controlled trial. Lancet. 2008;371:2109–19.
26. Celum C, Wald A, Lingappa JR, et al. Acyclovir and transmission of HIV-1 from persons infected with HIV-1 and HSV-2. N Engl J Med. 2010;362: 427–39.
27. Xu F, Sternberg MR, Kottiri BJ, et al. Trends in herpes simplex virus type 1 and type 2 seroprevalence in the United States. JAMA. 2006;296:964–73.

28. Koutsky L. The epidemiology behind the HPV vaccine discovery. Ann Epidemiol. 2009;19:239–44.
29. Daley MF, Crane LA, Markowitz LE, et al. Human papillomavirus vaccination practices: a survey of US physicians 18 months after licensure. Pediatrics. 2010;126:425–33.
30. Markowitz LE, Hariri S, Unger ER, Saraiya M, Datta SD, Dunne EF. Post-licensure monitoring of HPV vaccine in the United States. Vaccine. 2010;28: 4731–7.
31. Marrazzo JM, Martin DH, Watts DH, et al. Bacterial vaginosis: identifying research gaps proceedings of a workshop sponsored by DHHS/NIH/NIAID. Sex Transm Dis. 2010;37:732–44.
32. Sutton M, Sternberg M, Koumans EH, McQuillan G, Berman S, Markowitz L. The prevalence of Trichomonas vaginalis infection among reproductive-age women in the United States, 2001–2004. Clin Infect Dis. 2007;45:1319–26.
33. Miller WC, Swygard H, Hobbs MM, et al. The prevalence of trichomoniasis in young adults in the United States. Sex Transm Dis. 2005;32:593–8.
34. Klebanoff MA, Carey JC, Hauth JC, et al. Failure of metronidazole to prevent preterm delivery among pregnant women with asymptomatic Trichomonas vaginalis infection. N Engl J Med. 2001;345:487–93.
35. Wellings K, Collumbien M, Slaymaker E, et al. Sexual behavior in context: a global perspective. Lancet. 2006;368:1706–28.
36. Centers for Disease Control and Prevention. Youth risk behavior surveillance – United States SS, June 4, 2010. MMWR Morb Mortal Wkly Rep. 2010;59(No. SS-5).
37. Chandra A, Mosher WD, Copen C, Sionean C (2011) Sexual behavior, sexual attraction, and sexual identity in the United States: data from the 2006–2008 National Survey of Family Growth. Natl Health Stat Report 2011;Number 36.
38. Diamant AL, Schuster MA, McGuigan K, Lever J. Lesbians' sexual history with men: implications for taking a sexual history. Arch Intern Med. 1999;159:2730–6.
39. Lindley LL, Barnett CL, Brandt HM, Hardin JW, Burcin M. STDs among sexually active female college students: does sexual orientation make a difference? Perspect Sex Reprod Health. 2008;40:212–7.
40. Goodenow C, Szalacha LA, Robin LE, Westheimer K. Dimensions of sexual orientation and HIV-related risk among adolescent females: evidence from a statewide survey. Am J Public Health. 2008;98:1051–8.
41. Koh A, Gomez C, Shade S, Rowley E. Sexual risk factors among self-identified lesbians, bisexual women, and heterosexual women accessing primary care settings. Sex Transm Dis. 2005;32:563–9.
42. Dean L, Meyer I, Robinson K, et al. Lesbian, gay, bisexual, and transgender health: findings and concerns. J Gay Lesbian Med Assoc. 2000;4:102–51.
43. Hassan WM, Lavreys L, Chohan V, et al. Associations between intravaginal practices and bacterial vaginosis in Kenyan female sex workers without symptoms of vaginal infections. Sex Transm Dis. 2007;34:384–8.
44. Myer L, Kuhn L, Stein ZA, Wright Jr TC, Denny L. Intravaginal practices, bacterial vaginosis, and women's susceptibility to HIV infection: epidemiological evidence and biological mechanisms. Lancet Infect Dis. 2005;5:786–94.
45. Mohllajee AP, Curtis KM, Martins SL, Peterson HB. Hormonal contraceptive use and risk of sexually transmitted infections: a systematic review. Contraception. 2006;73:154–65.
46. Morrison CS, Richardson BA, Mmiro F, et al. Hormonal contraception and the risk of HIV acquisition. AIDS. 2007;21:85–95.
47. Baeten JM, Benki S, Chohan V, et al. Hormonal contraceptive use, herpes simplex virus infection, and risk of HIV-1 acquisition among Kenyan women. AIDS. 2007;21:1771–7.
48. Overton ET, Shacham E, Singhatiraj E, Nurutdinova D. Incidence of sexually transmitted infections among HIV-infected women using depot medroxyprogesterone acetate contraception. Contraception. 2008;78:125–30.
49. Shafii T, Stovel K, Holmes K. Association between condom use at sexual debut and subsequent sexual trajectories: a longitudinal study using biomarkers. Am J Public Health. 2007;97:1090–5.
50. Martino SC, Elliott MN, Collins RL, Kanouse DE, Berry SH. Virginity pledges among the willing: delays in first intercourse and consistency of condom use. J Adolesc Health. 2008;43:341–8.
51. Rosenbaum JE. Patient teenagers? A comparison of the sexual behavior of virginity pledgers and matched nonpledgers. Pediatrics. 2009;123:e110–20.
52. O'Hanlan KA, Crum CP. Human papillomavirus-associated cervical intraepithelial neoplasia following lesbian sex. Obstet Gynecol. 1996;88:702–3.
53. Kellock D, O'Mahony CP. Sexually acquired metronidazole-resistant trichomoniasis in a lesbian couple. Genitourin Med. 1996;72:60–1.
54. Marrazzo JM, Stine K, Koutsky LA. Genital human papillomavirus infection in women who have sex with women: a review. Am J Obstet Gynecol. 2000;183:770–4.
55. Tao G. Sexual orientation and related viral sexually transmitted disease rates among US women aged 15 to 44 years. Am J Public Health. 2008;98:1007–9.
56. Marrazzo JM, Stine K, Wald A. Prevalence and risk factors for infection with herpes simplex virus type-1 and -2 among lesbians. Sex Transm Dis. 2003;30: 890–5.
57. Marrazzo JM, Koutsky LA, Kiviat NB, Kuypers JM, Stine K. Papanicolaou test screening and prevalence of genital human papillomavirus among women who have sex with women. Am J Public Health. 2001; 91:947–52.
58. Kwakwa HA, Ghobrial MW. Female-to-female transmission of human immunodeficiency virus. Clin Infect Dis. 2003;36:e40–1.

59. Marrazzo JM, Koutsky LA, Eschenbach DA, Agnew K, Stine K, Hillier SL. Characterization of vaginal flora and bacterial vaginosis in women who have sex with women. J Infect Dis. 2002;185:1307–13.

60. Singh D, Fine D, Marrazzo. *C. trachomatis* infection among women reporting sex with women screened in family planning clinics in the Pacific Northwest, 1997–2005. Am J Public Health. 2010.

61. Gorgos L, Fine D, Marrazzo J. Chlamydia positivity in American Indian/Alaska Native women screened in family planning clinics, 1997–2004. Sex Transm Dis. 2008;35:753–7.

62. Cochran SD, Mays VM, Bowen D, et al. Cancer-related risk indicators and preventive screening behaviors among lesbians and bisexual women. Am J Public Health. 2001;91:591–7.

63. Mercer CH, Bailey JV, Johnson AM, et al. Women who report having sex with women: British national probability data on prevalence, sexual behaviors, and health outcomes. Am J Public Health. 2007;97:1126–33.

64. Einhorn L, Polgar M. HIV-risk behavior among lesbians and bisexual women. AIDS Educ Prev. 1994;6:514–23.

65. Marrazzo JM, Coffey P, Bingham A. Sexual practices, risk perception and knowledge of sexually transmitted disease risk among lesbian and bisexual women. Perspect Sex Reprod Health. 2005;37:6–12.

66. Kurth AE, Martin DP, Golden MR, et al. A comparison between audio computer-assisted self-interviews and clinician interviews for obtaining the sexual history. Sex Transm Dis. 2004;31:719–26.

67. Lemp GF, Hirozawa AM, Givertz D, et al. Seroprevalence of HIV and risk behaviors among young homosexual and bisexual men. The San Francisco/Berkeley Young Men's Survey. JAMA. 1994;272:449–54.

68. Marrazzo J, Cassells S, Ringwood K. Characteristics of young bisexual women's relationships with their male partners. In: 2006 National STD Prevention Conference, Centers for Disease Control and Prevention; 2006; Jacksonville, FL; 2006.

69. Friedman SR, Neaigus A, Jose B, et al. Sociometric risk networks and risk for HIV infection. Am J Public Health. 1997;87:1289–96.

70. Fethers K, Marks C, Mindel A, Estcourt CS. Sexually transmitted infections and risk behaviours in women who have sex with women. Sex Transm Infect. 2000;76:345–9.

71. Saewyc EM, Bearinger LH, Blum RW, Resnick MD. Sexual intercourse, abuse and pregnancy among adolescent women: does sexual orientation make a difference? Fam Plann Perspect. 1999;31:127–31.

72. Bevier P, Chiasson M, Heffernan H, Castro K. Women at a sexually transmitted disease clinic who reported same-sex contact: their HIV seroprevalence and risk behaviors. Am J Public Health. 1995;10:1366–71.

73. Johnson RE, Nahmias AJ, Magder LS, Lee FK, Brooks CA, Snowden CB. A seroepidemiologic survey of the prevalence of herpes simplex virus type 2 infection in the United States. N Engl J Med. 1989;321:7–12.

74. Xu F, Sternberg MR, Markowitz LE. Women who have sex with women in the United States: prevalence, sexual behavior and prevalence of herpes simplex virus type 2 infection-results from national health and nutrition examination survey 2001–2006. Sex Transm Dis. 2010;37(7):407–13.

75. Mosher WD, Chandra A, Jones J. Sexual behavior and selected health measures: men and women 15–44 years of age, United States. Adv Data. 2002;2005:1–55.

76. Ness RB, Randall H, Richter HE, et al. Condom use and the risk of recurrent pelvic inflammatory disease, chronic pelvic pain, or infertility following an \ episode of pelvic inflammatory disease. Am J Public Health. 2004;94:1327–9.

77. Weller S, Davis K. Condom effectiveness in reducing heterosexual HIV transmission. Cochrane Database Syst Rev. 2002:CD003255.

78. Gottlieb SL, Douglas Jr JM, Foster M, et al. Incidence of herpes simplex virus type 2 infection in 5 sexually transmitted disease (STD) clinics and the effect of HIV/STD risk-reduction counseling. J Infect Dis. 2004;190:1059–67.

79. Wald A, Langenberg AG, Link K, et al. Effect of condoms on reducing the transmission of herpes simplex virus type 2 from men to women. JAMA. 2001;285:3100–6.

80. Nielson CM, Harris RB, Nyitray AG, Dunne EF, Stone KM, Giuliano AR. Consistent condom use is associated with lower prevalence of human papillomavirus infection in men. J Infect Dis. 2010;202:445–51.

81. Winer RL, Hughes JP, Feng Q, et al. Condom use and the risk of genital human papillomavirus infection in young women. N Engl J Med. 2006;354:2645–54.

82. Manhart LE, Koutsky LA. Do condoms prevent genital HPV infection, external genital warts, or cervical neoplasia? A meta-analysis. Sex Transm Dis. 2002;29:725–35.

83. Hogewoning CJ, Bleeker MC, van den Brule AJ, et al. Condom use promotes regression of cervical intraepithelial neoplasia and clearance of human papillomavirus: a randomized clinical trial. Int J Cancer. 2003;107:811–6.

84. Bleeker MC, Hogewoning CJ, Voorhorst FJ, et al. Condom use promotes regression of human papillomavirus-associated penile lesions in male sexual partners of women with cervical intraepithelial neoplasia. Int J Cancer. 2003;107:804–10.

85. Martin ET, Krantz E, Gottlieb SL, et al. A pooled analysis of the effect of condoms in preventing HSV-2 acquisition. Arch Intern Med. 2009;169:1233–40.

86. Gallo MF, Grimes DA, Lopez LM, Schulz KF. Nonlatex versus latex male condoms for contraception. Cochrane Database Syst Rev. 2006. Last reviewed 26 May 2008.

87. Proposed guidance for condom labeling. http://www.fda.gov/ForConsumers/ByAudience/ForPatientAdvocates/HIVandAIDSActivities/ucm124512.htm. Accessed 28 Aug 2009.

88. Vijayakumar G, Mabude Z, Smit J, Beksinska M, Lurie M. A review of female-condom effectiveness: patterns of use and impact on protected sex acts and STI incidence. Int J STD AIDS. 2006;17:652–9.

89. Minnis AM, Padian NS. Effectiveness of female controlled barrier methods in preventing sexually transmitted infections and HIV: current evidence and future research directions. Sex Transm Infect. 2005;81:193–200.

90. Macaluso M, Blackwell R, Jamieson DJ, et al. Efficacy of the male latex condom and of the female polyurethane condom as barriers to semen during intercourse: a randomized clinical trial. Am J Epidemiol. 2007;166:88–96.

91. http://www.accessdata.fda.gov/scripts/cdrh/cfdocs/cfAdvisory/details.cfm?mtg=708. Accessed 30 Dec 2008.

92. Padian NS, van der Straten A, Ramjee G, et al. Diaphragm and lubricant gel for prevention of HIV acquisition in southern African women: a randomised controlled trial. Lancet. 2007;370:251–61.

93. Ramjee G, van der Straten A, Chipato T, et al. The diaphragm and lubricant gel for prevention of cervical sexually transmitted infections: results of a randomized controlled trial. PLoS One. 2008;3:e3488.

94. Sawaya GF, Chirenje MZ, Magure MT, et al. Effect of diaphragm and lubricant gel provision on human papillomavirus infection among women provided with condoms: a randomized controlled trial. Obstet Gynecol. 2008;112:990–7.

95. Cates W, Feldblum P. HIV prevention research: the ecstasy and the agony. Lancet. 2008;372:1932–3.

96. Padian NS, Buve A, Balkus J, Serwadda D, Cates Jr W. Biomedical interventions to prevent HIV infection: evidence, challenges, and way forward. Lancet. 2008;372:585–99.

97. Karim SA, Coletti A, Richardson BA, et al. Safety and effectiveness of vaginal microbicides BufferGel and 0.5% PRO 2000/5 gel for the prevention of HIV infection in women: results of the HPTN 035 trial. In: 16th conference on retroviruses and opportunistic infections; February 8–11, 2009; Montreal, Canada; 2009.

98. McCormack S, Ramjee G, Kamali A, et al. PRO2000 vaginal gel for prevention of HIV-1 infection (Microbicides Development Programme 301): a phase 3, randomised, double-blind, parallel-group trial. Lancet. 2010;376:1329–37.

99. Skoler-Karpoff S, Ramjee G, Ahmed K, et al. Efficacy of Carraguard for prevention of HIV infection in women in South Africa: a randomised, double-blind, placebo-controlled trial. Lancet. 2008;372:1977–87.

100. Austin MN, Rabe LK, Hillier SL. Limitations of the dye-based method for determining vaginal applicator use in microbicide trials. Sex Transm Dis. 2009;36:368–71.

101. Van Damme L, Govinden R, Mirembe FM, et al. Lack of effectiveness of cellulose sulfate gel for the prevention of vaginal HIV transmission. N Engl J Med. 2008;359:463–72.

102. Halpern V, Ogunsola F, Obunge O, et al. Effectiveness of cellulose sulfate vaginal gel for the prevention of HIV infection: results of a Phase III trial in Nigeria. PLoS One. 2008;3:e3784.

103. Peterson L, Nanda K, Opoku BK, et al. SAVVY (C31G) gel for prevention of HIV infection in women: a phase 3, double-blind, randomized, placebo-controlled trial in Ghana. PLoS One. 2007;2:e1312.

104. Feldblum PJ, Adeiga A, Bakare R, et al. SAVVY vaginal gel (C31G) for prevention of HIV infection: a randomized controlled trial in Nigeria. PLoS One. 2008;3:e1474.

105. Cohen MS, Chen YQ, McCauley M, Gamble T, Hosseinipour MC, Kumarasamy N, et al. HPTN 052 Study Team. Prevention of HIV-1 infection with early antiretroviral therapy. N Engl J Med. 2011;365(6):493–505. Epub 18 Jul 2011.

106. Anglemyer A, Rutherford G, Egger M, Siegfried N. Antiretroviral therapy for prevention of HIV transmission in HIV-discordant couples. Cochrane Database Syst Rev. 2011. Issue 5.

107. Cohen MS, Kashuba AD. Antiretroviral therapy for prevention of HIV infection: new clues from an animal model. PLoS Med. 2008;5:e30.

108. Peterson L, Taylor D, Roddy R, et al. Tenofovir disoproxil fumarate for prevention of HIV infection in women: a phase 2, double-blind, randomized, placebo-controlled trial. PLoS Clin Trials. 2007;2:e27.

109. Karim QA, Karim SS, Frohlich JA, et al. Effectiveness and safety of tenofovir gel, an antiretroviral microbicide, for the prevention of HIV infection in women. Science. 2010;10:1126.

110. Grant RM, Lama JR, Anderson PL, et al. Preexposure chemoprophylaxis for HIV prevention in men who have sex with men. N Engl J Med. 2010.

111. Grant R, Lama JR, Glidden DV, Team iS. Pre-exposure chemoprophylaxis for prevention of HIV among trans-women and MSM: iPrEx study. In: CROI; Boston, MA; 2011.

112. Liu AY, Vittinghoff E, Irby R, et al. BMD loss in HIV – men participating in a TDF PrEP clinical trial in San Francisco. In: CROI. Boston, MA; 2011.

113. Interim guidance: preexposure prophylaxis for the prevention of HIV infection in men who have sex with men. MMWR Morb Mortal Wkly Rep. 2011;60:65–8.

114. FHI statement on the FEM-PrEP HIV preventions study. 2011. http://www.fhi.org/en/AboutFHI/Media/Releases/FEM-PrEP_statement041811.htm. Accessed 18 Apr 2011.

115. Safety and effectiveness of tenofovir 1% gel, tenofovir disproxil fumarate, and emtricitabine/tenofovir disoproxil fumarate tablets in preventing HIV in

women. Clinical trial. http://clinicaltrials.gov/ct2/show/NCT00705679.

116. Abu-Raddad LJ, Magaret AS, Celum C, et al. Genital herpes has played a more important role than any other sexually transmitted infection in driving HIV prevalence in Africa. PLoS One. 2008;3:e2230.

117. Freeman EE, Weiss HA, Glynn JR, Cross PL, Whitworth JA, Hayes RJ. Herpes simplex virus 2 infection increases HIV acquisition in men and women: systematic review and meta-analysis of longitudinal studies. AIDS. 2006;20(1):73–83

118. Watson-Jones D, Weiss HA, Rusizoka M, et al. Effect of herpes simplex suppression on incidence of HIV among women in Tanzania. N Engl J Med. 2008;358:1560–71.

119. Lingappa JR, Baeten JM, Wald A, et al. Daily acyclovir for HIV-1 disease progression in people dually infected with HIV-1 and herpes simplex virus type 2: a randomised placebo-controlled trial. Lancet. 2010;375:824–33.

120. Karim QA, Karim SS, Frohlich JA, et al. Effectiveness and safety of tenofovir gel, an antiretroviral microbicide, for the prevention of HIV infection in women. In: 18th international AIDS conference; July 18–23, 2010; Vienna, Austria; 2010.

121. McClelland RS, Richardson BA, Hassan WM, et al. Improvement of vaginal health for Kenyan women at risk for acquisition of human immunodeficiency virus type 1: results of a randomized trial. J Infect Dis. 2008;197:1361–8.

122. Schwebke JR, Desmond R. A randomized trial of metronidazole in asymptomatic bacterial vaginosis to prevent the acquisition of sexually transmitted diseases. Am J Obstet Gynecol. 2007;196:517.e1–6.

123. Cheng L, Gulmezoglu AM, Piaggio G, Ezcurra E, van Look PF. Interventions for emergency contraception. Update of 2004 document. Cochrane Database Syst Rev. 2008;16:CD001324.

124. Hatcher RA, Trussell J, Nelson AL, Cates W, Stewart FS, Kowal D. Contraceptive technology. 19th ed. New York: Ardent Media; 2007.

125. Antiretroviral postexposure prophylaxis after sexual, injection-drug use, or other nonoccupational exposure to HIV in the United States. MMWR Morb Mortal Wkly Rep. 2005;54:1–20.

126. Markowitz LE, Dunne EF, Saraiya M, Lawson HW, Chesson H, Unger ER. Quadrivalent human papillomavirus vaccine: recommendations of the Advisory Committee on Immunization Practices (ACIP). MMWR Recomm Rep. 2007;56:1–24.

127. Food and Drug Administration. Product approval information – package insert. Gardasil (quadrivalent human papillomavirus types 6, 11, 16, 18). Merck & Co., Whitehouse Station, NJ. 2008. http://www.fda.gov/cber/products/gardasil.htm.

128. Munoz N, Manalastas Jr R, Pitisuttithum P, et al. Safety, immunogenicity, and efficacy of quadrivalent human papillomavirus (types 6, 11, 16, 18) recombinant vaccine in women aged 24–45 years: a randomised, double-blind trial. Lancet. 2009;373:1949–57.

129. Petaja T, Keranen H, Karppa T, et al. Immunogenicity and safety of human papillomavirus (HPV)-16/18 AS04-adjuvanted vaccine in healthy boys aged 10–18 years. J Adolesc Health. 2009;44:33–40.

130. Giuliano AR, Lazcano-Ponce E, Villa LL, et al. The human papillomavirus infection in men study: human papillomavirus prevalence and type distribution among men residing in Brazil, Mexico, and the United States. Cancer Epidemiol Biomarkers Prev. 2008;17:2036–43.

131. Cutts FT, Franceschi S, Goldie S, et al. Human papillomavirus and HPV vaccines: a review. Bull World Health Organ. 2007;85:719–26.

132. Paavonen J, Jenkins D, Bosch FX, et al. Efficacy of a prophylactic adjuvanted bivalent L1 virus-like-particle vaccine against infection with human papillomavirus types 16 and 18 in young women: an interim analysis of a phase III double-blind, randomised controlled trial. Lancet. 2007;369:2161–70.

133. Daniels D, Grytdal S, Wasley A. Surveillance for acute viral hepatitis – United States, 2007. MMWR Surveill Summ. 2009;58:1–27.

134. Mast EE, Weinbaum CM, Fiore AE, et al. A comprehensive immunization strategy to eliminate transmission of hepatitis B virus infection in the United States: recommendations of the Advisory Committee on Immunization Practices (ACIP) Part II: immunization of adults. MMWR Recomm Rep. 2006;55:1–33.

135. Fiore AE, Wasley A, Bell BP. Prevention of hepatitis A through active or passive immunization: recommendations of the Advisory Committee on Immunization Practices (ACIP). MMWR Recomm Rep. 2006;55:1–23.

136. Flynn NM, Forthal DN, Harro CD, Judson FN, Mayer KH, Para MF. Placebo-controlled phase 3 trial of a recombinant glycoprotein 120 vaccine to prevent HIV-1 infection. J Infect Dis. 2005;191:654–65.

137. Pitisuttithum P, Gilbert P, Gurwith M, et al. Randomized, double-blind, placebo-controlled efficacy trial of a bivalent recombinant glycoprotein 120 HIV-1 vaccine among injection drug users in Bangkok, Thailand. J Infect Dis. 2006;194:1661–71.

138. Fauci AS, Johnston MI, Dieffenbach CW, et al. HIV vaccine research: the way forward. Science. 2008;321:530–2.

139. Johnston MI, Fauci AS. An HIV vaccine – challenges and prospects. N Engl J Med. 2008;359:888–90.

140. Rerks-Ngarm S, Pitisuttithum P, Nitayaphan S, et al. Vaccination with ALVAC and AIDSVAX to prevent HIV-1 infection in Thailand. N Engl J Med. 2009;361:2209–20.

141. Gray RH, Kigozi G, Serwadda D, et al. Male circumcision for HIV prevention in men in Rakai, Uganda: a randomised trial. Lancet. 2007;369:657–66.

142. Weiss HA, Halperin D, Bailey RC, Hayes RJ, Schmid G, Hankins CA. Male circumcision for HIV

prevention: from evidence to action? AIDS. 2008;22:567–74.

143. Auvert B, Taljaard D, Lagarde E, Sobngwi-Tambekou J, Sitta R, Puren A. Randomized, controlled intervention trial of male circumcision for reduction of HIV infection risk: the ANRS 1265 Trial. PLoS Med. 2005;2:e298.

144. Bailey RC, Moses S, Parker CB, et al. Male circumcision for HIV prevention in young men in Kisumu, Kenya: a randomised controlled trial. Lancet. 2007;369:643–56.

145. UNAIDS and WHO. New data on male circumcision and HIV prevention: policy and programme implications; WHO/UNAIDS technical consultation male circumcision and HIV prevention: research implications for policy and programming montreux. Geneva: Joint United Nations Programme on HIV/AIDS and World Health Organization; 2007.

146. Auvert B, Sobngwi-Tambekou J, Cutler E, et al. Effect of male circumcision on the prevalence of high-risk human papillomavirus in young men: results of a randomized controlled trial conducted in orange farm, South Africa. J Infect Dis. 2009;199:14–9.

147. Sobngwi-Tambekou J, Taljaard D, Nieuwoudt M, Lissouba P, Puren A, Auvert B. Male circumcision and Neisseria gonorrhoeae, Chlamydia trachomatis, and Trichomonas vaginalis: observations in the aftermath of a randomised controlled trial for HIV prevention. Sex Transm Infect. 2009;85:116–20.

148. Tobian AA, Serwadda D, Quinn TC, et al. Male circumcision for the prevention of HSV-2 and HPV infections and syphilis. N Engl J Med. 2009;360:1298–309.

149. Mehta SD, Moses S, Agot K, et al. Adult male circumcision does not reduce the risk of incident Neisseria gonorrhoeae, Chlamydia trachomatis, or Trichomonas vaginalis infection: results from a randomized, controlled trial in Kenya. J Infect Dis. 2009;200:370–8.

150. Warner L, Ghanem KG, Newman DR, Macaluso M, Sullivan PS, Erbelding EJ. Male circumcision and risk of HIV infection among heterosexual African American men attending Baltimore sexually transmitted disease clinics. J Infect Dis. 2009;199:59–65.

151. Millett GA, Flores SA, Marks G, Reed JB, Herbst JH. Circumcision status and risk of HIV and sexually transmitted infections among men who have sex with men: a meta-analysis. JAMA. 2008; 300:1674–84.

152. Gray RH, Kigozi G, Serwadda D, et al. The effects of male circumcision on female partners' genital tract symptoms and vaginal infections in a randomized trial in Rakai, Uganda. Am J Obstet Gynecol. 2009;200:42.e1–7.

153. Behavioral counseling to prevent sexually transmitted infections: U.S. Preventive Services Task Force recommendation statement. Ann Intern Med. 2008;149:491–6, W95.

154. Lin JS, Whitlock E, O'Connor E, Bauer V. Behavioral counseling to prevent sexually transmitted infections: a systematic review for the U.S. Preventive Services Task Force. Ann Intern Med. 2008;149:497–508. W96–9.

155. Recommendations for incorporating human immunodeficiency virus (HIV) prevention into the medical care of persons living with HIV. Clin Infect Dis. 2004;38:104–21.

156. McClelland RS, Baeten JM. Reducing HIV-1 transmission through prevention strategies targeting HIV-1-seropositive individuals. J Antimicrob Chemother. 2006;57:163–6.

157. Centers for Disease Control and Prevention. Recommendations for partner services programs for HIV infection, syphilis, gonorrhea, and chlamydial infection. MMWR Recomm Rep. 2008;57:1–83. quiz CE1-4.

158. Golden MR, Whittington WL, Handsfield HH, et al. Effect of expedited treatment of sex partners on recurrent or persistent gonorrhea or chlamydial infection. N Engl J Med. 2005;352:676–85.

159. Gaydos CA, Wright C, Wood BJ, Waterfield G, Hobson S, Quinn TC. Chlamydia trachomatis reinfection rates among female adolescents seeking rescreening in school-based health centers. Sex Transm Dis. 2008;35:233–7.

160. Peterman TA, Tian LH, Metcalf CA, et al. High incidence of new sexually transmitted infections in the year following a sexually transmitted infection: a case for rescreening. Ann Intern Med. 2006;145:564–72.

161. Gatski M, Mena L, Levison J, et al. Patient-delivered partner treatment and Trichomonas vaginalis repeat infection among human immunodeficiency virus-infected women. Sex Transm Dis. 2010;37:502–5.

162. Kelly JA, Sikkema KJ, Holtgrave DR. Behavioral interventions for prevention of STDs and HIV infection at the community level. In: Holmes KK, Sparling PF, Stamm WE, et al., editors. Sexually transmitted diseases. 4th ed. New York: McGraw Hil; 2008. p. 1849–56.

Prevention of HIV and Other Blood-Borne and Sexually Transmitted Diseases in People Who Inject Drugs: Current Status and Future Prospects

12

Richard Needle, Sasha Mital, and Andrew Ball

Introduction

Scientific consensus has emerged that introducing and scaling up core interventions of a comprehensive HIV prevention program—linked with an enabling environment of laws, policies, and regulations supportive of prevention, treatment, and care—can stabilize and halt the spread of, and even reverse, the HIV epidemic among persons who inject drugs (PWID) [1–4]. Yet, the global burden of HIV and other diseases among persons who inject drugs (heroin, cocaine, and amphetamine-type stimulants) is high and growing in many regions of the world. Availability and access to evidence-based core interventions are low; profound obstacles persist, limiting the nature, scope, and quality of prevention, treatment, and care services. Despite the fact that every country reporting persons who inject drugs has made commitments to protect human rights in relation to HIV [5],[1] many do not enforce their policies and violate the human rights of persons who inject drugs [6, 7].

It has been estimated that there are about 15.9 million male and female persons who inject drugs (PWIDs) globally, with as many as 2.59 million PWIDs in the USA [8]. Among the 148 countries in which injecting drug use has been documented, 120 (81%) reported HIV among PWIDs in 2007. Globally, an estimated 3.0 million people who inject drugs are HIV positive, which accounts for about 10% of total HIV infections [8]. Drug use, particularly injection drug use, plays a major role

The findings and conclusions in this report are those of the authors and do not necessarily represent the official position of the U.S. Government

R. Needle (✉)
Office of the Global Aids Coordinator, 2100 Pennsylvania Avenue Washington, DC 20037, USA
e-mail: needlerh@state.gov

S. Mital
Division of Global HIVAIDS, U.S. Centers for Disease Control and Prevention, 1600 Clifton Rd., NE, MS E-04, Atlanta, GA 30333, USA
e-mail: smital@cdc.gov

Λ. Ball
HIV Department, World Health Organization, Avenue Appia 20 1211, Geneva 27, Switzerland
e-mail: balla@who.int

[1] …to "enact, strengthen or enforce, as appropriate, legislation, regulations and other measures to eliminate all forms of discrimination and against and to ensure the full enjoyment of all human rights and fundamental freedoms by people living with HIV/AIDS and members of vulnerable populations" [5].

S.O. Aral, K.A. Fenton, and J.A. Lipshutz (eds.), *The New Public Health and STD/HIV Prevention: Personal, Public and Health Systems Approaches*, DOI 10.1007/978-1-4614-4526-5_12,
© Springer Science+Business Media New York 2013

in the transmission of not only HIV but also other blood-borne infections, hepatitis B (HBV), and hepatitis C (HCV), contributing significantly to the global burden of disease [9]. HBV and HIV also can be transmitted through risky sexual practices [10, 11][2]. Burden of other sexually transmitted infections (STIs)[3] is also high among persons who use drugs [15].

The proportion of persons who inject drugs and could benefit from core interventions, to those who access and receive the interventions (coverage rates), is very low [6, 16, 17]. A 2009 report describes that globally, only 26% of PWIDs were reached with HIV prevention services of any kind [18]. Fewer than 10% of all PWIDs have access to syringe and needle programs. Only 8% of opioid users have access to essential and proven effective medication-assisted treatment. Four percent of PWIDs living with HIV infection are receiving antiretroviral treatment (ART) [16, 19]. Services are even more limited for persons who inject drugs and are incarcerated—a common event for between 56 and 90% of people who inject drugs [7]. Many factors account for the gap between need and actual coverage—legal, policy, fiscal, and human resources as well as operational barriers. To a great extent, low coverage rates and high burden of disease in PWIDs reflects a country-level struggle to resolve the tension between responding with criminal justice versus a public health approach. A criminal justice approach uses punitive laws, policies, and law enforcement practices resulting in high rates of incarceration while a public health, human rights-based approach with

harm reduction strategies provides for supportive laws, policies, and environment that enable PWIDs to access comprehensive, low-threshold services [20–24].

This chapter focuses on creating and implementing a new public health approach to reduce the burden of disease among persons who use drugs, and address the challenges ahead. It starts with documenting the public health and human and social consequences and costs of not acting on informed and science-based policies, and establishing programs for scaling up comprehensive HIV prevention. The next section of this chapter is a review of global, regional, and country-level epidemiological data, including a focus on the USA, and on the current status of injection drug use and the global burden of HIV and other blood-borne and sexually transmitted infections among people who use drugs. The chapter focuses primarily on low- and middle-income countries and also includes a focus on the USA and some high-income countries that have achieved high intervention coverage rates for PWIDs. The only regions of the world with increasing HIV incidence according to the 2010 UNAIDS report are Central Asia and Eastern Europe, countries with drug-driven epidemics [25].

The second section reviews some of the macro-level structural determinants—policies, regulations, and associated law enforcement practices, and high rates of incarceration of PWIDs—that shape vulnerability, risk, transmission, and country-level programmatic response to these infections. In the third section, we discuss evidence-based findings and best practices related to the prevention of HIV and other infections among PWID. This section also focuses on coverage and scaling up of HIV, Hepatitis, and STI prevention, treatment, and care for PWIDs, including new approaches to deliver services. The final section highlights the challenges ahead for a new public health approach to prevention of HIV and other blood-borne and sexually transmitted infections for persons who inject drugs. The challenges are clear.

---

[2]While sexual transmission of HCV is considered unlikely (only 10% of people in the U.S. with acute HCV infections report sexual contact and a known HCV-infected person as their only risk) [12], outbreaks have been reported among men who have sex with men and partners of PWIDs [11, 13, 14].

[3]In this article, sexually transmitted infections (STIs) include bacterial infections, syphilis, gonorrhea and Chlamydia unless otherwise noted.

Box 12.1: Key Messages

- The global scale of opiate, cocaine, and amphetamine-type stimulant use, the globalization of the drug trade and trafficking, and the growing burden of HIV, hepatitis B and C, sexually transmitted infections and tuberculosis associated with injection and non-injection drug use is a major public health concern.

- In many countries, there are unresolved and unbalanced policy and resource allocation tensions between governmental sectors related to drug control and public health approaches to prevention, treatment, and care of PWIDs who are at risk for HIV other blood-borne and sexually transmitted diseases. This tension limits the nature, scope, availability, quality, and effectiveness of health services for PWIDs.

- There is strong evidence that a comprehensive package of interventions—including needle and syringe programs,

medication-assisted treatment, and anti-retroviral therapy—can prevent the further spread of HIV and other blood-borne diseases among persons who use drugs. These interventions are not available in many countries and, where available, access is limited and coverage rates are very low.

- To reduce the burden of disease from HIV, HCV, HBV, and STIs by closing the gap between those who would benefit from these interventions and those who actually receive them, a public health harm reduction approach that links legal and human rights is needed. This approach ensures an enabling environment to support implementing and scaling up a comprehensive package of low-threshold services.

- Among persons who use drugs, burden of STI is also high as the type of drug used can facilitate high-risk sexual practices and put persons in high-risk environments.

Epidemics of Drug Use and Epidemiology of HIV, Other Blood-Borne Infections, and STIs Among Drug Users

Global Overview of Illicit Drug Use

The global scale of illicit drug use and the burden of HIV and other diseases associated with injection drug use represents a major international public health concern. The globalization of the drug trade and resulting increases in the availability of drugs due to trafficking from source countries, and navigating through and to destination countries (particularly heroin, cocaine, and amphetamines), greatly contributes to demand for these drugs in countries with high-level consumption; increasing demand for drugs in countries with historically low levels of consumption, as new trafficking patterns are established; and conditions that introduce and/or sustain HIV epidemics. HIV prevalence has been reported to follow drug trafficking patterns, suggesting that emerging trafficking routes can predict HIV spread among PWIDs [26].

Worldwide, it was estimated that between 155 and 250 million persons used drugs at least once in 2008, including 12.8–21.9 million who used opiates, 15–19 million who used cocaine, and 13.7–52.9 who used amphetamine type stimulants [27].[4] Of these, 16–38 million people were identified as problem drug users, defined as regular or frequent users of drugs who face social or health consequences because of their drug use [27].[5]

There is considerable regional, country, and subnational variation in patterns of drug use (types of drugs available, drugs used, and modes of administration, e.g., smoked, sniffed, snorted, or injected), the sizes of the drug-using populations, and prevalence of use. Prevalence of drug use and demand for treatment for specific drugs

---

[4]Not all drug users inject drugs, and the proportion of injecting drug users to non-injection drug users varies by the type of drug used.

[5]A major challenge to understanding the burden of drug use comes from the data as definitions of drug use and methods of calculation vary.

are all closely linked with geographic proximity to cultivation (notably opium and coca), production, distribution, trafficking, and transit of the illicit drugs. Table 12.1 shows that the proportion of drug users varies geographically by region and by drug used. Opiate use, which consists mostly of injection of heroin, is highest in Europe, and particularly in Eastern European and Central Asian countries. Cocaine use is highest in the Americas, mostly reflecting high prevalence of use and demand (about 40% of global demand) in North America, particularly the USA [27]. In recent years, the trafficking of drugs from Mexico to the USA in response to demand has resulted in considerable violence and deaths associated with drug distribution and efforts to police and limit the supply to the USA. Finally, the highest numbers of amphetamine users are found in Asian countries. Some persons who use drugs inject amphetamine-type stimulants. In reality, a range of drugs are used by persons who inject drugs in most countries—with some users limiting their use to a single drug, and many using a range of different drugs. The use of multiple drugs in Asian countries and increasingly in Eastern European countries, particularly amphetamine-type stimulants and opiates, undermines the potential effectiveness of medication-assisted treatment of opioid dependence with methadone.

The countries with the largest estimated numbers of PWIDs are China (2.35 million in 2005), the USA (1.86 million in 2002), and the Russian Federation (1.825 million in 2007) [8].

Illicit Drug use in the USA

Drug use patterns in the USA have changed over time. New drugs have emerged, and familiar drugs such as heroin have cycles of popularity, following epidemiological curves of rising incidence and prevalence, stability, and declining incidence [28, 29]. Epidemics of heroin use were reported in the late 1940s and again in the late 1960s (with the highest incidence occurring between 1971 and 1977), followed by epidemic-level use of cocaine, which in turn was followed by the emergence of the "crack" cocaine epidemic and, most recently, epidemics of

amphetamine-type stimulants. Use of heroin, cocaine hydrochloride (particularly injection use), and "crack" cocaine have resulted in upward swings in incidence of HIV and other blood-borne infections resulting from the reuse of syringes.

In the US, 21.8 million persons are estimated to use illicit substances (including marijuana) and 7.1 million drug users had a diagnosis of drug dependence in 2009 [30]. Cocaine and crack were used by 1.6 million people, while heroin was used by 200,000 people [30]. Most persons who use drugs who need treatment do not receive it. Only 10–33% of those with drug dependencies receive treatment; however, the number of people receiving treatment has increased steadily from 2002 to 2009 [30, 31].

Drug Treatment Admissions

In 2007, 1.8 million annual admissions into drug treatment facilities were reported and listed by primary substance abused. The largest percentage of admissions were for alcohol (40.3%), followed by opiates consisting primarily of heroin (18.6%), marijuana/hashish (15.8%), cocaine and crack (12.9%), amphetamine-type stimulants including methamphetamines (7.9%), and other drugs (1.4%) [32].

Treatment Admissions by Race

In the USA, drug use disproportionately impacts racial and ethnic minority populations, particularly African American men and women. African Americans make up about 12.3% of the U.S. population [33], while more than 22% of treatment admissions for heroin were among African Americans, 48.8% of smoking "crack" admissions, and 23.2% of cocaine admissions. Unlike heroin and "crack," which are disproportionately used by African Americans, methamphetamines are used most frequently by Hispanic populations [32]. These data are limited to those in treatment and do not represent the overall drug-using population, most of whom cannot access or are not seeking treatment. This pattern of disproportionate impact of drug use on racial minorities is reflected in HIV and other blood-borne infection surveillance data, incarceration rates, and data from treatment admissions for drug dependence [34–37].

Table 12.1 Global prevalence and estimated number (in millions) of users of opiates, heroin, cocaine, and amphetamines among population aged 15–64, 2008

	Opiates				Cocaine				Amphetamines			
	Estimated number of annual users[a]		Percent of population 15–64		Estimated number of annual users[a]		Percent of population 15–64		Estimated number of annual users[a]		Percent of population 15–64	
	Low	High	Low	High	Low	High	Low	High	Low	High	Low	High
Africa	0.68	2.93	0.1	0.5	1.02	2.67	0.2	0.5	0.35	1.93	0.1	0.4
Americas	2.29	2.44	0.4	0.4	8.72	9.08	1.4	1.5	3.04	3.28	0.5	0.5
Asia	6.46	12.54	0.2	0.5	0.43	2.27	<0.1	0.1	2.37	15.62	0.1	0.6
Europe	3.29	3.82	0.6	0.7	4.57	4.97	0.8	0.9	3.85	4.08	0.7	0.7
Oceania	0.12	0.15	0.5	0.6	0.33	0.39	1.4	1.7	0.84	0.91	3.6	4.0
Global	12.84	21.88	0.3	0.5	15.07	19.38	0.3	0.4	10.45	25.82	0.2	0.6

Source: UNODC. World Drug Report. New York: United Nations; 2010
[a] In millions

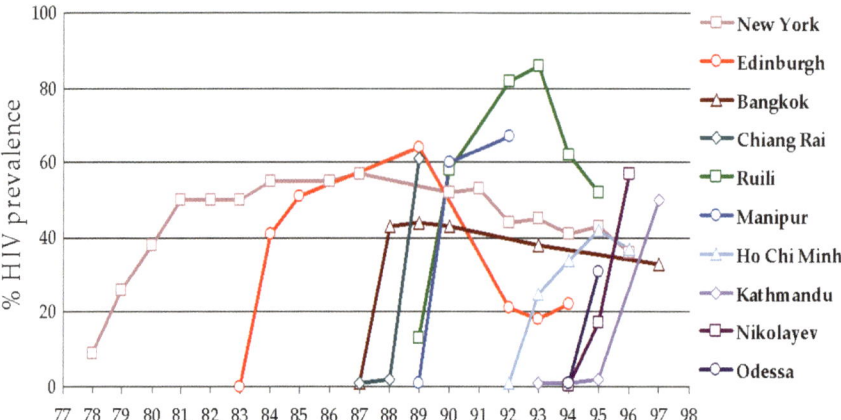

Fig. 12.1 Rapid Increase in HIV prevalence among injection drug users in 10 cities, 1977–1998 [38]. Source: Ball AL, Rana S, Dehne KL. HIV prevention among injecting drug users: responding in developing and transitional countries. Public Health Rep 1998;113(Supp 1) 170–81

Epidemiology of HIV Among Persons Who Inject Drugs

Global Overview

Epidemics of HIV among PWIDs have been characterized by explosive growth, sustained high prevalence, and geographic spread from the epicenter to other regions within a country over time. The number of countries reporting HIV among PWIDs, as reported earlier, continues to grow, and epidemics among PWIDs are now occurring in countries with generalized heterosexual HIV epidemics. Figure 12.1 shows the rapid increase in HIV prevalence in a number of countries, starting with the first reported epidemic in New York City; HIV seroprevalence among PWIDs in New York City increased from under 10% in 1978 to more than 50% by 1983 [38, 39]. This type of outbreak has also been documented in other countries, and more recently in Eastern Europe and Central Asia [40]. Rapid spread is associated with high-risk injection practices—primarily multiperson reuse of drug injection equipment and, specifically, HIV-contaminated syringes and needles. Not all countries with injection drug use and HIV among PWIDs experienced rapid increase in HIV prevalence. This will be discussed more fully in the section on HIV prevention.

Around 30% of global HIV infections outside of sub-Saharan Africa are caused by use of contaminated injecting equipment by PWIDs, accounting for an increasing proportion of those living with the virus [15]. Injection drug use is the major route of HIV transmission in Eastern Europe, Central Asia and Canada, and is driving the epidemic in parts of South and Southeast Asia, the Middle East, Latin America, and North Africa. Of the estimated three million drug users living with HIV globally, 32% live in Eastern Europe, 22% in East and Southeast Asia, 19% in Latin America, and 27% in all other regions [8]. HIV is reported in 8.74–22.4% of estimated 1.29–2.59 million PWIDs in the US. [8].

In some countries where the major mode of HIV transmission is heterosexual sex, drug use-driven epidemics are emerging. In addition to facing the enormous burden of heterosexually transmitted HIV, some sub-Saharan countries are experiencing changes in patterns of drug use, both IDU and non-IDU, which have implications for the potential spread of HIV and other STIs [41]. For example, there are more than 30,000 PWIDs in Kenya with an HIV prevalence of 36.3–49.5%, and approximately 262,975 PWIDs in South Africa with an HIV prevalence of 4.8–20% [8].Drug trafficking, specifically heroin and cocaine, to and through these countries has created and led to increased use [42, 43]. Southern and Eastern Africa currently has the second highest growth in opiate use, and Western Africa has emerged as a major trafficking route for cocaine and opiates [27].

Other changes in epidemic patterns of HIV among PWIDs have also been reported. HIV epidemics among PWIDs have high potential to spread rapidly between those who inject drugs and the wider community through sexual transmission [44, 45]. Des Jarlais and colleagues [46] report that a number of countries with historically drug-driven HIV epidemics, specifically Ukraine and Russia, are reporting increasing rates of heterosexual transmission, though this shift is most likely based on transmission from persons who inject drugs to their non-injection sexual partners. These countries also experience high HIV prevalence among overlapping high-risk populations of sex workers, men who have sex with men (MSM), and people who use drugs (injection and non-injection).

HIV in the USA

The HIV epidemic in the USA reflects the high burden of disease across most-at-risk populations—primarily MSM, with a small percentage of MSM who inject drugs, and among male and female heterosexual persons who inject drugs. HIV among PWIDs was first officially reported in the USA in 1981, but in New York it can be traced back to 1976 [39]. According to the centers for Disease Control of Prevention, of the 1.1 million people in the USA living with HIV in 2006, persons who inject drugs made up 19% (204,600) of all HIV infections. PWID accounted for 10% (4,110) of the estimated 41,087 new HIV infections in 2008 in 37 states, while PWIDs and MSM accounted for an additional 3% of new HIV infections [47]. Persons who inject drugs (40%) are also significantly more likely than MSM (35%) and persons who engage in high-risk heterosexual contact to receive a late HIV diagnosis [36]. Though HIV incidence among PWID has fallen by 80% since its peak in the early 1990s, and risk behaviors have declined, injection drug use was still the third highest reported risk factor for HIV infection in the USA in 2007 (after male-to-male sexual contact and high-risk heterosexual contact); reuse of syringes and high-risk sexual practices persist [44].

During 2004–2007, a total of 152,917 persons received a diagnosis of HIV infection in 34 states reporting data, including 19,687 (12.9%) persons who inject drugs. These data reveal, as did the data on race and drug use by treatment admissions, the disproportionate burden of disease among African Americans. African Americans accounted for 11,321 (57.5%) of HIV-infected PWIDs, while

---

Box 12.2. Epidemiology of Drug Use: Overview

- The prevalence of drug use—injection and non-injection use of opiates and cocaine, amphetamine-type stimulants, crack, and other drugs—varies by region and country.
- China, Russia, and the USA have the highest numbers of PWID in the world.
- HIV incidence and prevalence among PWIDs varies by geographic region and country and is highest in Eastern Europe, Central Asia and some countries in Southeast Asia. It is lowest, and declining, in Western Europe, New Zealand and Australia, and the USA. HIV in persons who inject drugs has also recently been reported in a number of sub-Saharan African countries.
- Persons who inject drugs are also at high risk for HBV and HCV, which share common modes of transmission—reuse of contaminated syringes and needles and other injection-related equipment, and high-risk

sexual practices. HCV is the most prevalent blood-borne infection among PWIDs throughout the world, and the coinfection rate among PWIDs with HIV is at least 90%.
- Burden of STI is also high among persons who use drugs as type of drug used can facilitate high-risk sexual practices and put persons in high-risk environments.
- Between 56 and 90% of drug users globally experience incarceration. Drug use and transmission of HIV and other blood-borne diseases occur in prisons and other closed settings. Incarcerated persons have higher rates for these diseases, even higher than rates in the communities in which they live before incarceration.
- Drug use, HIV and other blood-borne and sexually transmitted infections, and incarceration disproportionately affect minority populations in the USA.

whites accounted for 4,216 (21.4%), and Hispanics or Latinos for 3,764 (19.1%) [36].

Epidemiology of Viral Hepatitis (HBV and HCV) and Injection Drug Use: Global and U.S. Overview

In addition to HIV, persons who inject drugs are also at high risk from other blood-borne infections, including HBV and HCV, through the sharing of injecting equipment (needles and other injection-related equipment such as cotton filters, water, and spoons/cookers) [48]. HCV is the most prevalent infection among PWIDs and injection drug use is the primary mode of HCV transmission in the developed world [49–51]. A growing body of evidence demonstrates transmission of HCV through high-risk, often traumatic, sexual practices among heterosexuals, HIV-infected individuals, and MSM where non-injection drug use is also occurring [13, 52, 53]. HBV is approximately 10 times more transmissible than HCV, and 20 times more transmissible than HIV [50].

Approximately 180 million people in the world are living with HCV; approximately 90% of all new infections are attributed to PWID [54]. Considerable variation in HCV prevalence exists within and across and regions [55]. HCV prevalence has been reported among PWIDs in 57 of the 131 countries with PWIDs. In 9 of these countries, HCV prevalence was estimated at between 20 and 50%; it ranged between 50 and 90% in 31 countries, with prevalence estimates of anti-HCV among PWIDs at least 90% in 17 countries. HIV/HCV coinfection among PWIDs has been found in 16 countries reporting PWID [56, 57]. Estimates show that at least 90% of HIV cases were coinfected with HCV in eight of these countries (China, Poland, Puerto Rico, Russia, Spain, Switzerland, Thailand, and Vietnam) [56]. Global prevalence rates of HBV among PWIDs are not available, however site-specific surveys show HBV prevalence among cohorts of PWIDs at 50–84% in the USA [58], 27% in Wales [59], 55% in Georgia [60], and 53.3% in Switzerland [61].

At the end of 2005, there were 3.2 million people in the USA living with chronic hepatitis C. Similar to reports of HIV incidence among PWIDs,

HCV incidence has been on the decline since the late 1980s reflecting increased awareness and access to needle and syringe programs. In 2007, there were 17,000 new infections, and injection drug use accounted for 48% of the cases [37] It is estimated that 50–90% of HIV-infected PWIDs are also infected with HCV [62]. It has been estimated that between 48,014 and 86,424 noninstitutionalized PWIDs are living with both HIV and HCV [12].

An estimated 800,000 to 1.2 million people in the USA are infected with HBV. In 2007, it was estimated that 43,000 new HBV infections occurred in the USA [37]. Though HBV incidence in the USA has declined in the last decade, high rates of HBV infection continue to occur among persons in identified risk groups, including PWIDs. In 15% of the cases, PWID was reported as a risk factor among those whose risk information was available. HBV rates in 2007 were highest among non-Hispanic blacks (2.3 per 100,000) [37].

Epidemiology of STIs (Syphilis, Gonorrhea, and Chlamydia) in Drug-Using Populations

Globally, surveillance data on sexually transmitted infections (STIs) are limited, and data on STIs among drug-using populations are limited to site-specific surveys. However, meta-analyses on STIs in drug-using populations reveal a high burden. Semaan and colleagues [63] found that in the USA, 1–6% of drug users are infected with syphilis, 1–3% with gonorrhea, and 2–4% with chlamydia, with variations in rates based on race, sex, age, drug-using behavior, and region. Without straightforward comparability across figures, rates of STIs among people who use drugs appear disproportionately high compared to rates among the general population demonstrates [52, 64].[6]

Among persons who use drugs, the prevalence of chlamydia was lower among whites (4% among white males and 6% among white females)

---

[6]In 2009, there were 4.4 syphilis cases, 99.1 gonorrhea cases and 409.2 Chlamydia cases per 100,000 population in the United States [64].

and older drug users (2% among <25 years old). It was higher among female "crack" users (14%), those who trade sex (8%), and those with more than five partners in a period of 4 weeks (9%). Studies conducted outside the USA reported rates similar to those in USA: 3% in Quebec City, Canada, 2% in Chiang Mai, Thailand; 6% in Melbourne, Australia [63].

Coffin and colleagues [65] found similar variations in syphilis prevalence among drug users in low- and middle-income countries by sex, risk behaviors, and region. In their review, an overall prevalence of 11.1% was reported while median syphilis prevalence was 4.0% among males and 19.9% among females [65]. Female drug users are consistently at higher risk for and have higher rates of STIs. Sex work could explain the relationship between female sex and syphilis prevalence as high prevalence was observed among female sex workers and their clients (10.8–64.7%) [65–69].

Risk Factors for STIs Among Persons Who Use Drugs

Overlapping and multiple risks are associated with drug use and STI transmission among people who use drugs, their partners and the larger community. Risk for STIs varies by the drug used, reflecting the pharmacology of the specific drug (cocaine hydrochloride, "crack," amphetamine-type stimulants, heroin, and other opioids), and the setting or context in which these drugs are used [70, 71]. While heroin is associated with reduced sexual arousal and activity, cocaine and amphetamine use has a strong relationship with STI risk behaviors such as increased impulsivity, unprotected sex, "rough" sex, multiple partners, and group sex [72–75]. "Shooting galleries," crack houses, and bathhouses are venues where overlapping high-risk groups (drug users selling sex and/or money for drugs, sex workers selling sex to drug users, and men who have sex with multiple male partners and use amphetamines) congregate and engage in sex and drug use, increasing the risk for sexual transmission of infections [76–81].

The co-occurrence of male-to-male sexual activity, use of amphetamine-type stimulants, and STI risk behaviors has been well documented.

Use of amphetamine-type stimulants, such as methamphetamine, is prevalent among some MSM communities [82–85], and are often used in sexual contexts to prolong pleasure and reduce inhibitions [86, 87], resulting in behaviors such as unprotected sex, multiple sex partners, and subsequent STI transmission [73, 88].

The exchange of sex for money and/or drugs often co-occurs with drug use among female drug users and results in high STI rates [89, 90]. Female drug users also play a key role in the transmission of STIs by creating a bridge between smaller populations with high prevalence of STIs/HIV and drug use to the larger general population via heterosexual sex and often, commercial sex [81, 91]. The relationship among crack, sex work, and STIs in the USA serves as an example [92, 93]. An association between crack use and risky sexual behaviors has been reported. Beginning in 1986, the rise in crack cocaine use coincided with the rise in primary and secondary syphilis among African Americans. In Baltimore, primary and secondary syphilis cases increased from 144 in 1993 to 669 in 1997 and were attributed to crack cocaine use and the exchange of sex for crack [94]. When crack enters a community, the number of sex sellers increases, therefore driving down the price of sex, often to the price of a "hit." The sex economy is elastic, meaning that demand increases as price decreases so the decreased price leads to more buyers of sex work. High competition among sex workers gives the consumer the upper hand to insist on riskier sex acts or further lower the price causing the sex worker to take on more clients [95, 96]. Additionally, consumers of sex work often come from outside the drug-using communities thereby creating a bridge for disease transmission beyond persons who use drugs and their regular sex partners.

Macro- and Micro-Environmental Factors and Vulnerability to HIV and Other Blood-Borne and Sexually Transmitted Infections

Many factors help explain why the burden of disease, especially HIV, is high and growing among PWIDs in many developed, low-, and middle-income countries. Rhodes and colleagues have developed a risk environment framework that focuses on the overlap and interaction of social, structural, and environmental factors, categorized as either macro- or micro-environmental factors that influence vulnerability and risk for HIV acquisition and transmission [97, 98].

High-risk injecting and sexual behaviors drive the spread of these infections and are affected by a number of structural factors, including economic, political, legal, social and policy environmental factors [97, 99]. This section briefly reviews some of the macro- and micro-environmental factors that shape vulnerability, risk, and transmission for persons who use drugs. Among the many factors increasing vulnerability of PWIDs and risks for spreading HIV and other blood-borne and sexually transmitted infections are globalization of the drug trade, restrictive laws and punitive drug policies, incarceration of persons who inject drugs, and gender norms around female PWIDs. Today, there is increasing recognition that health should be the core focus of drug policy; drug dependence is a treatable health problem; treatment and other alternatives are more effective for health and social outcomes than incarceration; universal access to drug treatment should be integrated into the health care system, and the human rights of persons who inject drugs have to be protected by ensuring equitable and voluntary access to services that can reduce harm and prevent HIV, morbidity, and mortality associated with drug use [6, 27].

Globalization of the Drug Trade

Though the supply of opioids and cocaine (the two main problem drugs) has declined, the amount produced and trafficked remains substantial. Along with reductions in cultivation, production, and use of heroin and cocaine, there has been an increase in the production and use of synthetic amphetamine-type stimulants and prescription drugs [27]. Drug markets are dynamic and evolve, and the availability of a range of drugs to meet demand is a factor. Crucial to the health of PWIDs is the resolution of multi-sector tensions

and nonaligned policies between criminal justice agencies in governments that favor interdiction to reduce supply and demand, laws and incarceration resulting from the possession of drugs, and the public health sector approach aimed at minimizing harm to PWIDs [20, 21].

Cocaine is produced largely in the Andean region of South America, which supplies the USA, the largest market. Recently, cocaine has been trafficked through and to Africa, notably West and Central Africa [22]. A high demand for amphetamine-type stimulants in the USA, particularly methamphetamines, reflects the drug's primary trafficking route to the USA through Mexico and a co-occurring methamphetamine epidemic in Mexico [22, 100][7]. Beyrer and colleagues reported that overland heroin export routes have been associated with co-occurring epidemics of injecting drug use and HIV infection in three Asian countries (India, China, and Myanmar) and along four trafficking routes: from Myanmar to cities in China, Laos, and Vietnam [26]. Outbreaks of injecting drug use and HIV in Myanmar, India, China, and Vietnam have been associated with Burmese and Laotian overland heroin trafficking routes. For the past 6 years, production has been declining in Myanmar and increasing in Afghanistan where, in 2008, about 82% of the opium was produced. With the trafficking from Afghanistan, increases in injection drug use and the associated spread of HIV have been reported in that region [101, 102]. There is considerable concern today regarding newly established cocaine and opiate trafficking routes, mostly through Africa, as countries in the region are reporting increased drug use, including injection drug use and HIV [103–105]. Only recently have some of these countries in sub-Saharan Africa been reporting use of cocaine (mostly crack) and heroin, injection drug use, high-risk sexual practices, and HIV infection among injection and non-injection drug users. This could create a second-wave epidemic of HIV and other sexually transmitted infections

---

[7]For more on ATS, trafficking, and patterns of use, see World Drug Report 2010 [27].

in countries currently experiencing enormous burden from heterosexually transmitted HIV.

Country-Level Laws and Drug Policies

In many countries drug control laws and policies are based on reducing supply and demand of drugs through interdiction, methods that often translate into policies that emphasize incarceration and punishment of drug users for possession and use, rather than facilitating access to treatment services. Drug users often report harassment by law enforcement staff, compulsory detention, high incarceration rates, fears of being arrested, stigma and discrimination, delayed or nonuse of health services by drug users, and interference with maintaining their ARV regimens [21, 106, 107]. More than 50 countries have compulsory treatment for people who use drugs and/or the death sentences for drug offenses [6]. Public health approaches provide an alternative to, or complement, drug control measures. For example, harm reduction interventions, including needle and syringe programs, and voluntary medication-assisted therapy (MAT) programs using methadone and/or buprenorphine, can prevent transmission of HIV, other blood-borne infections, and associated morbidity and mortality [19, 108].

Though a number of countries have changed laws and policies to support harm reduction programs, many countries maintain drug paraphernalia laws that prevent drug users from accessing clean needles.[8] [109]. Some countries forbid the use of medication assisted therapy (particularly methadone treatment).[9] Even in many countries that have made considerable progress in changing their laws and policies to create an enabling environment for the introduction and scaling-up of harm reduction services for PWIDs, tensions between drug control and public health approaches continue to occur, limiting access and support for services [110].

Recognition is growing that drug control policies to reduce the supply of illicit drugs and criminal justice approaches to responding to the needs of drug users have in many instances increased the marginalization of drug users and diminished the capacity of countries to offer treatment to those who need it most [22].

In U.S. drug policy, a repeated pattern of passing laws after new epidemics of drug use have emerged has resulted in increased incarceration rates for drug users. Each of the U.S. drug epidemics described in the earlier section (heroin, cocaine, crack, and ATS) resulted in increased media and political attention, and the introduction of harsher legislation for drug users that favors incarceration over treatment for drug dependence. Since 2009, this approach has been under review, and policy debate has seen a shift from a criminal justice approach to responding to drug use as a public health issue [111].[10] The criminal justice approach favors the investment of resources in public security, drug control activities, and law enforcement rather than in public health, which focuses on drug dependence treatment and the prevention and treatment of other drug-related health problems, including HIV infection [106].

---

[8]After the 21 years of banning the use of Federal funds for needle and syringe programs, in 2009 the law changed although some states still challenge Federal allowance of these programs. Subsequently, the Congress of the United States reinstated the ban on using federal funds to support needle exchange programs by adding restrictive language to the spending bill of 2012. The ban was reinstated despite strong evidence and the endorsement of major scientific bodies that needle exchange programs as a component of a comprehensive HIV prevention programs are highly effective in preventing the spread of HIV among persons who inject drugs. This ban impacts both domestic and global programs

[9]In this document, medication assisted therapy (MAT), methadone maintenance therapy (MMT), and opioid substitution therapy (OST) all define similar treatment modalities. The text reports the data according to the terms used by the study authors.

[10]Gostin and Lazzarini (1997) provide a fuller discussion of the theory and science and consequences of public health and criminal justice approaches [66].

Drug Use and Incarceration: A Global and U.S. Overview

Many studies report injection drug use in prisons, along with a high prevalence of both HIV and HBV, and evidence of HIV and HCV transmission among incarcerated populations [7, 55, 112]. Studies in a range of countries reveal that between 56 and 90% of PWIDs have been incarcerated, and it is estimated that 10–48% of male prisoners and 30–60% of female prisoners are drug users or drug dependent [7, 113].

At the end of 2007, the USA reported 1,595,034 persons incarcerated, more than any other country in the world. Drug-related offenses accounted for 49% of the growth in the prison population between 1995 and 2003 [114], an alarming figure as increases in incarceration rates correspond with increases in new AIDS infections [115]. Of those incarcerated, 38.2% were non-Hispanic black, 34% were white, 20.8% were Hispanic, and 7% were of other races [116]. Non-Hispanic blacks make up approximately 12–13% of the population [33], yet they make up just under 40% of those arrested for drug violations and 53% of those sentenced to prison for a drug offense [117]. Non-Hispanic blacks make up more than 80% of the defendants sentenced for crack offenses [118]. These data highlight again how drugs disproportionately affect minorities. The number of non-Hispanic black persons incarcerated for drug offenses in state prisons had fallen from 145,000 in 1999 to 113,500 in 2005, a 22% decline. During this same period, the number of white drug offenders increased 43%, from about 50,000 to more than 72,000 [117].

Data on drug use patterns of incarcerated populations in the USA, dating back to reports in 2004, reveal that in the month before the criminal offense was committed, cocaine/crack was the most frequently reported drug used (21% for state prisoners and 18% for federal prisoners) [119]. Stimulants were used by 12.5% of state prisoners and 11% of federal prisoners in the month before the offense was committed. Eight percent of the state prisoners and 6% of the federal prisoners used heroin and other opioids in the month before the offense.

Drug use within prisons is common [7]. Many people who use drugs within the community where they live continue their drug use once imprisoned, although the prevalence and frequency of drug use tends to decline during the period of incarceration. Prison is also a setting for drug initiation among non-drug users as they are exposed to drug-using situations, which may result in the initiation and continuation of drug use after their release. Prisons pose a high-risk environment for injecting drug use. The lack of sterile injecting equipment, limited access to prevention and treatment services, overcrowding, and lack of privacy result in very high-risk injecting practices. In particular, sharing of injecting equipment is common among a population where HIV, viral hepatitis, and other blood-borne infections are already high [7, 55].

Most PWIDs return to their respective communities after their sentences. A majority of those who inject in prison report sharing syringes, and high-risk sexual behavior is common among drug users while incarcerated [7, 120, 121]. The return of previously incarcerated PWIDs to home communities has significant implications for the spreading of HIV and other blood-borne and sexually transmitted infections [122].

Prevention of HIV, HBV, HCV, and STIs

For more than 25 years, scientific evidence has been accumulating that comprehensive HIV prevention programs can help avert, halt, and reverse HIV epidemics among PWIDs [1–3, 135]. Early in the HIV epidemic among PWIDs, a number of cities (Glasgow, Scotland; Lund, Sweden; Sydney, Australia; Tacoma, Washington; and Toronto, Canada) implemented effective programs to prevent significant HIV epidemics from emerging and maintained low and stable HIV seroprevalence rates in the population of PWIDs. Core multi-component prevention interventions—community-based outreach, large-scale provision of sterile injection equipment through syringe exchange programs, pharmacies[11] and, in one city, large-scale drug dependence treatment—can reverse and contain epidemics among PWIDs, reducing incidence and prevalence [46]. New York City, with the largest epidemic of HIV among PWIDs in the world, legalized and implemented a large-scale expansion of syringe exchange programs in the early 1990s, including outreach and testing and counseling services [136]. Hartel and Schoenbaum [137] reported that HIV among injecting heroin users in the Bronx, who were in methadone maintenance therapy (MMT) in the late 1970s when the epidemic began, had a lower prevalence rate (34%) than those who enrolled in MMT in 1980 and 1984 (44%); the HIV prevalence rate was highest for PWIDs who enrolled after 1985 (53%).

Over time, evidence continues to accumulate that these interventions—outreach, needle and syringe programs (NSPs) and MAT—singularly and in combination affect risk behaviors and can reduce incidence and prevalence of HIV among persons who inject drugs. Community-based outreach provides a range of services to persons who inject drugs in their natural environments. Outreach workers in the community in fixed and/ or mobile sites and street locations provide access to risk-reduction information, enable people who use drugs to reduce their drug use and needle-sharing behaviors by providing alcohol wipes, bleach, water, condoms, and referral to services [2, 138]. Some outreach programs train PWIDs in overdose prevention—teaching them how to administer naloxone—and some outreach workers provide sterile needles and syringes. Outreach has been demonstrated to enable PWIDs to access the means to reduce their risk behaviors.[12] Through referral mechanisms, outreach increases the likelihood that persons who inject drugs will have access to a range of other complementary services essential to reduce risk of acquisition and transmission of HIV and other blood-borne infections [138]. The evidence is

strong that NSPs result in reduced risk behaviors, lower HIV prevalence, greater use of services, and, importantly, reduced injection drug use [139]. Consistent findings from evaluation studies of NSPs reveal that they increase the availability of sterile injection equipment, reduce the number of contaminated needles in circulation, and reduce the risk of new HIV infections [1, 140]. Des Jarlais and Semaan [136] reported that most NSPs provide a range of other services, including referral to drug dependence treatment programs, specifically MAT and other programs. Medication-assisted treatment with methadone or buprenorphine has been shown to be effective for opioid dependence, reducing risk behaviors related to injection drug use, preventing HIV transmission, and improving PWIDs' adherence to antiretroviral therapy [3][13]. In a recent review of evidence on MMT, the Institute of Medicine concluded, based on randomized clinical trials and a number of observation studies, that persons receiving MAT report reductions in drug-related risk behaviors, including the frequency of injecting and sharing equipment [142]. Metzger found that persons who inject drugs and remained in methadone treatment had a lower HIV incidence than those who were not enrolled in MAT [143]. Other interventions, not unique to persons who inject drugs, are also now part of a comprehensive HIV response, including ART (see Box 12.3).

The core interventions discussed above and listed elsewhere in the text are potentially important strategies for limiting the spread of HCV and HBV. Specifically for HCV, NSPs with risk reduction emphasis on not sharing or reusing injection equipment, MAT, and other drug dependence treatment, condom programming and safer sex practices and prevention and treatment of STIs are effective. HCV can be transmitted sexually, particularly in the context of HIV coinfection [144]. Because background prevalence is much higher for HCV than HIV, and it is more infectious, though it varies regionally, the need to

---

[11]Pharmacies only in some cities.

[12]See IOM for a review of the evidence and discussion of the limitations of the studies.

[13]Methadone maintenance treatment has been available in the United States since 1964 [141].

Box 12.3. Key Messages on Prevention for PWIDs

- A comprehensive package of evidence-based harm reduction interventions implemented in a range of venues including the community, public health facilities, and prisons and other closed settings can be highly effective in preventing HIV, other blood-borne and sexually transmitted infections, and tuberculosis.
- The combination of NSPs, MAT, and ART implemented at high coverage rates has been demonstrated to reduce incidence and prevalence among PWIDs.
- Providing colocated, comprehensive, gender-friendly and integrated low threshold services in multiple venues for PWIDs can

result in higher coverage, equity, timely use, efficiencies, and higher quality HIV/AIDS services.

- Structural interventions are critical to reduce the impact of punitive laws, regulations, policies, law enforcement practices, and other legal barriers that contribute to the vulnerability, marginalization, discrimination and stigmatization and impede the scaling up of harm reduction interventions among PWIDs.
- Policies and interventions should follow the principles affirmed in the UN General Assembly's 2006 Political Declaration of HIV/AIDS that address stigma and discrimination as critical elements in combating HIV/AIDS.

reach more at-risk populations earlier is of critical importance. For HBV, vaccination is an additional intervention that can have an impact on transmission and interventions to increase safer sex practices for PWID, MSM, and those who have not been vaccinated for hepatitis B [52]. Most important is that NSPs and outreach provide information about HCV and ways to prevent transmission by providing sterile cotton swabs, alcohol wipes for cleaning injection sites, sterile water, cookers, and other disinfection supplies and skills to promote adherence [140]. Evidence suggests NSPs have less impact on the transmission and acquisition of HCV than on HIV, though one study found that NSPs had a significant effect on decreasing HCV and HBV acquisition [145]. Substance dependence treatment has been shown to reduce the incidence of HCV [51]. In a study in Seattle, those who remained in MMT longer had a lower HCV prevalence than those who interrupted or dropped out of treatment [146].

In addition to MAT for the treatment of opioid dependence, non-pharmacologic therapies are effective strategies at treating cocaine and amphetamine dependence and preventing HIV, hepatitis, and STI risk behaviors associated with drug use. It is important to consider these strate-

gies in addition to MAT, as the number of cocaine, amphetamine, and poly-drug users grow [27, 147]. In addition, many opioid users engage in cocaine use while on drug treatment [148, 149]. Effective psychosocial interventions including cognitive-behavioral therapies and contingency management are currently available to treat cocaine and methamphetamine dependence [150, 151] and pharmacologic therapy may be available in the future [152, 153].

Combination Interventions

Combination prevention programs consist of a mix of structural, biomedical, and behavioral interventions. Findings from recent mathematical modeling studies reveal that combination interventions—NSPs and MAT (if coverage reaches 50% of the persons who inject drugs)—in 5 years could lead to a 20% reduction in HIV incidence depending on the setting [19]. And, when ART is combined with MAT and NSPs, reaching 50% of the persons who inject drugs and are HIV positive, after 5 years the incidence will be a 50% median reduction of 29%. Strathdee and colleagues [108] modeled changes in risk environments in regions with different types of HIV epidemics among persons who inject drugs. Consistent with the work of Degenhardt and colleagues [19], they report that by reducing unmet needs by 60% in MAT, NSPs, and ART, there are reductions in HIV prevalence ranging from 30 to 41% over 5 years. They also reported that structural level changes like changing laws in Kenya to allow MAT in public clinics and needle syringe programs or reducing changing police practices related to harassment and violence in Odessa, Ukraine, can further contribute to reducing HIV incidence.

Structural Interventions

Optimizing the impact of core interventions to prevent the further spread of HIV requires implementation of structural interventions to help create an enabling environment supportive of an effective HIV response in a range of settings (community, clinics, jail/prisons, and other detention settings) [55].

Structural interventions seek to create contextual changes in the social, physical, economic, and political environments to remove or reduce barriers that contribute to HIV/AIDS vulnerabilities and risks, and that impede access to services, and to create an enabling environment supporting implementation with evidence- and human rights-based laws, policies, and regulations, facilitating the scaling up of prevention interventions. The rationale for the potential value of structural interventions is clear [19, 97]. Laws, policies, regulations, resulting stigma and discrimination, incarceration without legal rights and violations of human rights to health are among the factors that account for the limited availability, inaccessibility, low coverage, and continuing high burden of disease. Among the structural strategies most often mentioned are efforts to improve the legal environment—laws and policies, law enforcement, and legal clinics—for persons who inject drugs and who are arrested. These reforms could include laws promoting protection from discrimination, gender-based violence, human rights violations, and laws to enable harm reduction services to operate effectively without impunity [23]. Other structural interventions and potential effects operating at macro and micro levels of the physical, social, economic, and policy environments described by Degenhardt and colleagues [19], can include scale-up of needle and syringe provision and legal reform enabling protection of drug-user rights.

HIV, HBV, and HCV Prevention in Prison and Other Closed Settings

Jurgens, Ball, and Verster [7] reviewed the effectiveness of interventions to reduce PWID risk behaviors and HIV, HBV, and HCV transmission in prison settings. Evidence of injection and high-risk sexual practices in these settings has been referred to earlier. There is substantial HIV transmission through drug use in prisons, and many studies have also reported HCV outbreaks among incarcerated populations [21]. More prisons are now recognizing the epidemiological realities of transmission in these settings and have begun to introduce core interventions; most countries, however, do not provide these services. NSPs have been introduced in more than 50 prisons in 12 western and eastern European and central Asian countries. In some countries, only a few prisons have NSPs, while in Kyrgyzstan and Spain, NSPs in prisons have been rapidly scaled up. With the exception of one study, evidence demonstrates that sharing of injecting equipment either stopped after implementation of the NSPs [154, 155] or substantially declined [156–158]. PWIDs in Moldovan prisons with NSPs also reported fewer incidents of sharing injecting equipment [159].

Since the early 1990s, there has been a marked increase in the number of prison systems providing opioid substitution therapy (OST) to prisoners. Jurgens, Ball, and Verster (2009) found that in all studies of prison-based MMT programs, prisoners who inject heroin and other opioids and who receive MMT inject substantially less frequently than those not receiving this therapy [7, 160–163]. Access to OST in prisons also reduces injection risks and syringe sharing [164]. Some countries, Spain in particular, has scaled up NSPs and OST in prisons and the seroconversion rates for HIV and hepatitis C virus have decreased substantially.

Prevention and Treatment of HCV

HCV is more infectious than HIV and more prevalent, especially among younger injectors, with modes of transmission including reuse of contaminated syringes, needles, and other injection equipment [12, 62, 165]. Due to shared risk factors and prevention strategies between HIV and hepatitis, HCV prevention is critical to an effective HIV prevention strategy among PWIDs. Modeling studies demonstrate that HIV and HCV prevalence among PWIDs are proportional and that reducing HCV prevalence below a threshold of 30% would substantially reduce any HIV risk and likely make HIV prevalence negligible [166].

Edlin and colleagues [167] have outlined and discussed the strategies for prevention and treatment of HCV. These include strategies for primary prevention (preventing exposure) by reducing injection drug use through evidence-based substance use prevention and expansion of substance dependence treatment. Most critical is preventing and/or reducing transition from non-injecting drug use to injecting drug use [168]. Edlin describes options in secondary prevention (preventing infection) of HCV transmission among PWIDs by providing access to sterile syringes and other injection equipment, repeal of paraphernalia and syringe prescription laws, establishment of syringe exchange and distribution programs, education of physicians and pharmacists to help PWIDs gain access to sterile injection equipment, community-based outreach to PWIDs, and client-centered HCV counseling and testing [169]. For tertiary prevention (preventing disease) and reducing liver diseases in the infected person, Edlin identifies potentially effective strategies, including medical treatment for HCV infection, integration of medical and social services, and provision of services to incarcerated populations [77]. Most important is that needle and syringe exchange programs and outreach provide information about HCV and ways to prevent transmission by providing sterile cotton swabs, alcohol wipes for cleaning injection sites, sterile water, cookers, and other disinfection supplies and skills to promote adherence [140]. Evidence suggests NSPs have less impact on the transmission and acquisition of HCV virus than on HIV, though one study found that NSPs had a significant effect on decreasing HCV and HBV acquisition [145]. Treatment for drug dependence has been shown to reduce the incidence of HCV [51]. In a study in Seattle, it was found that those who remained in MMT longer had a lower HCV prevalence than those who interrupted or dropped out of treatment [146].

STI Prevention Among Persons Who Use Drugs

Historically, prevention for drug users has centered on injection-related risk, overlooking the fact that drug users are at high risk for sexual transmission of infections, including HIV and STIs. STI control among drug users is an important public health strategy as the presence of an STI infection increases susceptibility and infectivity of HIV [170–173]. HIV positive women are significantly more likely to be coinfected with multiple STIs compared to those who are HIV negative [174]. Presence of an STI may also facilitate HCV transmission [175].

STI control is a public health priority for drug users for several reasons. First, it has implications for persons who use drugs as well as those who do not use drugs but may have sex with drug users [176]. As STI treatment decreases transmission, identification of STI cases among drug users would give treatment options to these individuals and would help reduce the spread of infection to others, both inside and outside of this population [177]. Since drug users face many individual and provider-level barriers to accessing STI prevention and control services, they are likely to go untreated and further transmit infections inside their networks. Clinical management of STIs also leads to reduced incidence of HIV over time [178], and provides an opportunity for health care providers to assess drug use as a risk behavior that can lead to vaccination for hepatitis A and B, screening for viral hepatitis, STIs and HIV, and appropriate treatment services for these infections along with linkages to other prevention strategies for drug users, including needle and syringe programs and drug dependence treatment [52].

As more biomedical interventions become available for the prevention and control of STIs, attention has shifted to improving health care-seeking behaviors and the behaviors of care providers [179]. Individual-level interventions can modify drug use or STI risk behaviors [180] but structural changes are also required for large-scale impact [181]. For example, routine STI screening and treatment at drug treatment admission and other primary care venues commonly frequented by drug users would facilitate access to these services [95, 182]. According to CDC, drug use is a risk factor for gonorrhea among women and routine screening is recommended [52]. STI infection is a marker for high-risk sexual behaviors, so screening for these infections presents an opportunity to provide risk reduction counseling and other effective behavioral interventions.

Gender Norms Around Female PWIDs

HIV infections are rising among female PWIDs in Asia, Eastern Europe, and other countries [123, 124] as females who use drugs face a greater risk of blood-borne and sexually transmitted infection [125]. Female PWIDs often rely on male partners to initiate drug use, procure drugs, and inject them with drugs [126–129]. As drug-using practices often follow social norms, women are more likely to use contaminated equipment as they inject after men, and refusal to use drugs or share injecting equipment results in increased risk of physical in sexual abuse, further increasing likelihood of infection [127, 130]. As stated earlier, sex work is common among females who use drugs, making them more vulnerable to infection [131].

Women who inject drugs face additional barriers to prevention and treatment services such as childcare duties, lack of power to negotiate service use and lack of access to resources [129, 132]. Men are the primary recipients of these interventions in many settings [132]. Despite evidence of their efficacy, drug treatment, harm reduction, and HIV prevention programs for women who use drugs are under-funded, and the programs that do exist rarely address intimate partner and sexual violence, reproductive health, empowerment strategies, and other risk factors among women who use drugs [133]. Provision of low-threshold services increases uptake among women and availability of gender-friendly services that include flexible hours, childcare services, social and psychological support, and programs for drug-using sex workers will further fill the coverage gap [132, 134].

Organizing and Delivering Core Intervention and Other Health Services to Persons Who Inject Drugs

New public health approaches in organizing and delivering services will require changes in their law enforcement approaches to injection drug use and HIV to be effective and have an impact on the epidemic.

Availability and Coverage of Core Interventions

Of the 151 countries reporting injection drug use, NSPs are available in 82 countries, while only 10 countries have NSPs in prisons [55]. It is estimated that about 8% of PWIDs accessed an NSP at least once in the past 12 months, and fewer than 5% of injections were covered by sterile syringes. In the 16 countries with PWIDs in Eastern Europe, it is estimated that there are 9 syringes distributed per PWID per year. The number is highest in Australia and New Zealand (213/year per PWID), comparatively high in Central Asia (92/year per PWID), and relatively low in the USA and Canada (23/year per PWID) [17]. For OST, available in 71 countries, which covers 65% of the estimated population of persons who inject drugs, only 8 PWIDs per every 100 were receiving OST. Again, there is considerable range by region with very low rates in Central Asia and Eastern Europe—about 1 per 100 PWIDs, about 4 per 100 PWIDs in East and

Southeast Asia, highest in Western Europe (61 per 100 PWIDs), and much less in the U.S and Canada (13 per 100 PWIDs) [17]. The same pattern prevails for ART coverage rates. In a limited number of countries reporting coverage rates for ART among persons who inject drugs, only 4 of every 100 HIV-positive PWIDs who were in need of ART were receiving it [19].

Barriers to Introducing and Scaling Up Services

There are many reasons for low coverage rates, including cultural, legal, policy, regulatory, technical, fiscal, human resource constraints, and operational barriers, and attitudes and beliefs of service providers. These factors are obstacles to introducing, scaling up and implementing innovative strategies to organize and deliver services [16, 55].[14] In many countries, persons who inject drugs are required to be registered by name and with law enforcement. This information is often shared with health providers before they are eligible for services. Mimiaga and colleagues [183] report that in one Eastern European country, harassment and discrimination by police with threats of arrest, and the need to bribe police to avoid arrest are major barriers to adherence to MAT and ART. Laws that criminalize nonmedical use of syringes, along with punitive laws for possession of small amounts of drugs, law enforcement harassment of PWIDs, detention without due process and subjecting persons who use drugs to non-evidence-based treatment interventions create obstacles to implementing and scaling up interventions and reducing vulnerability to HIV and other blood-borne and sexually transmitted infections. Carrying condoms is often used as evidence by law enforcement of engaging in sex work [184]. The public health consequences can

be observed in high incarceration rates, unavailability of services, low and often delayed utilization of services, and limited progress in the prevention of HIV, hepatitis, and STIs.

Policy and service providers' personal beliefs affect the availability and quality of services. Despite evidence from neurosciences that drug addiction is a chronic and relapsing condition that is treatable, like other diseases such as diabetes and hypertension, controversies continue relative to the treatment of addiction and providing NSP services [139, 140, 185]. Medication-assisted treatment consistently has been proven to be an effective treatment for opioid addiction and the prevention of HIV. As more PWIDs access and remain in MAT, less crime is committed and fewer drug-related arrests are conducted, meaning fewer criminal justice costs. In addition, the demand for drugs is reduced, and less money is spent on illegal drugs, meaning less money in the informal market [186]. However, myths persist that providing medication such as methadone is substituting one addiction for another, rather than a treatment.

Coordination and Integration of a Comprehensive Package of Interventions to Address Needs of Persons Who Inject Drugs

It is critically important that all public health services or facilities that have contact with persons who inject drugs have the capacity to provide a full range of integrated, colocated direct services and/or linked referrals to other services [187]. The rationale for the recommendation is clear. Persons who use drugs are at increased risk for multiple comorbid conditions, including problems associated with drug use, such as addiction and mental health issues; multiple infections, such as HIV, STIs, and hepatitis; and adverse social conditions, such as stigma, poverty, and incarceration [188–191]. Additionally, persons who use drugs are less likely to use health services due to fear of arrest or discrimination, exacerbating negative health outcomes [97, 192, 193]. Integration of prevention, care, and treatment

---

[14]See the following reports for more elaborate discussion: International Harm Reduction Association. Global State of Harm reduction, 2010; Needle & Zhao, HIV Prevention among Injection Drug Users: Closing the Coverage Gap, 2010.

services for persons who use drugs addresses both comorbidities and low service utilization. Ideally, integrated services are colocated and share client records to increase efficiency, access to services, the level of prevention and care for clients, and reduce costs. Services can also be integrated through a system of coordinated referrals. Programs that have provided integrated services for persons who use drugs report successful outcomes including increased testing rates, medication adherence, entry into drug treatment services and attendance of PWID at services [194–197]. And these services should be offered in multiple venues including prisons, in the community, and a range of public health clinics and other facilities. The services should include priority interventions for persons who inject drugs—NSP, MAT, and ART—sexual risk reduction services and others that include screening, risk reduction and treatment for prevalent and co-occurring conditions. Not only can these services reduce burden of disease in individual drug users and their networks of sex- and drug-using partners, they also serve as an entry point into other prevention and treatment services specific to drug users, such as syringe exchange and drug treatment. Health services in communities where drug use takes place can assess patients for drug use. In addition to prevention strategies specific to persons who use drugs, members of this population also benefit from access to health interventions such as vaccination for hepatitis A and B, and screening and treatment of HIV, STIs and hepatitis (see new CDC guidelines: www.cdc.gov/std/treatment/2010/) using standardized assessment tools, and providing relevant linkages as necessary [52].

Low Threshold Services

According to a report from the Open Society Institute (OSI), low threshold programs are flexible in their organization, delivery of services and eligibility requirements to access services [198]. The overall objective is to make services available to the greatest number of persons who inject drugs and rely on strategies that recognize

that these populations are often hard to reach and retain in services. Colocation and integration of services can be effective, as referenced earlier; however, the extent to which this new service delivery strategy works depends on adopting principles related to low threshold programs. The list that follows is illustrative and not exhaustive, and provides examples of strategies that can remove barriers and expand availability and utilization of services. Some overarching low threshold principles include not restricting eligibility for services based on current drug-using practices or not requiring persons who inject drugs to have failed other "treatment interventions" (detoxification in detention centers); active or previous injection drug use should not be a reason not to provide ART; ART should not be dependent on enrolling in MAT (often not available); and access to ART should not require "proof" that PWIDs can be adherent with the prescribed MAT regimen.

All who seek treatment should be eligible. As reported by OSI, some specific low threshold strategies for MAT include quick service on demand and without complex paperwork, no waiting lists, service delivery by medical and nonmedical staff, limited or no urine screening without being used for disqualification from the program, abstinence from drugs not required, treatment by prescription (both buprenorphine and methadone), no registration of users, no biological testing, no requirement for any type of counseling or directly observed dose-taking before beginning unsupervised administration, flexible eligibility requirements, treatment in prisons, and take-home doses [198]. For MAT and other services, most critical is a nonjudgmental harm-reduction philosophy that does not insist on complete abstinence from drug use. Also important is reducing operational constraints, such as hours of operation, location of facilities, costs for services and ensuring multiple models of service availability in multiple venues. For NSPs, OSI reports that this means multiple service delivery models and maximizing the number of needles and syringes distributed by supporting secondary exchange of syringes, and with no limits on the number of syringes to be distributed.

Other strategies that will contribute to coverage and effectiveness include ensuring there are no stock outs of commodities like syringes and needles, and that the types of syringes and needles distributed reflect the needs of the persons who use drugs. Ensuring that services are responsive to PWIDs requires that these persons participate in planning, program development and implementation [6].

Public Health Role of the USA

The USA plays an important role on the issues mentioned above through its international influence on drug control policies related to reducing supply and demand for drugs and protecting the safety and public health of persons who inject drugs, through their financial and technical support to the Global Fund, and the President's Emergency Plan for AIDS Relief (PEPFAR) program. PEPFAR provides technical and fiscal resources to countries with HIV epidemics, including those with concentrated epidemics of HIV among persons who inject drugs, and countries with expanding rates of injection drug use and HIV among persons who inject drugs [199]. In 2010, the USA issued a new drug control strategy through the Office of National Drug Control Policy, a new domestic HIV/AIDS policy through the Office of the National AIDS Policy in the White House, and policy and program guidelines through PEPFAR [200–202]. Implementing evidence-based law enforcement strategies—scaling up and increasing access to treatment for addiction, integrating addiction services into the health system with support through health services, recognizing and acting on the public health consequences of use of drugs, such as overdose deaths and HIV/AIDS, and recognizing the evidence supporting interventions in the comprehensive package of services—allows for better coordination and collaboration with the PEPFAR program.

On July 10, 2010, PEPFAR released a revised technical guidance document titled *Comprehensive HIV Prevention for People Who Inject Drugs*

(www.pepfar.gov).[15] This document affirmed PEPFAR's support for comprehensive, evidence-based, and human rights-based HIV prevention programs for persons who inject drugs. Along with the guidance, PEPFAR explicitly allowed funds to be used for needle and syringe exchange programs (NSPs) for the first time as one component of comprehensive HIV prevention programs among PWIDs [202]. The policy shift was announced following congressional lifting of the domestic ban on NSPs as part of the Consolidated Appropriations Act of 2010 in December 2009. As mentioned earlier, studies have consistently shown that NSPs—providing clean, unused syringes and a range of other services, including referrals and linkages with drug treatment, HIV testing and counseling and antiretroviral (ARV) treatment for PWIDs—result in marked decreases in drug-related risk behaviors (e.g., sharing of contaminated injection equipment, other unsafe injection practices and frequency of injections) and decrease the risk of HIV transmission. PEPFAR also supports procurement of methadone and buprenorphine and provides funds for interventions along with technical assistance to host governments and partners. The USG policy and programs are consistent with the 2009 World Health Organization, United Nations Office on Drugs and Crime, and UNAIDS Technical Guide for countries to set targets for universal access to HIV prevention, treatment and care for PWIDs. PEPFAR works with partner governments and civil societies to address the imbalance between the high levels of HIV risk and disease burden among PWIDs and the low level of coverage of a comprehensive package of prevention, treatment and care services. The PEPFAR policy and comprehensive HIV prevention package, including NSP, is now accepted by The Office of National Drug Control Policy for the first time, and

---

[15]The U.S. President's Emergency Plan for AIDS Relief (PEPFAR), works in more than 80 developing countries-those with generalized and concentrated HIV epidemics. The program focuses on prevention strategies to decrease new infections, and life-saving treatment and care for those already living with HIV.

endorsed in the 2010 National Drug Control Strategy [200, 201]. The PEPFAR 5-year strategy seeks to expand prevention, treatment and care services for PWIDs in both concentrated and generalized epidemics.

In 2009, President Obama committed additional funds through the Global Health Initiative (GHI) to support the work of PEPFAR with an additional focus on women and children through infectious diseases, nutrition, maternal and child health, and safe water programs (http://www.pepfar.gov/ghi/index.htm). GHI activities initially focused on eight countries and have now spread to include over 20 more, many of which are countries with emerging epidemics of HIV among persons who use drugs [42, 203]. Increasing impact through strategic coordination and integration, strengthening and leveraging of key multilateral organizations, global health partnerships and private sector engagement, a women, girls and gender equality-centered approach, and promoting research and innovation are four key principles underlying implementation of GHI. These principles align with the a public health approach to addressing HIV and other blood-borne and sexually transmitted infections among drug users, in terms of providing a comprehensive package of evidence-based services and coordinated participation across public and private sectors.

Box 12.4. The USA: Problems, Challenges and Opportunities

- The demand for drugs is significant in the USA and the country represents a huge market with heroin, cocaine and other drugs being trafficked from South America and Mexico. Domestic production of amphetamine-type stimulants also occurs.
- Twenty millions persons in the U.S have used an illicit drug; most prevalent is marijuana with substantial numbers using cocaine, crack, heroin and methamphetamines. Seventeen million have a diagnosable drug disorder. Drug dependence is a chronic and treatable condition.
- The USA, Russia, and China have the greatest number of persons who inject drugs.
- More than seven million Americans are in the criminal justice system with two million incarcerated and five million on parole. Fifty percent of these people are dependent on drugs.
- PWIDs make up less than 1.3% of the U.S. population and account for 19% of HIV infections and 90% of hepatitis C infections.

- African American males and females are disproportionately impacted by drug dependence, HIV, and are greatly overrepresented in the criminal justice system.
- The USA, compared to other high-income countries, has lower coverage rates for HIV core prevention interventions—MAT and NSPs—and PWIDs and who are living with HIV have lower rates of ART enrollment than other groups living with HIV.
- The USA is the largest donor to the Global Fund for AIDS, Tuberculosis and Malaria. Through PEPFAR, there is financial, technical and programmatic support for counties with HIV epidemics among PWIDs.
- The USA plays a powerful role in influencing drug and HIV policy globally. There is great need to harmonize domestic and global drug and HIV policies to ensure that the tensions between criminal justice and public health approaches to responding to epidemics that have impeded prevention are resolved.

The New Public Health Approach

Public Health Challenges

Persons who use drugs are at increased risk for multiple, comorbid conditions, including problems associated with drug use, such as addiction and mental health issues, multiple infections such as HIV, STIs and hepatitis, overdose, and adverse social conditions such as stigma, poverty, discrimination, and incarceration. While burden of disease is high in persons who inject drugs, availability and access to needle and syringe programs, medication-assisted treatment, and antiretroviral therapy (ART) services are limited, particularly in many low- and middle-income countries. In large part, services are limited because of structural barriers (laws, policies, and regulations and other and programmatic and operational barriers) and strongly held but unfounded beliefs by many about drug users. All of these can impede the implementation of prevention, treatment, and care services.

New Public Health Response

The challenge for the public health community is to embrace the concept that harm reduction should be a core element of a public health response to HIV/AIDS where injecting drug use exists. A 'comprehensive package of harm reduction' has been described in this chapter as outlined by the WHO, UNODC and UNAIDS, and provides guidance to countries on the selection of evidence-based policies and interventions, including interventions for reducing HIV transmission and treatment of HIV/AIDS and associated comorbidities [204]. For these interventions to have an impact on HIV epidemics in different countries, political will and leadership are necessary across government and nongovernment sectors to align drug control policies with public health goals, in accordance with human rights principles for the prevention, treatment and care of persons who inject drugs and are at risk for or currently are living with HIV and other blood-borne and sexually transmitted diseases. More specifically, supportive policy, legal and social environments that facilitate rather than impede the implementation of appropriate models of service delivery need to be created.

References

1. Wodak A, Cooney A. Effectiveness of sterile needle and syringe programming in reducing HIV/AIDS among injecting drug users. Geneva: World Health Organization; 2005.
2. Needle R, Burrows D, Friedman S, et al. Effectiveness of community-based outreach in preventing HIV/AIDS among injection drug users. Geneva: World Health Organization; 2004.
3. Farrell M, Marsden J, Ling W, Ali R, Gowing L. Effectiveness of drug dependence treatment in preventing HIV among injecting drug users. Geneva: World Health Organization; 2005.
4. Piot P, Zewdie D, Turmen T. HIV/AIDS prevention and treatment. Lancet. 2002;360(9326):86–8.
5. UNGASS. Declaration of commitment on HIV/AIDS. New York: United Nations; 2001.
6. UNAIDS. Call for urgent action to improve coverage of HIV services for injecting drug users. *UNAIDS* 2010 March 10; Available from: http://www.unaids.org/en/KnowledgeCentre/Resources/FeatureStories/archive/2010/20100309_IDU.asp.
7. Jurgens R, Ball A, Verster A. Interventions to reduce HIV transmission related to injecting drug use in prison. Lancet Infect Dis. 2009;9(1):57–66.
8. Mathers BM, Degenhardt L, Phillips B, et al. Global epidemiology of injecting drug use and HIV among people who inject drugs: a systematic review. Lancet. 2008;372(9651):1733–45.
9. Gordon RJ, Lowy FD. Bacterial infections in drug users. N Engl J Med. 2005;353(18):1945–54.
10. Hoffmann CJ, Thio CL. Clinical implications of HIV and hepatitis B co-infection in Asia and Africa. Lancet Infect Dis. 2007;7(6):402–9.
11. Roy KM, Goldberg DJ, Hutchinson S, et al. Hepatitis C virus among self declared non-injecting sexual partners of injecting drug users. J Med Virol. 2004;74:62–6.
12. Centers for Disease Control and Prevention. Surveillance for acute viral hepatitis—United States, 2006. MMWR Recomm Rep. 2008;57(SS-2):1–24.
13. Urbanus AT, van de Laar TJ, Stolte IG, et al. Hepatitis C virus infections among HIV-infected men who have sex with men: an expanding epidemic. AIDS. 2009;23(12):F1–7.
14. Danta M, Brown D, Bhagani S, et al. Recent epidemic of acute hepatitis C virus in HIV-positive men who have sex with men linked to high-risk sexual behaviours. AIDS. 2007;21(8):983–91.

15. Des Jarlais C, Semaan S. HIV and other sexually transmitted infections in injection drug users and crack cocaine smokers. In: Holmes KK, Sparling PF, Stamm WE, Piot P, Wasserheit JN, Corey L, et al., editors. Sexually transmitted diseases. 4th ed. New York: McGraw-Hill; 2008. p. 237–55.

16. Needle R, Zhao L. HIV prevention among injection drug users: closing the coverage GAP. Washington, DC: Center for Strategic and International Studies Global Health Policy Center; 2010.

17. Mathers BM, Degenhardt L, Ali H, et al. HIV prevention, treatment, and care services for people who inject drugs: a systematic review of global, regional, and national coverage. Lancet. 2010;375(9719):1014–28.

18. Mathers BM, Degenhardt L, Adam P, et al. Estimating the level of HIV prevention coverage, knowledge and protective behavior among injecting drug users: what does the 2008 UNGASS reporting round tell us? J Acquir Immune Defic Syndr. 2009;52 Suppl 2:S132–42.

19. Degenhardt L, Mathers B, Vickerman P, Rhodes T, Latkin C, Hickman M. Prevention of HIV infection for people who inject drugs: why individual, structural, and combination approaches are needed. Lancet. 2010;376(9737):285–301.

20. Gostin LO, Lazzarini Z. Prevention of HIV/AIDS among injection drug users: the theory and science of public health and criminal justice approaches to disease prevention. Emory Law J. 1997;46(2):587–696.

21. Jurgens R, Csete J, Amon JJ, Baral S, Beyrer C. People who use drugs, HIV, and human rights. Lancet. 2010;376(9739):475–85.

22. UNODC. World Drug Report. New York: United Nations; 2008.

23. International HIV/AIDS Alliance. Global commission on HIV and the law. International HIV/AIDS Alliance 2010. Available from: http://www.worldaidscampaign.org/en/Global-Programmes/Global-Commission-on-HIV-and-the-Law.

24. International HIV/AIDS Alliance, Commonwealth HIV and AIDS Action Group. Enabling legal environments for effective HIV responses: a leadership challenge for the Commonwealth. 2010.

25. UNAIDS. Report on the Global AIDS Epidemic. Geneva: World Health Organization; 2010.

26. Beyrer C, Razak MH, Lisam K, Chen J, Lui W, Yu XF. Overland heroin trafficking routes and HIV-1 spread in south and south-east Asia. AIDS. 2000;14(1):75–83.

27. UNODC. World Drug Report. New York: United Nations; 2010.

28. Ditton J, Frischer M. Computerized projection of future heroin epidemics: a necessity for the 21st century? Subst Use Misuse. 2001;36(1–2):151–66.

29. Hughes PH, Rieche O. Heroin epidemics revisited. Epidemiol Rev. 1995;17(1):66–73.

30. Substance Abuse and Mental Health Services Administration. Results from the 2009 National Survey on Drug Use and Health: National Findings. Rockville, MD: US Department of Health and Human Services; 2010. Report No.: Publication No. SMA 10-4586.

31. Wiessing L, Likatavicius G, Klempova D, Hedrich D, Nardone A, Griffiths P. Associations between availability and coverage of HIV-prevention measures and subsequent incidence of diagnosed HIV infection among injection drug users. Am J Public Health. 2009;99(6):1049–52.

32. Substance Abuse and Mental Health Services Administration OoAS. Treatment Episode Data Set (TEDS). Highlights—2007. National Admissions to Substance Abuse Treatment Services. Rockville, MD, Department of Health and Human Services; 2009. Report No.: DHHS Publication No. (SMA) 09-4360.

33. U.S. Census Bureau. State and County QuickFacts: Data derived from Population Estimates. httt://www.census.gov 2009. Available from: http://quickfacts.census.gov/qfd/states/00000.html

34. Centers for Disease Control and Prevention. Sexually transmitted disease surveillance, 2007. Atlanta, GA: Department of Health and Human Services; 2008.

35. Centers for Disease Control and Prevention. HIV/AIDS Surveillance Report, 2007. Atlanta, GA: U.S. Department of Health and Human Services; 2009.

36. Centers for Disease Control and Prevention. HIV infections among injection-drug users—34 states, 2004–2007. MMWR Recomm Rep. 2009;58(46):1291–5.

37. Centers for Disease Control and Prevention. Surveillance for acute viral hepatitis—United States 2007. MMWR Recomm Rep 2009;58:1–37.

38. Ball AL, Rana S, Dehne KL. HIV prevention among injecting drug users in developing and transitional countries. Pub Health Rep 1998; 113(Supp 1) 170–81.

39. Des Jarlais DC, Friedman SR, Novick DM, et al. HIV-1 infection among intravenous drug users in Manhattan, New York City, from 1977 through 1987. JAMA. 1989;261(7):1008–12.

40. Wolfe D, Malinowska-Sempruch K. Illicit drug policies and the global HIV epidemic: Effects of UN and national government approaches. New York: Open Society Institute; 2004.

41. Needle RH, Kroeger K, Belani H, Hegle J. Substance abuse and HIV in sub-Saharan Africa: introduction to the special issue. Afr J Drug Alcohol Stud. 2006;5(2):83–91.

42. Beckerleg S, Telfer M, Hundt GL. The rise of injecting drug use in East Africa: a case study from Kenya. Harm Reduct J. 2005;2:12.

43. Parry CD, Pithey AL. Risk behaviour and HIV among drug using populations in South Africa. Afr J Drug Alcohol Stud. 2006;5(2):140–57.

44. Centers for Disease Control and Prevention. HIV-associated behaviors among injecting-drug users—23 cities, United States, May 2005–February 2006. MMWR Recomm Rep. 2009;58(13):329–32.

45. Strathdee SA, Sherman SG. The role of sexual transmission of HIV infection among injection and non-injection drug users. J Urban Health. 2003;80(4 Suppl 3):iii7–14.

46. Des Jarlais DC, Arasteh K, Semaan S, Wood E. HIV among injecting drug users: current epidemiology, biologic markers, respondent-driven sampling, and supervised-injection facilities. Curr Opin HIV AIDS. 2009;4(4):308–13.

47. Centers for Disease Control and Prevention. Diagnoses of HIV infection and AIDS in the United States and dependent areas, 2008. Atlanta, GA: Department of Health and Human Services; 2011.

48. Thorpe LE, Outlett LJ, Hershow R, et al. Risk of hepatitis C virus infection among young adult injection drug users who share injection equipment. Am J Epidemiol. 2002;15:645–53.

49. Shepard CW, Finelli L, Alter MJ. Global epidemiology of hepatitis C virus infection. Lancet Infect Dis. 2005;5(9):558–67.

50. Simonsen L, Kane A, Zaffran M, Kane M. Unsafe injections in the developing world and transmission of blood-borne pathogens: a review. Bull World Health Organ. 1999;77(10):789–801.

51. Crofts N, Nigro L, Oman K, Stevenson E, Sherman J. Methadone maintenance and hepatitis C virus infection among injecting drug users. Addiction. 1997;92(8):999–1005.

52. Centers for Disease Control and Prevention. Sexually transmitted disease treatment guidelines, 2010. MMWR Recomm Rep. 2010;59(12):1–10.

53. van de Laar TJ, van der Bij AK, Prins M, et al. Increase in HCV incidence among men who have sex with men in Amsterdam most likely caused by sexual transmission. J Infect Dis. 2007;196(2):230–8.

54. Hellard M, Sacks-Davis R, Gold J. Hepatitis C treatment for injection drug users: a review of the available evidence. Clin Infect Dis. 2009;49(4):561–73.

55. International Harm Reduction Association. The Global State of Harm Reduction 2010: Key issues for broadening the response. London: International Harm Reduction Association; 2010.

56. Aceijas C, Rhodes T. Global estimates of prevalence of HCV infection among injecting drug users. Int J Drug Policy. 2007;18(5):352–8.

57. Aceijas C, Stimson GV, Hickman M, Rhodes T. Global overview of injecting drug use and HIV infection among injecting drug users. AIDS. 2004;18(17):2295–303.

58. Murrill CS, Weeks H, Castrucci BC, et al. Age-specific seroprevalence of HIV, hepatitis B virus, and hepatitis C virus infection among injection drug users admitted to drug treatment in 6 US cities. Am J Public Health. 2002;92(3):385–7.

59. Craine N, Walker AM, Williamson S, Brown A, Hope VD. Hepatitis B and hepatitis C seroprevalence and risk behaviour among community-recruited drug injectors in North West Wales. Commun Dis Public Health. 2004;7(3):216–9.

60. Shapatava E, Nelson KE, Tsertsvadze T, del Rio C. Risk behaviors and HIV, hepatitis B, and hepatitis C seroprevalence among injection drug users in Georgia. Drug Alcohol Depend. 2006;82 Suppl 1:S35–8.

61. Gerlich M, Gschwend P, Uchtenhagen A, Kramer A, Rehm J. Prevalence of hepatitis and HIV infections and vaccination rates in patients entering the heroin-assisted treatment in Switzerland between 1994 and 2002. Eur J Epidemiol. 2006;21(7):545–9.

62. Centers for Disease Control and Prevention. Coinfection with HIV and Hepatitis C Virus. Centers for Disease Control and Prevention 2005;Available at URL: http://www.cdc.gov/hiv/resources/Factsheets/coinfection.htm.

63. Semaan S, Des J, Malow R. STDs among Illicit Drug Users in the United States: The need for interventions. In: Aral SO, Douglas JM, editors. Behavioral Interventions for Prevention and Control of Sexually Transmitted Diseases. New York: Springer Science Business Media, LLC; 2007. p. 397–430.

64. Centers for Disease Control and Prevention. Sexually Transmitted Disease Surveillance 2009. Atlanta, GA: Department of Health and Human Services; 2010.

65. Coffin LS, Newberry A, Hagan H, Cleland CM, Des J, Perlman DC. Syphilis in drug users in low and middle income countries. Int J Drug Policy. 2010;21:20–7.

66. Platt L, Rhodes T, Judd A, et al. Effects of sex work on the prevalence of syphilis among injection drug users in 3 Russian cities. Am J Public Health. 2007;97(3):478–85.

67. Altaf A, Shah SA, Zaidi NA, Memon A, Nadeem uR, Wray N. High risk behaviors of injection drug users registered with harm reduction programme in Karachi, Pakistan. Harm Reduct J. 2007;4:7.

68. Rhodes T, Platt L, Maximova S, et al. Prevalence of HIV, hepatitis C and syphilis among injecting drug users in Russia: a multi-city study. Addiction. 2006;101(2):252–66.

69. Carey MP, Ravi V, Chandra PS, Desai A, Neal DJ. Screening for sexually transmitted infections at a DeAddictions service in south India. Drug Alcohol Depend. 2006;82(2):127–34.

70. Rawson RA, Washton A, Domier CP, Reiber C. Drugs and sexual effects: role of drug type and gender. J Subst Abuse Treat. 2002;22(2):103–8.

71. Ross L, Kohler CL, Grimley DM, Bellis J. Intention to use condoms among three low-income, urban African American subgroups: cocaine users, noncocaine drug users, and non-drug users. J Urban Health. 2003;80(1):147–60.

72. Booth RE, Watters JK, Chitwood DD. HIV risk-related sex behaviors among injection drug users, crack smokers, and injection drug users who smoke crack. Am J Public Health. 1993;83(8):1144–8.

73. Reback CJ, Larkins S, Shoptaw S. Changes in the meaning of sexual risk behaviors among gay and bisexual male methamphetamine abusers before and

after drug treatment. AIDS Behav. 2004;8(1): 87–98.

74. Shoptaw S, Reback CJ. Methamphetamine use and infectious disease-related behaviors in men who have sex with men: implications for interventions. Addiction. 2007;102 Suppl 1:130–5.

75. Semple SJ, Zians J, Grant I, Patterson TL. Impulsivity and methamphetamine use. J Subst Abuse Treat. 2005;29(2):85–93.

76. Donoghoe MC. Sex, HIV and the injecting drug users. Br J Addict. 1992;87(3):405–16.

77. Edlin BR, Irwin KL, Faruque S, et al. Intersecting epidemics–crack cocaine use and HIV infection among inner-city young adults. Multicenter Crack Cocaine and HIV Infection Study Team. N Engl J Med. 1994;331(21):1422–7.

78. Tross S, Abdul-Quader A, Silvert H, Des J. Condom use among male injecting-drug users—New York City, 1987–1990. MMWR Recomm Rep. 1992; 41(34):617–20.

79. Greenberg J, Schnell D, Conlon R. Behaviors of crack cocaine users and their impact on early syphilis intervention. Sex Transm Dis. 1992;19(6): 346–50.

80. UNODC. World Drug Report. New York: United Nations; 2005.

81. Aral SO. Determinants of STD epidemics: implications for phase appropriate intervention strategies. Sex Transm Infect. 2002;78 Suppl 1:i3–13.

82. Cochran SD, Ackerman D, Mays VM, Ross MW. Prevalence of non-medical drug use and dependence among homosexually active men and women in the US population. Addiction. 2004;99(8):989–98.

83. Celentano DD, Valleroy LA, Sifakis F, et al. Associations between substance use and sexual risk among very young men who have sex with men. Sex Transm Dis. 2006;33(4):265–71.

84. Bolding G, Hart G, Sherr L, Elford J. Use of crystal methamphetamine among gay men in London. Addiction. 2006;101(11):1622–30.

85. Colfax GN, Mansergh G, Guzman R, et al. Drug use and sexual risk behavior among gay and bisexual men who attend circuit parties: a venue-based comparison. J Acquir Immune Defic Syndr. 2001;28(4):373–9.

86. Colfax G, Santos GM, Chu P, et al. Amphetamine-group substances and HIV. Lancet. 2010;376(9739):458–74.

87. Semple SJ, Zians J, Strathdee SA, Patterson TL. Sexual marathons and methamphetamine use among HIV-positive men who have sex with men. Arch Sex Behav. 2009;38(4):583–90.

88. Wong W, Chaw JK, Kent CK, Klausner JD. Risk factors for early syphilis among gay and bisexual men seen in an STD clinic: San Francisco, 2002–2003. Sex Transm Dis. 2005;32(7):458–63.

89. Weber MP, Schoenbaum EE. Heterosexual transmission of HIV infection in intravenous and non-intravenous drug-using populations. Arch AIDS Res. 1991;5:45–7.

90. Stockman JK, Strathdee SA. HIV among people who use drugs: a global perspective of populations at risk. J Acquir Immune Defic Syndr. 2010;55 Suppl 1:S17–22.

91. Gollub EL. A neglected population: drug-using women and women's methods of HIV/STI prevention. AIDS Educ Prev. 2008;20(2):107–20.

92. Marx R, Aral SO, Rolfs RT, Sterk CE, Kahn JG. Crack, sex, and STD. Sex Transm Dis. 1991;18(2):92–101.

93. CDC. Relationship of syphilis to drug use and prostitution—Connecticut and Philadelphia, Pennsylvania. Morb Mortal Wkly Rep. 1988;37(49):755–8.

94. Williams PB, Ekundayo O. Study of distribution and factors affecting syphilis epidemic among inner-city minorities of Baltimore. Public Health. 2001;115(6):387–93.

95. Ross MW, Hwang LY, Zack C, Bull L, Williams ML. Sexual risk behaviours and STIs in drug abuse treatment populations whose drug of choice is crack cocaine. Int J STD AIDS. 2002;13(11):769–74.

96. Baseman J, Ross M, Williams M. Sale of sex for drugs and drugs for sex: an economic context of sexual risk behavior for STDs. Sex Transm Dis. 1999;26(8):444–9.

97. Rhodes T, Singer M, Bourgois P, Friedman SR, Strathdee SA. The social structural production of HIV risk among injecting drug users. Soc Sci Med. 2005;61(5):1026–44.

98. Rhodes T, Simic M. Transition and the HIV risk environment. BMJ. 2005;331(7510):220–3.

99. Gupta GR, Parkhurst JO, Ogden JA, Aggleton P, Mahal A. Structural approaches to HIV prevention. Lancet. 2008;372(9640):764–75.

100. National Council Against Addictions, National Institute on Psychiatry Ramon de la Fuente, National Institute on Public Health. 2008 National Household Survey on Addictions, Mexico. 2009.

101. Todd CS, Safi N, Strathdee SA. Drug use and harm reduction in Afghanistan. Harm Reduct J. 2005;2:13.

102. Fallahzadeh H, Morowatisharifabad M, Ehrampoosh MH. HIV/AIDS epidemic features and trends in Iran, 1986–2006. AIDS Behav. 2009;13(2): 297–302.

103. Needle R, Kroeger K, Belani H, Achrekar A, Parry CD, Dewing S. Sex, drugs, and HIV: rapid assessment of HIV risk behaviors among street-based drug using sex workers in Durban, South Africa. Soc Sci Med. 2008;67(9):1447–55.

104. Parry CD, Carney T, Petersen P, Dewing S, Needle R. HIV-risk behavior among injecting or non-injecting drug users in Cape Town, Pretoria, and Durban, South Africa. Subst Use Misuse. 2009;44(6):886–904.

105. Reid SR. Injection drug use, unsafe medical injections, and HIV in Africa: a systematic review. Harm Reduct J. 2009;6:24.

106. Gable L, Gamhartner K, Gostin LO, Hodge JG, van Puymbroeck RV. Legal aspects of HIV/AIDS: a

guide for policy and law reform. Washington, DC: The World Bank; 2007.

107. Wolfe D, Cohen J. Human rights and HIV prevention, treatment, and care for people who inject drugs: key principles and research needs. J Acquir Immune Defic Syndr. 2010;55 Suppl 1:S56–62.

108. Strathdee SA, Hallett TB, Bobrova N, et al. HIV and risk environment for injecting drug users: the past, present, and future. Lancet. 2010;376(9737): 268–84.

109. Clark PA, Fadus M. Federal funding for needle exchange programs. Med Sci Monit. 2010;16(1): H1–13.

110. Kamarulzaman A. Impact of HIV prevention programs on drug users in Malaysia. J Acquir Immune Defic Syndr. 2009;52 Suppl 1:S17–9.

111. Fields G. While house czar calls for end to 'war on drugs'. Wall Street Journal 2009 May 14.

112. Macalino GE, Vlahov D, Sanford-Colby S, et al. Prevalence and incidence of HIV, hepatitis B virus, and hepatitis C virus infections among males in Rhode Island prisons. Am J Public Health. 2004;94(7):1218–23.

113. Jurgens R, World Health Organization, UNODC, UNIADS. Interventions to address HIV in prisons: HIV care, treatment and support. Geneva: World Health Organization; 2007.

114. Okie S. Sex, drugs, prisons, and HIV. N Engl J Med. 2007;356(2):105–8.

115. Johnson RC, Raphael S. The effects of male incarceration dynamics on acquired immune deficiency syndrome infection rates among African American women and men. J Law Economics. 2009;52(May):251–93.

116. Sabol WJ, Couture H. Prison inmates at midyear 2007. Washington, DC: Department of Justice Bureau of Justice Statistics; 2008.

117. Mauer M. Racial disparities in the criminal justice system. Washington, DC: The Sentencing Project; 2009.

118. U.S. Sentencing Commission. Sourcebook of federal sentencing statistics, Tables 33-36 and Table 38. U S Sentencing Commission 2009;Available at: URL: http://www.ussc.gov/ANNRPT/2008/table33.pdf, http://www.ussc.gov/ANNRPT/2008/table34.pdf, http://www.ussc.gov/ANNRPT/2008/table35. pdf,http://www.ussc.gov/ANNRPT/2008/table36.pdf, http://www.ussc.gov/ANNRPT/2008/table38.pdf.

119. Bureau of Justice Statistics. Drug use and dependence, state and federal prisoners, 2004. Washington, DC: U.S. Department of Justice; 2006. Report No.: NCJ 213530.

120. Werb D, Kerr T, Small W, Li K, Montaner J, Wood E. HIV risks associated with incarceration among injection drug users: implications for prison-based public health strategies. J Public Health (Oxf). 2008;30(2):126–32.

121. Milloy MJ, Buxton J, Wood E, Li K, Montaner JS, Kerr T. Elevated HIV risk behaviour among recently incarcerated injection drug users in a Canadian setting: a longitudinal analysis. BMC Public Health. 2009;9:156.

122. Clarke JG, Stein MD, Hanna L, Sobota M, Rich JD. Active and Former Injection Drug Users Report of HIV Risk Behaviors During Periods of Incarceration. Subst Abus. 2001;22(4):209–16.

123. UNAIDS Reference Group on HIV and Human Rights. Statement on Human Rights and Universal Access to HIV, Prevention, Treatment, Care & Support. 2008.

124. Wechsberg WM, Luseno W, Ellerson RM. Reaching women substance abusers in diverse settings: stigma and access to treatment 30 years later. Subst Use Misuse. 2008;43(8–9):1277–9.

125. UNODC. HIV/AIDS prevention and care for female injecting drug users. Austria: UNODC; 2006.

126. Cleland CM, Des J, Perlis TE, Stimson G, Poznyak V. HIV risk behaviors among female IDUs in developing and transitional countries. BMC Public Health. 2007;7:271.

127. Bryant J, Brener L, Hull P, Treloar C. Needle sharing in regular sexual relationships: an examination of serodiscordance, drug using practices, and the gendered character of injecting. Drug Alcohol Depend. 2010;107(2–3):182–7.

128. el-Bassel N, Gilbert L, Wu E, Go H, Hill J. HIV and intimate partner violence among methadone-maintained women in New York City. Soc Sci Med. 2005;61(1):171–83.

129. el-Bassel N, Terlikbaeva A, Pinkham S. HIV and women who use drugs: double neglect, double risk. Lancet. 2010;376(9738):312–4.

130. el-Bassel N, Gilbert L, Wu E, Go H, Hill J. Relationship between drug abuse and intimate partner violence: a longitudinal study among women receiving methadone. Am J Public Health. 2005;95(3):465–70.

131. Kumar MS, Virk HK, Chaudhuri A, Mittal A, Lewis G. A rapid situation and response assessment of the female regular sex partners of male drug users in South Asia: factors associated with condom use during the last sexual intercourse. Int J Drug Policy. 2008;19(2):148–58.

132. Pinkham S, Malinowska-Sempruch K. Women, harm reduction and HIV. Reprod Health Matters. 2008;16(31):168–81.

133. Carael M, Marais H, Polsky J, Mendoza A. Is there a gender gap in the HIV response? Evaluating national HIV responses from the United Nations General Assembly Special Session on HIV/AIDS country reports. J Acquir Immune Defic Syndr. 2009;52 Suppl 2:S111–8.

134. Dolan K, Salimi S, Nassirimanesh B, Mohsenifar S, Mokri A. The establishment of a methadone treatment clinic for women in Tehran, Iran. J Public Health Policy. 2011;32:219–30.

135. Ball AL. HIV, injecting drug use and harm reduction: a public health response. Addiction. 2007;102(5):684–90.

136. Des Jarlais DC, Semaan S. HIV prevention for injecting drug users: the first 25 years and counting. Psychosom Med. 2008;70(5):606–11.

137. Hartel DM, Schoenbaum EE. Methadone treatment protects against HIV infection: two decades of experience in the Bronx, New York City. Public Health Rep. 1998;113 Suppl 1:107–15.

138. Coyle SL, Needle RH, Normand J. Outreach-based HIV prevention for injecting drug users: a review of published outcome data. Public Health Rep. 1998;113 Suppl 1:19–30.

139. Preventing HIV transmission: The role of sterile needles and bleach. Washington, DC: National Academy Press; 1995

140. Institute of Medicine. Preventing HIV transmission: The role of sterile needles. Institute of Medicine: National Academy Press; 1994.

141. Dole VP, Nyswander M. A medical treatment for diacetylmorphine (Heroin) addiction. A clinical trial with methadone hydrochloride. JAMA. 1965;193: 646–50.

142. Institute of Medicine. Preventing HIV Infection among Injecting Drug Users in High-Risk Countries. Washington, DC: The National Academies Press; 2007.

143. Metzger DS, Navaline H, Woody GE. Drug abuse treatment as AIDS prevention. Public Health Rep. 1998;113 Suppl 1:97–106.

144. Walsh N, Higgs P, Crofts N. Recognition of hepatitis C virus coinfection in HIV-positive injecting drug users in Asia. J Acquir Immune Defic Syndr. 2007;45(3):363–5.

145. Hagan H, Jarlais DC, Friedman SR, Purchase D, Alter MJ. Reduced risk of hepatitis B and hepatitis C among injection drug users in the Tacoma syringe exchange program. Am J Public Health. 1995; 85(11):1531–7.

146. Thiede H, Hagan H, Murrill CS. Methadone treatment and HIV and hepatitis B and C risk reduction among injectors in the Seattle area. J Urban Health. 2000;77(3):331–45.

147. Substance Abuse and Mental Health Services Administration OoAS. The NSDUH report: Methamphetamine use, abuse, and dependence: 2002, 2003, and 2004. Washington, DC: Substance Abuse and Mental Health Services Administration; 2005.

148. Magura S, Kang SY, Nwakeze PC, Demsky S. Temporal patterns of heroin and cocaine use among methadone patients. Subst Use Misuse. 1998;33(12): 2441–67.

149. Thula MA. Cocaine use and dependence in clients attending a drug treatment centre in Dublin. The Psychiatrist. 2009;33:88–91.

150. Dutra L, Stathopoulou G, Basden SL, Leyro TM, Powers MB, Otto MW. A meta-analytic review of psychosocial interventions for substance use disorders. Am J Psychiatry. 2008;165(2):179–87.

151. Lee NK, Rawson RA. A systematic review of cognitive and behavioural therapies for methamphetamine dependence. Drug Alcohol Rev. 2008;27(3): 309–17.

152. Oliveto A, Poling J, Mancino MJ, et al. Randomized, double blind, placebo-controlled trial of disulfiram for the treatment of cocaine dependence in methadone-stabilized patients. Drug Alcohol Depend. 2011;113(2–3):184–91.

153. Kuehn BM. Scientists target cocaine addiction. JAMA. 2009;302(24):2641–2.

154. Nelles J, Fuhrer A, Hirsbrunner H, Harding T. Provision of syringes: the cutting edge of harm reduction in prison? BMJ. 1998;317(7153):270–3.

155. Stark K, Herrmann U, Ehrhardt S, Bienzle U. A syringe exchange programme in prison as prevention strategy against HIV infection and hepatitis B and C in Berlin, Germany. Epidemiol Infect. 2006;134(4):814–9.

156. Menoyo C, Zulaica D, Parras F. Needle exchange programs in prisons in Spain. Can HIV AIDS Policy Law Rev. 2000;5(4):20–1.

157. Stover H. Evaluation of needle exchange pilot projects shows positive results. Can HIV AIDS Policy Law Newsl. 2000;5(2–3):60–9.

158. Nelles J, Fuhrer A, Vincenz I. Evaluation der HIV- und Hepatitis-Prophylaxe in der Kantonalen Anstalt Realta. Berne: Universitare Psychiatrische Dienste Bern; 1999.

159. Pintilei L. Harm reduction in prisons of Republic of Moldova. Ukraine: Kiev; 2005.

160. Dolan KA, Wodak AD, Hall WD. Methadone maintenance treatment reduces heroin injection in New South Wales prisons. Drug Alcohol Rev. 1998;17(2):153–8.

161. Dolan KA, Shearer J, MacDonald M, Mattick RP, Hall W, Wodak AD. A randomised controlled trial of methadone maintenance treatment versus wait list control in an Australian prison system. Drug Alcohol Depend. 2003;72(1):59–65.

162. Boguna J. Methadone maintenance programmes. In: O'Brien O, editor. *Report of the 3rd European Conference on Drug and HIV/AIDS Services in Prison*. London: Cranstoun Drug Services; 1997. p. 68–70.

163. Heimer R, Catania H, Newman RG, Zambrano J, Brunet A, Ortiz AM. Methadone maintenance in prison: evaluation of a pilot program in Puerto Rico. Drug Alcohol Depend. 2006;83(2):122–9.

164. Larney S. Does opioid substitution treatment in prisons reduce injecting-related HIV risk behaviours? A systematic review. Addiction. 2010;105(2): 216–23.

165. Hagan H, Des J, Stern R, et al. HCV synthesis project: preliminary analyses of HCV prevalence in relation to age and duration of injection. Int J Drug Policy. 2007;18(5):341–51.

166. Vickerman P, Hickman M, May M, Kretzschmar M, Wiessing L. Can hepatitis C virus prevalence be used as a measure of injection-related human immunodeficiency virus risk in populations of injecting drug users? An ecological analysis. Addiction. 2010;105(2):311–8.

167. Edlin BR, Kresina TF, Raymond DB, et al. Overcoming barriers to prevention, care, and treatment of hepatitis C in illicit drug users. Clin Infect Dis. 2005;40 Suppl 5:S276–85.

168. Mateu-Gelabert P, Treloar C, Calatayud VA, et al. How can hepatitis C be prevented in the long term? Int J Drug Policy. 2007;18(5):338–40.

169. Edlin BR. Prevention and treatment of hepatitis C in injection drug users. Hepatology. 2002;36 (5 Suppl 1):S210–9.

170. Rottingen JA, Cameron DW, Garnett GP. A systematic review of the epidemiologic interactions between classic sexually transmitted diseases and HIV: how much really is known? Sex Transm Dis. 2001;28(10):579–97.

171. Cohen MS. HIV and sexually transmitted diseases: lethal synergy. Top HIV Med. 2004;12(4):104–7.

172. Institute of Medicine. The Hidden Epidemic: Confronting Sexually Transmitted Diseases. Washington, DC: National Academy Press; 1997.

173. Hayes R, Watson-Jones D, Celum C, van de Wasserheit J. Treatment of sexually transmitted infections for HIV prevention: end of the road or new beginning? AIDS. 2010;24 Suppl 4:S15–26.

174. Miller M, Liao Y, Wagner M, Korves C. HIV, the clustering of sexually transmitted infections, and sex risk among African American women who use drugs. Sex Transm Dis. 2008;35(7):696–702.

175. Jin F, Prestage GP, Matthews G, et al. Prevalence, incidence and risk factors for hepatitis C in homosexual men: data from two cohorts of HIV-negative and HIV-positive men in Sydney, Australia. Sex Transm Infect. 2010;86(1):25–8.

176. Tyndall MW, Patrick D, Spittal P, Li K, O'Shaughnessy MV, Schechter MT. Risky sexual behaviours among injection drugs users with high HIV prevalence: implications for STD control. Sex Transm Infect. 2002;78 Suppl 1:i170–5.

177. Wasserheit JN, Aral SO. The dynamic topology of sexually transmitted disease epidemics: implications for prevention strategies. J Infect Dis. 1996;174 Suppl 2:S201–13.

178. Grosskurth H, Mosha F, Todd J, et al. Impact of improved treatment of sexually transmitted diseases on HIV infection in rural Tanzania: randomised controlled trial. Lancet. 1995;346(8974):530–6.

179. Aral SO, Holmes KK. Social and behavioral determinants of the epidemiology of STDs: Industrialized and developing countries. In: Holmes KK, Sparling PF, Mardh P, Lemon SM, Stamm WE, Piot P, et al., editors. Sexually transmitted diseases. 3rd ed. New York: McGraw-Hill; 1999. p. 39–76.

180. Semaan S, Des J, Sogolow E, et al. A meta-analysis of the effect of HIV prevention interventions on the sex behaviors of drug users in the United States. J Acquir Immune Defic Syndr. 2002;30 Suppl 1:S73–93.

181. Blankenship KM, Friedman SR, Dworkin S, Mantell JE. Structural interventions: concepts, challenges and opportunities for research. J Urban Health. 2006;83(1):59–72.

182. Lally MA, Alvarez S, Macnevin R, et al. Acceptability of sexually transmitted infection screening among women in short-term substance abuse treatment. Sex Transm Dis. 2002;29(12):752–5.

183. Mimiaga MJ, Safren SA, Dvoryak S, Reisner SL, Needle R, Woody G. "We fear the police, and the police fear us": structural and individual barriers and facilitators to HIV medication adherence among injection drug users in Kiev, Ukraine. AIDS Care. 2010;22(11):1305–13.

184. Blankenship KM, Koester S. Criminal law, policing policy, and HIV risk in female street sex workers and injection drug users. J Law Med Ethics. 2002; 30(4):548–59.

185. Wright-De AL, Weinstein B, Jones TS, Miles J. Impact of the change in Connecticut syringe prescription laws on pharmacy sales and pharmacy managers' practices. J Acquir Immune Defic Syndr Hum Retrovirol. 1998;18 Suppl 1:S102–10.

186. Open Society Institute. Harm Reduction: Public Health and Public Order. International Harm Reduction Development Program; 2007 Oct.

187. The Reference Group to the UN of HIV and Injection Drug Use. Consensus Statement of the Reference Group to the United Nations on HIV and Injecting Drug Use. 2010.

188. Des Jaralis DC, Semaan S. HIV and other sexually transmitted infections in injection drug users and crack cocaine smokers. In: Holmes KK, Sparling PF, Stamm WE, Piot P, Wasserheit JN, Corey L, et al., editors. Sexually transmitted diseases. 4th ed. New York: McGraw-Hill; 2008. p. 237–55.

189. Gebo KA, Keruly J, Moore RD. Association of social stress, illicit drug use, and health beliefs with nonadherence to antiretroviral therapy. J Gen Intern Med. 2003;18(2):104–11.

190. Chander G, Himelhoch S, Moore RD. Substance abuse and psychiatric disorders in HIV-positive patients: epidemiology and impact on antiretroviral therapy. Drugs. 2006;66(6):769–89.

191. Gunn RA, Murray PJ, Ackers ML, Hardison WG, Margolis HS. Screening for chronic hepatitis B and C virus infections in an urban sexually transmitted disease clinic: rationale for integrating services. Sex Transm Dis. 2001 March;28(3):166–70.

192. Latkin CA, Knowlton RA. Micro-social structural approaches to HIV prevention: A social ecological perspective. AIDS Care. 2005;17 Suppl 1:S102–13.

193. Cottrell CA, Neuberg SL. Different emotional reactions to different groups: A sociofunctional threat-based approach to "prejudice". J Pers Soc Psychol. 2005;88(5):770–89.

194. Sylla L, Bruce RD, Kamarulzaman A, Altice FL. Integration and co-location of HIV/AIDS, tuberculosis and drug treatment services. Int J Drug Policy. 2007;18(4):306–12.

195. Sylvestre DL, Zweben JE. Integrating HCV services for drug users: a model to improve engagement and outcomes. Int J Drug Policy. 2007;18(5):406–10.

196. Birkhead GS, Klein SJ, Candelas AR, et al. Integrating multiple programme and policy approaches to hepatitis C prevention and care for injection drug users: a comprehensive approach. Int J Drug Policy. 2007;18(5):417–25.

197. Hennessy RR, Weisfuse IB, Schlanger K. Does integrating viral hepatitis services into a public STD clinic attract injection drug users for care? Public Health Rep. 2007;122 Suppl 2:31–5.
198. Keeny E, Saucier R. Lowering the threshold: Models of accessible methadone and buprenorphine treatment. New York: Open Society Institute; 2010.
199. Zhao M, Du J, Lu GH, et al. HIV sexual risk behaviors among injection drug users in Shanghai. Drug Alcohol Depend. 2006;82 Suppl 1:S43–7.
200. U.S. Office of National Drug Control Policy. National Drug Control Strategy. 2010.
201. U.S. Office of National AIDS Policy. Nation HIV/AIDS Strategy for the United States. 2010.
202. PEPFAR. Comprehensive HIV prevention for people who inject drugs, revised guidance. 2010.
203. Sharma M, Oppenheimer E, Saidel T, Loo V, Garg R. A situation update on HIV epidemics among people who inject drugs and national responses in South-East Asia Region. AIDS. 2009;23(11):1405–13.
204. World Health Organization, UNODC, UNAIDS. WHO, UNODC, UNAIDS technical guide for countries to set targets for universal access to HIV prevention, treatment and care for injecting drug users. Geneva: WHO/UNAIDS/UNODC; 2009.

Health, Sexual Health, and Syndemics: Toward a Better Approach to STI and HIV Preventive Interventions for Men Who Have Sex with Men (MSM) in the United States

13

Thomas E. Guadamuz, Mark S. Friedman,
Michael P. Marshal, Amy L. Herrick, Sin How Lim,
Chongyi Wei, and Ron Stall

STI and HIV Prevention Among Gay Men: The Need for a Broader Vision to Support Prevention Action

HIV was first discovered in the United States 30 years ago. Since then, one characteristic of the epidemic has remained constant: gay men, or men who have sex with men (MSM), have been among the most severely impacted of any social group in the nation. While MSM account for less than 5% of all men in most behavioral surveys, they currently account for nearly 60% of all new HIV infections in the United States [1]. A recent CDC analysis calculated that MSM are 60 and 61 times more likely to be infected with HIV and syphilis, respectively, than heterosexual men and are 54 and 93 times more likely to be infected with HIV and syphilis, respectively, than women [2].

Health disparities involving other sexually transmitted infections (STI), such as Hepatitis, have also been documented for MSM [3]. Together, these ongoing sexually transmitted epidemics constitute an important health problem among Americans. Thus, we need to continue to explore ways to better manage HIV and other STI epidemics among MSM.

Lay and professional discussion about gay men's health and lifestyle seem to inevitably lead to discussions of HIV and STI, even though other important health disparities involving other dangerous health conditions also exist among MSM [4]. This is due in part to the substantial health disparities involving STI epidemics between gay and heterosexual men. It should also be noted that public health discussions of gay men's health and health promotion programs targeted at gay men focus, almost exclusively, on HIV [5]. What researchers and public health practitioners often do not fully appreciate is that other health disparities faced by gay men, whether they are infectious or noninfectious disease epidemics, may play an important role in HIV prevention efforts. Previous studies have shown that other non-HIV/STI health outcomes among gay men (e.g., depression, substance use, suicidal ideation) are significantly correlated with high-risk behaviors for HIV/STI

T.E. Guadamuz • M.S. Friedman • A.L. Herrick
C. Wei • R. Stall (✉)
Department of Behavioral and Community Health
Sciences, University of Pittsburgh Graduate School
of Public Health, 208 Parran Hall, 130 DeSoto Street,
Pittsburgh, PA 15261, USA

M.P. Marshal
Department of Psychiatry, University of Pittsburgh
School of Medicine, Pittsburgh, PA, USA

S.H. Lim
Centre of Excellence for Research in AIDS (CERiA),
Faculty of Medicine, University of Malaya,
Kuala Lumpur, Malaysia

S.O. Aral, K.A. Fenton, and J.A. Lipshutz (eds.), *The New Public Health and STD/HIV Prevention:*
Personal, Public and Health Systems Approaches, DOI 10.1007/978-1-4614-4526-5_13,
© Springer Science+Business Media New York 2013

infection, thus pointing to the need to consider other outcomes of gay men's health in order to effectively prevent HIV infection [6]. In other words, by ignoring the complexity of forces that impact gay men's general health and well-being, we may actually be doing a disservice to HIV and STI prevention efforts among gay men.

Moreover, recent studies have shown that the causal pathway for HIV and STI risks is not limited to one dimensional, individual-level indicators (as often evaluated in risk-factor epidemiology), but instead involves complex interrelated domains [7, 8] that, for gay men, may include gay culture and norms, substance use, peer pressure, social and sexual networks, social support, access to care, and general sociocultural (e.g., race, ethnicity, educational attainment, socioeconomic position, and religion) and environmental contexts (e.g., poverty, violence, opportunities for social mobility, migration to gay ghettos, acculturation to the gay community, racial and ethnic discrimination, and homophobia). These multilevel factors are most likely to interact throughout the life course, from childhood to adolescence to adulthood and to older age [4]. Therefore, to really understand how to prevent HIV and STIs, one must consider other psychosocial health outcomes that are common among high-risk gay men (e.g., depression, violence and victimization, suicidal ideation, childhood sexual abuse, substance use, and sex work/ survival sex), how these outcomes interrelate with one another and with multilevel factors to produce HIV and STI transmission and acquisition risks.

Current HIV and STI prevention for gay men can be described as limited in terms of both theoretical scope and potency. Certainly, many existing interventions have been proven efficacious in controlled settings, but they are almost exclusively designed to operate at the level of the individual [9, 10]. Drawing on dominant cognitive behavioral theories, these prevention models emphasize, to varying degrees, changes in knowledge, self-efficacy, intentions, peer group norms, safe sex negotiation, and condom use skills in order to increase rates of safe sex practice among gay men. As such, these interventions are designed to primarily manipulate individual-level variables without consideration of variables that go beyond individual-level determinants of HIV/ STI risk. This approach has become the dominant behavioral intervention method to reduce HIV/ STI transmission among gay men [9, 10].

Although interventions that operate primarily at the level of the individual have strong evidence for efficacy [9, 10], HIV and STI incidence continue to persist among MSM in the United States. For this reason, it may be a good time to enhance our prevention approach to include strategies that might yield more effective results within MSM communities. This chapter will summarize the evidence for variables that operate beyond the level of the individual and suggest approaches that might draw on these domains to improve the efficacy and effectiveness of HIV/STI prevention practice among MSM in the United States.

STI and HIV/AIDS Epidemics Among MSM in the United States: A Grim Portrait

STI affect MSM disproportionately, compared to their heterosexual counterparts. Rates of gonorrhea, syphilis, and HPV-associated anal cancer have been two, three, and almost five times higher, respectively, among MSM than men who have sex with women (MSW) [3, 11–13]. Herpes simplex virus type 2, the virus responsible for genital herpes, is two times higher among MSM than MSW [14]. And while there is a significant decreasing national trend of general STI in the US population over the past decade, this is not the case for MSM [1]. The situation is even more serious for Black MSM. A recent meta-analysis found that Black MSM were two times more likely to be diagnosed with current STI than White MSM (95% confidence interval [CI]: 1.68–2.67) [15].

Similarly, the prevalence of HIV and AIDS among MSM is *disproportionately increasing*, as compared to MSW. In the United States, MSM still comprise the highest proportion of newly diagnosed HIV and AIDS cases than any other risk group [1]. In 2004–2005, the National HIV Behavioral Surveillance survey, conducted by the U.S. Centers for Disease Control and Prevention (CDC) among 1767 MSM in five U.S. cities, found an overall HIV prevalence of 25% (CI: 23–28%) [16]. Using confidential, name-based data obtained from 33 states from 2001–2004, the CDC reported the rate of HIV diagnosis for White, Hispanic, and Black MSM to be 14.6, 39.0, and 70.8 per 100,000, respectively. Given these rates, Black and Hispanic MSM are five times and three times higher than White MSM, respectively, to be diagnosed with HIV infection [17]. And among those diagnosed with AIDS, Black MSM were less likely than White MSM to survive 3 years from date of diagnosis. These data point to the urgency for quick and effective response to the HIV crisis among MSM, particularly Black and Hispanic MSM.

The HIV Incidence Surveillance Group at the CDC released 2006 incidence data which estimated that 45% of new infections are among Black individuals and that 53% of new infections are among MSM [18]. A comprehensive community-based study conducted by the CDC in 7 U.S. cities found HIV incidence to be 2.5% among whites (CI=1.4–4.6%), 3.5% among Hispanics (CI=1.4–8.6%), and 14.7% among blacks (CI=7.9–27.1%) [19].

Remarkably, these estimates are not dissimilar to those of historical past. In 1984, before any formal AIDS prevention programs, the San Francisco Men's Health Study found a prevalence of 48.5% among gay men aged 25–54 in that city [20]. And that was before the availability of antiretroviral medications, mass condom promotion campaigns, and availability of community-based voluntary counseling and testing.

Therefore, it is time to recognize that current HIV and STI prevention programs have not significantly succeeded in decreasing HIV and STI incidence rates that have been sustaining for more than a decade among MSM, especially among Black and Hispanic MSM. We believe that the reasons for the intractable nature of the HIV/STI epidemics among MSM are multifactorial and therefore require that the prevention response include interventions that operate beyond the level of the individual.

Why Are STI and HIV Prevalence Among MSM So High?

As argued above, factors contributing to STI and HIV acquisition and transmission are complex and are not limited to individual-level indicators,

but instead involve a web of interrelated biologic, behavioral, social, and cultural factors at the individual (e.g., race, genetics, circumcision status, social class, education, substance use), community (e.g., social and sexual networks, violence and victimization, social and community support, community norms), and societal and structural levels (e.g., homophobia, racism, poverty, policy, and laws) [7, 8, 20]. Further, these factors may not be static and one dimensional, but instead contribute to an individual's risk distinctively, across and between levels, and at different magnitudes throughout an individual's life course. STI and HIV research among MSM that examines factors that operate beyond the level of the individual is still limited. With these limitations in mind, we will discuss the current evidence to explain high STI and HIV prevalence among MSM at the individual, community, and societal levels.

Individual-Level Variables

A plethora of individual-level risk factors for STI and HIV infection have been studied and documented since the beginning of the HIV epidemic 30 years ago. These variables can be organized into demography, biology, behaviors, and psychological factors.

Demography

Correlational studies have found HIV and STI prevalence among MSM to be significantly associated with Black race [16, 21–23], Hispanic ethnicity [21–24], lower education [24, 25], and older age [24–26]. In addition, Black race [19, 27] and younger age [13, 19, 27, 28] have been shown to be associated with HIV incidence. However, focusing on these demographic determinants alone is insufficient.

Biology

Biological factors have also been shown to be associated with HIV and STI infections. One notable example is the role of the CCR5 receptors that aid HIV to infect human cells. Persons who have a mutation by which these receptors are not expressed are resistant to HIV infection [29–33]. Circumcision may also protect MSM from HIV and STI infection; however, current findings do not support this hypothesis for MSM [34]. Finally, having an STI is a significant correlate of HIV infection in a number of population-based studies [35, 36].

Behaviors

It is not surprising that unprotected anal intercourse is the most cited correlate of STI and HIV infection [21, 22, 37–39]. Anal intercourse between men whereby the penis penetrates the anal canal has been shown as the most efficient way to transmit STI, as compared to penal-vaginal sex [40]. Furthermore, having more than one sexual partner has also been shown to increase STI and HIV risks [21, 23, 37]. Sexual intercourse between men, in reality, is more complicated and sometimes involves the use of alcohol and illicit substances like marijuana, poppers, cocaine, hallucinogens, amphetamines, and opiates [22, 24, 38, 41–45]. For instance, a major outbreak of syphilis among MSM was connected to the use of crystal methamphetamine in the US West coast [45, 46]. Being high on these substances may directly impact sexual behavior itself by prolonging sex (e.g., amphetamines), enhancing sex (e.g., hallucinogens), or simply coping with the pain of anal sex (e.g., poppers). However, an indirect effect of alcohol and substances is that they inhibit or impair usual decision-making and safer sex norms, which may result in unprotected, prolonged, or unwanted sex. Additionally, substance use by way of injection in itself is directly associated with HIV infection [21–24]. Conversely, a behavior that has a direct protective effect on STI and HIV transmission is HIV testing. Studies have shown that MSM who know their HIV positive status are less likely to engage in risky behaviors [46–51]. Thus, manipulating risky behaviors have been widely shown to reduce STI and HIV infections among MSM [9, 10].

Psychological Factors

There are several psychological factors that directly and indirectly affect HIV and STI transmission and acquisition risks and they may be developmental in nature. For example, early sexual debut and having had experiences of abuse (physical, mental, and sexual) in childhood have been shown as significant predictors of high-risk behaviors in adulthood [52–54]. Moreover, certain attitudes and personalities are also associated with increased risky behaviors. These include having reduced concern about HIV/AIDS in the era of highly active antiretroviral therapy (HAART), sexual sensation seeking, and sexual compulsivity [55–60].

Moreover, mental health-related variables including lower self-esteem, major depression, and suicidal ideation are significant correlates of high-risk behaviors for STI and HIV infection [61, 62]. Another psychological variable that transcends categories is internalized homophobia. This individual-level variable is highly correlated with non-White race, using alcohol and substances, having lower self-esteem, major depression, and suicidal thoughts [63–65].

Interpersonal, Social, and Sexual Network-Level Variables

Recently, interpersonal, social, and network-level variables have gained attention in the field. One important variable that operates at the interpersonal-level is disclosure of HIV status, also known as serodisclosure [24, 66, 67]. As a result, there have been a number of strategies that MSM have applied based on this principle. One strategy is negotiated safety whereby two men in a seroconcordant relationship "negotiate" or agree on a set of rules whereby unprotected anal intercourse can only occur in the primary relationship and that either no anal intercourse at all or anal intercourse with condoms can occur outside the primary relationship [68]. Another strategy is serosorting whereby MSM choose to have unsafe sex with partners of the same serostatus and use condoms with partners of a different or unknown status [69]. Another practice is seropositioning whereby MSM take on a sexual position depending upon the serostatus of the sexual partner (e.g., an HIV-negative man may take the insertive role with a HIV-positive or unknown status man since transmission risks are lessened for the insertive partner) [70]. These activities are not uncommon and are being practiced by some MSM today, particularly in large urban settings [71]. While some of the logic underlying these strategies may make sense, there is currently not enough empirical evidence to declare certain strategies as efficient or effective, mostly because of the complicated assumptions about true serostatus, HIV viremia, and community viral load (this term will be discussed in detail below) [72].

Failure to negotiate condoms under different conditions and contexts is an important correlate of STI and HIV infection. Sexual intercourse between MSM often occurs under circumstances that impair negotiation. As discussed earlier, behaviors such as alcohol and substance use can impair decision-making abilities and communication skills. Additionally, being in a high-risk sexual network may affect condom negotiation and ultimately, lead to STI and HIV infection. Sexual networks are clusters of sexual partner types within a certain geographical residential area, or certain social groups, or even based on private, virtual or public venues [73–75]. The latter may include public sex environments like public restrooms, rest stops, bathhouses, sex clubs, and circuit parties—all of which have been shown to be associated with increased risk of STI and HIV infection [76, 77].

Among racial and ethnic minority MSM, some studies have suggested that social and sexual networks, specifically sexual partner selection, HIV testing and disclosure are important factors related to HIV and STI acquisition [78–80]. For example, African-American MSM tend to have anal sex partners of a different age group (younger or older), of African American race, and of an unknown HIV status or unrecognized HIV infection, which may then contain or isolate HIV infections within that community [78, 79]. Among Latino MSM, culturally specific factors

such as machismo and acculturation are related to substance use and unprotected anal sex [80]. Currently, the mechanism by which racism transcends and mediates the relationship between social and cultural factors and HIV transmission and acquisition risks among African American and Latino MSM is not well understood.

Community/Community Viral Load

A concept related to interpersonal and sexual network is that of community viral load, which postulates that HIV transmission efficiency depends on the number of infected individuals with acute and longer term infections, infected individuals on antiretroviral therapy (ART) and uninfected individuals in a sexual network. Thus STI and HIV transmission dynamics may be enhanced or reduced if MSM in the community have access to and are adherent of ART, or if they practice seroadaptive behavioral strategies [66, 67]. Studies that take into account community viral load in modeling individual's STI and HIV risks are still scarce.

Other community-related variables are social support, gay community engagement, and peer norms [3, 79]. These variables at high levels have been shown to be protective of STI and HIV infection whereby individual-level risk behaviors discussed previously are reduced.

Policy and Structural-Level Variables

Structural-level variables, particularly social and economic policies, have been shown to affect the health and well being of the individual [81–83]. Some examples are legislation restricting the access and supply of tobacco and alcohol and the subsequent decrease in tobacco and alcohol use, as well as tobacco and alcohol-related morbidities [84, 85].

How gay-related social policies affect STI and HIV risks, however, are less studied. Indirectly, there is some empirical evidence. A recent study found that individuals living in states that do not extend protection laws (hate crimes and employment discrimination laws, in particular) to sexual minorities had significantly higher psychiatric disorders in the past 12 months [86], a known correlate of STI and HIV risk [87]. Another study, using data from the Massachusetts Youth Risk Behavior Survey, found that lesbian, gay or bisexual (LGB) adolescents in schools with LGB support groups were less likely to be threatened or injured with a weapon by another student or to attempt suicide compared with LGB adolescents in schools without these groups [88]. In the same study, LGB adolescents who attended schools with anti-bullying programs were also less likely to attempt suicide [88]. Hence, measuring the effects of similar structural-level programs on MSM health may have important implications for gay-friendly public policies.

Another important societal-level variable that explains health disparities among MSM is homophobia. While homophobia is socially constructed and culturally reproduced, it may also be internalized within an individual or institutionalized at the structural level. Experiences of homophobia, whether from family members, peers, or classmates at schools, can be complicated and involve many levels. These experiences often occur within lager social and cultural realms of a community (e.g., racial, ethnic, cultural, religious, and socioeconomic). Further, these processes may also be sustained, reinforced, or driven by specific social policies and laws (e.g., Don't Ask Don't Tell, Defense of Marriage Act). Similarly, social processes by which homophobia is developed can change overtime, from early adolescence to adulthood and beyond [4].

Young MSM who are more visible because they do not conform to traditional gender roles or who are "out" (disclose their sexual orientation identity to others) are often picked on, bullied, or victimized by their peers, authorities, and even family members [4]. These early gay-related events have been shown to predict risky sexual and substance using behaviors in adulthood [3, 6, 20, 53]. Moreover, young MSM are more likely than young heterosexual men to drop out of high school and to attempt suicide [89]. For those that dropped out, they are limited in the jobs they can

find and subsequently may not have access to adequate health insurance and preventative health. Additionally, some men who drop out of school or who are "kicked out" of their homes (often by their families) may migrate to urban gay centers where they may be exposed to different social norms that involve risk-taking activities like substance and alcohol use, survival sex and/or unsafe sexual practices with multiple partners in a high STI and HIV prevalent setting [90]. Similarly, for MSM who are "out" at work, they may find themselves hitting the glass ceiling, find that their opportunities are limited or are not placed in leadership and high-profile positions because of their sexual orientation.

Moreover, masculine norms and traditional gender roles, which are culturally and socially constructed, are dictated by and replicated within the community very early in childhood and particularly in school environments throughout adolescence. Homophobia can thus be exacerbated and reproduced when one does not conform to certain gender role that society expects. Young men who do not meet these socially determined standards face consequences like bullying, violence (verbal, physical, and sexual), and victimization [91], which are known correlates of HIV infection. Indirectly, not meeting gender-specific norms may exclude these men from their gender-conforming peers, thus keeping MSM from forming interpersonal relationships with their male peers, and subsequently having inadequate social and peer support networks, and may affect normal adolescent development, in general. Even MSM who are gender role conforming may still observe the adverse consequences of not meeting these social expectations and are thus forced to keep their same-sex desires in silence, or may use alcohol and drugs to cope. Alternatively, gender role conforming MSM may even participate in inflicting abuse to their gender role nonconforming peers in order to fulfill or establish their masculinity in front of their peers. Social stigma also affect sexual partner seeking among both gender role conforming and nonconforming MSM by forcing them to meet one another anonymously through the Internet or through public sex environments where unsafe sexual activities with multiple partners and/or substance use is commonplace. Therefore, homophobia transcends and affects individual-community- and societal-level factors in gay and bisexual men's health.

Moreover, the availability and disbursement of funding that target MSM research and prevention programs is highly politicized, limited, and not always driven by science. Holtgrave, for example, has shown that while the epidemiologic surveillance data have shown a continual increase in the prevalence of HIV, the CDC HIV prevention funding has remained stagnant since the early 1990s [92]. Structural-level factors, like disbursement of funding, are important to STI and HIV risk and need to be modeled with other factors working at different risk levels: the behaviors of an individual (e.g., condom use, types of sexual activities, serosorting strategies), the prevalence of HIV infection within the group that one finds sexual partners, the proportion of individuals in that group who know that they are infected and so less likely to engage in high risk behaviors, the proportion of infected individuals in that group who have accessed and adhere to antiretroviral medications and are no longer efficient HIV transmitters, among others. Thus, risk for STI and HIV transmission for gay men can be thought as an *interaction* between risks that exist at the individual level, risks at the community level, and also the social and cultural contexts of these risks at the societal level. For racial and ethnic minority MSM, culturally specific issues may compound all the aforementioned risk factors at multiple levels and differently throughout the life course.

Syndemics Theory: One Way to Conceptualize Multilevel Variables to STI and HIV Risks

It is therefore not surprising that MSM find themselves juggling several risks for numerous health outcomes at multiple levels throughout the life course. One way to improve our prevention approach is to rethink the way we understand and conceptualize STI and HIV transmission and acquisition risks. While STI and HIV infection is

the focus of this chapter, other health outcomes such as depression, suicidal ideation, violence and victimization, childhood sexual abuse, substance use, and risky sexual behaviors are all intertwined and interact to produce a syndemic condition for MSM that ultimately leads to STI and HIV infection [6]. Stall and colleagues developed the syndemics theory as one way to organize the multilevel predictors, correlates, mediators, and moderators of gay-specific factors at multiple levels and throughout the life course [127]. The theory states that a set of psychosocial health conditions (or distinct epidemics) interact to enhance the harmful effects of each other and together operate to raise STI and HIV risk levels (Fig. 13.1).

Developmental Basis for Syndemic Production

A central premise underlying syndemics theory is that it is a developmental process that begins early in life when discrimination and victimization increase with frequency as youth traverse regular gay-related developmental milestones and their sexual orientation and identity crystallize. While there is a growing body of cross-sectional research showing that LGB psychosocial health disparities begin early in life, there is a dearth of longitudinal studies that examine individual trajectories of adolescent psychosocial health problems over time. Two recent studies however have begun to examine disparities across time using this longitudinal framework. Corliss and colleagues [93] used survival analysis and multivariate generalized estimating equations repeated-measures linear regression to compare alcohol use among heterosexual, mostly heterosexual, bisexual, and gay/lesbian youth using participants in the "Growing Up Today" study. They found that compared with heterosexual youth, LGB youth reported an earlier age of initiation of alcohol use. Further, compared with their same-gender heterosexual peers, "mostly heterosexual" males and females, and bisexual females reported higher rates of past month drinking, number of drinks consumed at one

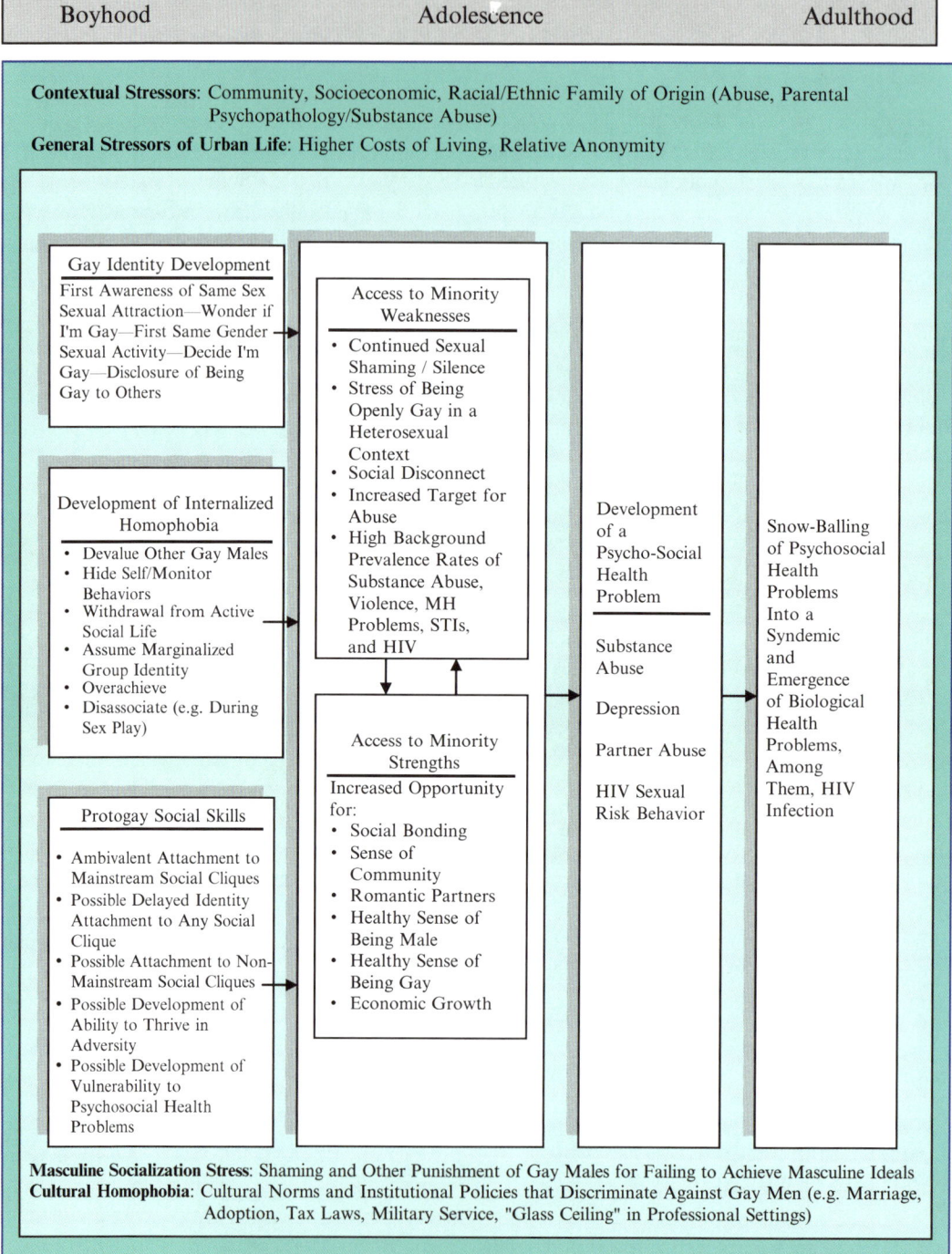

Fig. 13.1 Conceptual framework of syndemic production among MSM

time, and binge drinking over time as they aged into young adulthood. Similar findings were reported by Marshal and colleagues [94], who expanded on Corliss's results by examining use of tobacco and marijuana using a large epidemiological sample of high school students followed for three waves into young adulthood. Using latent curve models, Marshal and colleagues showed that mostly heterosexual and bisexual youth reported significantly higher alcohol, tobacco, and marijuana use across all time points, compared with heterosexual youth. Youth who identified as gay or lesbian reported similar levels of substance use at baseline, however, they reported sharper growth in substance use frequency across time than did heterosexual youth, and significantly higher use at the final time point. In sum, these two studies demonstrate that there may be significant scientific value to examining and understanding how health disparities, and in particular syndemic processes, unfold over time in the context of adolescent development and gay-related developmental milestones.

Additional evidence has recently emerged to further support the syndemics approach to HIV infection risks among young MSM. One of the first empirical studies to quantitatively test the syndemic process in adolescents was conducted by Mustanski and colleagues [95] among an urban, ethnically diverse (approximately 70% non-White) community-based sample of 310 self-identified MSM age 16–24 years in Chicago. The investigators found a significant independent association between regular binge drinking, street drug use, regular marijuana use, psychological distress, intimate partner violence, and sexual assault with (1) multiple anal sex partners (Odds Ratio [OR] = 1.24; CI: 1.05–1.47) (2) unprotected anal sex (OR = 1.42; CI: 1.19–1.68) and (3) HIV infection (OR = 1.42; CI: 1.12–1.80). The authors conclude that existing co-occurring epidemics of psychosocial health problems additively magnify the sexual behavioral risks and HIV infection itself among this urban sample of young MSM.

Moreover, Friedman et al. [96] found that the timing of gay-related developmental milestones (e.g., age of first awareness of same-sex sexual attractions and disclosure of sexual orientation) was associated with early abuse and with negative health outcomes in adulthood among gay/bisexual men in the Urban Men's Health Study. Participants who reached these gay-related developmental milestones earlier were more likely to experience forced sex and gay-related harassment prior to adulthood and to be HIV seropositive and experience partner abuse, depression, and gay-related victimization during adulthood. Early forced-sex, physical abuse, and gay-related harassment were associated with several negative health outcomes in adulthood including HIV infection, partner abuse, and depression.

In a meta-analysis, Friedman and colleagues [97] found that gay and bisexual males, compared to heterosexuals, have greater odds of experiencing childhood (before age 18) sexual abuse, parental physical abuse, and peer victimization. Most strikingly, gay and bisexual males, compared to heterosexual males, were 4.9 times more likely to report experiencing childhood sexual abuse.

Marshal and colleagues [98] recently conducted a meta-analysis examining depression and suicide disparities between gay and heterosexual youth. Results showed that sexual minority youth were almost three times as likely to report a history of suicidality (ideation, intent/plans, and/or attempts), and reported higher rates of depression symptoms on average than did heterosexual youth (Cohen's $d = 0.33$). Their results demonstrate the significant amount of psychological distress experienced by sexual minority youth, which may contribute to other short-term and long-term health problems including substance use and abuse, interpersonal problems, and risky sexual behavior.

Finally, Herrick and colleagues [99] conducted a meta-analysis to examine if sexual minority youth reported higher rates of having sex while under the influence of drugs and alcohol. Results indicated that sexual minority youth were almost twice as likely to report sex while intoxicated compared to their heterosexual peers (OR = 1.91, $p < 0.001$). These results suggest that sexual minority youth are engaging in HIV sexual risk behaviors at higher rates than their nonsexual minority peers.

Current STI and HIV Prevention Programs

While there is scientific evidence for the reduction of STI and HIV risks at the individual and small-group level [9, 10], these efforts may not be enough to manage these epidemics among MSM [72]. Additionally, empirical studies are limited to controlled settings and while efficacious, may not be effective in real-world settings over time [92, 100]. Furthermore, MSM that are targeted for current HIV prevention efforts often ignore prevention messages and instead practice their own "prevention" strategies, including seroadaptive behaviors like partner serosorting, seropositioning, and taking antiretrovirals before unprotected anal intercourse [66, 67, 72].

A review of the current CDC's compendium of evidence-based HIV behavioral interventions for MSM yielded nine tier 1 best-evidence interventions (*Brief Group Counseling; Choosing Life: Empowerment, Actions, Results (CLEAR); EXPLORE; Healthy Living Project; Healthy Relationships; Many Men Many Voices; Positive Choice: Interactive Video Doctor; Seropositive Urban Men's Intervention Trial (SUMIT); Personalized Cognitive Risk-Reduction Counseling (PCRC Enhanced Peer Led Intervention)* and five tier 2 good-evidence interventions (*Community Promise, Mpowerment, Partnership for Health, Peer Opinion Leader (POL) and Together Learning Choices (TLC)*) [101] (Table 13.1). Almost all of these interventions focus on changing individual-level variables, involve either one-on-one or small group sessions and, for the most part, do not directly address interpersonal, community-level, or structural-level factors (Table 13.2). For example, of the tier 1 interventions—which are considered as having the strongest science, there are no community-level interventions. The three interventions that are at the community level are placed into tier 2 because they did not have high enough retention rates, too few communities randomized and/or differential retention rates across study arms, which is not uncommon since individuals and families alike move in and out of communities [101]. Moreover, many of these interventions,

while under the risk category of MSM, were not initially developed or intentionally aimed at MSM populations. But because they had some MSM in the original intervention efficacy study, they are categorized as interventions for MSM in the Compendium. It is thus not surprising that many of the gay-specific variables in Table 13.2 (e.g., internalized, cultural, and institutional homophobia; gay community engagement) were not checked. Yet, among interventions developed for gay men (e.g., Brief Group Counseling, EXPLORE, POL, Many Men Many Voices, SUMIT, Mpowerment), few directly dealt with changing gay community-specific social and cultural norms, partly because many of these interventions were one-on-one or focused on changing variables at the individual level. Interestingly, most of these interventions focused primarily on reducing sexual risk-taking behaviors and very few interventions addressed multiple health outcomes (e.g., depression, suicidality, substance abuse, violence).

While these evidence-based behavioral interventions tend to be based primarily on individual-level variables, there is an average reduction of unprotected anal sex by 27%, compared to minimal or no interventions [9, 10]. But if these interventions were to also include other variable levels, then there may be larger risk-reduction effects.

Additionally, theories that underlie these interventions assume that men are free actors to respond to HIV prevention messages regarding risk. However, if men are mired in the effects of depression, substance abuse, and partner violence, the assumption underlying HIV prevention programs that men are free to act may well be flawed. To the extent, then, that men are freed from the confines created by high prevalence of coexisting psychosocial problems, their ability to respond successfully to HIV prevention efforts may well be enhanced. Thus, by raising health levels of gay men across multiple fronts, the effectiveness of HIV prevention as well as other health promotion efforts may well be improved. It is this disconnect that keeps STI and HIV prevention programs from effectively responding to the epidemic among MSM.

Table 13.1 List of CDC's Compendium of Evidenced-Based HIV Behavioral Interventions for MSM (as of June 2009) [101]

Name	Target population	Theoretic basis	Goals of intervention	Intervention targets
Tier 1 best-evidence interventions				
Brief Group Counseling [102]	API MSM	HBM, TRA, SCT	– Increase positive ethnic and sexual identity – Increase acknowledgement of HIV risk behaviors – Eliminate or reduce sex risk behaviors	– Development of positive self-identity – Social support – Safer sex education – Eroticizing and negotiating safer sex
CLEAR [113]	Young HIV-pos substance abusers	CBT, SAT	– Reduce sexual and substance use risk behaviors – Improve mental and physical health	– Promotion of healthy routines, medication adherence, and coping – Identification situations that elicit risky behaviors – Strategies to reduce emotional stress and increase quality of life
EXPLORE [103–105]	HIV-neg MSM	IMB, ME, SLT	– Prevent new HIV infections, reduce UAI, serodiscordant UAI and serodiscordant URAI	– Risk assessment – Sexual communication – Knowledge of HIV serostatus – Alcohol and drug use – Triggers for unsafe sex – Motivational interviewing
Healthy Living Project [114]	HIV-pos persons at risk of transmitting HIV	SAT	– Eliminate/reduce HIV sexual and injecting risk behaviors – Improve health care practices and quality of life	– Quality of life education – Managing co-occurring symptoms – Promotion of healthy behaviors
Healthy Relationships [115, 116]	HIV-pos men and women	SCT	– Reduce risk behaviors	– Skills to cope with HIV-related stressors and risky sexual situations – Enhance decision-making skills – Develop strategies to maintain relationships while protecting themselves and partners.
Many Men, Many Voices [106, 107]	HIV-neg or HIV-unknown Black MSM	SCT, BSA, TTBC	– Reduce UAII and UARI, sex partners Increase CCU and increase STI and HIV testing	– Self-esteem – Educate about HIV risk and sensitize to personal risk – Interactions of HIV and other STI and sensitize to personal risk – Risk-reduction strategies – Enhance self-efficacy, partner communication, and negotiation – Social support and relapse prevention
PCRC [109]	HIV-neg MSM who went through repeat testing	Gold, RP	– Reduce UAS with non-primary partners or discordant status	– Self-justifications – Diary of sexual activity
Positive Choice: Interactive Video Doctor [117]	HIV-pos clinic patients	MIP	– Reduce partners, unprotected intercourse, and illicit drug use	– Clinic patients are taught patient-tailored harm reduction strategies – Health care providers receive cuing sheets with patients risk profiles and suggested counseling statements

(continued)

Table 13.1 (continued)

Name	Target population	Theoretic basis	Goals of intervention	Intervention targets
SUMIT Enhanced Peer Led [112]	HIV-pos MSM	IMB, SCT, TPB	– Reduce UAI with HIV-negative or unknown partners – Reduce unprotected insertive oral sex with HIV-neg or unknown status partners – Increase condom use during insertive anal sex with HIV-neg or unknown partners – Increase HIV status disclosure to sex partners	– Increase knowledge of sex risk practices – Increase motivation to adopt reduced risk practices – Encourage disclosure of HIV status to partners, – Promote personal responsibility to prevent HIV transmission – Increase awareness of substance use and mental health issues – Encourage identification and management of personal risk triggers
Tier 2 good-evidence interventions				
Community Promise [120]	IDUs, non-gay identified MSM, high-risk youth, female sex workers, residents in areas with high rates of STDs	TMBC, HBM, TRA, SCT	– Increase consistent condom use – Increase disinfecting of injection equipment	– Community mobilization – Distribution of small-media materials and risk-reduction supplies
Mpowerment [108]	HIV-neg or HIV-unknown young MSM	Diffusion of Innovations	– Reduce UAI	– Community-level peer-led outreach – Small groups – Publicity campaign/social support/social outlets
Partnership for Health [118, 119]	HIV-pos clinic patients	MFT, MP, SC	– Eliminate or reduce unprotected anal and vaginal sex	– Cultivate patient–provider relationship – Emphasize loss-framed messages in counseling and identifying goals
POL [110, 111]	Men who frequent gay bars	Diffusion of Innovations	– Reduce UAI	– Popular opinion leaders trained to endorse behavior change to peers in gay clubs – Focus on changing norms in social networks
TLC [121–123]	HIV-pos adolescent and young adult clinic patients	SAT	– Enhance health behaviors – Increase condom use – Eliminate or reduce unprotected sex or refuse to have unsafe sex – Eliminate or reduce drug and alcohol use	– Small group discussions (disclosure, living with HIV and safer sex and substance use practices)

Abbreviation: PCRC Personalized Cognitive Risk-Reduction Counseling, *POL* Peer Opinion Leader, *SUMIT* Seropositive Urban Men's Intervention Trial, *API* Asian-Pacific Islander, *HBM* Health Belief Model, *TRA* Theory of Reasoned Action, *SCT* Social Cognitive Theory, *IMB* Information-Motivation-Behavior skill model, *ME* Motivational Enhancement, *SLT* Social Learning Theory, *BSA* Behavioral Skills Acquisition Model, *TMBC* Trans-theoretical Model of Behavioral Change, *UAII* Unprotected Anal Insertive Intercourse, *Gold* Gold's model of "on-line" vs. "off-line" self-appraisal of risk behavior, *RP* Model of Relapse Prevention, *TPB* Theory of Planned Behavior, *MIP* Motivational Interviewing Principals, *SAT* Social Action Theory, *CBT* Cognitive Behavioral Therapy, *MFT* Message Framing Theory, *MP* Mutual Participation, *SC* Stages of Change, *TLC* Together Learning Choices, *CLEAR* Choosing Life: Empowerment, Actions, Results

Table 13.2 CDC's Compendium of Effective Behavioral Interventions for MSM and Levels of HIV/STI risks

Levels of HIV/STI risks	Tier 1 best-evidence interventions for MSM								
	Brief group counseling	CLEAR	EXPLORE	Healthy living project	Healthy relationships	Many men many voices	Positive choice: interactive video doctor	SUMIT	PCRC
Individual									
Biology (e.g., circumcision, CCR5,)	X								
Internalized homophobia	X					X			
Demography (e.g., race, SES)	X					X			
Psychology and mental health									
Depression		X		X				X	
Suicidal ideation		X		X				X	
Victimization									
Sexual abuse							X		
Substance abuse		X	X	X				X	
Alcohol abuse		X	X	X				X	
Sexual sensation-seeking	X	X	X	X	X	X	X	X	X
Attending saunas, circuit parties, and public sex environments									
Interpersonal									
Condom negotiation	X	X	X	X	X	X	X	X	X
Negotiated safety					X			X	X
HIV disclosure (e.g., serosorting, seropositioning)					X			X	
Community									
Community viral load									
Social support	X					X			
Gay community engagement									
Peer Norms									
Culture and Society									
Cultural Homophobia									
Institutional Homophobia									
Policy									
Protection laws (from hate crimes, etc.)									
Employment rights and protections									
Marriage rights									
Funding for MSM programs									

(continued)

Table 13.2 (continued)

Levels of HIV/STI risks	Tier 2 Good-Evidence Interventions				
	Community promise	Mpowerment	Partnerships for health	POL	TLC
Individual					
Biology (e.g., circumcision, CCR5,)					
Internalized homophobia		X			
Demography (e.g., race, SES)					
Psychology and mental health					
Depression					
Suicidal ideation					
Victimization					
Sexual abuse					
Substance abuse	X				X
Alcohol abuse					X
Sexual sensation-seeking	X	X	X	X	X
Attending saunas, circuit parties, and public sex environments		X			
Interpersonal					
Condom negotiation	X	X		X	X
Negotiated safety					
HIV disclosure (e.g., serosorting, seropositioning)					X
Community					
Community viral load					
Social support		X			
Gay community engagement		X		X	
Peer Norms		X		X	
Culture and Society					
Cultural Homophobia		X			
Institutional Homophobia					
Policy					
Protection laws (from hate crimes, etc.)					
Employment rights and protections					
Marriage rights					
Funding for MSM programs					

Moving the Field Forward

This chapter has summarized the contextual complexities of HIV infection risks and the many shortcomings of current STI and HIV prevention approaches for MSM, and in the process has attempted to outline the multiple opportunities for the field to move forward to enhance health promotion programs for MSM. In addition, there exist multiple opportunities to make our research agendas more innovative.

An important theme of this chapter has been to emphasize the need to integrate multiple levels of intervention action—at the level of the individual, the dyad, the community, the culture and at the level of policy—in our approaches to epidemiological investigations and public health practice. At present, the field primarily emphasizes intervention action at the level of the individual and in general has not learned to effectively address variables that drive risk beyond the level of the individual, much less to integrate intervention action at multiple levels in order to increase overall intervention efficacy. Part of this research agenda may include new ways to measure community-level and network-level (e.g., sexual, social, cultural) indicators related to MSM health; the effects of changing structural-level policies like protection laws and legal recognition of same-sex relationships on the health and well-being of adolescent and adult MSM; the effects of racism, discrimination, and homophobia at multiple levels (internalized, cultural and institutional) beyond, and within MSM communities (particularly with respect to racial and ethnic minority MSM); the extent to which MSM have access to health care, in general, or utilize certain health care sectors, in particular; and the effects of anti-bullying school-based programs on levels of gay-related violence and victimization among young MSM. Existing innovative programs that address multiple levels of prevention action that are already implemented by front-line community-based organizations need to be properly evaluated. This community-based evaluation research will generate some insights as to the effectiveness of these strategies, even though

these data will fall short of the rigor of an RCT experimental study.

It is also clear that while gay men are attempting multiple strategies to reduce their sexual risk, they are doing so in a historical moment when there are few data to help inform them about the epidemiological wisdom of these strategies. That is, while many MSM are engaging in a set of sexual practices that they believe will lower their risk for HIV transmission (e.g., serosorting strategies, negotiated safety, positional strategies, withdrawal, and viral load serosorting), men are engaging in these behaviors without strong evidence to guide their decisions about which strategies would serve them best. The time is long overdue for the field to conduct studies on the relative epidemiological risks of each of these strategies, not only in terms of HIV transmission but also in terms of the risks for other STIs. In short, it is time for science to catch up with the sexual risk-reduction strategies currently being practiced by MSM.

Not only must we rethink how to address the multilevel determinants of health among MSM in public health practice, we also must be mindful of the possibility that multiple psychosocial epidemics exist among MSM, which in turn drive STI and HIV risk in gay male communities. Hence, a one-disease "siloed" prevention program of research and public health practice will probably fall short of the goal of supporting gay men's health efforts. In response to this situation, we might consider evaluating a prevention cocktail approach whereby multiple disease outcomes are screened and dealt with concurrently [72], with a view to measuring whether the effects of this approach are greater than if each psychosocial and HIV/STI disease outcome was approached individually. In short, work to create a broader gay men's health agenda, which addresses the epidemics of depression, substance abuse, and violence victimization might not only raise levels of health in terms of these dangerous epidemics but also work to increase the effectiveness of our HIV/STI prevention programs. Again, the time is long overdue to test the efficacy of this approach to raising levels of health among gay men.

Moreover, research on resilience and protective factors related to STI and HIV risks for MSM is urgently needed. While we tend to study MSM who are at highest risks—who are actually only the minority of all MSM, we must also learn from MSM who have endured and successfully overcome similar obstacles and averted STI and HIV infections. The behavioral literature is full of examples of resilience of gay men to health threats, be it in regard to high levels of smoking cessation, self-resolution of substance abuse careers, the ability to stay seronegative for decades on end even while having a very active sex life. Clearly there are strong themes of resilience among gay men, and men who have evidenced these patterns in the face of the AIDS epidemic are very likely to have a great deal to teach us about the creation of effective prevention programs. Some research questions to consider might include describing the sources for MSM's strength in high-risk situations, how and through what mechanisms do social capital and social cohesion within MSM communities (virtual or physical) effect STI and HIV risks, and what are the multilevel factors, for example, that have kept men safe and healthy over long periods of time. In addition, studying how it is that men resolve substance abuse careers on their own (a not-uncommon pattern among MSM with a substance abuse history) might also lend us important insights in terms of intervention design. Learning how to avert infections, prevent syndemic production, and raise levels of resilience among MSM will be critical for the field.

With respect to migration of MSM to urban centers, two recommendations may improve wellbeing as structural-level interventions. First, in established urban gay communities, programs that support positive gay community building are needed. In contexts where heavy alcohol and substance use are commonplace or sex clubs and high-risk sexual activities with multiple partners are highly prevalent, communities might consider fielding alternative outlets for MSM to socialize and meet one another. Second, for other smaller cities across the United States where most MSM still reside and work, the promotion of gay-friendly communities may well yield important

dividends. Efforts to build safe communities within smaller cities may work to keep men from migrating to larger cities that have higher prevalence rates of HIV and STIs. By virtue of keeping men out of high prevalence sexual networks, community-building in smaller, low HIV prevalence cities would work as a structural HIV prevention effort. But by creating positive and healthy spaces for MSM in both large urban centers and smaller cities, there may be an opportunity to disrupt the production of high prevalence/high incidence HIV/STI clusters and so raise levels of health among MSM regardless of where men reside.

Finally, longitudinal and dynamic approaches to the prevention of STI and HIV infection that take into account the life course perspective might also serve us well in terms of deepening our understanding of health and well-being among MSM. A life course research agenda might start by studying why it is that adolescent MSM have a much worse health profiles in terms of numerous psychosocial health conditions than their heterosexual peers even before they reach the age of 18. However, as important as this question is, understanding the production of health and disease across the life course from youth to middle age and from middle age to late life will undoubtedly generate important insights toward improved intervention design. This tradition of research among MSM has barely begun and will likely be an important focus as our research designs and research questions become more sophisticated. This agenda will become even more complex as we move to questions of understanding the production of health and illness in minority communities of MSM, as well as communities outside of the largest urban centers.

Furthermore, current prevention programs that target gay youth are limited and out-of-date. For example, gay youth are telling us that in order to prevent the transmission of HIV, programs need to go beyond talking about just sexuality and HIV and to include issues as diverse as intimacy; substance abuse; self-esteem; violence and victimization; sexual identity development; safe havens; how to have fun in a positive and safe way; provision of older gay mentors; and greater support from schools, religious organizations, families, communities of color, and the gay community itself [124]. Therefore, we suggest that positive youth development programs that focus on multiple problems during critical development periods at multiple levels for at-risk youths be developed, implemented, and evaluated. Similar programs that focus on constructs such as bonding, self-confidence, competence, character development, empowerment, and resilience have been shown to be effective [124–126].

In summary, while it is disheartening that we have so far to go in terms of raising levels of health among MSM after over a quarter century of HIV prevention work, it is also exciting to consider the many innovative ways that might be attempted to raise levels of health in MSM communities. This broader gay men's health agenda, while important to MSM, is also likely to inform prevention and care efforts in other marginalized communities and so yield additional dividends in terms of the research investment required to meet this agenda. Thus, while we have a long road ahead of us in terms of improving the health of MSM, this road will be full of exciting and useful challenges and is therefore a challenge that should be taken up with enthusiasm.

References

1. CDC. HIV/AIDS and men who have sex with men (MSM). Centers for Disease Control and Prevention [Web site]. www.cdc.gov/hiv/topics/msm/. Accessed May 6, 2010.
2. Purcell DW, Johnson C, Lansky A, Prejean J, Stein R, Denning P, Gaul Z, Weinstock H, Su J, Crepaz N. Calculating HIV and Syphilis Rates for Risk Groups: Estimating the National Population Size of Men Who Have Sex with Men. Latebreaker Abstract 22896; 2010 National STD Prevention Conference; Atlanta, GA.
3. Valdiserri RO. Sexually transmitted infections among gay and bisexual men. In: Wolitski RJ, Stall R, Valdiserri RO, editors. Unequal opportunity: health disparities affecting gay and bisexual men in the United States. New York, NY: Oxford University Press; 2008. p. 159–93.
4. Wolitski RJ, Stall R, Valdiserri RO, editors. Unequal opportunity: health disparities affecting gay and bisexual men in the United States. New York, NY: Oxford University Press; 2008.
5. Gay and Lesbian Medical Association and LGBT health experts. Healthy People 2010: Companion document for lesbian, gay, bisexual, and transgender (LGBT) health. San Francisco, CA: Gay and Lesbian Medical Association; 2001.
6. Stall R, Mills TC, Williamson J, Hart T, Greenwood G, Paul J, Pollack L, Binson D, Osmond D, Catania JA. Association of co-occurring psychosocial health problems and increased vulnerability to HIV/AIDS among urban men who have sex with men. Am J Public Health. 2003;93:939–42.
7. Aral SO, Padian NS, Holmes KK. Advances in multi-level approaches to understanding the epidemiology and prevention of sexually transmitted infections and HIV: An overview. J Infect Dis. 2005;191:S1–6.
8. Poundstone KE, Strathdee SA, Celentano DD. The social epidemiology of human immunodeficiency virus/acquired immunodeficiency syndrome. Epidemiol Rev. 2004;26:22–35.
9. Johnson WD, Diaz RM, Flanders WD, Goodman M, Hill AN, Holtgrave D, Malow R, McClellan WM. Behavioral interventions to reduce risk for sexual transmission of HIV among men who have sex with men. Cochrane Database Syst Rev. 2008;3:CD001230.
10. Herbst JH, Beeker C, Mathew A, McNally T, Passin WF, Kay LS, Crepaz N, Lyles CM, Briss P, Chattopadhyay S, Johnson RL, Task Force on Community Preventive Services. The effectiveness of individual-, group-, and community-level HIV behavioral risk-reduction interventions for adult men who have sex with men: a systematic review. Am J Prev Med. 2007;32:S38–67.
11. CDC. Trends in primary and secondary syphilis and HIV infections in men who have sex with men—San Francisco and Los Angeles, California, 1998–2002. MMWR Morb Mortal Wkly Rep. 2004;53:575–8.
12. CDC. HIV/STD risks in young men who have sex with men who do not disclose their sexual orientation—six U.S. cities, 1994–2000. MMWR Morb Mortal Wkly Rep. 2003;52:81–6.
13. Buchacz K, Greenberg A, Onorato I, Janssen R. Syphilis epidemics and human immunodeficiency virus (HIV) incidence among men who have sex with men in the United States: implications for HIV prevention. Sex Transm Dis. 2005;32:S73–9.
14. Siegel D, Golden E, Washington AE, Morse SA, Fullilove MT, Catania JA, Marin B, Hulley SB. Prevalence and correlates of herpes simplex infections. The population-based AIDS in Multiethnic Neighborhoods Study. JAMA. 1992;268:1702–8.
15. Millett GA, Flores SA, Peterson JL, Bakeman R. Explaining disparities in HIV infection among black and white men who have sex with men: a meta-analysis of HIV risk behaviors. AIDS. 2007;21:2083–91.
16. CDC. HIV prevalence, unrecognized infection, and HIV testing among men who have sex with men—five U.S. cities, June 2004–April 2005. MMWR Morb Mortal Wkly Rep. 2005;54:597–601.

17. Hall HI, Byers RH, Ling Q, Espinoza L. Racial/ethnic and age disparities in HIV prevalence and disease progression among men who have sex with men in the United States. Am J Public Health. 2007;97:1060–6.

18. Hall HI, Song R, Rhodes P, Prejean J, An Q, Lee LM, Karon J, Brookmeyer R, Kaplan EH, McKenna MT, Janssen RS, rHIV Incidence Surveillance Group. Estimation of HIV incidence in the United States. JAMA. 2008;300:520–9.

19. CDC. HIV incidence among young men who have sex with men—seven U.S. cities, 1994–2000. MMWR Morb Mortal Wkly Rep. 2001;50:440–4.

20. Winkelstein Jr W, Lyman DM, Padian N, Grant R, Samuel M, Wiley JA, Anderson RE, Lang W, Riggs J, Levy JA. Sexual practices and risk of infection by the Human Immunodeficiency Virus: The San Francisco Men's Health Study. JAMA. 1987;257:321–5.

21. Valleroy LA, MacKellar DA, Karon JM, Rosen DH, McFarland W, Shehan DA, Stoyanoff SR, LaLota M, Celentano DD, Koblin BA, Thiede H, Katz MH, Torian LV, Janssen RS. HIV prevalence and associated risks in young men who have sex with men. Young Men's Survey Study Group. JAMA. 2000;284:198–204.

22. Harawa NT, Greenland S, Bingham TA, Johnson DF, Cochran SD, Cunningham WE, Celentano DD, Koblin BA, LaLota M, MacKellar DA, McFarland W, Shehan D, Stoyanoff S, Thiede H, Torian L, Valleroy LA. Associations of race/ethnicity with HIV prevalence and HIV-related behaviors among young men who have sex with men in 7 urban centers in the United States. J Acquir Immune Defic Syndr. 2004;35:526–36.

23. Celentano DD, Sifakis F, Hylton J, Torian LV, Guillin V, Koblin BA. Race/ethnic differences in HIV prevalence and risks among adolescent and young adult men who have sex with men. J Urban Health. 2005;82:610–21.

24. Xia Q, Osmond DH, Tholandi M, Pollack LM, Zhou W, Ruiz JD, Catania JA. HIV prevalence and sexual risk behaviors among men who have sex with men: results from a statewide population-based survey in California. J Acquir Immune Defic Syndr. 2006;41:238–45.

25. Catania JA, Osmond D, Stall RD, Pollack L, Paul JP, Blower S, Binson D, Canchola JA, Mills TC, Fisher L, Choi KH, Porco T, Turner C, Blair J, Henne J, Bye LL, Coates TJ. The continuing HIV epidemic among men who have sex with men. Am J Public Health. 2001;91:907–14.

26. Buchacz KA, Siller JE, Bandy DW, Birjukow N, Kent CK, Holmberg SD, Klausner JD. HIV and syphilis testing among men who have sex with men attending sex clubs and adult bookstores–San Francisco, 2003. J Acquir Immune Defic Syndr. 2004;37:1324–6.

27. Ackers M, Greenbery A, Lin C, Batholow B, Hirsch A, Longhi M, Gurwith M. High HIV incidence among men who have sex with men participating in an HIV vaccine efficacy trial, United States, 1998–2002. Abstract 857; 11th Conference on Retroviruses and Opportunistic Infections; San Francisco, CA.

28. Penkower L, Dew MA, Kingsley L, Becker JT, Satz P, Schaerf FW, Sheridan K. Behavioral, health and psychosocial factors and risk for HIV infection among sexually active homosexual men: the Multicenter AIDS Cohort Study. Am J Public Health. 1991;81:194–6.

29. Samson M, Libert F, Doranz BJ, Rucker J, Liesnard C, Farber CM, Saragosti S, Lapoumeroulie C, Cognaux J, Forceille C, Muyldermans G, Verhofstede C, Burtonboy G, Georges M, Imai T, Rana S, Yi Y, Smyth RJ, Collman RG, Doms RW, Vassart G, Parmentier M. Resistance to HIV-1 infection in caucasian individuals bearing mutant alleles of the CCR-5 chemokine receptor gene. Nature. 1996;382:722–5.

30. Paxton WA, Kang S, Koup RA. The HIV type 1 coreceptor CCR5 and its role in viral transmission and disease progression. AIDS Res Hum Retroviruses. 1998;14:S89–92.

31. Marmor M, Sheppard HW, Donnell D, Bozeman S, Celum C, Buchbinder S, Koblin B, Seage 3rd GR. HIV Network for Prevention Trials Vaccine Preparedness Protocol Team. Homozygous and heterozygous CCR5-Delta32 genotypes are associated with resistance to HIV infection. J Acquir Immune Defic Syndr. 2001;27:472–81.

32. O'Brien TR, Padian NS, Hodge T, Goedert JJ, O'Brien SJ, Carrington M. CCR-5 genotype and sexual transmission of HIV-1. AIDS. 1998;12:444–5.

33. Huang Y, Paxton WA, Wolinsky SM, Neumann AU, Zhang L, He T, Kang S, Ceradini D, Jin Z, Yazdanbakhsh K, Kunstman K, Erickson D, Dragon E, Landau NR, Phair J, Ho DD, Koup RA. The role of a mutant CCR5 allele in HIV-1 transmission and disease progression. Nat Med. 1996;2:1240–3.

34. Millett GA, Flores SA, Marks G, Reed JB, Herbst JH. Circumcision status and risk of HIV and sexually transmitted infections among men who have sex with men: a meta-analysis. JAMA. 2008;300:1674–84.

35. Koblin BA, Husnik MJ, Colfax G, Huang Y, Madison M, Mayer K, Barresi PJ, Coates TJ, Chesney MA, Buchbinder S. Risk factors for HIV infection among men who have sex with men. AIDS. 2006;20:731–9.

36. Hanson J, Posner S, Hassig S, Rice J, Farley TA. Assessment of sexually transmitted diseases as risk factors for HIV seroconversion in a New Orleans sexually transmitted disease clinic, 1990-1998. Ann Epidemiol. 2005;15:13–20.

37. Samuel MC, Hessol N, Shiboski S, Engel RR, Speed TP, Winkelstein Jr W. Factors associated with human immunodeficiency virus seroconversion in homosexual men in three San Francisco cohort studies, 1984-1989. J Acquir Immune Defic Syndr. 1993;6:303–12.

38. Seage 3rd GR, Mayer KH, Horsburgh Jr CR, Holmberg SD, Moon MW, Lamb GA. The relation

between nitrite inhalants, unprotected receptive anal intercourse, and the risk of human immunodeficiency virus infection. Am J Epidemiol. 1992;135:1–11.

39. Williamson LM, Hart GJ. HIV prevalence and undiagnosed infection among a community sample of gay men in Scotland. J Acquir Immune Defic Syndr. 2007;45:224–30.

40. Henderson RH. Improving sexually transmitted disease health services for gays: a national prospective. Sex Transm Dis. 1977;4:58–62.

41. Ostrow DG, DiFranceisco WJ, Chmiel JS, Wagstaff DA, Wesch J. A case-control study of human immunodeficiency virus type 1 seroconversion and risk-related behaviors in the Chicago MACS/CCS Cohort, 1984-1992. Multicenter AIDS Cohort Study. Coping and Change Study. Am J Epidemiol. 1995;142:875–83.

42. Skinner WF. The prevalence and demographic predictors of illicit and licit drug use among lesbians and gay men. Am J Public Health. 1994;84:1307–10.

43. Cochran SD, Ackerman D, Mays VM, Ross MW. Prevalence of non-medical drug use and dependence among homosexually active men and women in the US population. Addiction. 2004;99:989–98.

44. Halkitis PN, Shrem MT, Martin FW. Sexual behavior patterns of methamphetamine-using gay and bisexual men. Subst Use Misuse. 2005;40:703–19.

45. Patterson TL, Semple SJ, Zians JK, Strathdee SA. Methamphetamine-using HIV-positive men who have sex with men: correlates of polydrug use. J Urban Health. 2005;82:i120–1126.

46. Hirshfield S, Remien RH, Walavalkar I, Chiasson MA. Crystal methamphetamine use predicts incident STD infection among men who have sex with men recruited online: a nested case-control study. J Med Internet Res. 2004;6:e41.

47. Wolitski RJ, MacGowan RJ, Higgins DL, Jorgensen CM. The effects of HIV counseling and testing on risk-related practices and help-seeking behavior. AIDS Educ Prev. 1997;9:52–6.

48. Higgins DL, Galavotti C, O'Reilly KR, Schnell DJ, Moore M, Rugg DL, Johnson R. Evidence for the effects of HIV antibody counseling and testing on risk behaviors. JAMA. 1991;266:2419–29.

49. Lauby JL, Millett GA, LaPollo AB, Bond L, Murrill CS, Marks G. Sexual risk behaviors of HIV-positive, HIV-negative, and serostatus-unknown Black men who have sex with men and women. Arch Sex Behav. 2008;37:708–19.

50. MacKellar DA, Valleroy LA, Behel S, Secura GM, Bingham T, Celentano DD, Koblin BA, LaLota M, Shehan D, Thiede H, Torian LV. Unintentional HIV exposures from young men who have sex with men who disclose being HIV-negative. AIDS. 2006;20: 1637–44.

51. Weinhardt LS, Carey MP, Johnson BT, Bickham NL. Effects of HIV counseling and testing on sexual risk behavior: a meta-analytic review of published research, 1985-1997. Am J Public Health. 1999;89: 1397–405.

52. Mimiaga MJ, Noonan E, Donnell D, Safren SA, Koenen KC, Gortmaker S, O'Cleirigh C, Chesney MA, Coates TJ, Koblin BA, Mayer KH. Childhood sexual abuse is highly associated with HIV risk-taking behavior and infection among MSM in the EXPLORE Study. J Acquir Immune Defic Syndr. 2009;51:340–8.

53. Paul JP, Catania J, Pollack L, Stall R. Understanding childhood sexual abuse as a predictor of sexual risk-taking among men who have sex with men: The Urban Men's Health Study. Child Abuse Negl. 2001;25:557–84.

54. Relf MV, Huang B, Campbell J, Catania J. Gay identity, interpersonal violence, and HIV risk behaviors: an empirical test of theoretical relationships among a probability-based sample of urban men who have sex with men. J Assoc Nurses AIDS Care. 2004; 15:14–26.

55. Adam PC, Teva I, de Wit JB. Balancing risk and pleasure: sexual self-control as a moderator of the influence of sexual desires on sexual risk-taking in men who have sex with men. Sex Transm Infect. 2008;84:463–7.

56. Crepaz N, Hart TA, Marks G. Highly active antiretroviral therapy and sexual risk behavior: a meta-analytic review. JAMA. 2004;292:224–36.

57. Kalichman SC, Heckman T, Kelly JA. Sensation seeking as an explanation for the association between substance use and HIV-related risky sexual behavior. Arch Sex Behav. 1996;25:141–54.

58. Difranceisco W, Ostrow DG, Chmiel JS. Sexual adventurism, high-risk behavior, and human immunodeficiency virus-1 seroconversion among the Chicago MACS-CCS cohort, 1984 to 1992. A case-control study. Sex Transm Dis. 1996;23:453–60.

59. Ostrow DE, Fox KJ, Chmiel JS, Silvestre A, Visscher BR, Vanable PA, Jacobson LP, Strathdee SA. Attitudes towards highly active antiretroviral therapy are associated with sexual risk taking among HIV-infected and uninfected homosexual men. AIDS. 2002;16:775–80.

60. Ostrow DG, Silverberg MJ, Cook RL, Chmiel JS, Johnson L, Li X, Jacobson LP. multicenter AIDS cohort study. Prospective study of attitudinal and relationship predictors of sexual risk in the multicenter AIDS cohort study. AIDS Behav. 2008;12: 127–38.

61. Alvy LM, McKirnan DJ, Mansergh G, Koblin B, Colfax GN, Flores SA, Hudson S, MIX Project Study Group. Depression is Associated with Sexual Risk Among Men Who Have Sex with Men, but is Mediated by Cognitive Escape and Self-Efficacy. AIDS Behav. 2011;15:1171–9.

62. De Santis JP, Colin JM. Provencio Vasquez E, McCain GC. The relationship of depressive symptoms, self-esteem, and sexual behaviors in a predominantly Hispanic sample of men who have sex with men. Am J Mens Health. 2008;2:314–21.

63. Shoptaw S, Weiss RE, Munjas B, Hucks-Ortiz C, Young SD, Larkins S, Victorianne GD, Gorbach PM.

Homonegativity, substance use, sexual risk behaviors, and HIV status in poor and ethnic men who have sex with men in Los Angeles. J Urban Health. 2009;86:77–92.

64. Hatzenbuehler ML, Nolen-Hoeksema S, Erickson SJ. Minority stress predictors of HIV risk behavior, substance use, and depressive symptoms: results from a prospective study of bereaved gay men. Health Psychol. 2008;27:455–62.

65. Grossman AH. Homophobia: a cofactor of HIV disease in gay and lesbian youth. J Assoc Nurses AIDS Care. 1994;5:39–43.

66. Snowden JM, Raymond HF, McFarland W. Prevalence of seroadaptive behaviours of men who have sex with men, San Francisco, 2004. Sex Transm Infect. 2009;85:469–76.

67. Eaton LA, Kalichman SC, O'Connell DA, Karchner WD. A strategy for selecting sexual partners believed to pose little/no risks for HIV: serosorting and its implications for HIV transmission. AIDS Care. 2009;21:1279–88.

68. Guzman R, Colfax GN, Wheeler S, Mansergh G, Marks G, Rader M, Buchbinder S. Negotiated safety relationships and sexual behavior among a diverse sample of HIV-negative men who have sex with men. J Acquir Immune Defic Syndr. 2005;38:82–6.

69. McConnell JJ, Bragg L, Shiboski S, Grant RM. Sexual seroadaptation: lessons for prevention and sex research from a cohort of HIV-positive men who have sex with men. PLoS One. 2010;5:e8831.

70. Van de Ven P, Kippax S, Crawford J, Rawstorne P, Prestage G, Grulich A, Murphy D. In a minority of gay men, sexual risk practice indicates strategic positioning for perceived risk reduction rather than unbridled sex. AIDS Care. 2002;14:471–80.

71. Bohl DD, Raymond HF, Arnold M, McFarland W. Concurrent sexual partnerships and racial disparities in HIV infection among men who have sex with men. Sex Transm Infect. 2009;85:367–9.

72. Stall R, Herrick A, Guadamuz TE, Friedman MS. Updating HIV prevention with gay men: Current challenges and opportunities to advance health among gay men. In: Mayer KH, Pizer H, editors. HIV prevention. London, UK: Academic Press; 2009. p. 267–80.

73. Aral SO. Sexual network patterns as determinants of STD rates: paradigm shift in the behavioral epidemiology of STDs made visible. Sex Transm Dis. 1999;26:262–4.

74. Doherty IA, Padian NS, Marlow C, Aral SO. Determinants and consequences of sexual networks as they affect the spread of sexually transmitted infections. J Infect Dis. 2005;191:S42–54.

75. Al-Tayyib AA, McFarlane M, Kachur R, Rietmeijer CA. Finding sex partners on the internet: what is the risk for sexually transmitted infections? Sex Transm Infect. 2009;85:216–20.

76. Binson D, Woods WJ, Pollack L, Paul J, Stall R, Catania JA. Differential HIV risk in bathhouses and public cruising areas. Am J Public Health. 2001;91:1482–6.

77. Lister NA, Smith A, Tabrizi S, Hayes P, Medland NA, Garland S, Fairley CK. Screening for Neisseria gonorrhoeae and Chlamydia trachomatis in men who have sex with men at male-only saunas. Sex Transm Dis. 2003;30:886–9.

78. Raymond HF, McFarland W. Racial mixing and HIV risk among men who have sex with men. AIDS Behav. 2009;13:630–7.

79. Bingham TA, Harawa NT, Johnson DF, Secura GM, MacKellar DA, Valleroy LA. The effect of partner characteristics on HIV infection among African American men who have sex with men in the Young Men's Survey, Los Angeles, 1999–2000.

80. Dolezal C, Carballo-Diequez A, Nieves-Rosa L, Diaz F. Substance use and sexual risk behavior: Understanding their association among four ethnic groups of Latino men who have sex with men. J Subst Abuse. 2000;11:323–36.

81. Kidder DP, Wolitski RJ, Royal S, Aidala A, Courtenay-Quirk C, Holtgrave DR, Harre D, Sumartojo E, Stall R. Housing and Health Study Team. Access to housing as a structural intervention for homeless and unstably housed people living with HIV: rationale, methods, and implementation of the housing and health study. AIDS Behav. 2007;11:149–61.

82. Kerrigan D, Moreno L, Rosario S, Gomez B, Jerez H, Barrington C, Weiss E, Sweat M. Environmental-structural interventions to reduce HIV/STI risk among female sex workers in the Dominican Republic. Am J Public Health. 2006;96:120–5.

83. Des Jarlais DC. Structural interventions to reduce HIV transmission among injecting drug users. AIDS. 2000;14:S41–6.

84. Frieden TR, Mostashari F, Kerker BD, Miller N, Hajat A, Frankel M. Adult tobacco use levels after intensive tobacco control measures: New York City, 2002–2003. Am J Public Health. 2005;95:1016–23.

85. Chaloupka FJ, Grossman M, Saffer H. The effects of price on alcohol consumption and alcohol-related problems. Alcohol Res Health. 2002;26:22–34.

86. Hatzenbuehler ML, Keyes KM, Hasin DS. State-level policies and psychiatric morbidity in lesbian, gay, and bisexual populations. Am J Public Health. 2009;99:2275–81.

87. Mills TC, Paul J, Stall R, Pollack L, Canchola J, Chang YJ, Moskowitz JT, Catania JA. Distress and depression in men who have sex with men: the Urban Men's Health Study. Am J Psychiatry. 2004;161:278–85.

88. Goodenow C, Szalacha L, Westheimer K. School support groups, other school factors, and the safety of sexual minority adolescents. Psychol Schools. 2006;43:573–89.

89. Suicide Prevention Resource Center. Suicide risk and prevention for lesbian, gay, bisexual, and transgender youth. Newton, MA: Education Development Center, Inc. 2008; Available at www.sprc.org/library/SPRC_LGBT_Youth.pdf. Accessed June 27, 2011.

90. Mills TC, Stall R, Pollack L, Paul JP, Binson D, Canchola J, Catania JA. Health-related characteristics of men who have sex with men: a comparison of those living in "gay ghettos" with those living elsewhere. Am J Public Health. 2001;91:980–3.

91. Herek GM. Hate crimes and stigma-related experiences among sexual minority adults in the United States: prevalence estimates from a national probability sample. J Interpers Violence. 2009;24:54–74.

92. Holtgrave DR. When "heightened" means "lessened": the case of HIV prevention resources in the United States. J Urban Health. 2007;84:648–52.

93. Corliss HL, Rosario M, Wypij D, Fisher LB, Austin SB. Sexual orientation disparities in longitudinal alcohol use patterns among adolescents: findings from the Growing Up Today Study. Arch Pediatr Adolesc Med. 2008;162:1071–8.

94. Marshal MP, Friedman MS, Stall R, Thompson AL. Individual trajectories of substance use in lesbian, gay and bisexual youth and heterosexual youth. Addiction. 2009;104:974–81.

95. Mustanski B, Garofalo R, Herrick A, Donenberg G. Psychosocial health problems increase risk for HIV among urban young men who have sex with men: preliminary evidence of a syndemic in need of attention. Ann Behav Med. 2007;34:37–45.

96. Friedman MS, Marshal MP, Stall R, Cheong J, Wright ER. Gay-related development, early abuse and adult health outcomes among gay males. AIDS Behav. 2008;12:891–902.

97. Friedman MS, Marshal MP, Guadamuz TE, Wei C, Wong CF, Saewyc E, Stall R. A Meta-Analysis to examine disparities in childhood sexual abuse, parental physical abuse, and peer victimization among sexual minority and non-sexual minority individuals. Am J Public Health. 2011;101:1481–94.

98. Marshal MP, Dietz L, Friedman MS, Stall R, Smith H, McGinley J, Murray P, D'Augelli A, Brent D. Depression and suicide disparities between heterosexual and sexual minority youth: A meta-analytic review. J Adolesc Health. 2011;49:115–23.

99. Herrick AL, Marshal MP, Smith HA, Sucato G, Stall RD. Sex while intoxicated: a meta-analysis comparing heterosexual and sexual minority youth. J Adolesc Health. 2011;48:306–9.

100. Holtgrave DR, Curran JW. What works, and what remains to be done, in HIV prevention in the United States. Annu Rev Public Health. 2006;27:261–75.

101. CDC. 2009 Compendium of Evidence-Based HIV Prevention Interventions. Centers for Disease Control and Prevention. [Web site] www.cdc.gov/hiv/topics/research/prs/evidence-based-interventions.htm. Accessed June 27, 2011.

102. Choi KH, Lew S, Vittinghoff E, Catania JA, Barrett DC, Coates TJ. The efficacy of brief group counseling in HIV risk reduction among homosexual Asian and Pacific Islander men. AIDS. 1996;10:81–7.

103. Chesney MA, Koblin BA, Barresi PJ, Husnik MJ, Celum CL, Colfax G, Mayer K, McKirnan D, Judson FN, Huang Y, Coates TJ. EXPLORE Study Team. An individually tailored intervention for HIV prevention: Baseline data from the EXPLORE study. Am J Public Health. 2003;93:933–8.

104. Koblin BA, Chesney MA, Husnik MJ, Bozeman S, Celum CL, Buchbinder S, Mayer K, McKirnan D, Judson FN, Huang Y, Coates TJ. EXPLORE Study Team. High-risk behaviors among men who have sex with men in 6 US cities: Baseline data from the EXPLORE study. Am J Public Health. 2003;93: 926–32.

105. The EXPLORE Study Team. Effects of a behavioural intervention to reduce acquisition of HIV infection among men who have sex with men: The EXPLORE Randomised Controlled Study. Lancet. 2004;364:41–50.

106. Kelly JA, St. Lawrence JS, Hood HV, Brasfield TL. Behavioral intervention to reduce AIDS risk activities. J Consult Clin Psychol. 1989;57:60–7.

107. Wilton L, Herbst JH, Coury-Doniger P, Painter TM, English G, Alvarez ME, Scahill M, Roberson MA, Lucas B, Johnson WD, Carey JW. Efficacy of an HIV/STI Prevention Intervention for Black Men Who Have Sex with Men: Findings from the many men, many voices (3MV) Project. AIDS Behav. 2009;13:532–44.

108. Kegeles SM, Hays RB, Coates TJ. The Mpowerment Project: A Community-level HIV Prevention Intervention for Young Gay Men. Am J Public Health. 1996;86:1129–36.

109. Dilley JW, Woods WJ, Sabatino J, Lihatsh T, Adler B, Casey S, Rinaldi J, Brand R, McFarland W. Changing sexual behavior among gay male repeat testers for HIV: A randomized, controlled trial of a single-session intervention. J Acquir Immune Defic Syndr. 2002;30:177–86.

110. Kelly JA, St Lawrence JS, Diaz YE, Stevenson LY, Hauth AC, Brasfield TL, Kalichman SC, Smith JE, Andrew ME. HIV Risk Behavior Reduction Following Intervention with Key Opinion Leaders of Population: An Experimental Analysis. Am J Public Health. 1991;81:168–71.

111. Kelly J. Popular Opinion Leaders and HIV Peer Education: Resolving Discrepant Findings, and Implications for the Implementation of Effective Community Programmes. AIDS Care. 2004;16: 139–50.

112. Seal DW, Kelly JA, Bloom FR, Stevenson LY, Coley BI, Broyles LA. HIV prevention with young men who have sex with men: What young men themselves say is needed. AIDS Care. 2000;12:5–26.

113. Rotheram-Borus M, Swendeman D, Comulada S, Weiss RE, Lee M, Lightfoot M. Prevention for Substance-using HIV positive young people: telephone and in-person delivery. J Acquir Immune Defic Syndr. 2004;37:S68–77.

114. Healthy Living Project Team. Effects of a behavioral intervention to reduce risk of transmission among people living with HIV: The Healthy Living Project randomized controlled study. J Acquir Immune Defic Syndr. 2007;44:213–21.

115. Kalichman SC, Rompa D, Cage M, et al. Effectiveness of an intervention to reduce HIV transmission risk in HIV-positive people. Am J Prev Med. 2001;21: 84–92.

116. Kalichman SC, Rompa D, Cage M. Group intervention to reduce HIV transmission risk behavior among persons living with HIV-AIDS. Behav Modif. 2005;29:256–85.

117. Gilbert P, Ciccarone D, Gansky SA, Bangsberg DR, Clanon K, McPhee SJ, et al. Interactive "Video Doctor" counseling reduces drug and sexual risk behaviors among HIV-positive patients in diverse outpatient settings. PLoS One. 2008;3:1–10.

118. CDC AIDS Community Demonstration Projects Research Group. Community-level HIV intervention in 5 cities: Final outcome data from the CDC AIDS Community Demonstration Projects. Am J Public Health. 1999;89:336–45.

119. Centers for Disease Control and Prevention. Community-level prevention of human immunodeficiency virus infection among high-risk populations: The AIDS Community Demonstration Projects. MMWR Recomm Rep. 1996;45:1–24.

120. Richardson JL, Milam J, McCutchan A, Stoyanoff S, Bolan R, Weiss J, et al. Effect of brief safer-sex counseling by medical providers to HIV-1 seropositive patients: A multi-clinic assessment. AIDS. 2004;18:1179–86.

121. Rotheram-Borus MJ, Lee MB, Murphy DA, Futterman D, Duan N, Birnbaum JM, et al. Efficacy of a preventive intervention for youths living with HIV. Am J Public Health. 2001;91:400–5.

122. Rotheram-Borus M, Murphy DA, Coleman C, Swendeman D. Counseling adolescents: Designing interventions to target routines, relationships, roles, and stages of adaptation. In: Chesney MA, Antoni MH, editors. *Innovative Approaches to Health Psychology: Prevention and Treatment Lessons from AIDS*. Washington, DC: American Psychology Association; 2002. p. 15–44.

123. Rotheram-Borus M, Murphy DA, Wight RG, Lee MB, Lightfoot M, Swendeman D, et al. Improving the quality of life among young people living with HIV. Eval Prog Planning. 2001;24:227–37.

124. Catalano RF, Berglund ML, Ryan JAM, Lonczak HS, Hawkins JD. Positive youth development in the United States: Research findings on evaluations of positive youth development programs. Ann Am Acad Polit Soc Sci. 2004;591:98–124.

125. Roth JL, Brooks-Gunn J. What exactly is a youth development program? Answers from research and practice. Appl Dev Sci. 2003;7:94–111.

126. Gavin LE, Catalano RF, David-Ferdon C, Gloppen KM, Markham CM. A review of positive youth development programs that promote adolescent sexual and reproductive health. J Adolesc Health. 2010;46:S75–91.

127. Stall R, Friedman MS, Catania JA. Interacting epidemics and gay men's health: A theory of syndemic production among urban gay men. In: Wolitski RJ, Stall R, Valdiserri RO, editors. Unequal opportunity: health disparities affecting gay and bisexual men in the United States. New York, NY: Oxford University Press; 2008. p. 251–74.

Social Determinants of Sexual Health in the USA Among Racial and Ethnic Minorities

14

Hazel D. Dean and Ranell L. Myles

Introduction

Despite improvements in the prevention, diagnosis, and treatment of HIV/AIDS and other sexually transmitted infections (STI), racial and ethnic minority populations continue to experience disproportionately higher rates and increasing numbers of persons diagnosed with STIs. For example, in 37 states with mature HIV surveillance systems, there were 35,526 persons ≥13 years old who received diagnoses of HIV in 2009, 71% of whom were racial and ethnic minorities [1]. Further disparities were also observed among persons reported with syphilis, gonorrhea, and Chlamydia. In 2009, more than 70% of syphilis, 82% of gonorrhea, and 71% of Chlamydia cases were among racial and ethnic minorities [2].

As the nation's population becomes more racially and ethnically diverse, there must be increased public health efforts to understand structural and social factors that place individuals

in these communities at elevated risks for STIs [3]. Public health officials are increasingly promoting the importance of measuring, monitoring, and linking social determinants of health variables to health outcome data [4, 5]. The results can then be used to understand structural and social influences on disease acquisition and transmission and develop impactful programs to reduce physical and sexual health disparities [3, 6].

In this chapter, we explore how the sexual health of various racial/ethnic groups is influenced by structural and social determinants and provide examples of the impact of key societal systems on the ability of racial and ethnic minorities to achieve optimal sexual health. First, we describe Federal government definitions of racial and ethnic groups and provide a synopsis of national standards for the collection and reporting of racial and ethnic data. We also define demographic and social characteristics of racial and ethnic minorities in the United States. Second, we use national surveillance data for the four reportable STIs—Chlamydia, HIV, gonorrhea, and syphilis—to highlight disparities among racial and ethnic groups. Third, we then discuss determinants of population health and focus specifically on structural and social determinants of health and the intersection with sexual health. In the fourth section, we introduce a framework to describe determinants of sexual health highlighting major systems influences on the sexual health of minorities. We then discuss how systems-based approaches can improve sexual health and reduce

Disclaimer
The findings and conclusions in this report are those of the authors and do not necessarily represent the official position of the Centers for Disease Control and Prevention.

H.D. Dean, Sc.D., M.P.H. (✉) • R.L. Myles, M.P.H.
National Center for HIV/AIDS, Viral Hepatitis, STD, and TB Prevention, Centers for Disease Control and Prevention, 1600 Clifton Rd., NE, MS E-07, Atlanta, GA 30333, USA
e-mail: hdd0@cdc.gov

S.O. Aral, K.A. Fenton, and J.A. Lipshutz (eds.), *The New Public Health and STD/HIV Prevention: Personal, Public and Health Systems Approaches*, DOI 10.1007/978-1-4614-4526-5_14,
© Springer Science+Business Media New York 2013

rates of the four reportable STIs among racial and ethnic minorities in the USA. Finally, we summarize the material presented and recommend actions to move forward to improve the sexual health of racial and ethnic minorities in the USA.

Demographic and Social Characteristics of Racial and Ethnic Minorities in the USA

The Collection and Reporting of Racial/Ethnic Data

In the USA, data on race and ethnicity are collected in part to describe distributions of social, demographic, health, and economic characteristics in racial/ethnic subgroups and changes in these distributions over time. In public health, racial/ethnic data are used to describe the current health of a population and the likelihood of various health outcomes among members of a population, and to identify populations in need of improved health services.

To promote consistency in how data for various racial and ethnic groups are collected and reported by federal agencies, the Office of Management and Budget (OMB) requires Federal agencies to use racial/ethnic classifications. These standards include five race groups—white, black or African-American, American Indian or Alaska Native, Asian, and Native Hawaiian or Other Pacific Islander—and a minimum of two categories for ethnicity: Hispanic or Latino and Not Hispanic or Latino. Hispanics/Latinos may be of any race. Respondents to self-administered surveys can select one or more races when they self-identify [7].

Standard Definitions for Racial and Ethnic Groups

Race categories as defined by OMB reflect racial self-identification according to the race or races with which the person most closely identifies. OMB defines race as follows: White persons originate from any of "the original peoples of Europe, the Middle East, or North Africa." Black or African Americans have "origins in any of the Black racial groups of Africa." American Indian and Alaska Natives have origins in any of the "original peoples of North and South America (including Central America) and who maintain tribal affiliation or community attachment." Asians have origins in any of "the original peoples of the Far East, Southeast Asia, or the Indian subcontinent." Native Hawaiian and Other Pacific Islanders have origins in any of "the original peoples of Hawaii, Guam, Samoa, or other Pacific Islands" [7].

Race and Hispanic Origin in the US 2010 Census

According to the US Census, 308,059,724 people were living in the USA in 2010. Of these, 63.7% were classified as white, 12.6% as black, 4.8% as Asian, 0.9% as American Indian or Alaska Native, and 0.2% Native Hawaiian or other Pacific Islander. People of Hispanic origin or ethnicity can be of any race. In 2010, 16.3% of the US population self-identified as Hispanic [8]. The 2010 Census indicates that between 2000 and 2010 the Hispanic population grew by 43%, accounting for more than half of the total population growth in the USA [9]. If these trends continue, by 2050, the Hispanic population is projected to make up 29% of the US population, and whites will become a minority group (47%) [10].

Social Characteristics of US Racial and Ethnic Minority Groups

Several interrelated social conditions associated with race/ethnicity have a significant impact on US residents' access to adequate housing, employment opportunities, voting power, education, public services, and environmental and social networks. These "conditions in which people are born, grow, live, work, and age, including (the quality of) the health system (available to them)" are commonly referred to as "social determinants of health" and are considered to be contributing factors for inequities in health [11]. Five major determinants of population health include: genes and biology, health behaviors, medical care, social/societal characteristics, and total ecology; more than half of population health is determined by social/societal characteristics and total ecology [12].

Social determinants of health can also be described in the context of the physical, social, and personal resources that people have to cope with the economic and social conditions that influence their health [13]. These resources include but are not limited to "conditions for early childhood development; education, employment, and work; food security, health services, housing, income, and income distribution; social exclusion; the social safety net; and unemployment and job security" [13]. Inequities in the distribution of these resources have contributed to health inequities among racial/ethnic groups in the USA. Social determinants not only differ by racial/ethnic minority groups, but these differences can have an adverse impact on them compared to whites. Because minorities experience greater disparities in most health outcomes, including STIs, these differential determinants affect some groups more adversely than others. Some of these conditions are explained below as they relate to the different racial/ethnic groups outlined in this chapter.

Heterogeneity Within Minority Groups

While racial/ethnic minority groups differ in many ways across groups and from whites, differences within groups are rarely acknowledged, discussed, or researched. Racial/ethnic minority groups are heterogeneous and within each group are varying socioeconomic status, geographical origins/locations, education, and religion [14–16]. Analyses that examine disparities across groups assume there is homogeneity within racial/ethnic groups, however not acknowledging the heterogeneity within each OMB designated racial category can impede research on health inequities [17]. For example, between 2003 and 2006, shorter HIV-to-AIDS diagnosis intervals were more common among Hispanics born in Mexico than those born in the USA [18]. Similarly, the epidemiology of HIV infection differs for foreign-born blacks compared to native-born blacks; foreign-born blacks are more likely than native-born blacks to be diagnosed with AIDS within 1 year of their HIV diagnoses [19].

According to the American Community Survey, in 2007, 12.6% of the US population was foreign born [20]. Of all foreign-born people, 48% were Hispanic, as were 10% of the native born population. Regardless of nativity, 64% of Hispanics in the USA reported being from Mexico, with the next most common countries of origin being from Cuba, El Salvador, the Dominican Republic, Guatemala, and Columbia. Eight percent of the US black population was foreign-born, with 54% from the Caribbean (including Jamaica, Haiti, and Trinidad and Tobago), 34% from Africa (including Nigeria, Ethiopia, and Ghana), and 5% from South America [20].

Among Asians, 67% reported being foreign-born, with China, the Philippines, India, Vietnam, and Korea being the most common countries or origin. Among the American Indian and Alaska Native (AI/AI) population, 77% were born in countries in Central America, mostly Mexico, but also Guatemala, El Salvador, Honduras, and others. An additional 5% of AI/AIs were from Canada. Of the Native Hawaiians and other Pacific Islanders, only 5% were foreign-born, primarily from the Philippines, Vietnam, Korea, or Canada. Among people who indicated being of some other race, 81% were from countries in Central America [20].

Geography, Segregation, and Home Ownership

Geographically, racial/ethnic minority populations are concentrated in the Western, South western, and Southern regions of the USA. Other states in which minorities accounted for at least 37% of the population in 2004–2005 included Illinois, Michigan, New York, and Maryland [21]. Racial/ethnic minorities also tend to be concentrated in certain neighborhoods as a result of residential segregation, which has several consequences that may contribute to poorer health among residents of these neighborhoods. These include fewer employment opportunities, lower income, poorer schools, lower test scores among students in these schools, higher dropout rates, and higher rates of teen pregnancy [22, 23]. Racial disparities in health might be influenced by the lack of infrastructures (employment, better schools, etc.) that would mitigate against these factors that impact good health. [24]

Segregation continues to be a predictor of significant health disparities. In addition, high-poverty neighborhoods disproportionately house poor blacks and Hispanics. Even though blacks make up just 12% of the population, one-third of people living in metropolitan high-poverty tracts are black and one-third are Hispanic who make up 16% of the population [25]. Research has found that, "although residential segregation is decreasing, the relationship between segregation and infant mortality disparities appears to have intensified in recent years." [24] LaVeist and colleagues found that with full racial integration, racial gaps in rates of infant mortality among blacks would decrease by 2.31 per 1,000 live births, and Hispanics would have a lower infant mortality than whites. [24] In another study about racial/ethnic segregation, Acevedo-Garcia and colleagues found that 76% of all black children and 9% of all Latino children in the USA (regardless of whether they were poor) lived in neighborhoods with higher poverty rates than those in neighborhoods where the poorest white children lived [23]. Many black and Latino children experience multiple disadvantages related to segregation that poor white children do not, including attending poor-performing schools, being exposed to high rates of crime, living in substandard housing, and having limited access to grocery stores with healthy food choices, all of which are factors associated with poor health [23].

Home ownership has also been associated with better general health and lower risk for STIs among adults and adolescents. Compared with renters, homeowners were more likely to be married or widowed, to have less frequent sexual intercourse, to have higher self-satisfaction and self-esteem, to have higher self ratings of health, and to be less likely to approve of premarital and teenage sexual intercourse [26]. Homeowners have also been found to have better overall physical and psychological health and a higher overall level of happiness [27]. According to the 2010 Census, the overall home ownership rate in the USA was 66.9% but differed substantially by race/ethnicity: 71% among whites, 52.3% among AI/ANs, 58.9% among Asians/Native Hawaiians/Other Pacific Islanders, 47.5% among Hispanics, and 45.4% among blacks [28].

Family Composition

The composition of families also varies by race/ethnicity. Using the National Survey of Family Growth, Taylor et al. found that married respondents across all racial/ethnic had the lowest rates of sexual risk behaviors [29]. In addition, they found that marital status attenuated the association between race and STI risk for blacks; however, even in marriage, the prevalence of some sexual risk behaviors was higher for blacks than other races [29]. In 2010, 51.3% of people over 15 were married. Marriage was highest among Asians (61.4%), whites (55.5%), and Hispanics (46.0%); and blacks were the least likely to be married (32.0%).

Incarceration

Of 785,586 people who were inmates in local US jails throughout the USA in 2007, 42.5% were white, 39.2% black, and 16.4% Hispanic [30]. Of the more than two million people who were inmates in the federal prison system in 2009, 39.4% were black, 34.2% were white, and 20.6% were Hispanic [31]. Because blacks and Hispanics constitute less than half of the US population but nearly two thirds of the incarcerated population, it is important to understand how incarceration and a criminal record affects their lives in many ways. A criminal history affects one's ability to get a job and to vote in elections, and directly impacts employment, financial stability, and becoming a contributing member of society. Imprisonment places economic, emotional, and physical constraints on the family and loved ones of those incarcerated.

Employment

According to the Bureau of Labor Statistics, the 2010 national unemployment rate was 9.6% and varied substantially by race/ethnicity: 16.0% among blacks, 12.5% among Hispanics, 8.7% among whites, and 7.5% among Asians [32]. Not only do blacks and Hispanics have substantially higher unemployment rates than whites and Asians, but they are also less likely to have relatively high-paying jobs classified as managerial or professional. In the 2010 workforce population, 47.0% of Asians and 37.9% of whites were employed in such occupations, compared with 29.1% of blacks and 18.9% of Hispanics. Conversely, 16.4% of Hispanics 15.0% of blacks were employed in generally lower paying jobs classified as "production" or "transportation," whereas only 11.3% of whites and 10.0% of Asians were employed in such jobs [32]. Unemployment rates are generally lower for people with bachelor's degrees or higher (4.7% in 2010). However, disparate rates of unemployment for people of color with a bachelor's degree or higher were: 7.9% for blacks, 6.0% for Hispanics, 5.5% for Asians, and 4.3% for whites. Intersected with gender, black men with higher education have the highest unemployment rate of all groups at 9.2% [32]. This poses a unique challenge for black men who pursue higher education because they are at a disadvantage for employment upon graduation compared to other groups and often have accumulated student loan debt.

Income and Wealth

Disparities in health are often associated racial/ethnic differences, but actually, differences in health by socioeconomic status (SES) are generally larger than differences by race/ethnicity and explain more of the variance in health status [33]. Historically, blacks have experienced disproportionately lower median incomes than any other group. While the recession has resulted in income losses for all groups, in 2010, disparities remained in the average earnings of Asians ($64,308), Whites ($54,620), Hispanics ($37,759), and blacks ($32,068) [34].

Looking at income alone does not paint a clear enough picture of how much money is actually available to use. Another way to determine a person's economic well-being is to look at their net worth, defined as the difference between assets and liabilities. The level of wealth alludes to the available resources for emergencies, sickness, job loss, etc. There are disparities in net worth by race and ethnicity. A recent study by the Pew Research Center revealed that wealth gaps between whites, blacks, and Hispanics are at record highs. In addition, the housing market crisis in 2006 followed by the recession took a greater toll on the wealth of minorities than whites. In 2009, the median net worth was $5,677 for blacks, $6,325 for Hispanics, $113,149 for whites. Declines in net worth from 2005 to 2009 were greatest for Hispanics (66%) and blacks (53%), and modest for whites whose net worth only fell 16% [35].

Healthcare

Racial/ethnic minorities were more likely to report being in fair or poor health, to have higher mortality rates than whites, and to be disproportionately affected by several other life conditions. In self-reports of health status, American Indians/Alaskan Natives (16.5%), blacks (14.6%), Hispanics (13.3%), and people of two or more races (12.6%) were more likely to report fair or poor health. At each stage of the life cycle, Hispanics, blacks, American Indians/Alaska Natives and whites have higher mortality rates than Asians and Native Hawaiians/Pacific Islanders. Blacks followed by American Indian/Alaskan Natives have the highest rates of mortality [36].

In 2010, 16.3% of the nation did not have health insurance but there were substantial variations in coverage among racial/ethnic minorities. As compared to 11.7% of whites without health insurance in 2010, the lack of health insurance was: 30.7% among Hispanics, 20.8% among blacks, and 18.1% among Asians [34]. These data were not reported for Native Hawaiians/Other Pacific Islanders or American Indian/Alaskan Natives for 2010, however 2008 data showed similar disproportions in lack of health insurance; 18% among Native Hawaiians/Other Pacific Islanders and 30.7% among American Indian/Alaskan Natives. [37] There are also similar substantial disparities in the accessibility, utilization, and quality of health care [38]. Smedley argued that in order to make access to high-quality health care in the USA more equitable, "policymakers must attend to structural and community-level problems, such as the misdistribution of health care resources, the lack of effective mechanisms for underserved communities to participate in health care planning, and the presence of cultural and linguistic barriers in health care settings." [39]

A study in 2004 revealed that all people of color were less likely than whites to have a usual place to receive health care and to have had a healthcare visit in the last year, and more likely to experience worse care than whites [40]. Similarly, Kaiser issued a report in 2006 indicating that most whites felt that blacks and Latinos received the same quality of medical care as did whites. Most blacks and Latinos, however, indicated that they feel the quality of medical care they receive compared to whites, is lower [36]. People of color are more likely to be unemployed, have lower income, and have lower paying jobs [36]. These intersections of race, class, and healthcare access are extremely important considerations that should not be overlooked when addressing sexual health.

In summary, members of US racial/ethnic minority groups (other than Asians) are in general more likely than whites to have life experiences associated with elevated risks for multiple health problems, including HIV/AIDS and other STIs.

Sexually Transmitted Infections Among Racial and Ethnic Minorities

This section highlights the disproportionate rates of HIV/AIDS and other STIs as well as other infections among racial/ethnic minorities. Unless otherwise indicated all statistics reported for the four reportable STIs in this section come from the 2009 STD Surveillance Report or the 2009 HIV/AIDS Surveillance Report; national surveillance data collected by the US Centers for Disease Control and Prevention [1, 2]. For diagnoses of HIV infection, we used data reported from 40

states with confidential name-based HIV infection surveillance since at least January 2006. Data for the three remaining reportable STIs were reported from the 50 states, the District of Columbia, and US Territories.

Disparities in rates of STIs were assessed by using rate ratios and relative percentage difference, two relative measures of disparity recommended by the Centers for Disease Control and Prevention [41]. Rate ratios are customarily used to describe disparities in rates of gonorrhea, syphilis, and chlamydia and relative percentage differences are used to describe disparities in rates of HIV diagnoses [2, 42]. Relative disparity measures are useful to assess the impact of disparity elimination programs and to inform policy development [41].

The rate ratio describes the rate for the group of interest as a multiple of the reference group rate. It is calculated by dividing the rate in the group of interest by the rate in the reference group. The relative percentage difference was calculated as the ([{rate of interest − rate among referent group}/rate among referent group] X100). For both disparities measures, we used rates among whites as the referent group because whites typically have the lowest or second-lowest STI diagnosis rates. Below we describe disparities in rates of rates of the four reportable STIs stratified by racial and ethnic group.

African-Americans/Blacks

Mostly blacks carry the burden of STIs in the USA as they have the highest STI case rates reported to the Centers for Disease Control and Prevention (Gonorrhea, Chlamydia, Syphilis, and HIV). Therefore, a special emphasis will be placed on the black experience throughout this chapter. In 2009, the gonorrhea rate among blacks was more than 20 times higher than that of whites (556.4 cases per 100,000 vs. 27.2 per 100,000). Considering all racial, ethnic, and age categories, gonorrhea rates were highest for blacks aged 15–19 (1955.8 per 100,000) and 20–24 (2356.7 per 100,000) in 2009. The highest rate ratio was among black women aged 15–19 years who also had the highest rate of gonorrhea compared to everyone (2,613.8 per 100,000), 16.7 times higher than the rate among white women in the same age group (156.7 per 100,000). Black men aged 15–19 years had the highest rate ratio of all men compared to whites, their rates were 38.3 times higher than whites (1,316.4 per 100,000 vs. 34.4 per 100,000). Among men and women aged 20–24 years, the gonorrhea rate among blacks was 17.8 times higher than the rate among whites (2,356.7 per 100,000 and 132.2 per 100,000, respectively) [2].

The chlamydia rate among blacks in 2009 was nearly nine times higher than that of whites (1,559.1 per 100,000 vs. 178.8 per 100,000). By gender, the rate of Chlamydia among black women was nearly eight times higher than the rate among white women (2,095.5 and 270.2 per 100,000 women, respectively). The Chlamydia rate among black men was almost 12 times as high as the rate among white men (970.0 and 84.0 cases per 100,000 men, respectively) [2].

The primary and secondary (P&S) syphilis rate among blacks was about nine times higher than that of whites in 2009 (19.2 cases per 100,000 versus 2.1 per 100,000). Rate ratios reveal that while the highest case rate of P&S is among black men and women aged 20–24, the highest disparities are among those aged 15–19. The 2009 rate among black men aged 15–19 years (28.3 per 100,000) was 26 times higher than for white men (1.1). In 2009, rates were 29 times higher for black women aged 15–19 years (17.1 per 100,000) than for white women (0.6 per 100,000) of the same age [2].

Lastly, in 2009, blacks were estimated to account for 52% of all diagnoses of HIV infection (recall in 2009 they only made up ~12% of the US population). The rate of diagnoses of HIV infection among blacks was 66.6 per 100,000, 9 times higher than the rate for whites (7.2 per 100,000). The estimated rate of diagnoses of HIV infection among black men (122.2 per 100,000 population) was more than 8 times higher than the rate for whites (14.8 per 100,000). The rate of diagnoses of HIV infection among black women (47.8 per 100,000) was nearly 20 times as high as the rate for white women (2.4 per 100,000) [1].

Hispanics

In 2009, Hispanics also experienced notable disparities across all reportable STDs. The rate of reported gonorrhea infections among Hispanics was more than twice that of whites (58.6 per 100,000 vs. 27.2 per 100,000). The overall rate of Chlamydia was almost three times higher among Hispanics than whites (504.2 per 100,000 vs. 178.8 per 100,000). The rate of reported P&S syphilis cases among Hispanics was double that of whites (4.5 per 100,000 vs. 2.1 per 100,000). The rate of diagnoses of HIV infection among Hispanics was 22.8 per 100,000, more than 3 times higher than the rate for whites (7.2 per 100,000) [1, 2].

American Indian/Alaska Natives

In 2009, American Indian/Alaska Natives were also disproportionately affected by STDs. Gonorrhea rates among American Indian/Alaska Natives were 4.2 times higher than those of whites (113.3 per 100,000 vs. 27.2 per 100,000). Chlamydia rates were 4.3 times higher among American Indian/Alaska Natives than among whites (776.5 per 100,000 vs. 178.8 per 100,000). The rate of reported P&S syphilis among American Indian/Alaska Natives was nearly comparable to that of whites (2.4 cases per 100,000 versus 2.1 per 100,000). The rate of diagnoses of HIV infection among American Indians/Alaska Natives was 9.8 per 100,000, 1.4 times higher than the rate for whites (7.2 per 100,000) [1, 2].

Asian and Pacific Islanders

In 2009, Asian and Pacific Islanders experienced more favorable rates than whites for most of the four reportable STIs. The rate of reported gonorrhea infections among Asian and Pacific Islanders was lower than whites (18.1 per 100,000 vs. 27.2). Chlamydia rates were also lower among Asian and Pacific Islanders than whites (149.9 per 100,000 vs. 178.8). The rate of reported P&S

syphilis cases among Asian and Pacific Islanders was 1.6 per 100,000 compared to 2.1 among whites. Reporting of HIV diagnosis disaggregates Asians and Pacific Islanders where Asians are reported as a single group and Pacific Islanders are grouped with Native Hawaiians. The rate of diagnoses of HIV infection among Asians was lower than the rate for whites (6.4 per 100,000 vs. 7.2). Conversely, Native Hawaiian and Pacific Islanders experienced a nearly 3 times higher rate of HIV diagnoses than whites (21.0 per 100,000) [1, 2].

Relative Percentage Difference

During 2009, the relative percentage difference in STI diagnosis rates among blacks compared to whites was higher across all STIs. For the four STIs, the relative percentage differences were 1945, 825, 814 and 772% for gonorrhea, primary and secondary syphilis, HIV, and Chlamydia, respectively. The next highest relative differences were for Chlamydia (334%) and gonorrhea (317%) among American Indian/Alaska Natives. Asians had STI diagnosis rates lower than whites for all STIs (decrease in relative percentage difference: 11% for HIV; 17% for Chlamydia; 24% for primary and secondary syphilis, and 34% for gonorrhea) [2]. (Table 14.1)

With the exception of blacks, disparities of racial/ethnic minorities compared to whites have been relatively stable over the past 4–5 years, or have decreased. For example, in 2006, the rate ratio indicated that for rates of HIV diagnoses, blacks were 8.9 times higher than whites, and in 2009 they were 9.3 times higher than whites. All other groups maintained stable disparity rates except for Native Hawaiian and Pacific Islanders who had 4.2 times higher HIV diagnoses rates than whites in 2006 and 2.9 times the rate of whites in 2009. There is a similar trend for blacks in gonorrhea and P&S syphilis disparities as well. In 2005, rates of gonorrhea and P&S syphilis among blacks were 17.6 and 5.4 times higher than whites, and in 2009 were 20.5 and 9.1 times higher than whites. This suggests that disparities are widening for blacks.

Table 14.1 Rates of human immunodeficiency virus (HIV) infections, Chlamydia, Gonorrhea, and Primary and Secondary Syphilis by Race/ethnicity, 2009

	2009 rate	Relative difference (%)
Human immunodeficiency virus (HIV)		
American Indian/Alaska Native	9.8	36.1
Asian	6.4	−11.1
Black/African American	66.6	825.0
Hispanic/Latino	22.8	216.7
Native Hawaiian/other Pacific Islander	21.0	191.7
White	7.2	–
Chlamydia		
American Indian/Alaska Native	776.5	334.3
Asian or Pacific Islander	149.0	−16.7
Black/African American	1559.1	772.0
Hispanic/Latino	504.2	182.0
White	178.8	–
Gonorrhea		
American Indian/Alaska Native	113.3	316.5
Asian/Pacific Islander	18.1	−33.5
Black/African American	556.4	1,945.6
Hispanic/Latino	58.6	115.4
White	27.2	–
Primary and Secondary Syphilis		
American Indian/Alaska Native	2.4	14.3
Asian/Pacific Islander	1.6	−23.8
Black/African American	19.2	814.3
Hispanic/Latino	4.5	114.3
White	2.1	–

Another important consideration in the discussion of STIs among racial/ethnic minorities is the geographic distribution of STI rates. In 2009, rates of HIV diagnosis were highest among the southeastern part of the USA ranging from 17.1 to 33 cases per 100,000 population. States with the highest rates include but are not limited to: Texas, Louisiana, Mississippi, Georgia, Florida, North Carolina, South Carolina, Tennessee, etc. Chlamydia, gonorrhea, and P&S syphilis rates are also highest in the southeastern pats of the USA. According to the US Census, The black population is concentrated largely in the southeastern states and urban areas [1, 2, 43]. In summary, national STI surveillance data from 2009 indicate persistent and severe racial disparities in STI rates among most racial and ethnic minority groups. Blacks/African-Americans experienced a disproportionate burden across all four reportable STIs.

Determinants of Population Health and Social Determinants of Sexual Health

Social Determinants of Health

The World Health Organization (WHO) defines social determinants of health as the social and economic factors and conditions that affect the health and well-being of people and communities. A number of these conditions are discussed in section II as they relate to the social characteristics and experiences of racial/ethnic minorities in the USA. Part of understanding how social determinants of health work is knowing that these conditions are shaped by the distribution of money, power, and resources, which are, in turn, influenced by policy choices [44]. Social determinants of health (hereafter referred to as SDH) are divided into three categories—social environment, physical environment, and health services.

The social environment includes employment status and occupation type, level of educational attainment, income, and country of birth. The social environment could also include race/ethnicity because social forces such as racism, discrimination, and segregation may mediate certain stages of the disease process—infection, diagnosis, treatment, and outcome. The second category of social determinants of health, the physical environment, includes housing status, incarceration status, area of residence, residential segregation, and population density. Lastly, the health services category includes factors such as health insurance status, access to care, quality of care, or vaccination status.

The World Health Commission on Social Determinants of Health Model

In an effort to reveal the impact of and address social determinants of health on a global scale, The WHO Commission on Social Determinants of Health (CSDH) was created. The WHO CSDH developed a model to describe the interaction of the following elements: socioeconomic and political context; structural determinants and socioeconomic position; intermediary determinants (includes material circumstances, social-environmental circumstances, behavioral and biological factors, and the healthcare system); a crosscutting determinant that incorporates social cohesion and social capital into the model; and finally the impact on health equity and wellbeing (measured as health outcomes) (Fig. 14.1) [44]. While this model has been used mostly to examine the impact of SDH on chronic diseases, it is adaptable to different diseases, including sexually transmitted infections, which is explained in the next section.

The CSDH model was designed to map specific entry points for intervention or policy development. It proposes a series of actions that could be taken at various operational levels to reduce health disparities. Beginning from the left side of the figure, structural determinants of health inequities are defined as structural social stratification mechanisms, joined to and influenced by institutions and processes embedded in the socioeconomic and political context which gives rise to a set of unequal socioeconomic positions. Within the socioeconomic position domain, groups are stratified according to proxy indicators such as income levels, education, and occupation. Socioeconomic positions then translate into specific determinants of individual health status reflecting the individual's social location within the stratified system. What this means is that a person's socioeconomic position affects his/her health, but this effect is not direct.

Socioeconomic position influences health through more specific intermediary determinants. In the model, they are represented as material circumstances, behaviors and biological factors,

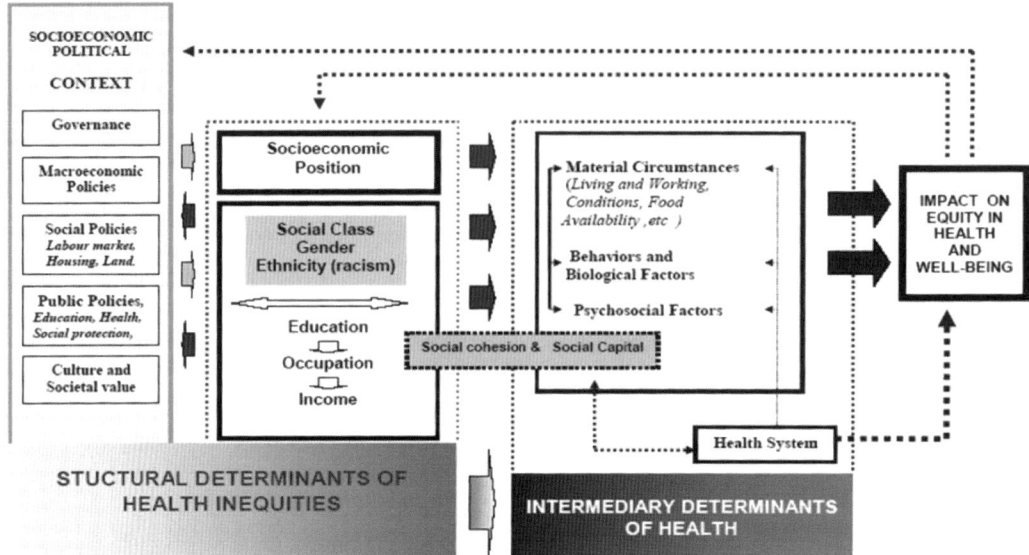

Fig. 14.1 World Health Organization Conceptual Framework for Action on Social Determinants of Health. WHO Commission on Social Determinants of Health, 2007 [44]

and psychosocial factors. This section of the model illustrates that the underlying social determinants of health disparities operate through a set of intermediary determinants of health to shape health outcomes. Included in the intermediary determinant are material circumstances such as living and working conditions and the financial means to buy food or warm clothing. Behavioral and/or biological include factors such as nutrition, physical activity, and tobacco and alcohol consumption. Biological factors also include genetics. Psychosocial factors include factors such as psychosocial stressors, stressful living situations, social support and coping skills.

In this model, the health system is viewed as an intermediary determinant because the health system plays a role in directly addressing differences in exposure and vulnerability by improving equitable access to care and in the promotion of intersectoral action to improve health status. Social cohesion and social capital are crosscutting determinants and cut across both the structural and intermediary dimensions. The dark solid arrows illustrate the impact of social position on each of the levels. The dotted arrows are feedback mechanisms signifying differential social, economic and health consequences.

The CSDH framework specifies entry points for intervention or policy development and proposes a series of actions that could be taken at various operational levels to reduce health disparities. For example, addressing structural determinants to reduce health disparities may require action at the governmental or multiagency level [45]. We adapt this model for use in describing determinants of sexual health associated with racial/ethnic disparities in rates of HIV/AIDS and other STIs. The next section of the chapter provides a definition for social determinants of sexual health and describes key attributes of a conceptual framework to address disparities in sexual health among racial and ethnic minorities in the USA.

Social Determinants of Sexual Health

Social determinants of sexual health are defined here as the range of the social and economic factors known to influence and contribute to sexual health. *The Conceptual Model of Social Determinants of Sexual Health and Health Inequities* illustrates key attributes and inputs to address health equity for populations most

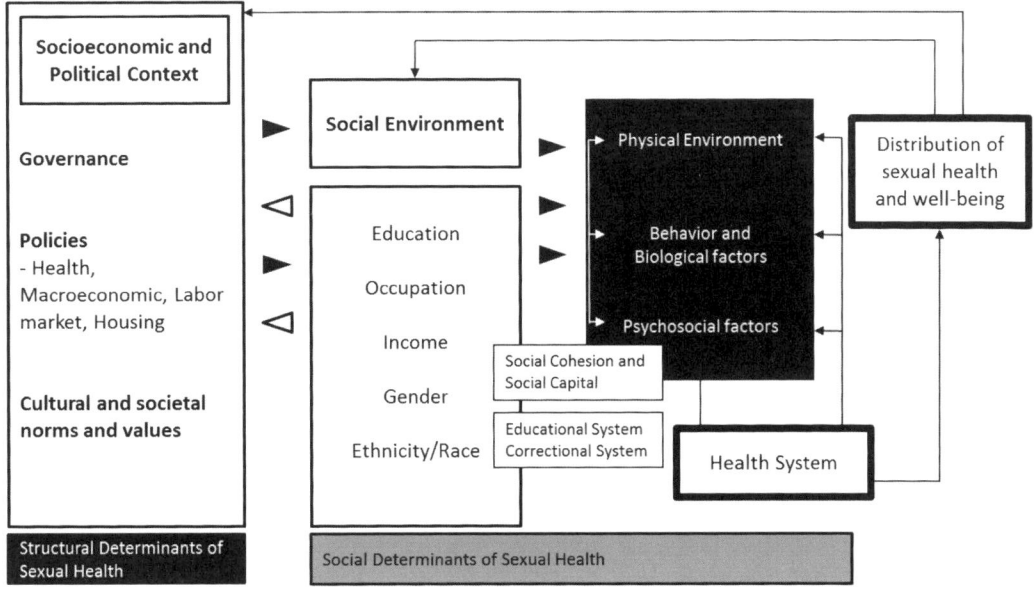

Fig. 14.2 Conceptual Model of Social Determinants of Sexual Health. Adapted from the World Health Organization's Model of Social Determinants of Health and Equity, 2007 (See Fig. 14.1)

adversely affected by STIs. For this section, we operationalize the model focusing on one population group—African Americans or blacks—because of the extremely high rates of all reportable STIs in this population. We then discuss specific systems-based interventions that may be implemented to reduce rates of STIs in this population.

The range of structural and social determinants contributing to sexual health include: laws and policies that influence the socioeconomic and political context of sexual health and well-being; social position, social cohesion and social capital, behavioral and biological factors, material circumstances, and psychosocial factors. There are three cross-cutting intermediary determinants—educational, correctional, and health system (Fig. 14.2).

Description of the Conceptual Model

The model begins with the structural determinants of sexual health on the left. The structural determinants of sexual health encompass the socioeconomic and political context, which includes

governance, the influence of policies, and the influence of cultural and societal norms and values. Examples of such policies include providing access to health care, encouraging HIV testing, implementing syringe exchange programs, and funding reproductive health services. Cultural and societal norms and values include stigma, discrimination, gender differences in health prevention, access, and treatment, and homophobia. Also included in this section is community empowerment, specifically, community participation, acceptance and ownership in the development of sustainable policies and practices.

The second part of the model illustrates the social determinants of sexual health which encompasses the social environment and other factors related to the physical environment, behavioral and biological factors, and psychosocial factors. The social environment includes: income, education, occupation, sexuality, gender, and ethnicity (racism). Within this section of the model, there are also intermediary determinants that mediate the effects of the social environment and include social cohesion and social capital, and the educational and correctional systems. Variations in each aspect of the model have an impact on the distribution of sexual health and well-being among the population. Examples for selected domains of the model are described below.

Structural Determinants of Sexual Health

Socioeconomic and Political Context

Issues related to governance and policies, as well as cultural and societal norms and values can play a significant role in sexual health. In recent years, there have been successful efforts to increase the enactment of laws and policies to improve the health of all Americans, many of which contain specific provisions that may influence sexual health. Government-led initiatives such as the Patient Protection and Affordable Care Act, National Prevention Strategy, and National HIV/AIDS Strategy all include key provisions related to reducing disparities and promoting health equity by addressing social determinants of health [46–48]. These major structural policy initiatives can have an impact on how health care is delivered in the USA, increase use of a social determinants of health approach in public health practice, and likely lead to overall improvements in sexual health among racial and ethnic minorities. A synopsis of initiatives most impactful for reducing sexual health disparities and promoting health equity is presented below.

- The *Patient Protection and Affordable Care Act* contains provisions related to health insurance reform, access to care and quality improvement, health disparities reduction, and a number of new initiatives aimed at reducing health disparities. These initiatives include efforts to strengthen Federal data collection and analysis of racial and ethnic data, primary language spoken, sex, and disability status. The law also provides the US Department of Health and Human Services the opportunity to collect additional demographic data to further improve our understanding of healthcare disparities [49]. Further, the law requires that a National Strategy for Quality Improvement be developed to improve the delivery of health care services, patient outcomes, and reduce health disparities and creates the Patient-Centered Outcomes Research Institute to conduct comparative effectiveness research on health care service outcomes to include impact on racial and ethnic minorities [50].

- The *National Prevention Strategy* was authorized by the Affordable Care Act to help transform the US health care system towards a more prominent focus on prevention and wellness. The Strategy outlines four key areas to foster prevention into communities: (1) building healthy and safe community environments; (2) expanding quality preventive services in clinical and community settings; (3) empowering people to make healthy choices and (4) eliminating health disparities. Additionally, the Strategy identifies sexual and reproductive health as one of seven priorities to improve health and wellness and presents a plan to include other key sectors such as education, transportation, and agriculture to promote health [47].

- The first ever *US National HIV AIDS Strategy (NHAS)* was launched by the White House in 2010. The NHAS seeks to ensure coordination across the federal government and among stakeholders to achieve three primary goals: to reduce the number of new infections; to increase access to care and optimize health outcomes for people living with HIV; and to reduce HIV-related health disparities. The NHAS calls for increased focus on culturally and linguistically appropriate interventions that include effective communication strategies, expansion of HIV testing and diagnosis, and improved access to prevention, care, and treatment services to reduce the number of new HIV infections [48].

Racial/ethnic minorities often view society through different cultural lenses than dominant racial groups or whites in the USA, and these differences translate into a variety of "structural" norms and values that may influence sexual health behavior, or one's sexual network for that matter. Researchers are well aware of the stigma associated with HIV/AIDS and how these attitudes can impact HIV prevention measures [51]. Other cultural and societal norms should also be explored as they relate to experiences of racial/ethnic minorities. For example, a study examining social barriers to STI treatment among respondents in Alabama found that blacks and church-goers were more likely to see STIs as a sign of immorality and that they were therefore more likely to delay or refuse treatment because of embarrassment. Black female church goers were less likely to seek treatment than any other group [52]. Another interesting and timely study illuminated important explicit and implicit ideologies among black heterosexual men and the implications for HIV risk. For explicit ideologies of masculinity among these men, the common theme was that black men should have sex with multiple partners (often concurrently), and should not be gay or bisexual. Implicit ideologies of masculinity included men's perception that they do not have the ability to decline sex, even risky sex, and that women should be held responsible for condom use [53]. While men in this study may not directly articulate these ideologies, and other cultural idioms may not be known among racial/ethnic minorities, it is important to know that these factors may shape positive or negative sexual risk behaviors.

Social Determinants of Sexual Health

Social Environment

The social environment involves several factors that were addressed in the social characteristics section: education occupation, income, gender, and race/ethnicity. For brevity and in light of the recent economic downturn, we focus on economic systems. Recently, there have been declines in the socioeconomic status of racial and ethnic minorities as evidenced by data on wealth among racial and ethnic groups. A recent study by the Pew Foundation found that the white–black wealth gap is the widest since the census began tracking such data in 1984 [35]. Recent Census data show that Whites on average have a net worth 20 times that of blacks and 18 times that of Hispanics [35]. These data further quantify the dismal impact of the economic downturn on racial and ethnic minority communities with

predominantly younger minorities being hit the hardest—the same group most disproportionately impacted by rates of STIs. Income has been shown to play a role in "progression from poor health to worse health." [54]

This intersection of race, class, and disease is very important in assessing sexual health outcomes among blacks. In a California study, Springer and colleagues found a strong positive association between poverty and rates of STIs. Rates among blacks were considerably higher than all other racial/ethnic groups regardless of income. Blacks in the highest poverty category had a six times greater rate of gonorrhea than their white counterparts, emphasizing the need for researchers and policy makers to consider how to address the compounding effects of both identities, being black and living in poverty, to ameliorate health disparities [55].

Physical Environment, Behavioral/Biological and Psychosocial Factors

The broken window theory posits that the appearance of the physical environment regulates individual behavior. In turn, negative physical appearances such as broken windows send a message that no one cares, so behaviors that are usually prohibited are tolerated. Cohen and colleagues found that the same could be said regarding sexual risk behaviors, gonorrhea in particular. They found that the in high poverty neighborhoods, blocks with high broken window scores had significantly higher gonorrhea rates than those with low broken windows scores, and this explained more of the variance in rates of infection than did a poverty index [56]. In another study, researchers examined whether neighborhood economic disadvantage was associated with inconsistent condom use among black youth. Investigators found that contrary to previous studies with aggregated national data, where higher neighborhood economic disadvantage is associated with poorer health, these youth exhibited more condom use [57]. Findings such as these suggest that further research is needed to explore protective structural factors among racial/ethnic minority groups that may be masked in general population studies not focused to measure true racial/ethnic differences.

Social and sexual networks of individuals influence risks of acquiring and transmitting infectious diseases. These networks can serve a supportive role in facilitating reductions in risk of STD acquisition and transmission or may facilitate riskier sexual behaviors [58, 59]. Studies suggest that there are differences between blacks and whites in the type and number of partners they include in their sexual networks [60–62]. In one analysis, the authors conclude that sexually transmitted infections remain high within the black population because they are more likely than other racial and ethnic groups to choose African Americans as partners [63]. Other potential pathways with direct relevance to sexual networks and the transmission of sexually transmitted infections include both factors that alter the ratio of women to men and forces that discourage long-term stable relationships and prevalence of STIs within sexual networks [64, 65].

Cross-Cutting Determinants

In our conceptual model (Fig. 14.2), there are two cross-cutting determinants that mediate the effects of the social environment; social cohesion and social capital, and the education and correctional systems. There are competing definitions for social capital and which type of social capital should be targeted to address health in the WHO model. However, in *The Conceptual Model of Social Determinants of Sexual Health and Health Inequities* social capital may be more concrete in its application. Essentially, there are three approaches that characterize social capital: communitarian (relation between individual health and society), network (resources that flow and emerge through social networks), and resource distribution (psychosocial aspects affecting population health are a consequence of material life conditions) [66]. All three types of approaches can impact sexual health. Though not easily defined, social cohesion is often characterized by social trust, reciprocity, and the concern for the well-being of one's community; it can be measured by voting participation, number of cultural voluntary associations, and can sometimes involve

social relations [67]. According to The WHO CSDH, income inequality can erode social cohesion; the "social bonds that allow people to work together, decrease social resources, resulting in less trust and civic participation, greater crime, and other unhealthy conditions." [66] The educational and correctional systems are also important examples of these cross-cutting determinants. Both of these mediating factors are explained below in reference to their impact on sexual health disparities among racial/ethnic minorities.

Social Cohesion and Social Capital

The social networks mentioned in the section above are related to the cross cutting determinants of social cohesion and social capital. Social capital has also been linked to health status. Holtgrave and Crosby found that social capital was significantly correlated with gonorrhea, syphilis, chlamydia, and AIDS case rates, and found it to be a stronger predictor than income. Social capital was measured using a combination of variables including community organizational life, involvement in public affairs, volunteerism, informal sociability, and social trust [68]. Another study identified neighborhood social cohesion (the trust, caring, and willingness to help among adults, as well as the collective monitoring of youth by neighborhood adults through informal supervision mechanisms) as a source of impact on risk for STIs and condom use among adolescents [69].

Educational and Correctional Systems

Higher levels of education are associated with more years of life and an increased likelihood of obtaining or understanding basic health information and services needed to make appropriate health decisions [70, 71]. Less education predicts higher levels of health risks, such as obesity, substance abuse, and violence [72–74]. Health risks such as teenage pregnancy, poor dietary choices, inadequate physical activity, physical and emotional abuse, substance abuse, and gang involvement have a significant impact on how well students perform in school. Herd and colleagues analyzed the role of education attainment in the onset versus progression to disease. The authors found that education "plays a more critical role" than income in delaying onset of ill health and concludes that "reducing racial and class disparities in education policy" would produce the most impact on reducing health disparities [54].

In regard to sexual health education, a report examining sex education programs around the world, found that "curriculum-based sex and STI/HIV education programs implanted in schools or communities can delay sex, reduce the frequency of sex, reduce the number of partners, increase condom use, increase overall contraceptive use, and reduce unprotected sex," and most importantly that these programs do not increase any measure of sexual activity as some people fear [75]. Based on the fact that few Americans abstain from sex until marriage and most sexual encounters are initiated during adolescence, researchers have concluded that abstinence-only programs as defined by federal funding requirements are "morally problematic" as they undermine more comprehensive sexuality education and other programs [76]. In considering black adolescents, sex education, and the impact on sexual health, one study found that adolescents not receiving sex education were mostly black, from low-income non-intact families, and from rural areas. Those receiving abstinence-only education were younger and from low-to-moderate income intact families. Those receiving comprehensive sex education were older, white, and from higher income families [77]. If black adolescents are disproportionately impacted by STIs as illustrated above, additional effort should be devoted to implementing comprehensive sex education in schools that are plagued by disinvestment, segregation, and low academic achievement.

Compared with other racial and ethnic groups, African Americans account for a greater percentage of incarcerated persons. Black males account for 10% of the US population, but made up 37% (or 1 in 21) of the jail and prison population in 2008. Four percent of African American males were in jail or prison in 2008, compared to 1.7% of Hispanic males and 0.7% of white males [78]. Correctional systems and social networks within which incarcerated persons interact can promote or encourage risky health behaviors and may account for some health disparities [79]. Compared with the general population, incarcerated persons have a disproportionately greater burden of HIV and STDs [80, 81]. In general, studies suggest that sex and drug use decrease overall among incarcerated persons; however, these activities are conducted in a riskier manner inside prison than outside in the community [82, 83].

Although it is difficult to assess whether African Americans and whites have different risks of transmitting sexually transmitted infections while in prison, some studies indicate that there are few differences in their risk behaviors while incarcerated [82, 84]. This suggests that any association between incarceration and black-white disparities in sexually transmitted infections that relates to prison as a risk environment results from the greater likelihood that African Americans will be exposed to this environment [85]. In regards to HIV and STIs, prison inmates have higher rates than the general population. While incarcerated, they are at risk for coercive and risky sexual partnerships, and incarceration disrupts and destabilizes intimate partnerships. In addition, because incarceration disproportionately affects the black community, the black male-to-female gender ratio is reduced, contributing to racial/ethnic disparities in STI rates among black women [60]. The implications of disproportionate rates of infection among the black male prison population include a decreased sexual partner pool for black women who desire black male partners, and an increased likelihood of concurrent sexual relationships among black men and women, which can increase the risk of STIs [86]. Additionally, if not addressed, this may lead to increased rates of HIV and STI transmission among black men who have sex with men (MSM).

In summary, understanding the influence of structural and social determinants of sexual health are key to designing and implementing more effective, culturally relevant prevention programs. The interconnectedness between these multifaceted, complex determinants, and individual risk behavior, create a complex set of conditions that test the responsiveness of the health system and its ability to reduce inequities among the most affected population groups—most often, racial and ethnic minorities.

Systems-Based Approaches: Additional Efforts are Needed to Reduce Sexual Health Disparities

In order to make lasting changes in reducing disparities among rates of STIs in racial and ethnic minority communities, addressing key social determinants of sexual health must be incorporated into prevention programs. For example, education and income are key determinants of sexual health that must be considered in developing sexual health programs. People who live and work in low socioeconomic circumstances and who are from low educational backgrounds are at increased risk for reduced access to health care, unhealthy behavior, and poor health outcomes. To make a sustainable difference in sexual health of racial and ethnic minority populations, several actions are necessary.

- In *Education Systems,* effective state and local public health and school health policies and practices that are designed to help reduce the prevalence of health-risk behaviors and improve health outcomes among sexually active minority youth should be developed. These should ensure universal access to age appropriate, comprehensive sexual health education and utilize school-based health centers to promote a balanced approach to sexual health and wellness education.
- *Intersectoral Governance Systems* must continue to galvanize inter- and intra-agency and intersectoral leadership to create a more coordinated response to addressing sexual health disparities; develop, implement and evaluate high impact activities to ensure maximum return on investments. These governance systems should encourage leaders in racial and ethnic minority communities to re-prioritize organizational efforts to respond to increases in STIs in their communities.
- *Health Systems* must leverage resources allocated to community-based health centers to

include a coordinated and integrated approach focusing on educational, programmatic, and clinical services that promote sexual health and wellness. There is a continuing need to increase support for operations and behavioral science research and surveillance to identify and address the social determinants of sexual health.
- *Correctional Systems* should include routine opt-out testing of inmates in jails and prisons and condom distribution in correctional settings which may have the potential to reduce STIs both in prison and upon release back to the community.

Sexual Health of Racial and Ethnic Minorities: Moving Forward

In recent years, a number of structural health policies have been launched in the USA. Successful implementation of policy changes, reinvigorated governance structures including inter/intra-agency partnerships, and community engagement and empowerment, are all important structural determinants necessary to reduce racial/ethnic disparities in sexual health. Major structural changes in how health care is delivered in the USA will also likely lead to overall improvements in American's sexual health, as well as a reduction in racial/ethnic disparities in sexual health.

Meaningful partnerships with the education and correctional systems are essential to achieving health equity and reducing sexual health disparities in the USA. Efforts to reduce STI disparities using a "social determinants of sexual health" approach are key to making a sustainable difference. In order to achieve this lofty goal, it will be important for public health agencies and partners to incorporate a social determinant of sexual health approach into existing activities, such as research and surveillance, health communication, policy formulation, program development, capacity building, and collaborations with partners.

Structural and social determinants of sexual health are products of specific political and historical factors. Changing these determinants will be the most effective way to improve the sexual health of racial and ethnic minorities. By doing so, the sexual health of all Americans will be improved which will then lead to sustainable declines in STI rates among racial and ethnic minorities in the USA. However, such structural changes are difficult to implement, and efforts to do so should be made in tandem with individual-level interventions and by addressing intermediary determinants of sexual health.

References

1. Centers for Disease Control and Prevention. *HIV Surveillance Report, 2009*; vol. 21. http://www.cdc.gov/hiv/topics/surveillance/resources/reports/. Published February 2011. Accessed July, 2011.
2. Centers for Disease Control and Prevention. *Sexually Transmitted Disease Surveillance 2009*. Atlanta: U.S. Department of Health and Human Services; 2010.
3. Dean HD, Fenton KA. Addressing social determinants of health in the prevention and control of HIV/AIDS, viral hepatitis, sexually transmitted infections and tuberculosis. Public Health Rep. 2010;125 Suppl 4:1–5.
4. Harrison KM, Dean HD. Use of data systems to address social determinants of health: a need to do more. Public Health Rep. 2011;126 Suppl 3:1–4.
5. Koh HK. The ultimate measures of health. Public Health Rep. 2011;126 Suppl 3:14–5.
6. Freiden T. A framework for public health action: the health impact pyramid. Am J Public Health. 2010;100(4):590–5.
7. Office of Management and Budget. Revisions to the Standards for the Classification of Federal Data on Race and Ethnicity. *Federal Register* Notice October 30, 1997. http://www.whitehouse.gov/omb/rewrite/fedreg/ombdir15.html. Accessed July 2011.
8. U.S. Bureau of the Census. Population Estimates Program, DP-1 general demographic characteristics. 2008. http://factfinder.census.gov/servlet/QTSelectedDatasetPageServlet?_lang=en&_ts=288526567286. Accessed July 2011.
9. Passel JS, Cohn D. U.S. Population Projections: 2005–2050. Washington DC: Pew Research Center; 2008.
10. Ennis SR, Rios-Vargas M, Albert NG. *The Hispanic Population: 2010*. 2010 Census Briefs, C2020BR-04. U.S. Census Bureau, Washington, DC. May 2011.
11. World Health Organization. Social determinants of health. http://www.who.int/social_determinants/en/. Accessed 15 Mar 2010.
12. Tarlov AR. Public policy frameworks for improving population health. Ann N Y Acad Sci. 1999;896:281–93.
13. Raphael D. Introduction to the social determinants of health. In: Raphael D, editor. Social determinants of

health: Canadian perspectives. Toronto, Canada: Canadian Scholar's Press; 2004. p. 1–18.
14. Earl CE, Penney PJ. The significance of trust in the research consent process with African Americans. West J Nur Res. 2001;23(7):753–62.
15. Braun L. Race, ethnicity, and health: Can genetics explain disparities? Perspec Bio Med. 2002;45(2):159–74.
16. Williams DR, Jackson JS. Race/ethnicity and the 2000 census: Recommendations for African American and other black populations in the United States. Am J Pub Health. 2000;90(11):1728–30.
17. Ford CL, Harawa NT. A new conceptualization of ethnicity for social epidemiologic and health equity research. Soc Sci Med. 2010;71:251–8.
18. Espinoza L, Hall HI, Selik RM, Hu X. Characteristics of HIV infection Among Hispanics, United States 2003–2006. JAIDS. 2008;49(1):94–101.
19. Johnson AS, Xiaohong H, Dean HD. Epidemiologic differences between native-born and foreign-born blacks diagnosed with HIV infection in 33 U.S. states, 2001–2007. Public Health Rep. 2010;125(S4):61–9.
20. Grieco EM. *Race and Hispanic Origin of the Foreign-Born Population in the United States: 2007*, American Community Survey Reports, ACS-11. Washington, DC: U.S. Census Bureau; 2010.
21. James C, Thomas M, Lillie-Blanton M, Garfield R. Key Facts Race, Ethnicity & Medical Care. The Henry J. Kaiser Family Foundation. January 2007.
22. Williams DR, Collins C. Racial residential segregation: a fundamental cause of racial disparities in health. Pub Health Rep. 2001;116:404–16.
23. Acevedo-Garcia D, Osypuk TL, McArdle N, Williams DR. Toward a policy-relevant analysis of geographic and racial/ethnic disparities in child health. Health Aff. 2008;27(2):321–33.
24. LaVeist TA, Gaskin D, Trujillo AJ. Segregated spaces, risky places: the effects of racial segregation on health inequalities. Washington, DC: Joint Center for Political and Economic Studies; 2011.
25. Pendall R, Davies E, Freiman L, Pitingolo R. A Lost Decade: Neighborhood Poverty and the Urban Crisis of the 2000s. Washington, DC: Joint Center for Political and Economic Studies; 2011.
26. Rossi PH, Weber E. The social benefits of homeownership: empirical evidence from national surveys. Housing Policy Debate. 1996;7(1):1–35.
27. Dietz R, Haurin D. The social and private micro-level consequences of homeownership. J of Urban Econ. 2003;54(3):401–50.
28. U.S. Bureau of the Census. Homeownership Rates by Race and Ethnicity of Householder: 1994 to 2010 http://www.census.gov/hhes/www/housing/hvs/annual10/ann10t_22.xls. Accessed 31 Aug 2011.
29. Taylor EM, Adimora AA, Schoenbach VJ. Marital status and sexually transmitted infections among African Americans. J Family Issues. 2010;31(9):1147–65.
30. U.S. Bureau of Justice Statistics. Jail Inmates at Midyear 2010. http://bjs.ojp.usdoj.gov/index.cfm?ty=pbdetail&iid=2375. Accessed 31 Aug 2011.

31. Bureau of Justice Statistics (US). Prison Inmates at Midyear 2009. http://bjs.ojp.usdoj.gov/index.cfm?ty=pbdetail&iid=2200. Accessed 31 Aug 2011.

32. U.S. Bureau of Labor Statistics. 2011. Labor force characteristics by race and ethnicity, 2010. U.S. Department of Labor. Report 1032.

33. Williams DR. Race, socioeconomic status, and health—the added effects of racism and discrimination. Ann NY Acad Sci. 1999;896:281–93.

34. DeNavas-Walt C, Proctor BD, Smith JC. U.S. Census Bureau, Current Population Reports, P60–239, *Income, Poverty, and Health Insurance Coverage in the United States: 2010*, U.S. Government Printing Office, Washington, DC, 2011.

35. Taylor P, Kochhar R, Fry R, Velasco G, Motel S. Twenty—to—One: Wealth Gaps Rise to Record Highs Between Whites, Blacks and Hispanics. Washington DC, Pew Research Center; 2011.

36. James C, Thomas M, Lillie-Blanton M, Garfield R. Key Facts Race, Ethnicity & Medical Care. Menlo Park, CA: The Henry J. Kaiser Family Foundation; 2007.

37. DeNavas-Walt C, Proctor BD, Smith JC. U.S. Census Bureau, Current Population Reports, P60-236, Income, Poverty, and Health Insurance Coverage in the United States: 2008. , Washington, DC: U.S. Government Printing Office; 2008.

38. Gottschalck AO. *Net Worth and Asset Ownership of Households: 2002*. Current Population Reports, P70-115. Washington, DC: U.S. Census Bureau; 2008.

39. Smedley BD. Moving beyond access: achieving equity in state health care reform. Health Aff. 2008;27(2):447–55.

40. Agency for Healthcare Research and Quality (AHRQ). National Healthcare Disparities Report, 2005. http://www.ahrq.gov/qual/nhdr05/nhdr05.htm. Accessed 10 Jan 2011.

41. Keppel K, Pamuk E, Lynch J, et al. Methodological issues in measuring health disparities. Vital Health Stat. 2005;141(2):1–6.

42. Hall I, Byers RH, Ling Q, Espinoza LH. Ethnic and Age disparities in HIV prevalence and disease progression among Men Who have Sex with Men in the united states. Am J Public Health. 2007;97(6):1060–6.

43. Rastogi S, Johnson TD, Hoeffel EM, Drewery MP. *The Black Population 2010.* Census Briefs, C2010BR-06. Washington, DC: U.S. Census Bureau; 2011.

44. Commission on the Social Determinants of Health. *Closing the gap in a generation: health equity through action on the social determinants of health.* Final Report of the Commission on Social Determinants of Health. Geneva, World Health Organization; 2008.

45. World Health Organization. *Towards a conceptual framework for analysis and action on social determinants of health.* Discussion paper for the Commission on Social Determinants of Health. 2007. www.who.int. Accessed: Jul 2011.

46. U.S. Congress. Senate. *H.R. 3590, Patient Protection and Affordable Care Act.* H.R. 3590. 111th cong., 1st sess. (March 23, 2010) http://democrats.senate.gov/reform/patient-protection-affordable-care-act.pdf. Accessed July 2011.

47. National Prevention Council, *National Prevention Strategy,* Washington, DC: U.S. Department of Health and Human Services, Office of the Surgeon General, 2011.

48. White House Office of National AIDS Policy (ONAP). National HIV/AIDS Strategy for the United States. July 2010. http://whitehouse.gov/sites/default/files/uploads/NHAS.pdf. Accessed: July 2011.

49. US Department of Health and Human Resources. Proposed Data Collection Standards for Race, Ethnicity, Primary Language, Sex, and Disability Status Required by Section 4302 of the Affordable Care Act. http://minorityhealth.hhs.gov/section4302/. Accessed July, 2011)

50. Andrulis D, Siddiqui N, Purtle J and Duchon L. *Patient Protection and Affordable Care Act of 2010: Advancing Health Equity for Racially and Ethnically Diverse Populations.* Joint Center for Political and Economic Studies, July 2010: pg. 6. Available online: http://www.jointcenter.org/hpi/sites/all/files/PatientProtection_PREP_0.pdf.

51. Holmes KK, Mardh P, Sparling PF, et al., editors. Sexually transmitted diseases. 3rd ed. New York, NY: McGraw-Hill; 1999.

52. Lichtenstein B, Hook III EW, Sharma AK. Public tolerance, private pain: stigma and sexually transmitted infections in the American deep south. Cult Health Sex. 2005;7(1):43–57.

53. Bowleg L, Teti M, Massie JS, et al. 'What does it take to be a man? What is a real man?': ideologies of masculinity and HIV sexual risk among Black heterosexual men. Cult Health Sex. 2011;i:1–15.

54. Herd P, Goesling B, House JS. Socioeconomic position and health: the differential effects of education versus income on the onset versus progression of health problems. J Health Soc Behav. 2007;48(3):223–38.

55. Springer YP, Samuel MC, Bolan G. Socioeconomic gradients in sexually transmitted diseases: A geographic information system-based analysis of poverty, race/ethnicity, and gonorrhea rates in California, 2004–2006. Am J Pub Health. 2010;100(6):1060–7.

56. Cohen D, Spear S, Scribner R, et al. "Broken windows" and the risk of gonorrhea. Am J Pub Health. 2000;90(2):230–6.

57. Bauermeister JA, Zimmerman MA, Caldwell CH. Neighborhood disadvantage and changes in condom use among African American adolescents. J Urban Studies. 2010;88(1):66–83.

58. Wingood GM, DiClemente RJ. Enhancing adoption of evidence-based HIV interventions: promotion of a suite of HIV prevention interventions for African American women. AIDS Educ Prev. 2006;18(4 Suppl A):161–70.

59. Lang DL, Salazar LF, Wingood GM, DiClimente RJ, Mikhail I. Associations between recent gender-based violence and pregnancy, sexually transmitted infections, condom use practices, and negotiation of sexual practices among HIV-positive women. JAIDS. 2007;46(2):216–21.

60. Adimora AA, Schoenbach VJ. Social context, sexual networks, and racial disparities in rates of sexually transmitted infections. J Infect Dis. 2005;191 Suppl 1:S115–22.

61. Adimora AA, Shcoenbach VJ, Doherty IA. HIV and African Americans in the southern United States: sexual networks and social context. Sexually Trans Dis. 2006;33(7 Suppl):S39–45.

62. Thomas JC. From slavery to incarceration: social forces affecting the epidemiology of sexually transmitted diseases in the rural south. Sexually Trans Dis. 2006;33(7 Suppl):S6–10.

63. Laumann EO, Youm Y. Racial/ethnic group differences in the prevalence of sexually transmitted diseases in the United States: a network explanation. Sexually Trans Dis. 1999;26(5):250–61.

64. Adimora AA, Schoenbach VJ, Martinson FE, et al. Social context of sexual relationships among rural African Americans. Sexually Trans Dis. 2001;28(2):69–75.

65. Doherty IA, Padian NS, Marlow C, Aral SO. Determinants and consequences of sexual networks as they affect the spread of sexually transmitted infections. J Infect Dis. 2005;191 Suppl 1:S42–54.

66. World Health Organization. Commission on Social Determinants of Health. *A Conceptual Framework for Action on the Social Determinants of Health* (Draft). http://www.who.int/social_determinants/resources/csdh_framework_action_05_07.pdf. Retrieved Accessed Sept 2011.

67. Muntaner C, Lynch J. Income inequality, social cohesion, and class relations: A critique of Wilkinson's neo-Durkheimian research program. Int J Health Serv. 1999;29(1):59–81.

68. Holtgrave DR, Crosby RA. Social capital, poverty, and income inequality as predictors of gonorrhea, syphilis, chlamydia and AIDS case rates in the United States. Sex Transm Infect. 2003;70(1):62–4.

69. Kerrigan D, Witt S, Glass B, Chung S, Ellen J. Perceived neighborhood social cohesion and condom use among adolescents vulnerable to HIV/STI. AIDS Behav. 2006;10(6):723–9.

70. Parker RM. Health literacy: a challenge for American patients and their health care providers. Health Prom Intl. 2000;15:277–91.

71. DeWalt DA, Boone RS, Pignone MP. Literacy and its relationship with self-efficacy, trust, and participation in medical decision-making. Am J Health Behav. 2007;31:S27–35.

72. Gfroerer JC, Greenblatt JC, Wright DA. Substance use in the US in the US college-age population:

differences according to educational status and living arrangement. Am J of Pub Health. 1997;87(1):62–5.

73. Feldman J, Makuc DM, Kleinman J, Cornoni-Huntley J. National trends in educational differentials in mortality. Am J of Epi. 1989;129:919–33.

74. Williams DR. Socioeconomic differentials in health: a review and redirection. Soc Psych Quart. 1990;53(2):81–99.

75. Kirby D. *Sex Education: Access and Impact on Sexual Behaviour of Young People.* New York, NY: Population Division, Department of Economic and Social Affairs, United Nations Secretariat; 2011.

76. Santelli J, Ott MA, Lyon M, et al. Abstinence and abstinence-only education: A review of U.S. policies. *J Adol.* Health. 2006;38:72–81.

77. Kohler PK, Manhart LE, Lafferty WE. Abstinence-only and comprehensive sex education and the initiation of sexual activity and teen pregnancy. J Adol Health. 2008;42:344–51.

78. Bureau of Justice Statistics. Prison Inmates at Midyear 2008—Statistical Tables and Jail Inmates at Midyear—Statistical Tables. NCJ 123456. March 31, 2009. http://bjs.ojp.usdoj.gov/index.cfm?ty=pbdetail&iid=361 Accessed Jul 2011.

79. National Commission on Correctional Health Care. *Health status of soon-to-be-released inmates: a report to Congress. Vol. 1.* Washington, DC: National Commission on Correctional Health Care, 2002.

80. Dean-Gaitor H, Fleming PL. Epidemiology of AIDS in incarcerated persons in the United States, 1994–1996. AIDS. 1999;13:2429–35.

81. Hammett T, Harmon MP, Rhodes W. The burden of infectious disease among inmates of and releases from US correctional facilities, 1997. Am J Pub Health. 2002;92(11):1789–94.

82. Wohl AR, Johnson D, Jordan W, Lu S, Beall G, Currier J, Kerndt PR. High-risk behaviors during incarceration in African-American men treated for HIV at three Los Angeles public medical centers. JAIDS. 2000;24(4):386–92.

83. Inciardi JA. Crack, crack house sex, and HIV risk. Arch of Sexual Behav. 1995;24(3):249–69.

84. Kassira EN, Bauserman RL, Tomoyasu N, Caldeira E, Swetz A, Solomon L. HIV and AIDS surveillance among inmates in Maryland prisons. J Urban Health. 2001;78(2):256–63.

85. Blankenship KM, Smoyer AB, Bray SJ, Mattocks K. Black-white disparities in HIV/AIDS: the role of drug policy and the corrections system. J Health Care Poor Underserved. 2005;16(4 Suppl B):140–56.

86. Centers for Disease Control and Prevention. *Consultation to Address STD Disparities in African American Communities: Meeting Report.* http://www.cdc.gov/std/general/STDHealthDisparities ConsultationJune2007.pdf Published October 2007. Accessed Nov 2011.

Adolescent Sexual Health and Sexually Transmitted Infections: A Conceptual and Empirical Demonstration

15

J. Dennis Fortenberry and Devon J. Hensel

Adolescents have a disproportionate burden of the negative outcomes of sexual activity, such as sexually transmitted infections (STI), unintended pregnancy, and sexual coercion. These outcomes contribute to short- and long-term poor health, fertility, and economics that may reverberate into adulthood. Traditional public health research appropriately addresses these outcomes of adolescent sexual behavior by focusing on promotion of abstinence, delay of initiation of sexual activity, and consistent use of condoms and contraception [1]. The proposed 2020 health objectives, which emphasize positive youth development, continue this public health focus on isolated adverse outcomes [2]. This isolated focus obscures the larger developmental significance of sexuality and sexual behavior, creating a perspective that adolescent sexual health is an oxymoron in that adolescents cannot be simultaneously *sexual* and *healthy*.

Learning to express and manage sexuality is a continuous developmental task during adolescence. Adolescents are exposed to a variety of sexual interactions, including managing physical, social, and emotional aspects of relationships (e.g., sexual communication/negotiation,

jealousy/love, or sexual desire) [3] and a range of behaviors (e.g., from kissing to sexual intercourse) [4]. Considerable variability exists in the developmental trajectory of these interactions in adolescent and adult sexual health. Public health focus on adolescent sexual health is therefore important even if average age of first sexual intercourse was delayed to age 18 or older as a result of public health interventions [5].

Thus, an important challenge to a new public health perspective is formulation of an approach that supports healthy sexual development while maintaining attention on primary prevention of adverse outcomes such as STI. In this chapter, we provide empirical support for the construct of adolescent sexual health as linked to three key public health indicators: number of recent sex partners, frequency of condom use, and STI. This type of analysis allows extension of the conceptual content of adolescent sexual health to an explicitly public health application.

Sexual health has gained prominence in recent years as a guiding concept for the understanding of STI, and for the organization of testing, treatment, and prevention services. The World Health Organization (WHO) gives the following definition of sexual health:

> Sexual health is a state of physical, emotional, mental and social well-being related to sexuality; it is not merely the absence of disease, dysfunction or infirmity. Sexual health requires a positive and respectful approach to sexuality and sexual

J.D. Fortenberry, M.D. M.S. (✉) • D.J. Hensel, Ph.D.
Section of Adolescent Medicine, Department of
Pediatrics, Indiana University School of Medicine,
410 W. 10th Street, Suite 1001, Indianapolis,
IN 46202, USA
e-mail: jfortenb@iu.edu

S.O. Aral, K.A. Fenton, and J.A. Lipshutz (eds.), *The New Public Health and STD/HIV Prevention:*
Personal, Public and Health Systems Approaches, DOI 10.1007/978-1-4614-4526-5_15,
© Springer Science+Business Media New York 2013

responses, as well as the possibility of having pleasurable and safe sexual experiences, free of coercion, discrimination and violence. For sexual health to be attained and maintained, the sexual rights of all persons must be respected, protected and fulfilled [6].

This admirable public health standard for sexual health does not explicitly identify age, legal status, or developmental limits and therefore provides a useful starting point for consideration of adolescent sexual health. Some issues with application of this definition of sexual health to adolescents are addressed below.

A somewhat different definition of adolescent sexual health was proposed in the Consensus Statement of the National Commission on Adolescent Sexual Health, endorsed by more than 50 national medical and policy organizations: "Sexual health encompasses sexual development and reproductive health, as well as such characteristics as the ability to develop and maintain meaningful interpersonal relationships; appreciate one's own body; interact with both genders in respectful and appropriate ways; and express affection, love, and intimacy in ways consistent with one's own values" [7].

The Consensus Statement additionally notes that "responsible adolescent intimate relationships" should be "consensual, non-exploitative, honest, pleasurable, and protected against unintended pregnancy and STD's if any type of intercourse occurs."

The WHO and the National Consensus statement raise some additional issues to consider in thinking about the sexual health of adolescents. First, adolescents' sexual behavior is substantially limited by legal proscriptions. Most states have specific age thresholds to distinguish illegal and legal sexual activity [8, 9]. For example, in our home state of Indiana, partnered sexual activity before age 14 is defined as child abuse. Whether the sexual activity is consensual is not considered by these laws. Other states establish different age thresholds, up to age 18 years. This means that the precept of individual sexual autonomy implicit in the WHO definition is legally restricted. Note that we do not argue pro or con the appropriateness of this restriction. We simply

note that adolescents do not have full sexual autonomy in most jurisdictions.

Second, access by adolescents to sexual health information is often restricted by local governmental or school board policy, as well as by state and national statutes. The content of sex education curricula is often skewed toward abstinence, pregnancy, and STI, with little or no mention of masturbation, sexual pleasure or orgasm [6, 10]. We suspect that few persons within public health would endorse purposeful under-education as a national health strategy but that is the de facto approach in much of the United States.

Third, adolescents' sexual health is likely more explicitly linked to developmental change than at any other point during the sexual life span, with the possible exception of menopause. The span of years from puberty to young adulthood—roughly one decade—encompasses the physical, psychological, social, and relational changes that become critical parameters of sexual health in the decades after adolescence [4, 11–20].

Finally, definitions of sexual health are difficult to apply to adolescents because the empirical basis for understanding adolescent sexual health is typically limited to issues such as coercion, pregnancy, and STI. For example, almost no studies describe issues related to sexual response, satisfaction and pleasure in persons under age 18. A small body of research, however, is beginning to link these concepts—often under the umbrella of the term "sexual agency"—to STI prevention behaviors such as condom use [21–23].

In addition to consideration of specific limitations in the definitions of sexual health as applicable to adolescents, there are also issues about the nature of the construct of sexual health itself. From one perspective, sexual health simply is an umbrella concept to organize a set of distinct and not necessarily related characteristics. The various definitions of sexual health simply synthesize a worldview from the political, cultural, religious, and evidence-based perspectives of the various contributors to the definitions. For example, viewing sexual health "as state of physical, emotional, mental and social well-being related to sexuality" could tap a range of individual characteristics as disparate as erotophilia on the one hand and women's reproductive health rights on the other. The available definitions do not identify parameters that distinguish *sexual health* from other types of health, nor what factors are excluded from the mantel of sexual health. From this perspective, sexual health is a broad rhetorical label used to guide public health approaches to potentially disparate problems. For example, a public sexual health philosophy that promotes a positive engagement with one's sexuality while reducing health risks associated with sexual behaviors could apply equally to a program to increase human papillomavirus vaccine uptake among young women and a prostate cancer screening program targeted for middle-aged men. In this sense, sexual health is *not* a characteristic marked by between-individual differences. Rather, the concept of sexual health links traditional disease prevention approaches of public health to health promotion and wellness practices.

A much less commonly expressed alternative perspective suggests that sexual health represents an identifiable individual characteristic marked by between-person differences (i.e., some persons are sexually healthier than others) and by within-person differences (i.e., a person's sexual health may change over time). This alternative perspective on sexual health suggests a predictable coherence among the several components of sexual health, with variation in the quantity possessed.

In order for this alternative perspective to be of value to public health, individual variation in sexual health should be associated with outcomes that are traditionally assessed in STI-related public health functions. In other words, people who are "sexually healthier" behave in ways that, from a public health perspective, are "healthier." It is important to note—consonant with the WHO definition of sexual health—that that "sexually healthier" from a public health perspective is not simply being free of STI. Some very common STI (e.g., genital herpes) require long-term sexual health in the presence of a life-long STI. In addition, people whose behavior corresponds to factors associated with increased STI risk would also be considered "less sexually healthy" simply because of their behavior, even if they never contract an STI.

The possibility that sexual health among adolescents can be operationalized and measured follows from this perspective on sexual health we have just presented. The idea of this type of coherence in adolescents' health-related behaviors is not without theoretical and empirical precedent. In fact, a remarkably robust body of research—based in Problem Behavior Theory—demonstrates a substantial degree of predictable covariance of beliefs and attitudes, parent and peer influences, and other social-environmental factors on a range of potentially health-harming behaviors such as earlier sexual activity, or marijuana and alcohol use, as well as engagement in health-protective behaviors such as healthy eating or exercise behaviors [24].

Some data support the extension of Problem-Behavior Theory to the study of sexual health. For example, adolescents' use of condoms should more reliably co-vary with other health-protective behaviors than with health-harming behaviors. Using data drawn from a sample of 793 sexually experienced male and female adolescents, the relationship of contraceptive use with alcohol use, marijuana and other drug use, aggressive behaviors, delinquency, diet behaviors, exercise, seatbelt use, and dental hygiene behaviors was examined. Contraceptive use was examined in three different latent variable models, hypothesized to be more related to health-harming behaviors (Model A), health-protective behaviors (Model B), or bot health-harming and health-protective behaviors (Model C). A second-order confirmatory factor analysis showed that inclusion of contraceptive behavior as a health-protective behavior provided the most parsimonious fit to the data [25].

The purpose of this chapter, then, is to explore the construct of sexual health in adolescent women. Consonant with the purpose of this book, the results demonstrate the potential of a new public health approach to STI/HIV prevention for adolescents. We are fully aware that these data do not assess development of sexual health among young men, and that the data are most closely applicable to young women's heterosexual behaviors. Our intent (metaphorically) is to shine a light on a path that is poorly lit and mostly untrodden.

To explore the structure of sexual health and link this structure to the commonly used sexual health indicators, we used data from 386 adolescent women participating in a longitudinal research study in Indianapolis. These young women were recruited from three urban adolescent health clinics, and were between 14 and 17 years of age at enrollment. Detailed measures of sexual behavior were obtained by face-to-face interview at enrollment and each three months subsequently. At each 3-month interval, participants provided self-obtained vaginal samples for nucleic acid amplification tests (NAAT) for diagnosis of chlamydia, gonorrhea, and trichomonas. Results were available within 72 h and treatment offered for all positive tests. Additional details regarding methods can be seen in other publications [26–29].

The analyses presented here represent a cross-sectional subset (N=242) of enrollment interviews from young women who reported only one partner in the previous 3 months and who were not pregnant. A second-order latent variable modeling approach (in a structural equation modeling framework using AMOS, 17.0) was used to organize sexual health constructs in association with specific outcomes. Latent variable and structural equation modeling approaches have been extensively developed in social and behavioral sciences, but are infrequently used in public health applications [30]. Latent variables are assumed to account for variation in a set of several observed (or manifest) variables. The strength of relationships between the latent variable and each of the observed variables is assessed by a "loading." Loadings vary in magnitude and valence (either positive or negative), and are typically standardized. Statistical significance of loadings assesses the probability that an observed loading is not different than zero.

In our application of latent variables, we have additionally hypothesized that the latent variables associated with observed variables (first-order latent variables) themselves vary according to an additional underlying factor (second-order latent variable). In our analyses, the second-order latent variable was "sexual health."

Operationalization of Sexual Health: See Fig. 15.1a–f

Our first task was to operationalize the first-order latent variables to represent the various components of "sexual health" suggested in the WHO and National Consensus definitions. Choice of observed variables representing the first-order latent variables was somewhat arbitrary because key words in the definitions had to be matched to the content of available measures: exact matches were not always possible because of imprecision in key words or lack of appropriate measures.

We developed six first-order latent variables. Two of the first-order latent variables—Relationship Quality and Sexual Relationship Satisfaction—recognize that adolescent sexual behavior is typically expressed within the context of a relationship with another person, and the qualities of a given relationship are integral to a person's sexual health. Two additional latent variables—Sexual Autonomy and Absence of Sexual Pain—reflect individual agency in the expressions of partnered sexuality. The final two latent variables—Pregnancy Prevention Attitudes and Condom Use Self-Efficacy—refer to the complex balance of fertility management and disease prevention. The six first-order latent variables evaluated in the measurement model are presented below, along with justification for focus on each latent variable.

Relationship quality addresses the emotional content of relationships with specific partners. A substantial body of research documents the influence of emotional and relational aspects of dyads in the occurrence of sex, on the stability of relationships, and of the use of contraceptive and STI prevention methods [14, 31–33]. These associations are not straightforward from the perspective of STI risk. For example, condom use typically declines in relationships over time as trust and affiliation increase [21, 29, 34–36].

For the current research, *Relationship Quality* was taken from previously published research [21], operationalized from six, 4-point Likert type items [strongly disagree to strongly agree;

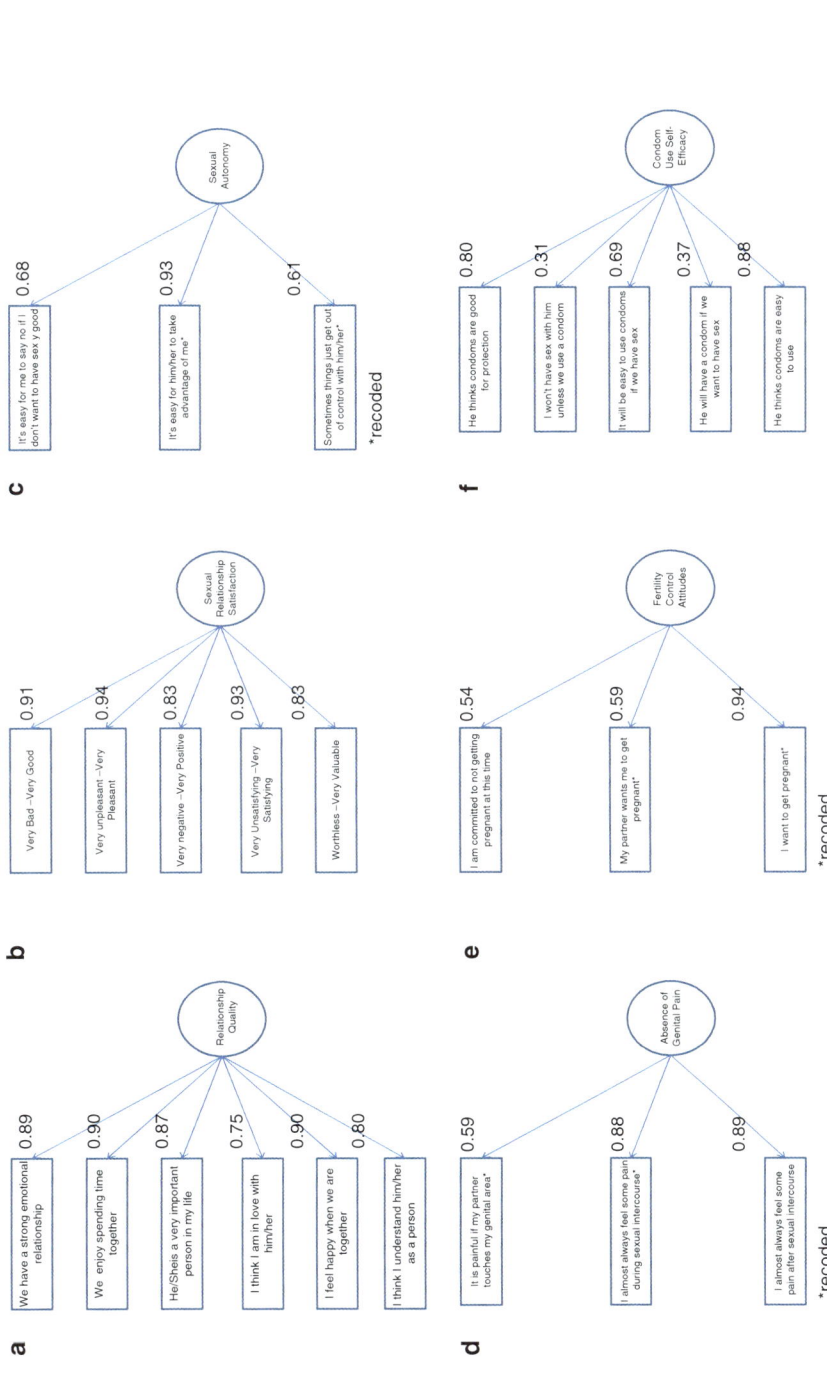

Fig. 15.1 First-order factor measurement model (**a**) Relationship Quality (**b**) Sexual Relationship Satisfaction (**c**) Sexual Autonomy (**d**) Absence of Genital Pain (**e**) Pregnancy Prevention Attitudes (**f**) Condom use self-efficacy

$\alpha=0.94$]—"We have a strong emotional relationship," 'We enjoy spending time together," "He/she is a very important person in my life," "I think I am in love with him/her," "I feel happy when we are together," and "I think I understand him/her as a person." Scale scores range for 6–24, with higher scores indicating higher quality.

Sexual Relationship Satisfaction specifically addresses young women's satisfaction with sexual interactions with a specific partner. Sexual satisfaction is an important aspect of adult relationships [37, 38] as well as those of younger women [39]. Satisfaction may be related to feeling that fertility and infection issues are adequately addressed as dual hormonal contraception/condom users have higher levels of sexual satisfaction than other women [40].

Sexual satisfaction was adapted from other research [37]. Sexual satisfaction was assessed by five, 7-point semantic differential items assessing a participant's feelings about the sexual relationship with that partner ($\alpha=0.95$): "very bad to very good," "very unpleasant to very pleasant," "very negative to very positive," "very unsatisfying to very satisfying," and "worthless to very valuable." Scores could range from 5 to 35, with higher score indicating higher satisfaction.

Sexual autonomy addresses a young woman's agency in sexual decision-making. In other words, her capacity to evaluate her own sexual interests and desires, and to engage in coercion-free sexual activity, or not, based on that evaluation [41–43].

Sexual autonomy was three 4-point Likert items (strongly disagree to strongly agree; $\alpha=0.80$): "It's easy for me to say no if I don't want to have sex," "It's easy for him/her to take advantage of me," (recoded) and "Sometimes things just get out of control with him/her" (recoded). These items were developed for the research project. Scores ranged from 3 to 12, with higher scored indicating greater autonomy.

Absence of sexual pain addresses an area of substantial difficulty and dysfunction among women. A recent national study reports that 52% of adolescent women ages 14–17 years reported at least some pain associated with their most recent coitus (JD Fortenberry; manuscript in preparation). Lubrication difficulties—that may be linked to pain—were also common. Studies of adult women link sexual pain to decreased sexual satisfaction, decreased relationship satisfaction, and lower rates of condom and contraceptive use [44–46].

Absence of pain was assessed using three, 4-point items ($\alpha=0.83$): "It is painful if my partner touches my genital area," "I almost always feel some pain during sexual intercourse," and "I almost always feel some pain after sexual intercourse." Higher scores indicated a greater degree of sexual pain. This scale was recoded for analysis, however, so that higher scores indicate *less* sexual pain.

Pregnancy Prevention attitudes represent a conceptually difficult area in the assessment of sexual health for adolescents. On the one hand, rates of early pregnancy and childbearing are associated with significant long-term health implications and are identified as a major target for public health intervention [47]. On the other hand, pregnancy and childbearing are celebrated aspects of many peoples' lives and as markers of physical health and continuity of family lineages [48–50].

Pregnancy prevention attitudes were assessed by was assessed using one 4-point Likert type item (strongly disagree to strongly agree): "I am committed to not getting pregnant at this time." We additionally used two, 3-point items examining pregnancy as a motivator for sex (not important to very important; reverse coded): "My partner wants me to get pregnant" and "I want to get pregnant." Internal reliability was good ($\alpha=0.80$). Scores ranged from 3 to 11, with higher scores indicating greater commitment to avoiding pregnancy.

Condom Use Self-efficacy

Self-efficacy is a core concept of social and psychological research related to health in general [51–54] and to sexual health in particular [55–59]. We chose to assess self-efficacy via a specific measure related to condoms because of the centrality of condoms as a method for contraception and STI prevention, and because of evidence that condom use is a common behavior among contemporary American adolescents [60].

Condom use self-efficacy was assessed by five 4-point Likert-type items (α=0.81): "He thinks condoms are good for protection," "I won't have sex with him unless we use a condom," "It will be easy to use condoms if we have sex," "He will have a condom if we have sex," and "He thinks condoms are easy to use." Scores ranged from 3 to 12, with higher scores indicating greater self-efficacy for condom use.

Establishing the Measurement Model for Sexual Health

We hypothesized that variation in these first-order latent variables could be accounted for by a second-order latent variable called "sexual health." Correlations among the six first-order factors are shown in Table 15.1. Examination of these correlations shows evidence of substantial intercorrelation, suggestive of a larger pattern of relationships.

The second-order confirmatory factor analysis assessing an underlying factor of sexual health and accounting for variation in the first-order latent variables is shown in Figure 15.2. Each of six first-order latent variables loaded positively and significantly on the second-order latent factor of Sexual Health. Overall model fit indices were above 0.90, and the RMSEA was 0.06. Model fit indices above 0.90 and RMSEA of 0.05 or less generally indicate that the hypothesized second-order factor structure provided an adequate fit to the data [61].

Table 15.1 Correlation matrix of first-order factors

	1.	2.	3.	4.	5.
1. Relationship quality	1.00				
2. Sexual satisfaction	0.98				
3. Sexual autonomy	0.86	0.83			
4. Absence of sexual pain	0.89	0.88	0.71		
5. Fertility control	0.97	0.97	0.82	0.91	
6. Condom use self-efficacy	0.97	0.96	0.88	0.85	0.96

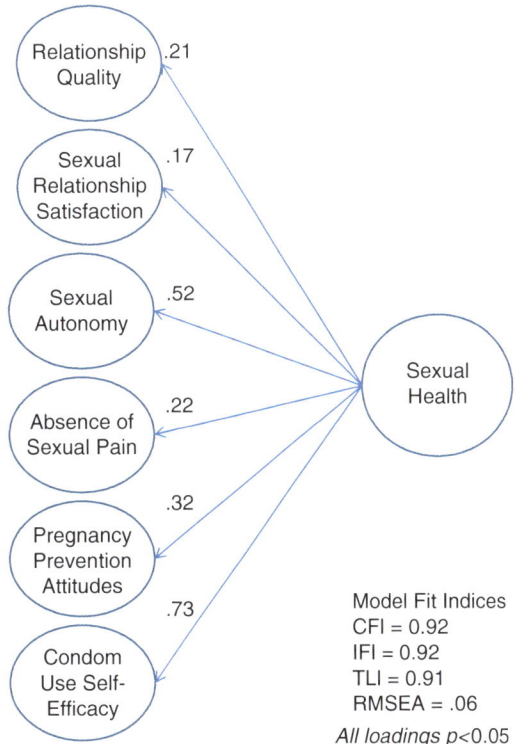

Fig. 15.2   Second-Order factor model of sexual health

Condom Use, Number of Partners, and STI as a Function of Sexual Health (Fig. 15.3a–c)

Having identified an adequate measurement model for the construct of sexual health, we next evaluated sexual health within the context of other variables assessed in traditional STI-related public health functions: condom use, number of partners, and STI. *Condom use* was measured as the proportion of penile-vaginal intercourse events in the previous 3 months that were condom-protected. For all participants and all time periods, the average proportion of condom-protected events was 0.48 (SD=0.42; median=0.50; range 0–100%). *Number of partners* was the lifetime number of sexual partners reported. The average number of lifetime partners was 5.92 (SD=4.03; median=5.00; range=0–23). *STI* was the identification of any chlamydia, gonorrhea, or trichomonas infection during the 3-month period.

Fig. 15.3 (**a**) Association of second-order latent variable for Sexual health and condom use (**b**) Association of second-order latent variable for Sexual health and lifetime sexual partners (**c**) Association of second-order latent variable for Sexual health and sexually transmitted infection

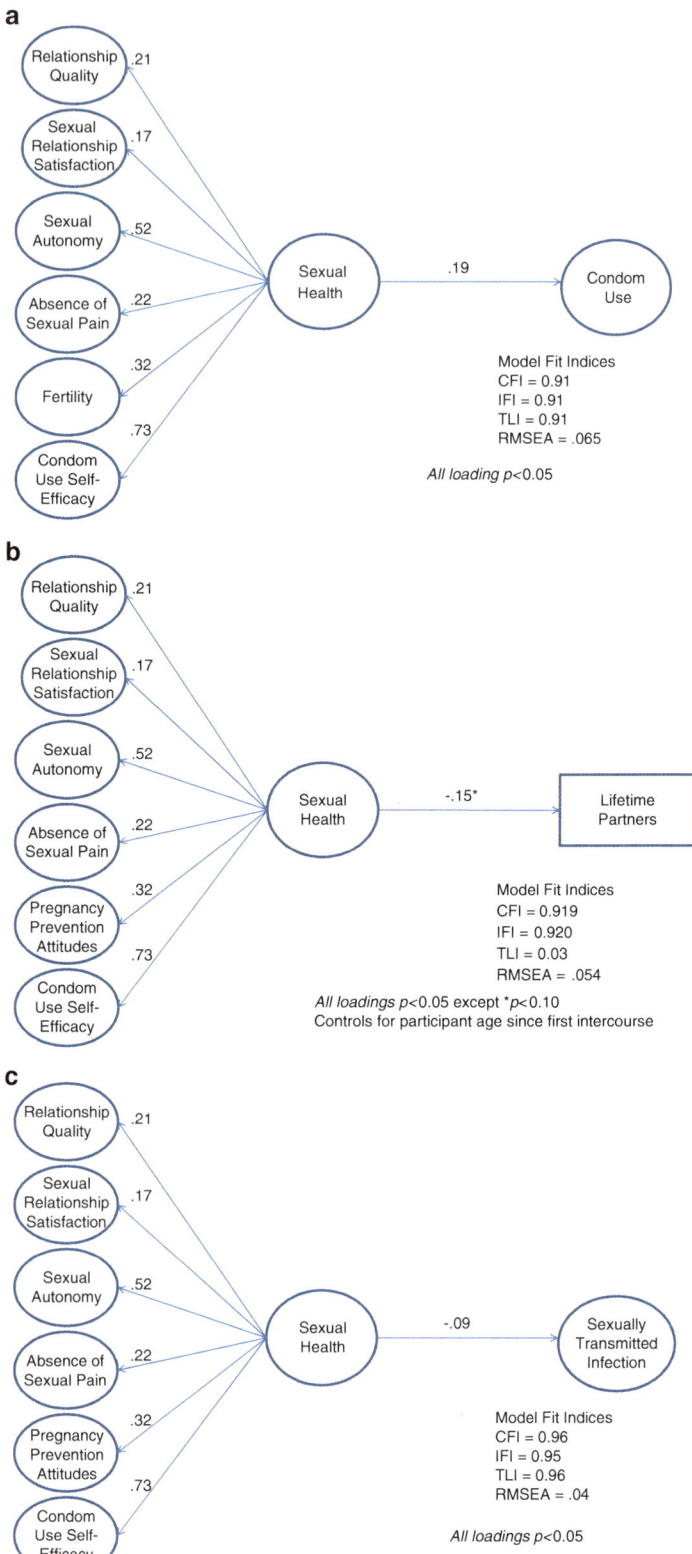

The average proportion of STI during any given 3-month period was 0.15 (SD=0.35; median=.00; range=0–100%).

Sexual Health and Condom Use

Sexual health for a given 3-month period significantly predicted the proportion of condom-protected events for that period (Figure 15.3a). Each of the fit indices was greater than 0.90 and the RMSEA was 0.065. These data suggest that this model of the relationship of a second-order construct of sexual health and condom use was a good fit to the data.

We also explored other models. Some theoretical perspectives such as Social Learning Theory suggest that the multi-item measure of condom self-efficacy should be strongly associated with condom use. Therefore, we compared a reduced model using condom self-efficacy as an indicator of sexual health with our full 6-factor model. Analyses using condom use self-efficacy as a single-item indicator of sexual health to predict condom use produced a significant path between sexual health and condom use. However, model fit of this simpler model was much worse (data not shown), suggesting the importance of the more detailed construct of sexual health presented above.

Sexual Health and Number of Sexual Partners

Sexual health was negatively associated with lifetime sex partners (Fig. 15.3b). This association was statistically significant only when a $p<0.10$ criterion was applied although it should be noted that each unit increase in the latent variable of sexual health was associated with decrease in one lifetime sexual partner. Model fit indices were adequate.

Sexual Health and STI

Sexual health was negatively associated with incident STI (Fig. 15.3c). All model fit indices were greater than 0.90, and the RMSEA was 0.04.

This suggests that the second-order construct of sexual health provides an excellent explanatory fit for incident STI, and is potentially an important element for understanding how people engage risk and protection more broadly.

We also considered other models to more thoroughly explore the relationship of sexual health and STI. Because sexual health is associated with condom use, we ran separate models of the association of sexual health and STI, controlling for condom use. These analyses showed that a direct path between sexual health and STI remained significant, even when controlling for level of condom use (data not shown). Moreover, model fit deteriorated, although it remained adequate.

Sexual Health and Abstinence

Abstinence from coitus is an important characteristic of adolescents' sexual behaviors. In fact, at any given time, most adolescents have either never had coitus or have not engaged in coitus in the previous 3 months [60]. Insight into the role of abstinence in sexual health would provide additional perspective on how a new approach to adolescent STI prevention could incorporate this developmentally appropriate construct.

We conducted a second set of second-order latent variable analyses that addressed abstinence as an outcome associated with sexual health. Additional details of these analyses can be obtained from the second author. In this expanded model, we added 3 first-order latent variables assessing dimensions of sexual health beyond those suggested by existing definitions: sexual communication, sexual self-esteem, and sexual anxiety. Fit indices of measurement models for these three multi-item scales were excellent. Incorporation of these new dimensions of sexual health into a second-order latent variable analysis showed that each of the new dimensions loaded significantly on the second-order latent factor of sexual health: sexual health was associated with higher sexual communication higher sexual self-esteem and lower sexual anxiety (all B: 0.16–0.88; all $p<0.05$). Using this expanded measure, greater sexual health was significantly associated with abstinence compared to coital experience ($B=0.08$; $p<0.05$). Among those with coital experience, sexual health predicted higher coital frequency, a wider noncoital sexual repertoire, condom use at last sex, higher ratio of condom protected events, using hormonal contraception, and using nonhormonal fertility control (all B: 0.02–0.07). Taken together, these data suggest that abstinence and non-abstinence — both of which are developmentally appropriate states during adolescence — can be usefully linked to a model of sexual health.

Discussion

Sexual health as a guiding paradigm for public health approaches to STI prevention among adolescents is a radical reorientation of perspective and effort. The data presented here provide empirical support for this reorientation by demonstrating that key STI-related public health indicators (condom use, number of partners, STI, abstinence) are best explained by an underlying construct of sexual health. Sexual health is thus a measurable construct in addition to an expression of public health ideals. This means that a key public health function — sentinel surveillance — could be implemented using measures that are reasonably easy to collect from diverse populations.

The finding of an association of adolescent women's sexual health with condom use, number of partners, STI, and abstinence is radical because prior approaches to adolescent sexual behavior and STI were almost exclusively based in the concept of risk associated with sexual behavior. The public health appeal of this risk-based perspective is based in its logical simplicity: adolescent sex is a necessary antecedent to adolescent STI; therefore, attempts to reduce adolescent sex are reasonable public health approaches to prevention of STI among adolescents. Advocacy of specific limits on sexual behaviors of specific groups have been characteristic of public health approaches to STI prevention for most of the past 130 years [62]. This fairly straightforward public health reasoning also resonates well with traditional social and religion-based approaches to control of sexual behavior of young people by

emphasizing sexual abstinence outside of marriage. Thus, abstinence-only until marriage emerged as a public health approach to sex education during much of the first decade of twenty-first century, despite lack of evidence for the effectiveness of this approach [63]. It is also possible that many Americans "fear" adolescent sexuality and believe that focus on healthy sexual behavior would only encourage additional risk [64].

Efforts to move away from solely risk-focused perspectives are also hampered by a lack of data with which to respond to the simple logical appeal of risk-based perspectives [11, 65]. For example, we demonstrated that satisfaction with the sexual aspects of a relationship is an important aspect of STI prevention (e.g., condom use and number of sexual partners) and STI incidence. However, the idea that young women can evaluate the sexual qualities of a relationship and that that evaluation affects STI risk is virtually unaddressed in a voluminous literature on adolescent STI. Adolescent STI prevention that emphasizes elements of sexual health such as sexual pleasure, sexual satisfaction, and relationships would possibly open a new era in public health approaches to prevention [66].

What would a sexual health perspective for prevention of adolescent STI look like? First, it would be based in a larger national strategy to improve sexual health [67]. Such a strategy could reinvigorate a national dialogue about the importance of sexual health in our nation's health [68]. One potential outcome of such renewed dialogue would be a reversal of a trend of *fewer* parents discussing sex and contraception with their children in 2002 than in 1985 [69]. The content of school-based sex education should shift to a sexual health perspective. Studies of the content of sex education curricula in other countries (the Netherlands, for example) show substantial more emphasis on health — including sexual wishes and desires — rather than risk [70, 71]. School curricula must contain thoughtful discussion of sexual pleasure in the context of life goals, pleasure, and relationships, as well as prevention of unhealthy consequences. A substantial body of evidence now supports the idea the comprehensive sex education is a far better approach to STI prevention than "abstinence-only until marriage" [6, 63, 72, 73].

The analyses presented here are intended as a "proof-of-concept." Other data are required to extend these analyses to more racially and geographically balanced samples of young women, and to samples of young men. We know almost nothing about application of the concept of sexual health to adolescents with same-sex partners, or those choosing both same- and different-sex partners. However, a public health infrastructure for obtaining diverse measures of sexual health from diverse adolescent samples does not currently exist. Substantial changes to surveys such as the Youth Risk Behavior Survey or the National Survey of Family Growth would be would be required to fully operationalize measures of sexual health such as we presented.

Our analyses provide a strong hint that such data would profitably contribute to a new public health perspective on adolescents and STI. The technical capacity to incorporate a sexual health perspective into prevention of adolescent STI is also quite obvious. The necessary social and political will to adopt such a perspective seems much more problematic.

References

1. U.S. Department of Health & Human Services. Healthy People 2010. 2nd ed. Washington DC: US Government Printing Office; 2000.
2. National Center for Health Statistics. http://www/cdc. gov/nchs/healthy_people.htm. Accessed 2/11/2011.
3. O'Sullivan LF, Brooks-Gunn J. The timing of changes in girls' sexual cognitions and behaviors in early adolescence: a prospective, cohort study. J Adolesc Health. 2005;37:211–9.
4. O'Sullivan LF, Cheng MM, Harris KM, Brooks-Gunn J. I wanna hold your hand: the progression of social, romantic and sexual events in adolescent relationships. Perspect Sex Reprod Health. 2007;39:100–7.
5. Santelli JS, Orr M, Lindberg LD, Diaz DC. Changing behavioral risk for pregnancy among high school students in the United States, 1991–2007. J Adolesc Health. 2009;45:25–32.
6. Koyama A, Corliss HL, Santelli JS. Global lessons on healthy adolescent sexual development. Curr Opin Pediatr. 2009;21:444–9.
7. Bacon JL. Adolescent sexuality and teen pregnancy prevention. J Pediatr Adolesc Gynecol. 1999;12:185–93.
8. Findholt N, Robrecht LC. Legal and ethical considerations in research with sexually active adolescents: The requirement to report statutory rape. Perspect Sex Reprod Health. 2002;34:259–64.
9. English A. The health of adolescent girls: does the law support it? Curr Womens Health Rep. 2002;2:442–9.
10. Santelli JS. Medical accuracy in sexuality education: ideology and the scientific process. Am J Public Health. 2008;98:1786–92.
11. Halpern CT. Reframing research on adolescent sexuality: Healthy sexual development as part of the life course. Perspect Sex Reprod Health. 2010;42:6–7.
12. Ott MA, Pfeiffer EJ, Fortenberry JD. Perceptions of sexual abstinence among high-risk early and middle adolescents. J Adolesc Health. 2006;39:192–8.
13. Miller BC, Benson B. Romantic and sexual relationship development during adolescence. In: Furman W, Brown BB, Feiring C, editors. The development of romantic relationships in adolescence. New York: Cambridge University Press; 1999. p. 99–121.
14. Furman W, Wehner EA. Adolescent romantic relationships: a developmental perspective. New Dir Child Dev. 1997;78:21–36.
15. Ehrhardt AA. Our view of adolescent sexuality—a focus on risk behavior without the developmental context. Am J Public Health. 1996;86:1523–5.
16. Rosenthal SL, Cohen SS, Biro FM. Developmental sophistication among adolescents of negotiation strategies for condom use. Develop Behav Pediatr. 1996;17:94–7.
17. Bolton Jr FG, MacEachron AE. Adolescent male sexuality: a developmental perspective. J Adolesc Res. 1988;3:259–73.
18. Christopher FS, Cate RM. Premarital sexual involvement: a developmental investigation of relational correlates. Adolescence. 1988;23:793–803.
19. Gfellner BM. Concepts of sexual behavior: construction and validation of a developmental model. J Adolesc Res. 1986;1:327–47.
20. Dornbusch SM, Carlsmith JM, Gross RT, et al. Sexual development, age, and dating: a comparison of biological and social influences upon one set of behaviors. Child Dev. 1981;52:179–85.
21. Sayegh MA, Fortenberry JD, Anderson JG, Orr DP. Effects of relationship quality on chlamydia infection among adolescent women. J Adolesc Health. 2005;37:163e161–8.
22. O'Sullivan LF, Udell W, Patel VL. Young urban adults' heterosexual risk encounters and perceived risk and safety: a structured diary study. J Sex Res. 2006;43:343–51.
23. O'Sullivan LF, Meyer-Bahlburg HFL, Watkins BX. Social cognitions associated with pubertal development in a sample of urban, low-income, African-American and Latina girls and mothers. J Adolesc Health. 2000;27:227–35.
24. Jessor R, Jessor SL. Problem behavior and psychosocial development: a longitudinal study of youth, vol. 1. New York: Academic; 1977.

25. Fortenberry JD, Costa FM, Jessor R, Donovan JE. Contraceptive behavior and adolescent lifestyles: a structural modeling approach. J Res Adolesc. 1997;7:307–29.

26. Hensel DJ, Fortenberry JD, Orr DP. Factors associated with event level anal sex and condom use during anal sex among adolescent women. J Adolesc Health. 2010;46:232–7.

27. Tanner AE, Hensel DJ, Fortenberry JD. A prospective study of the sexual, emotional, and behavioral correlates associated with young women's first and usual coital events. J Adolesc Health. 2010;47:20–5.

28. Hensel DJ, Fortenberry JD, Orr DP. Variations in coital and noncoital sexual repertoire among adolescent women. J Adolesc Health. 2008;42:170–6.

29. Fortenberry JD, Temkit M, Tu W, Katz BP, Graham CA, Orr DP. Daily mood, partner support, sexual interest and sexual activity among adolescent women. Health Psychol. 2005;24:252–7.

30. Chavance M, Escolano S, Romon M, Basdevant A, de Lauzon-Guillain B, Charles MA. Latent variables and structural equation models for longitudinal relationships: an illustration in nutritional epidemiology. BMC Med Res Methodol. 2010;10:37.

31. Buhrmester D, Furman W. The development of companionship and intimacy. Child Dev. 1987;58: 1101–13.

32. Collins WA, Welsh DP, Furman W. Adolescent romantic relationships. Annu Rev Psychol. 2009;60: 631–52.

33. Graber JA, Britto PR, Brooks-Gunn J. What's love got to do with it? Adolescents' and young adults' beliefs about sexual and romantic relationships. In: Furman W, Brown BB, Feiring C, editors. The Development of Romantic Relationships in Adolescence. New York: Cambridge University Press; 1999. p. 364–95.

34. Fortenberry JD, Brizendine EJ, Katz BP, Orr DP. The role of notification self-efficacy, anticipated consequences and relationship quality in adolescents' partner notification for sexually transmitted infections. Arch Pediatr Adolesc Med. 2002;156:1133–7.

35. Fortenberry JD, Tu W, Harezlak J, Katz BP, Orr DP. Condom use as a function of time in new and established adolescent sexual relationships. Am J Public Health. 2002;92:211–3.

36. Katz BP, Fortenberry JD, Zimet GD, Blythe MJ, Orr DP. Partner-specific relationship characteristics and condom use among young people with sexually transmitted infections. J Sex Res. 2000;37:69–75.

37. Byers ES. Evidence for the importance of relationship satisfaction for women's sexual functioning. Women Ther. 2001;24:23–6.

38. Sprecher S, Cate RM. Sexual satisfaction and sexual expression as predictors of relationship satisfaction and stability. In: Harvey JH, Wenzel A, Sprecher S, editors. The handbook of sexuality in close relationships. Mahwah, NJ: Lawrence Erlbaum Associates; 2004. p. 235–56.

39. Auslander BA, Rosenthal SL, Fortenberry JD, Biro FM, Bernstein DI, Zimet GD. Predictors of sexual satisfaction in an adolescent and college population. J Pediatr Adolesc Gynecol. 2007;20:25–8.

40. Higgins JA, Hoffman S, Graham CA, Sanders SA. Relationships between condoms, hormonal methods, and sexual pleasure and satisfaction: an exploratory analysis from the Women's Well-Being and Sexuality Study. Sex Health. 2008;5:321–30.

41. O'Sullivan LF. Sexual coercion in dating relationships: Conceptual and methodological issues. Sexual Res Soc Policy. 2005;20:3–11.

42. Auslander BA, Perfect MM, Succop PA, Rosenthal SL. Perceptions of sexual assertiveness among adolescent girls: initiation, refusal, and use of protective behaviors. J Pediatr Adolesc Gynecol. 2007;20:157–62.

43. Tolman DL. Object lessons: Romance, violation and female adolescent sexual desire. J Sex Educ Ther. 2000;25:70–9.

44. Landry T, Bergeron S. Biopsychosocial factors associated with dyspareunia in a community sample of adolescent girls. Arch Sex Behav. 2010;40(5): 877–89.

45. Tripp DA, Nickel JC, Ross S, Mullins C, Stechyson N. Prevalence, symptom impact and predictors of chronic prostatitis-like symptoms in Canadian males aged 16-19 years. BJU Int. 2009;103(8):1080–4.

46. Boardman LA, Stockdale CK. Sexual pain. Clin Obstet Gynecol. 2009;52:682–90.

47. Santelli JS, Melnikas AJ. Teen fertility in transition: recent and historic trends in the United States. Annu Rev Public Health. 2010;31:371–83.

48. Meade CS, Kershaw TS, Ickovics JR. The intergenerational cycle of teenage motherhood: an ecological approach. Health Psychol. 2008;27:419–29.

49. Heavey EJ, Moysich KB, Hyland A, Druschel CM, Sill MW. Female adolescents' perceptions of male partners' pregnancy desire. J Midwifery Womens Health. 2008;53:338–44.

50. White E, Rosengard C, Weitzen S, Meers A, Phipps MG. Fear of inability to conceive in pregnant adolescents. Obstet Gynecol. 2006;108:1411–6.

51. Cervone D. Thinking about self-efficacy. Behav Modif. 2000;24:30–56.

52. O'Leary A. Self-efficacy and health: behavioral and stress-physiological mediation. Cogn Ther Res. 1992;16:229–45.

53. O'Leary A. Self-efficacy and health. Behav Res Ther. 1985;23:437–51.

54. Bandura A. Self-efficacy: toward a unifying theory of behavioral change. Psychol Rev. 1977;84:191–215.

55. Barkley Jr TW, Burns JL. Factor analysis of the condom use self-efficacy scale among multicultural college students. Health Educ Res. 2000;15:485–9.

56. Jemmott III JB, Jemmott LS. HIV risk reduction behavioral interventions with heterosexual adolescents. AIDS. 2000;14 Suppl 2:S40–52.

57. Jemmott III JB, Jemmott LS, Fong GT, McCaffree K. Reducing HIV risk-associated sexual behavior among

African American adolescents: testing the generality of intervention effects. Am J Community Psychol. 1999;27:161–87.

58. O'Leary A, Ambrose TK, Raffaelli M, et al. Effects of an HIV risk reduction project on sexual risk behavior of low-income STD patients. AIDS Educ Prev. 1998;10:483–92.

59. Bryan AD, Aiken LS, West SG. Young women's condom use: the influence of acceptance of sexuality, control over the sexual encounter, and perceived susceptibility to common STDs. Health Psychol. 1997;16:468–79.

60. Fortenberry JD, Schick V, Herbenick D, Sanders SA, Dodge B, Reece M. Sexual behaviors and condom use at last vaginal intercourse: a national sample of adolescents ages 14 to 17 years. J Sex Med. 2010;7 Suppl 5:305–14.

61. Browne MW, Cudeck R. Alternative ways of assessing model fit. In: Bollen KA, Long JS, editors. Testing structural equation models, vol. 1. Newbury Park: Sage Publications; 1993. p. 136–62.

62. Brandt AM. No magic bullet: a social history of venereal diseases in the United States since 1880, vol. 1. New York: Oxford University Press; 1985.

63. Ott MA, Santelli JS. Abstinence and abstinence-only education. Curr Opin Obstet Gynecol. 2007;19:446–52.

64. Schalet A. Must we fear adolescent sexuality? Medscape General Med. 2004;6(4):44–4.

65. Fortenberry JD. Beyond validity and reliability: meaning-in-context of adolescents' self-reports of sexual behavior. J Adolesc Health. 2009;44:199–200.

66. Philpot A, Knerr W, Maher D. Promoting protection and pleasure: Amplifying the effectiveness of barriers against sexually transmitted infections and pregnancy. Lancet. 2006;368:2028–31.

67. Swartzendruber A, Zenilman JM. A national strategy to improve sexual health. J Am Med Assoc. 2010;304:1005–6.

68. Fenton KA. Time for a change: Rethinking and reframing sexual health in the United States. J Sex Med. 2010;7 suppl 5:250–2.

69. Robert AC, Sonenstein FL. Adolescents' reports of communication with their parents about sexually transmitted diseases and birth control: 1988, 1995, and 2002. J Adolesc Health. 2010;46:532–7.

70. Ferguson RM, Vanwesenbeeck I, Knijn T. A matter of facts… and more: an exploratory analysis of the content of sexuality education in The Netherlands. Sex Educ: Sex, Soc Learn. 2008;8:93–106.

71. Brugman M, Caron SL, Rademakers J. Emerging adolescent sexuality: a comparison of American and dutch college women's experiences. Int J Sex Health. 2010;22:32–46.

72. Isley MM, Edelman A, Kaneshiro B, Peters D, Nichols MD, Jensen JT. Sex education and contraceptive use at coital debut in the United States: results from Cycle 6 of the National Survey of Family Growth. Contraception. 2010;82:236–42.

73. Hogben M, Chesson H, Aral SO. Sexuality education policies and sexually transmitted disease rates in the United States of America. Int J STD AIDS. 2010;21:293–7.

Part IV

Critical Reviews:
New Public Health STD/HIV Prevention

Preventing HIV/AIDS in the United
States, 1981–2009: History
in the Making

16

Ronald Valdiserri

Introduction

The history of HIV/AIDS prevention is, without question, a great, unfinished work. True, there have been important milestones in the three decades since the epidemic was first described in the United States [1]—accomplishments in science, advances in policy and the evolution of organized efforts to prevent the spread of the human immunodeficiency virus [2]. Yet, the epidemic is far from over, either in the United States or elsewhere in the world. According to the UNAIDS, there were 33 million people living with HIV in 2007 and almost 3 million new infections that same year [3]. In the United States, an estimated 56,300 persons became newly infected with HIV in 2006—roughly 40% higher than previous estimates of HIV incidence [4]. Continued gaps in knowledge, notably in the domains of vaccine and microbicide development, have blunted efforts to prevent continued HIV transmission [5] and failure to bring proven HIV prevention interventions and programs to scale [6] has impeded optimal progress.

Unanswered questions and programmatic limitations notwithstanding, there is real benefit in reviewing the HIV/AIDS prevention experiences of the past three decades in the United States. A critical review of programmatic responses to the HIV/AIDS epidemic will help elucidate efforts that have resulted in successful prevention outcomes, deconstruct and analyze attempts that have failed, and continue to refine our knowledge of the various determinants that influence program success and failure. Consistent with the theme of this volume, this chapter explores a variety of prevention approaches spanning those that target individuals, focus on communities, or strive to alter the systems that serve the individuals, families, and communities at risk for acquiring or transmitting HIV.

Throughout this chapter, the term "program" is used broadly to refer to any organized effort to prevent the spread of human immunodeficiency virus [7]. As such, it encompasses efforts that serve a variety of target populations, employ various modalities, both biomedical and behavioral, and intervene at different levels, whether individual, community, or societal. Further, the term "program" is used without regard to sponsorship. Namely, this historic review considers programmatic responses that have arisen within communities, programs that have been sponsored by governmental public health organizations, and HIV prevention interventions that

Note that the author wrote this chapter while employed by the Department of Veteran's Affairs. The findings and conclusions of this chapter are those of the author and do not necessarily reflect the views of the United States government.

R. Valdiserri, M.D., M.P.H. (✉)
Office of HIV/AIDS and Infectious Disease Policy,
U.S. Department of Health and Human Services,
200 Independence Ave, S.W., Room 443H,
Washington, DC 20201, USA
e-mail: ron.valdiserri@hhs.gov

S.O. Aral, K.A. Fenton, and J.A. Lipshutz (eds.), *The New Public Health and STD/HIV Prevention:*
Personal, Public and Health Systems Approaches, DOI 10.1007/978-1-4614-4526-5_16,
© Springer Science+Business Media New York 2013

have been implemented and evaluated, using experimental or quasi-experimental designs, to determine their ability to effectively prevent the transmission of HIV.

Epidemiologic Overview of the US HIV/AIDS Epidemic

From an epidemiologic report of an unusual cluster of five cases of *Pneumocystis carinii* (since rechristened *Pneumocystis jerovecii*) pneumonia among five previously healthy young men in Los Angeles in 1981 [1, 8], HIV has grown into a national epidemic—and a global pandemic [3]. The Centers for Disease Control and Prevention (CDC) estimates that at the end of 2006, 1.1 million adults and adolescents in the United States were living with diagnosed or undiagnosed HIV infection [9] and that over 580,000 Americans have died as a result of the virus, since its first description in 1981 [10].

Even before the discovery of the causative agent, case–control studies suggested that AIDS was sexually transmissible [11] and reports of AIDS cases among injection drug users, persons with hemophilia and transfusion recipients supported blood-borne transmission [12]. Based on the evidence at hand, albeit incomplete, a number of community-based and professional organizations issued statements on the prevention and control of AIDS, followed in early March, 1983, by the US government's recommendations on steps that should be taken to prevent the spread of AIDS [13]. Groups at increased risk for AIDS were asked to refrain from donating plasma and/or blood and sexual contact with persons "known or suspected to have AIDS" (p. 102) was to be avoided [13].

During the first decade of the HIV/AIDS epidemic in the United States, incident AIDS cases increased, reaching over 106,000 reported cases in 1993 [14]. By 1993, AIDS had become the leading cause of death in men and women aged 25–44 years of age [15]. In the earliest years of the American epidemic, most AIDS cases were reported in men-who-have-sex-with-men (MSM), but cases reported in injection drug users (IDU) and cases attributed to heterosexual transmission

increased steadily through the early 1990s [16]. Initially, the majority of AIDS cases were reported among whites, but cases among black Americans increased throughout the epidemic and by 1996, there were more reported AIDS cases among blacks than among any other racial/ethnic group in the United States [16].

A tremendous advance in the fight against AIDS occurred in May 1983, when researchers at the Institute Pasteur in Paris reported the isolation of a T-lymphotropic retrovirus named "lymphadenopathy-associated virus" (LAV) from a homosexual male presenting with generalized lymphadenopathy [17]. Twenty five years later, in 2008, Barre-Sinoussi and Montagnier, two key authors of this original report, would be awarded the Nobel Prize for their discovery of the virus responsible for causing AIDS [18]. One year following the French report, researchers at the US National Cancer Institute reported isolating a similar virus (designated HTLV-III) from 48 individuals, including patients with AIDS, "pre-AIDS," and asymptomatic high-risk patients [19].

In early March 1985, the Food and Drug Administration (FDA) licensed a commercial test kit to detect antibodies to HTLV-III using enzyme-linked immunosorbent technology [20]. The availability of this test was a substantial prevention milestone in that it allowed a more accurate assessment of the spread of the virus among various populations—without having to limit surveillance activities to the symptomatic, end-stage of viral infection, i.e., the constellation of conditions collectively known as AIDS [21]. Rapidly implemented in blood banks across the United States, the test was used to screen all donated blood for the presence of antibodies to HIV—as the virus had come to be known in 1986 [22]—thus removing infected blood supplies. The incidence of transfusion-associated AIDS cases peaked shortly thereafter, in 1988 [23], and transfusion-associated AIDS has since been virtually eliminated in the United States [24].

The changing epidemiology of perinatal HIV infection in the United States reflects the evolution of efforts to prevent the transmission of HIV from infected mothers to their newborns. Using dried-blood specimens obtained from neonates for routine metabolic screening, the CDC implemented a population-based national survey in the late 1980s to measure the prevalence of HIV among child-bearing women and to estimate the incidence of HIV infection in newborns in the United States [25]. Early results indicated that approximately 1,800 newborns acquired HIV infection during 1989 [25]. By 1992 the survey had been expanded to 44 states, the District of Columbia, Puerto Rico and the US Virgin Islands; data indicated that in 1991–1992 there had been approximately 7,000 live births to HIV seropositive women with an estimated 1,400–2,100 newborns infected with HIV [26]. But these numbers would soon change.

An important prevention breakthrough occurred on February 21, 1994, when the National Institutes of Health (NIH) announced preliminary results from a randomized controlled trial (AIDS Clinical Trials Group Protocol 076) demonstrating that zidovudine given to pregnant women infected with HIV and their newborns significantly reduced the risk of HIV transmission [27]. A detailed analysis demonstrated that the zidovudine regimen, given ante-partum, intra-partum, and to the newborn for 6 weeks following birth, reduced maternal–infant transmission risk by approximately two-thirds [28]. US Public Health Service Guidelines for the use of zidovudine to reduce the risk of perinatal HIV transmission followed shortly after the NIH announcement [29]. The next year, in 1995, the Public Health Service recommended that health care providers should ensure that all pregnant women be routinely counseled about HIV and encouraged to be tested, so that those found to be infected could be provided information about zidovudine therapy to reduce the risk for perinatal HIV transmission [30]. Earlier prevention guidelines, promulgated before the findings of AIDS Clinical Trials Group Protocol 076, had focused on offering HIV counseling and testing only to those women in high-risk groups [31].

An analysis of trends in perinatal AIDS cases through June 1998 revealed a peak in 1992, followed by substantial declines that were associated with the increased uptake of zidovudine to prevent vertical transmission of HIV [32]. However, in 1999, the Institute of Medicine reported that despite substantial declines in peri-natally transmitted cases of AIDS in the United

States, the number of newborns infected remained "far above what is potentially achievable" (p. 6) and issued recommendations calling for universal HIV screening of all pregnant women with patient notification and the ability to decline (so-called "opt-out" testing) [33]. Available estimates suggest that currently, some 144–236 HIV infected infants are born annually in the United States—a 95% decrease since 1992 [34].

Arguably, one of the most prominent of changes in the epidemiology of HIV/AIDS in the United States has been the increase in the life expectancy of persons with HIV/AIDS that has occurred as a result of advances in treatment. Deaths among persons with AIDS, which had increased steadily through the mid-1990s, declined, for the first time, in 1996 [35]. This decline has been attributed to the use of more intensive antiretroviral therapies [36], including the introduction in late 1995 of a new class of antiretroviral agents, the protease inhibitors [2]. An analysis of 14 cohort studies involving over 43,000 HIV infected patients from the United States, Canada, and Western Europe demonstrated a marked decrease in mortality rates and corresponding increases in life expectancy between 1996 and 2005, brought about by improved treatment with combination antiretroviral therapy [37]. In addition to the obvious individual, community, and societal benefits of decreased mortality, improved survival with HIV disease also translates into increasing HIV/AIDS prevalence [38] and a need to enhance medical and prevention services for an ever growing population of Americans living with HIV [39].

In summary, approximately 1.1 million adults and adolescents are living with HIV/AIDS in the United States and reductions in mortality secondary to improved antiretroviral treatments are a major factor contributing to increasing HIV/AIDS prevalence [9]. Although HIV incidence is lower than the estimated 130,000 new infections that occurred in 1984–1985, at the peak of the US epidemic, it is estimated that over 56,000 persons become newly infected with HIV every year in America [4]. The majority of new HIV infections (73%) occur in males and nearly three-quarters of those are among men who have sex with men; among US women, high-risk heterosexual contact is the predominant mode of transmission [40]. Nearly half of all new HIV infections occur among blacks [40].

Evolution of Community and Governmental Prevention Response

Approaches to HIV prevention continue to evolve, based on advances in science, available resources, and the attitudes and values of providers, clients (i.e., the recipients of the prevention services) and other stakeholders [41]. This review of the evolution of community and governmental responses will touch upon each of these three major determinants in constructing a narrative of HIV prevention in the United States from 1981 through 2009.

Early Years

The earliest years of the AIDS epidemic in America were characterized by a mixture of fear and indifference [2]. In the months following the initial case report in June 1981 [1], the public health community read, with growing anxiety, a number of scientific publications describing the seemingly sudden onset of profound cellular immune dysfunction among young, previously healthy, homosexual men and drug users [42–44]. The next year, in 1982, a 20 month old infant from San Francisco who had received multiple transfusions developed an unexplained immunodeficiency and opportunistic infection [12]. Shortly thereafter, several other infants—without any history of blood transfusion—were reported with the same unexplained immunodeficiency and opportunistic infections [45]. Fear about this mysterious, fatal disease, referred to by some as "gay cancer" [46], began to spread in the gay community and among those who provided health care and social services to members of the gay community [47]. However, the mainstream media largely ignored the emerging epidemic [48] until the disclosure in July 1985 that the world-famous, Hollywood actor Rock Hudson had developed AIDS [49].

As chronicled by Andriote in his history of the impact of AIDS on gay community life in America, community-based organizations (CBOs) sprang up in New York and San Francisco and other metropolitan areas where homosexual populations were struggling to cope with the deadly new disease [46]. Like the Gay Men's Health Crisis in New York and the San Francisco AIDS Foundation (originally designated as the Kaposi's Sarcoma Foundation), these organizations tended to be multifunctional: disseminating information about AIDS as it became available; providing care to those who were stricken; advocating for additional governmental resources to support research into the cause and treatment of AIDS; and creating prevention materials targeted to gay men.

Lacking definitive information about the cause of AIDS, these earliest prevention efforts were, understandably, often imprecise. For example, some early community-developed materials urged gay men to reduce their number of sexual partners and assess their partners' overall health status as a means of reducing risk, while others more specifically advocated "avoiding the exchange of potentially infectious bodily fluids" ([46], p. 74).

The first prevention guidelines issued by the US government were published in November 1982, and were targeted to individuals who might be exposed to AIDS as a result of caring for the sick, including laboratorians [50]. Precautions included wearing gloves when handling blood specimens or bodily fluids from AIDS patients and labeling blood and other specimens with special warning labels such as "blood precautions" or "AIDS precautions" [50]. Since these guidelines were developed prior to the discovery of the causative virus, they were based on the assumption that a "transmissible agent" was responsible for AIDS. In March 1983, a scant few months before the publication by the French researchers on the T-lymphotropic virus [17], guidelines developed by CDC, FDA, and NIH recommended avoiding sexual contact with "persons known or suspected to have AIDS" [13].

For the most part, the discovery of the causative virus [17, 19] ended any credible question that AIDS was due to a noninfectious cause. However, the significance of a positive antibody test was initially unknown. Did it mean that the person was currently infected with or immune to the virus? [51]. In fairly short-order, mounting evidence suggested that individuals with antibodies to the virus were, indeed, infectious and capable of transmitting the virus "through intimate sexual contact," sharing needles, before or during childbirth, and through donated whole blood or blood products [52].

The US Public Health Service (PHS) published a plan for the prevention and control of AIDS in 1985 with several underlying assumptions: that more persons were infected with the virus than had developed AIDS; that AIDS could take up to several years to develop following infection; and that infected persons (i.e., those with "repeatedly reactive" antibody tests) could transmit the virus over many years—even though they remained asymptomatic [53]. Such epidemiologic circumstances called for "broad scale prevention and control activities" [53].

Community-Centered AIDS Prevention

In the absence of a vaccine or curative treatment, the PHS plan emphasized national, state, and community-level risk reduction and education programs to curtail viral transmission. Of note, the PHS plan called for the development of "specific prevention and control recommendations through consensus building among key individuals and groups" including "homosexual and bisexual men and IV drug users" ([53], p. 454). In particular, the PHS plan identified the need to provide risk reduction programs for "high-risk groups and individuals" through the implementation of "community risk reduction and health education programs to effect behavior change" ([53], p. 454). The prevention recommendations outlined in this early plan are consistent with accepted standards for high quality health promotion programs which dictate that such programs must reflect the special characteristics, needs and preferences of the populations for whom they are intended [54]. However, as described below, implementing these recommendations would soon lead to conflict with those who saw "community-centered" prevention for high-risk groups as synonymous with the promotion of homosexuality and drug use [46].

An early, groundbreaking example of community-centered prevention can be found in a formative study conducted by the Research and Decisions Corporation on behalf of the San Francisco AIDS Foundation. Five hundred, 30-min telephone interviews were conducted on a random probability sample of self-identified gay and bisexual men in the city and county of San Francisco in August and September of 1984 [55]. The researchers, who asked detailed questions about specific sexual practices, determined that most of the respondents already had high levels of knowledge about what behaviors carried the highest risk of transmission. Instead of focusing on the dissemination of information, the social marketing researchers who conducted the study advised that future prevention efforts should motivate people "to act on the information they already have" ([55], p. 116). Other research from San Francisco, conducted some 9 months earlier, had also found high levels of knowledge about risk reduction in gay men, but documented discrepancies between beliefs and actual behaviors [56]. In addition to knowledge, factors such as tension, gay identity, and knowing someone with advanced AIDS, were associated with the type and frequency of sexual behavior reported by the respondents [56].

Relying on their innate knowledge of the communities which they represented, community leaders implemented grassroots prevention efforts in New York, Los Angeles, San Francisco, and other metropolitan areas with large gay populations [46, 57–60]. Consistent with research demonstrating fairly high levels of existing knowledge within gay communities, these "home-grown" prevention efforts attempted, instead of just increasing information about AIDS, to influence the adoption of safer sexual practices—often by "eroticizing" safer sexual practices through workshops, graphic educational materials, and even film [61–63]. These approaches were described pejoratively by critics—typically not members of the high-risk populations for whom these efforts were intended—as "pornographic" or worse [62].

In the earliest years of the US AIDS epidemic, resources for prevention and education activities came largely from affected communities and, in some instances, from local governments [60]. In 1985, CDC announced funding for community-based AIDS demonstration projects and innovative projects for AIDS risk reduction [59]. Public health organizations and other public or nonprofit organizations, including community-based organizations, were eligible to apply. Over time, federal funding for HIV/AIDS has increased substantially, growing from $8 million dollars in 1982 to over $23.3 billion dollars in fiscal year 2008 [64]. Of note, the largest proportion (63%) of the fiscal year 2008 HIV/AIDS budget was devoted to treatment, with a much smaller portion, 14%, devoted to prevention [64].

Federal funding for HIV prevention activities, though essential, has periodically generated controversy among those who tend to view more explicit prevention information—including graphic visual approaches—as tantamount to the US government endorsing homosexuality, premarital sexual relations, or the use of illicit drugs [46, 62, 65]. As a result of these concerns, Congress enacted legislation in 1987 that specifically limited use of federal funds so they may not be used "to provide education or information designed to promote or encourage, directly, homosexual or heterosexual sexual activity or intravenous substance use"; these limitations remain in effect at the time of this writing [66]. These restrictions have particular relevance for HIV prevention efforts that embrace a philosophy of harm reduction.

HIV Prevention for Injection Drug Users

A brief review of efforts to reduce HIV transmission among injection drug users (IDU) highlights the inherent tensions between proponents of prevention approaches that remove or preclude risk versus those who embrace a continuum of prevention approaches, including strategies to reduce risk, when it cannot be completely eliminated. Providing sterile injection equipment to IDUs who cannot or will not stop injecting illicit drugs is an example of a harm reduction strategy that has generated substantial controversy among policy makers and community leaders.

In 1986, the US Public Health Service Plan for Prevention and Control of AIDS ("The Coolfont Report") identified increased treatment capacity for intravenous (IV) drug abuse as a major strategy for preventing AIDS transmission among IDUs [67]. However, the report also opined that "until treatment capacity is adequate…studies are needed to evaluate the efficacy and feasibility of promoting safer use of drug paraphernalia (for example, increased availability of sterile needles or 'works')" ([67], pp. 346–347).

The earliest known program to provide clean syringes to IDUs as a means of preventing hepatitis and HIV was organized by drug users in Amsterdam in 1984 [68]. In the United States, the first needle exchange programs for injecting drug users began in 1988 in Tacoma, Washington [69] and Brooklyn, NY [2], supported by nongovernmental organizations. Because of syringe prescription laws and drug paraphernalia statutes [70], many of these early programs operated in defiance of state law [71]. In 1988, Congress prohibited the use of federal funds for syringe exchange programs, even in those localities where such activities were deemed to be lawful [70].

It is important to not portray access to sterile injection equipment as an HIV prevention panacea for injecting drug users—and to recognize that there are valid concerns about unintended, negative consequences [72]. However, the preponderance of evidence shows that when IDUs participate in multicomponent HIV prevention programs that include syringe exchange (i.e., provision of sterile needles and syringes) they reduce drug-related HIV risk behaviors; furthermore, such programs neither expand drug use nor increase the frequency of injection [73, 74]. A number of observational studies have demonstrated lower rates of HIV seroprevalence among IDUs in communities with needle and syringe exchange programs (SEPs) compared to IDUs in communities without such programs [75, 76].

As of November 2007, a total of 185 syringe exchange programs were operating in 36 states, the District of Columbia and Puerto Rico [77]. These programs were supported by individuals, foundations, and state and local governments [77] because prior to fiscal year 2010, the specific prohibition on the use of federal funds to support access to sterile injection equipment remained in place. However, when the President signed the Fiscal Year 2010 Consolidated Appropriations Act in late December 2009, for the first time since 1988, the ban on federal funding for needle exchange programs was lifted [78]. Although the language in the appropriations bill did not provide increases in funding specifically for needle and syringe exchange programs, it does allow existing federal HIV prevention funds to be used to support these activities. Understandably, prevention advocates and activists who represent the psychological and medical needs of injection drug users hailed the policy change as a major victory.

An alternative to SEPs is the removal of barriers to the legal purchase of sterile needles and syringes at pharmacies. An early example of this approach was undertaken by Connecticut, which enacted laws in July 1992 to allow for the purchase (without prescription) and possession of up to ten needles/syringes; before the law was enacted, purchase and possession of needles/syringes without a prescription was illegal [79]. Subsequent analyses demonstrated decreases in self-reported syringe sharing among IDUs and increases in pharmacy purchases of sterile syringes by IDUs [80, 81]. Even in the absence of laws that restrict pharmacy sales of syringes, pharmacists' attitudes can influence IDUs access to sterile syringes [82, 83]. However, education and small group training has been shown to decrease negative opinions and attitudes toward pharmacy syringe sales to IDUs among both pharmacists and community members [84].

Drug treatment—especially pharmacological interventions for persons addicted to opioids—has proven to be highly effective in reducing illicit opioid use and, as such, high-risk drug injection practices [67]. However, comparable pharmacological interventions are not available for

stimulants and other injectable drugs. A variety of studies have shown that methadone maintenance treatment (MMT) reduces HIV risk behaviors (i.e., those behaviors directly or indirectly related to drug use) and/or HIV seroconversion [85–88]. Yet, it is estimated that fewer than 10% of individuals who are addicted to heroin and prescription opioids are receiving MMT [89]. While some addicted individuals who are not receiving methadone maintenance therapy are probably not yet ready to stop their drug use, it is likely that many more could be treated with MMT if treatment could be expanded [73, 89]. Yet, like access to sterile injection equipment, MMT still carries a stigma, in part related to the notion that it enables continued drug use [89, 90].

Certainly, transmission of HIV among injection drug users continues in the United States, but declines in the number of reported HIV/AIDS diagnoses among IDUs [91, 92] are consistent with reports of decreases in HIV incidence [93]. A more recent analysis comparing HIV prevalence among injecting and non-injecting drug users in New York City found "nearly identical" rates of HIV prevalence in both groups, suggesting that sexual risk behaviors may be taking on greater importance as a mode of HIV transmission among drug users [94].

AIDS Education Campaigns

As cited above, the earliest AIDS prevention plan developed by the US Public Health Service in 1985, called for "broad scale prevention and control activities, emphasizing educational and informational exchange" ([53], p. 453). By most accounts, past educational campaigns to prevent and control other sexually transmissible diseases, notably syphilis, had not been very successful [95]—likely because they had been based on a leitmotif of fear and guilt, typically portraying sexually transmissible diseases as the outcome of moral turpitude [96]. Many of these same, stigmatizing, themes arose again in the policy debates that surrounded early efforts to educate both the public and the so-called "high-risk groups" about the dangers of AIDS [97–99]. As previously noted, a major recurrent theme was the assertion, by some, that frank discussions of sexual and drug-using risk behaviors—in terms understandable and acceptable to target populations—was tantamount to endorsing those high-risk, and sometimes illegal, behaviors.

To its credit, the US Public Health Service, working through the CDC, strived to avoid the errors of past health campaigns that had deliberately or inadvertently stigmatized affected persons. In October 1987, CDC launched "America Responds to AIDS" (ARTA), part social marketing campaign and part public information campaign [100, 101]. The first phase of the campaign consisted of posters, brochures and public service announcements for television and radio and had as its theme general awareness of the epidemic and humanizing of people with AIDS [100]. In the late Spring of 1988, this effort was followed-up by a US-wide mailing of approximately 107 million English-language versions of the brochure "Understanding AIDS" [102]. This unprecedented mailing by the Federal government of a health-related document to every known US household had three main objectives:

- To make clear how AIDS is and is not transmitted.
- To make clear that what puts people at risk for AIDS are certain behaviors, not identification with "risk groups."
- To stimulate informed discussions about AIDS within families, with friends and among sexual partners [102].

In addition to AIDS information and education campaigns developed in the late 1980s for the general public, the federal government also supported, through grant programs from the CDC, AIDS education programs for school-aged youth, racial/ethnic minority populations, and individuals and groups engaged in high-risk sexual and drug use behaviors [103]. Shortly after the CDC entered into cooperative funding agreements with state and local education agencies, they published "Guidelines for Effective School Health Education to Prevent the Spread of AIDS" [104]. These guidelines were developed in collaboration with a number of national medical, public health, education, and youth-serving organizations. Reflecting a comprehensive approach to HIV prevention, the guidelines stated that "the principal purpose of education about AIDS is to prevent HIV infection" ([104], p. 4). Further, the guidelines recognized that different prevention approaches would be necessary for youth who had not yet engaged in sexual intercourse nor used illicit drugs versus those who had engaged in sexual intercourse or who had injected illicit drugs.

Theory Driven Behavioral Interventions

Several objective assessments have documented that in the earliest years of the American epidemic, funding to support HIV prevention activities lagged behind actual need—especially in the area of behavioral and social science research [97, 105–107]. This may explain, in part, the 1988 findings in the Government Accounting Office (GAO) report to Congress on ongoing AIDS educational campaigns in New York, San Francisco and Los Angeles [108]. GAO reported that "most exemplary campaigns had not systematically collected the data by which their outcomes could be measured" ([108], p. 5).

While the fields of health education and health promotion had progressed in the years following World War II [109–111], providing an evidence base upon which interventions to prevent HIV transmission could be modeled [112], the reality is that interventions specific to the prevention of HIV transmission remained largely untested throughout most of the first decade of the epidemic. Consider that when the CDC published its first "Compendium of HIV Prevention Interventions with Evidence of Effectiveness" in March 1999 [113], only two of the intervention studies included had been published in the first decade of the epidemic; both of the 1989 studies had evaluated risk reduction interventions for MSM [114, 115]. This situation would begin to improve in the 1990s, spurred on by the urgent need to identify effective interventions and by a mounting host of expert recommendations calling for expanded research into the behaviors resulting in HIV transmission [116–121].

The advancement of theory-driven behavioral interventions is well exemplified by the evolution of the federally funded AIDS Community Demonstration Projects [122]. When these projects were originally funded in 1985 in six US cities (Albany, Chicago, Dallas, Denver, Long Beach, and Seattle), they were envisioned as "flexible" and "broadly directed" programs that would help evaluate AIDS prevention activities at the community level ([103], p. 259). In the first 4 years of their funding, they focused largely on one-on-one risk reduction counseling for MSM and IDUs, both in clinical and community-based settings [123].

Important though these early efforts were, they brought to the fore a number of unanswered questions about the fundamental nature of programs designed to reduce high-risk sexual and drug-use behaviors. What is the optimal location and venue for AIDS prevention activities? What are the specific elements of a risk-reduction intervention that are effective in changing behaviors? How can public health workers reach high-risk individuals who do not perceive themselves to be at risk for HIV? Because of these and related questions, in late 1988, the CDC convened a group of experts in social and behavioral science, community interventions, and evaluation methodology to strategize about how best to design and implement community-level AIDS prevention interventions. As a result of their deliberations, the AIDS Community Demonstration Projects were wholly reconfigured [122, 123].

The newly designed AIDS Community Demonstration Projects (ACDPs) were predicated on the following, bedrock principles: interventions must be based on theoretically derived models of behavior change; intervention design must entail formative work, including close collaboration with the target community; social networking approaches should be used to access hard-to-reach populations; and AIDS prevention should be viewed as a social diffusion process in which both mass media and interpersonal communication channels play important roles [122].

Elements from a variety of behavioral models were incorporated into the design of the interventions, including the following: the Health Belief Model; the Theory of Reasoned Action; Social Cognitive Theory; and the Stages of Change (SOC) continuum of the Transtheoretical Model [124]. Operationalizing the construct that different interventions would be required for individuals engaged in risky sexual or drug use behaviors—depending upon where they might fall along a continuum of pre-intentions/intentions related to the behavior(s) of interest—represented a tremendous leap forward in the development of HIV prevention interventions. The mode by which prevention messages were transmitted was "small media," i.e., community newsletters, pamphlets, and baseball cards [125]. It is noteworthy that the content of these materials was based on actual stories of successful behavior change (including movement from pre-contemplation to contemplation of behavior change) from persons living in those communities, identified through careful formative work [125]. To support the intervention, key community members were mobilized to reinforce prevention messages while condoms and bleach kits (containing bleach, water and alcohol pads—along with instructions) were made widely available.

Cross-sectional surveys conducted over a 3 year period revealed that intervention communities, compared to comparison communities, had significantly higher levels of condom carrying (i.e., having a condom on one's person) as well as higher levels of consistent condom use with main and non-main partners [125]. At an individual level, respondents who had been recently exposed to the intervention were "more likely to carry condoms and to have higher stage-of-change scores for condom and bleach use" (p. 336, 125). The researchers did not find a community-level impact of the intervention on bleach use, which they attributed, in part, to a stated change in federal policy regarding the use of bleach which had been announced during the course of the study [125]. New federal guidelines, issued in 1993 [126], placed less emphasis on bleach use as an HIV prevention strategy than had earlier iterations.

While the AIDS Community Demonstration Projects have been highlighted as exemplars of advances in theory-based HIV prevention interventions, they are not the only examples. Throughout the decade of the 1990s, researchers published the results of a number of well-designed, theory-driven studies showing positive behavioral and/or health outcomes in response to interventions developed to reduce the risk of HIV transmission. Examples include risk reduction interventions for adolescents [127–130], drug users—both in and out of treatment [131–134], men-who-have-sex-with-men [135, 136], and women [137–139].

Institution-Based HIV Prevention

Although a strong argument can be made that all HIV prevention efforts entail distinctive circumstances, the category of institution-based HIV prevention deserves special mention in this review of HIV prevention program development. In short, the characteristics, culture and context of the institutions in which prevention services are embedded can have a profound impact on the planning, implementation and delivery of subsequent HIV prevention services. This premise is aptly demonstrated by a brief consideration of HIV prevention in schools and in correctional facilities.

In 1986, the Institute of Medicine's report "Confronting AIDS" endorsed the importance of educating the nation's youth about AIDS, but simultaneously recognized that "sex education in schools still must overcome considerable political opposition and political intransigence" ([97], p. 102). Two years later, the first Presidential Commission on the Human Immunodeficiency Virus Epidemic opined that "the provision of HIV education in our schools is of vital importance and must be introduced immediately" ([140], p. 88). The Commission stated that decisions about appropriate content should be determined locally and that school-based education "should highlight the benefits of character development, abstinence and monogamy" [140]. Several years later, the National Commission on AIDS, a group established by legislative action to develop and support national policy on HIV/AIDS,

made the following recommendation about school-based HIV prevention:

> School-based prevention should be presented in an integrated, comprehensive health curriculum that includes discussion of sexuality and that teaches general prevention skills, while still providing HIV-specific information. Schools and other youth-serving institutions should select curricula and teaching strategies that have been tested for efficacy through research and evaluation. ([141], p. C-24)

A majority of American adults report that they are in favor of teaching school students about abstinence as well as other methods for preventing pregnancy, HIV, and other sexually transmitted diseases [142]. Yet, surveys indicate that, over time, there has been an increasing emphasis on teaching abstinence as the *only* method of preventing pregnancy and STDs, including HIV [143–145]. Certainly, there is widespread consensus that early sexual initiation is associated with a host of health problems, in addition to HIV, and that delaying the onset of sexual activity is an important and appropriate prevention strategy for young people [146, 147]. Nevertheless, serious concerns have been raised about public funding policies that favor "abstinence only" approaches to HIV education [148, 149] in light of studies suggesting that these approaches may not be any more effective in delaying the initiation of sex than are comprehensive sex education programs [150].

Schools represent a complex nexus of beliefs, values, and attitudes of the students, their parents, the teachers, and the administrators, as well as the community at large. While schools provide a unique opportunity to deliver HIV prevention interventions, we must also recognize the tensions that exist across a variety of differing perspectives. Case in point, a systematic review of behavioral interventions to reduce HIV, STD, and pregnancy among adolescents found that one of the characteristics of successful programs was a strong focus on skills to reduce specific sexual risk behaviors [151]. However, the experts who conducted this review also noted that school systems may be more inclined to support "broad based programs" that don't delve into specific sexual risk behaviors—because they are less likely to raise community objections [151].

This supposition is supported by the results of a 2006 national survey of elementary, middle and high schools which revealed that only 21% of middle schools and 38.5% of high schools taught students how to correctly use a condom [152]. Compare this to 2007 data documenting that nearly half (47.8%) of all high school students report "ever" having sexual intercourse [153]. These observations are presented not to minimize different opinions and perspectives, but to underscore the institutional challenges of providing evidence-based HIV prevention interventions in school-based settings.

Correctional facilities represent another unique institutional setting for HIV prevention. Although information on the actual incidence of HIV infection among US inmates continues to remain elusive, cases of AIDS among inmates of US correctional facilities have been reported since the early years of the US epidemic [154]—often associated with a history of injection drug use [155] or high-risk sexual behaviors prior to arrest [156]. Once inside correctional facilities, tattooing, injection drug use (with sharing of injection equipment) and sex—both consensual and forced—provide further opportunities for HIV transmission among inmates [157, 158]. In 2006, an extensive epidemiologic investigation of 88 inmates who had seroconverted while incarcerated in a US state prison system, found strong associations between HIV positivity and reported male-to-male sex while in prison and reports of having received a tattoo while in prison [159].

In the summer of 1990, the National Commission on AIDS conducted a site visit and hearing to consider the myriad issues associated with HIV/AIDS among detainees of US federal, state, and local correctional facilities. Their subsequent report detailed continued discrimination towards inmates with HIV disease and a failure to educate inmates and staff about how to eliminate the risks of HIV transmission. The Commission noted that:

> Whether to distribute condoms in prison and whether to teach inmates how to sterilize needles and works have proven to be controversial questions for correctional officers. Both these questions have important political, social and moral dimensions. From a public health perspective, however, it is clear that where unprotected sexual and drug behavior are known to occur, the availability of condoms and bleach and water can reduce the risk. ([160], pp19–20)

As spelled-out above, competing ideologies of public health and public safety officials [161, 162] can impact the content and availability of HIV prevention services in US correctional facilities. Specifically, while harm reduction is a well-accepted value in the public health culture, access to condoms for inmates [163, 164] remains controversial among public safety officials, because of both security concerns and a hesitancy to recognize that sex behind bars is taking place. Even more divisive is the issue of making injection practices "safer" by providing sterile injection equipment to inmates who cannot or will not stop injecting drugs [165]. There are no officially sanctioned programs in the United States that provide sterile injection equipment to inmates of correctional facilities, although several countries in western and eastern Europe as well as central Asia have implemented such programs [165]. Thus, layered over the complexities of human sexuality, addiction and HIV prevention science are the cultural and organizational characteristics of correctional facilities. As with our discussion of HIV prevention in school-based settings, these controversies are not raised to cast blame or vilify, but to highlight the fact that institutional values and practices can have a profound impact on the development and delivery of HIV prevention services.

HIV Counseling & Testing Programs

As previously noted, when an antibody test for HIV first became commercially available, the implications of a positive test result were uncertain [51]. A group of experts convened by the National Institutes of Health in early July 1986 noted "we cannot precisely predict who among persons with antibody positivity will be ill or fatally ill in the future" [166]. Even in light of these uncertainties, public health officials anticipated that many persons at risk might desire antibody testing [167]. As such, in April 1985, the

US Centers for Disease Control and Prevention began providing funds to health departments to offer antibody testing in so called "alternate test sites" [168]. Public Health Service guidelines issued in 1986 recommended that counseling and testing should be "routinely offered to all persons at increased risk when they present to health care settings" [169]. Subsequent PHS recommendations expanded on the importance of including counseling before and after testing and detailed groups who should be routinely counseled and tested, including the following: persons who might have a sexually transmitted disease, IV drug users, women of childbearing age, persons with signs and symptoms of HIV, and persons who consider themselves at risk [170].

Traditionally, public health programs for the prevention and control of bacterial STDs have relied on models of enhanced screening for disease detection and subsequent treatment of infected individuals and their partners as a means of interrupting transmission [171]. It was into this historical and operational milieu that HIV counseling and testing programs were embedded. Of course, there are substantial differences between HIV and bacterial STDs—most notably the fact that syphilis and gonorrhea are curable with antibiotics. Nevertheless, shortly after the commercial licensure of test kits to detect HIV antibodies, hundreds of publicly funded test sites sprung up across the nation and tens of thousands of persons were tested for HIV [167]. It short order, HIV CTRPN (counseling, testing, referral, and partner notification) became recognized as an essential component of comprehensive HIV prevention programs [172].

A 1990 review, conducted by the Government Accounting Office (GAO) highlighted a number of gaps in the federally funded HIV counseling and testing program [173]. The GAO report found that only about 40% of those tested in public programs returned for their test results and that efforts to provide HIV counseling and testing for IDUs were only reaching small numbers of drug users. Finally, the report concluded that monitoring and evaluation of HIV counseling and testing programs was subpar, with very little information available on the impact of these services on subsequent risk behaviors [173].

Questions about the impact of HIV counseling and testing on subsequent risk behaviors began to surface shortly after the federal program was first implemented [174]. An early review of 50 studies noted substantial risk reduction in some populations following HIV counseling and testing—especially among serodiscordant heterosexual couples [175]. A larger review, published several years later, reported that individuals who learned they were HIV positive reduced risk behaviors while persons who learned that they were HIV negative did not [176]. However, these analysts hastened to add that details about the content of counseling were typically absent from the published studies, thereby limiting their ability to determine the independent behavioral effects of the counseling, in addition to the impact of learning of a positive or a negative HIV test result [176].

Based on expert opinion, including HIV counselor feedback, in the early 1990s, the CDC shifted its policy on HIV counseling from a didactic, information-driven process, to one that was "client-centered" and focused on developing a personalized risk reduction plan [177]. A randomized controlled trial, published later in the decade, supported this policy change when it demonstrated reductions in incident STDs among HIV negative heterosexual clients of STD clinics who had received "interactive client centered counseling," compared to those who had received traditional, didactic counseling [178].

As discussed later in this chapter, improvements in HIV therapy and continued emphasis on the importance of early diagnosis of HIV infection have continued to influence the evolution of national HIV testing policies. In its earliest programmatic incarnation, prevention specialists saw HIV counseling and testing as a strategy to empower individuals to adopt behaviors that would prevent the acquisition or transmission of HIV. Increasingly, prevention practitioners have come to emphasize the role of HIV counseling and testing as the gateway into lifesaving treatment. This subtle, albeit perceptible, shift in philosophy has substantial implications in a number of program domains, including the following: how and where to offer HIV counseling and testing; the relative contribution of counseling in the HIV counseling and testing paradigm; and how to improve linkages between programs and systems that diagnose HIV infection and those responsible for treating HIV disease.

HIV Prevention Community Planning

Throughout the course of the US epidemic there have been a number of changes in HIV prevention policy, in response to epidemiologic trends, advances in knowledge, and other factors. Historically, one of the most significant *programmatic* changes occurred in the mid-1990s, when the CDC implemented HIV Prevention Community Planning. This new approach required state and local health departments to prioritize HIV prevention funds based on local epidemiologic circumstances and with the active involvement of community representatives [179]. Prior to the implementation of HIV Prevention Community Planning, priorities for federal HIV prevention program funds were set nationally—with the largest share of resources mandated to be spent on CTRPN programs. For example, in 1993, the year before community planning was implemented, over 70% of the total funding awarded to state and local health departments was earmarked to be spent on CTRPN [180].

A convergence of factors influenced this change from centralized decision-making about HIV prevention priorities to local-level determination. A number of opinion leaders, both governmental and nongovernmental, questioned the disproportionate focus on CTRPN and criticized Congress and the federal government for mandating how prevention resources should be spent at the state and local levels [181, 182]. The CDC's own federal Advisory Committee on the Prevention of HIV Infection had come to a similar conclusion, based on a 7 month external review of CDC's HIV prevention activities [183]. Although the Committee recognized the benefits of CTRPN as a diagnostic tool, they recommended "shifting the emphasis away from testing as the main prevention intervention toward ongoing individual behavior-change interventions for those at highest risk of HIV infection" ([183], p. 5).

In response to these critiques, in December 1993, the CDC profoundly restructured the process by which HIV prevention programs were planned [179], formalizing the role of community representatives in the process [184] and elucidating evidence-based criteria to be used when setting HIV prevention priorities [179, 185]. Internal and external evaluations of the earliest years of "community planning" revealed a host of operational and methodological challenges attendant upon implementing an evidence-based, shared (i.e., governmental and community) decision making process for determining HIV prevention priorities [186–190]. Challenges notwithstanding, an analysis comparing the relative allocation of federal HIV prevention funds in fiscal year (FY) 1996 versus FY 1993 documented that fewer prevention dollars were spent on counseling and testing programs and that more federal funds were allocated to health education and risk reduction programs following the implementation of community planning [191].

HIV Prevention Community Planning is certainly not the first attempt to strengthen public health outcomes by empowering evidence-based, community decision making [192]. Nor should it be viewed as the solution for all of the challenges that attend the development and maintenance of effective, community-based, HIV prevention programs. Over a decade after its implementation, public health and policy analysts continue to grapple with complexities inherent in the process [193–195]. Arguably, one of the most important legacies of HIV Prevention Community Planning has been its extensive documentation of the difficulties that are encountered when attempting to operationalize HIV prevention science into real-world prevention programs.

Implementing HIV Prevention Science

HIV prevention science is not a homogeneous entity. A variety of scientific disciplines (e.g., behavioral, biomedical, organizational, etc.) comprise the knowledge base of HIV prevention. Not all of these disciplines are at the same stage of maturation and productivity in terms of their HIV prevention findings and outcomes. Further, consider the mix of factors that must be addressed in order to create a truly comprehensive, evidence-based HIV prevention program for a city, state or geographic region. What are the local epidemiologic circumstances of the HIV epidemic in that area? Where are most new infections occurring and what behaviors are resulting in HIV transmission? What are the unique cultural and developmental characteristics of the various at-risk populations that must be taken into consideration when developing consumer-oriented prevention interventions? What other significant determinants of health impact the various populations at risk for HIV infection?

Given the complexity of translating HIV prevention science into practice, it should come as no surprise that one of the recurrent themes of HIV prevention programming in the United States has been the gap between science and action.

Capacity Issues

As described elsewhere in this chapter, community-based organizations (CBOs) have often been ahead of organized governmental efforts in attempting to address the HIV prevention needs of their constituent populations. Furthermore, because of their unique position within the communities they serve, CBOs typically have more credibility with and understanding of the very populations whom we wish to reach with HIV prevention interventions [196, 197]. That is not to say that all CBOs automatically take up the challenge of HIV prevention—or, that when they have determined to do so, they have the requisite capacity to effectively plan and deliver effective HIV prevention interventions. A variety of individual, organizational, structural, and cultural constraints can act as barriers to taking on the responsibility of planning and delivering effective HIV prevention services, not the least of which is adequate resources [198, 199].

A nationwide sample of 77 community-based organizations providing AIDS services, surveyed in 1996–1997, revealed that while the majority of Directors and frontline staff favored "the inclusion of science-based group and workshop interventions as part of their overall repertoire of HIV prevention programs," many respondents also

believed that their organizations lacked either the resources or the technical skills to properly implement these interventions ([200], p. 83). Another analysis from that same sample found that most of the HIV prevention services then being offered to both MSM and women were primarily educational in nature (e.g., brochures and "AIDS 101" factual talks)—rather than the theory-driven, skills-based training that would be required to modify high-risk behaviors [201]. These findings echo an earlier analysis which summarized evaluations of AIDS prevention programs in the United States.

> With a few notable exceptions, the evaluated programs were generally too simplistic or too superficial to be able to make a significant impact on the continued transmission of infection or too unique to be replicable. ([202], p. 300)

Nor are these shortcomings limited to nongovernmental organizations. In 1992, following an assessment of national STD and HIV prevention programs, CDC program staff reported the following implementation gaps: inadequate use of data to delineate program direction, sporadic training and quality assurance for HIV counselors, and a reliance on "rote, form-driven prevention messages" [203]. Not surprisingly, health departments report that resource constraints impede their ability both to develop comprehensive, evidence-based HIV prevention programs and to provide adequate technical assistance to nongovernmental organizations offering HIV prevention services within their jurisdictions [204]. Another significant contributor to shortcomings in prevention capacity owes to the fact that during the first decade of the US AIDS epidemic, most health departments did not have substantial technical capacity in behavioral or social sciences [205]—given their historical reliance primarily on biomedical models to control and prevent sexually transmitted diseases.

Although the challenge of developing and sustaining HIV prevention capacity within governmental and nongovernmental organizations is ongoing [206], progress has been made in the three decades since the epidemic began [207]. Efforts to define and quantify the specific dimensions of HIV prevention program capacity should greatly help to tailor and target needed technical assistance [208]. And the explication of broad models [209], as well as specific strategies [210], that promote the incorporation of HIV prevention science into practice further inform the field. A recurrent and important theme in the consideration of HIV prevention capacity is the absolute necessity of ensuring that HIV prevention researchers collaborate closely with the communities for whom prevention services are intended and with the organizations that will ultimately deliver the interventions that are being tested by the researchers [211, 212].

HIV Prevention Issues of the Current Decade

As the previous discussion highlighted, shortcomings in the capacity to develop and deliver HIV prevention services at the scale and frequency required to have a demonstrable impact on HIV incidence will likely continue to impact national efforts. But gaps in prevention capacity are not the only challenges facing organized efforts to prevent HIV. This section briefly summarizes the key prevention issues facing us in this current decade of the US HIV epidemic.

Complacency

References to "HIV/AIDS complacency" first began appearing in the American press in the mid-1990s, describing diminished societal mobilization around and support for organized efforts to prevent and treat HIV [213]. A nationally representative telephone survey of over twenty-five hundred American adults, conducted in early 2009, revealed that only 6% named HIV/AIDS as the most urgent health problem facing the nation—down from 17% in 2006 [214]. Further, less than half of the surveyed adults reported that they had "heard, seen or read a lot or some about the problem of HIV/AIDS in the US" in the past year—45% in 2009 compared to 70% in 2004 [214]. While not unreasonable to assume that some level of HIV/AIDS complacency would

develop among the general population because of improvements in treatments for HIV disease [37, 38], the real concern is that individuals who are at increased risk for HIV infection or transmission may be less likely to engage in protective behaviors (including health-seeking behaviors for early HIV diagnosis) because they minimize the risk of the disease or its consequences.

Continuing Racial Disparities

At the time of this writing, the most recent estimates of HIV incidence in the US suggest that nearly half (46%) of all new HIV infections occur among African Americans [40]—despite the fact that African Americans account for only 14% of the US population [215]. Compared to whites, black men and black women have HIV incidence rates that are 5.9 and 14.7 times higher, respectively [40]. Although not as dramatically disparate, Hispanic males and females are also reported to have higher HIV incidence rates than white males and females: 2.2 and 3.8 times higher, respectively [40].

The higher prevalence of concurrent sexual partnerships (i.e., sexual partnerships that overlap in time) among non-Hispanic Black and Hispanic men, compared to white men, has been identified as a likely contributor to higher rates of heterosexually transmitted HIV infection among non-Hispanic Black and Hispanic women in the United States [216]. While sexual concurrency is associated with an increased risk for heterosexual HIV infection among racial/ethnic minorities, one must acknowledge the Gordian knot of other, interrelated factors that likely also contribute to higher rates of infection, including the following: residential segregation related to poverty, a shrinking pool of sexual partners for African American women (associated, in part, with higher rates of incarceration among African American men), economic inequality of women compared to men, and higher background rates of untreated sexually transmitted diseases related to fewer opportunities for timely diagnosis and treatment [217, 218].

Among black men-who-have-sex-with-men, higher HIV prevalence compared to white MSM does not appear to be the result of differences in individual risk behaviors [219]. Other factors, including sexual partner and network characteristics, high prevalence of untreated STDs, and individuals' lack of awareness of their positive HIV serostatus likely contribute to these disparities [219, 220]. A sobering analysis of 1,767 MSM recruited from community venues in five US cities revealed an overall HIV prevalence of 25%, with 46% of the African American MSM testing positive for HIV [221]. Among the HIV-infected men, 48% were unaware of their HIV infections; of the MSM with unrecognized HIV infection, 64% were black [221].

Exploring, in detail, the multifaceted issue of HIV/AIDS disparities within minority communities is beyond the scope of this chapter. But by any reckoning, the disproportionate burden of HIV infection among America's racial/ethnic minority populations represents a substantial, ongoing challenge to HIV prevention efforts in the United States [222].

Unanswered Questions in HIV Prevention Science

As stated at the beginning of this chapter, HIV/AIDS prevention is a great, unfinished work. Despite impressive advances over three decades, scientifically speaking, there remain major gaps in the knowledge base supporting HIV prevention. Perhaps the most obvious is the lack of an effective HIV vaccine, notwithstanding intensive research efforts [223]. Likewise, although a variety of topical microbicide agents (for vaginal or rectal application) remain under investigation [224], an effective agent has not yet been identified [225].

To date, the following biomedical interventions have been proven to be effective in preventing HIV transmission: male condoms, male circumcision, and the prophylactic use of antiretrovirals or contraception to prevent unwanted pregnancies to reduce mother-to-child HIV transmission [223]. Although laboratory tests have shown that polyurethane female condoms provide

an effective barrier against HIV transmission, the ability of the female condom to prevent HIV infection has not been directly assessed [223]. Based on three studies conducted in Africa, there is strong evidence that male circumcision, when performed by medically trained operators, can substantially reduce the acquisition of HIV by heterosexual men [226]. Although observational data in the United States show that circumcision is associated with substantially reduced HIV risk in patients with known heterosexual HIV exposure [227], there are major differences between the HIV epidemic in the United States and the epidemic in sub-Saharan Africa [228]. Because most sexual transmission of HIV in the United States occurs as a result of male-to-male sex and given the already relatively high prevalence of circumcision among US men, the role of male circumcision as an HIV prevention strategy in the United States remains under discussion [229].

Early detection and treatment of curable STDs has long been advocated as an essential component of comprehensive HIV prevention programs [230]. Certainly, timely detection and treatment of STDs is an important public health priority in its own rite. However, questions remain about the role of broad-scale STD prevention efforts as specific strategies to prevent HIV transmission, at a population-level, given mixed results from community level trials [223, 231]—including two recent trials showing no effect of HSV suppressive therapy on reducing HIV acquisition among African women and MSM from Peru and the United States [232, 233]. Some have interpreted these inconsistent results to suggest that the ability of broad-scale STD treatment programs to decrease HIV incidence is dependent upon the stage of the HIV epidemic at the time they are implemented [223, 234].

Underway at the time of this writing are trials to determine the effectiveness of using antiretrovirals prophylactically—as a means of preventing HIV infection among those who are at high, ongoing risk of acquiring the virus. PrEP (pre-exposure prophylaxis) is, at present, undergoing safety and efficacy testing among a variety of high-risk populations in the United States, Asia, and Africa [235]. Questions about PrEP abound, starting with the obvious: "Will it work?" If the trials are successful, a host of other issues will need to be resolved [236]. What systems of finance could be mobilized to pay for PrEP? Will access to PrEP result in an unintended rebound of unsafe sexual behaviors? Will widespread use of antiretrovirals result in increased drug resistance and toxicity? How should PrEP services be delivered—to whom and for how long? What is the best way to integrate PrEP into existing, traditional approaches to HIV prevention? Models suggest that PrEP could substantially reduce lifetime risk of HIV infection for certain high-risk individuals, although cost-effectiveness considerations will need to be taken into account as the trial results develop [237].

The unanswered questions in HIV prevention science highlighted in this section have been largely biomedical in nature. Equally relevant are unanswered questions that relate to the ongoing role of stigma as an impediment to successful HIV prevention efforts [238] and how best to ameliorate the deleterious effects of stigma. Although frequently invoked as a major barrier to successful HIV program efforts (including prevention, care and treatment programs), there is "little consensus among policy-makers and program implementers about how best to define, measure and diminish" stigma ([239], p. S 75). A 2008 review of the published scientific literature on HIV/AIDS-related stigma resulted in a number of specific recommendations for advancing the knowledge base underpinning this important, albeit poorly understood, phenomenon [239]. Recommendations included: developing a comprehensive conceptual framework for HIV/AIDS-related stigma; encouraging the use of valid and reliable stigma measures; and identifying and evaluating potential interventions to reduce stigma at a structural and institutional level [239]. Given that HIV/AIDS is first and foremost a "social disease," involving social and political science researchers in the mix of experts addressing unanswered questions in HIV prevention science, such as stigma, will certainly improve the quality of outcomes [240].

Balancing biomedical and non-biomedical approaches to HIV prevention

HIV viral load is one of the chief predictors of HIV transmission [241]. Given that combined antiretroviral therapy can successfully reduce viral load, and hence infectiousness [242–245], the notion that universal HIV testing and widespread antiretroviral therapy might be an effective approach to stopping the spread of HIV is gaining adherents [246, 247]. Some have even asserted that individuals under treatment who have undetectable plasma viral loads cannot transmit HIV sexually [248].

In the United States and Canada, evidence continues to mount that widespread antiretroviral treatment with subsequent decreases in "community viral load" are associated with reductions in new HIV diagnoses [249, 250]. No question, the early diagnosis and subsequent treatment of all who are infected with HIV is a worthwhile goal, prevention benefits aside. But given that HIV shedding in genital secretions can occur even in the face of undetectable HIV levels in the blood [251, 252] and recognizing that perceptions about the protective benefit of antiretroviral therapy might result in increased rates of unsafe sexual behavior [253, 254], it will be necessary to carefully evaluate "test and treat" strategies for unintended consequences such as behavioral disinhibition and increased resistance to antiviral drugs [255, 256].

Although not completely comparable, the experience with mass treatment as a strategy to prevent continued syphilis transmission is certainly instructive. A mass treatment intervention to interrupt heterosexual syphilis transmission in British Columbia was associated with an initial decrease in transmission followed by a rebound [257, 258]. Other program analysts have reported that increased rates of syphilis screening do not necessarily translate into decreased rates of syphilis transmission [259] and that it is essential to also address social determinants of health in order to successfully prevent the continued spread of sexually transmitted diseases [260].

These observations underscore the primary point of this discussion, namely, that biomedical approaches, by themselves, may not be adequate to reduce HIV incidence. In fact, there are those who believe that the current prevention response to HIV/AIDS has become overly "medicalized," meaning that prevention interventions based on social and political science have become undervalued and underutilized compared to those relying on biotechnology [240]. As such, a very real challenge facing us in this fourth decade of the epidemic is how best to balance and integrate biomedical and non-biomedical approaches to HIV prevention so as to optimize prevention outcomes.

Closer Alignment of HIV Prevention and HIV Care

Many would agree that "test and treat" biomedical approaches should not be viewed as a panacea capable of resolving all of the nation's unmet HIV prevention needs. But having stated that caution, there is no denying that in recent times the domain of HIV prevention has become more closely aligned with the domain of HIV care, largely driven by improvements in HIV treatments. While early intervention for those infected with HIV is not a new idea [261], it has gained in currency over the course of the epidemic [262], especially with the growing awareness that untreated HIV infection is associated with a host of negative consequences beyond AIDS, itself, including the development of many non-AIDS-defining diseases as well as the further spread of the virus [263].

Coupled with the drive to diagnose persons with HIV infection and to get them into medical care in a timely manner has been an increasing emphasis on the importance of tailoring prevention for persons living with HIV/AIDS, especially as those persons are living longer, productive and sexually active lives [39, 264–266]. Behavioral interventions targeted to persons living with HIV/AIDS have been shown to be effective in reducing unprotected sex and the acquisition of new STDs [267]. Furthermore,

high-risk sexual practices typically decrease after persons learn they are infected with HIV [268] and models suggest that a majority of new HIV infections in the United States are transmitted by persons who are unaware of their positive serostatus [269].

Because HIV testing is both a gateway into treatment as well as an increasingly important component of HIV prevention, we can expect to see continued emphasis on timely diagnosis of HIV. To that point, the CDC revised its policies on HIV testing in late 2006, recommending HIV screening for all adult patients in all health care settings across the United States [270]. This movement away from "risk-based" to "routine" HIV testing was taken to destigmatize the HIV testing process and to promote early diagnosis of HIV infection. Currently, it is estimated that there are more than 230,000 HIV infected persons in the United States who have not yet been diagnosed [9]. Equally concerning, nearly 40% of persons newly diagnosed with HIV in the United States develop AIDS within 12 months of their diagnosis—suggesting that they have been infected with the virus for many years prior to diagnosis [10].

Despite a broad public health consensus that early HIV diagnosis is beneficial to individuals and to society, barriers to promoting expanded HIV screening in health care settings exist, including the following: lack of insurance coverage for HIV screening, state laws that require pretest counseling and signature consent for HIV testing, and competing priorities among busy primary care providers [271–274]. Challenges notwithstanding, mounting evidence that early initiation of antiretroviral therapy has a positive impact on survival [275] will continue to fuel efforts to expand routine HIV testing in both health care and community settings. As these efforts unfold, it would be prudent to anticipate the need to strengthen referral mechanisms to assure individuals' smooth and timely movement from HIV diagnostic services into HIV care programs and to promote and sustain the incorporation of client-friendly HIV prevention services into HIV treatment programs [276, 277].

Conclusion

To quote Gertrude Stein, "History takes time." As such, any historical review of US HIV prevention efforts must, by definition, be considered a "work in progress." Even so, the lessons of the last three decades are highly relevant to future efforts to prevent the transmission of HIV and other related pathogens. Some of the most important lessons in HIV prevention are still being learned. For example, reliance on a single strategy to curtail the epidemic, no matter how effective that strategy might be, is unlikely to succeed. This observation is not offered as cynicism. Instead, it acknowledges the complex array of contextual factors, such as social networks, that mediate health outcomes [278–283]. Simply stated, a multifaceted public health problem requires a multipronged solution. Another lesson learned from our dealings with this virus is the recognition that new circumstances will continue to emerge and modify risk—both in context and practice. In the recent history of the American HIV/AIDS epidemic, the use of the Internet to meet sexual partners [284, 285] and changes in drug use—namely, the methamphetamine epidemic [286–288]—are two highly relevant examples of circumstances that have profoundly influenced HIV-related risk. Thus, to be effective, HIV prevention programs must not only be comprehensive, they must also be agile, able to adapt to emerging circumstances and needs.

Finally, we must never underestimate the importance of developing the capacity of communities to implement and sustain effective HIV prevention strategies. While policy makers and the technical experts who engage in HIV prevention are understandably drawn to the era's unanswered scientific questions, there is typically less interest in day-to-day implementation issues. Yet, the "post-discovery" issues of how to effectively move HIV prevention from the pages of grant reports and peer-reviewed journals and into the neighborhoods where individuals are being exposed to the virus is a tremendous, ongoing challenge [41, 289, 290]. In the opinion of some cognoscenti, this failure to bring effective HIV prevention interventions to scale is the reason why HIV incidence in the United States has not declined in recent years [212].

What we can say with certainty is this. HIV/AIDS, unlike any other health problem in recent times, has forced the United States and other nations of the world to confront the richly complex interplay between people, communities, systems, and circumstances to produce what we simplistically refer to as "health."

References

1. Centers for Disease Control and Prevention. Pneumocystis pneumonia—Los Angeles. MMWR Morb Mortal Wkly Rep. 1981;30:250–2.
2. Valdiserri RO. HIV/AIDS in historical profile. In: Valdiserri RO, editor. Dawning answers: How the HIV/AIDS epidemic has helped to strengthen public health. Oxford: Oxford University Press; 2003. p. 3–32.
3. UNAIDS. 2008 epidemiology slides. http://data.unaids.org/pub/GlobalReport/2008. Accessed 30 Dec 2008.
4. Hall HI, Song R, Rhodes P, et al. Estimation of HIV incidence in the united states. JAMA. 2008;300:520–9.
5. Merson MH, O'Malley J, Serwadda D, Apisuk C. The history and challenge of HIV prevention. Lancet. 2008;372:475–88.
6. Global HIV Prevention Working Group. Bringing HIV prevention to scale: an urgent global priority. http://www.globalhivprevention.org/pdfs/PWG-HIV_prevention_report-FINAL.pdf. Accessed 30 Dec 2008.
7. Valdiserri RO. Preventing AIDS: the design of effective programs. New Brunswick, NJ: Rutgers University Press; 1989.
8. Gottlieb MS. AIDS—past and future. N Engl J Med. 2001;344:1788–90.
9. Centers for Disease Control and Prevention. HIV prevalence estimates—United States, 2006. MMWR Morb Mortal Wkly Rep. 2008;57:1073–6.
10. Centers for Disease Control and Prevention. HIV/AIDS Surveillance Report, 2007, vol. 19. Atlanta: U.S. Department of Health and Human Services, Centers for Disease Control and Prevention; 2009. p. 1–63.
11. Centers for Disease Control and Prevention. A cluster of Kaposi's sarcoma and Pneumocystis carinii pneumonia among homosexual male residents of Los Angeles and orange counties, California. MMWR Morb Mortal Wkly Rep. 1982;31:305–7.
12. Centers for Disease Control and Prevention. Possible transfusion-associated acquired immune deficiency

syndrome (AIDS)—California. MMWR Morb Mortal Wkly Rep. 1982;31:652–4.

13. Centers for Disease Control and Prevention. Prevention of acquired immune deficiency syndrome (AIDS): report of inter-agency recommendations. MMWR Morb Mortal Wkly Rep. 1983;32(8): 101–4.

14. Centers for Disease Control and Prevention. HIV/AIDS Surveillance Report 1994;5(4):1–33.

15. Hariri S, McKenna MT. Epidemiology of human immunodeficiency virus in the United States. Clin Microbiol Rev. 2007;20:478–88.

16. Centers for Disease Control and Prevention. HIV and AIDS—United States, 1981–2000. MMWR Morb Mortal Wkly Rep. 2001;50:430–4.

17. Barre-Sinoussi F, Chermann JC, Rey F, et al. Isolation of a T-lymphotropic retrovirus from a patient at risk for acquired immune deficiency syndrome (AIDS). Science. 1983;220:868–71.

18. Lite J. Montagnier, Barre-Sinoussi and zur Hausen Share Nobel. Scientific American, Oct 6 2008. http://www.sciam.com/article.cfm?id=montagnier-barre-sinoussi&print=true. Accessed 6 Jan 2009.

19. Gallo RC, Salahuddin SZ, Popovic M, et al. Frequent detection and isolation of cytopathic retroviruses (HTLV-III) from patients with AIDS and at risk for AIDS. Science. 1984;224:500–3.

20. Centers for Disease Control and Prevention. Results of human T-lymphotropic virus type III test kits reported from blood collection centers—United States, April 22–May 19 1985. MMWR Morb Mortal Wkly Rep. 1985;34:375–6.

21. Buehler JW. HIV and AIDS surveillance: public health lessons learned. In: Valdiserri RO, editor. Dawning answers: How the HIV/AIDS epidemic Has helped to strengthen public health. Oxford, England: Oxford University Press; 2003. p. 33–55.

22. Coffin J, Haase A, Levy JA, et al. Human immunodeficiency viruses. Science. 1986;232:697.

23. Klevens RN, Hughes D. The impact of transfusion-associated AIDS in the United States. Abstract 769-W. 9th Conference on Retroviruses and Opportunistic Infections. 2002. http://www.retroconference. org/2002/Abstract/13540.htm. Accessed 21 Jan 2009.

24. Selik RM, Ward JW, Buehler JW. Trends in transfusion-associated acquired immune deficiency syndrome in the United States, 1982 through 1991. Transfusion. 1993;33:890–3.

25. Gwinn M, Pappaioanou M, George RJ, et al. Prevalence of HIV infection in childbearing women in the United States: surveillance using newborn blood samples. JAMA. 1991;265:1704–8.

26. Centers for Disease Control and Prevention. National HIV serosurveillance summary: results through 1992, vol. 3. Atlanta, GA: U.S. Department of Health and Human Services; 1994.

27. Centers for Disease Control and Prevention. Zidovudine for the prevention of HIV transmission from mother to infant. MMWR Morb Mortal Wkly Rep. 1994;43:285–7.

28. Connor EM, Sperling RS, Gelber R, et al. Reduction of maternal-infant transmission of human immunodeficiency virus type 1 with zidovudine treatment. N Engl J Med. 1994;331:1173–80.

29. Centers for Disease Control and Prevention. Recommendations for the use of zidovudine to reduce perinatal transmission of human immunodeficiency virus. MMWR Morb Mortal Wkly Rep. 1994;43(No. RR-11):1–20.

30. Centers for Disease Control and Prevention. U.S. Public Health Service recommendations for human immunodeficiency virus counseling and voluntary testing for pregnant women. MMWR Morb Mortal Wkly Rep. 1995;44(No. RR-7):1–15.

31. Centers for Disease Control and Prevention. Recommendations for assisting in the prevention of perinatal transmission of human T-lymphotropic virus type III/lymphadenopathy-associated virus and acquired immunodeficiency syndrome. MMWR Morb Mortal Wkly Rep. 1985;34(48):721–32.

32. Lindegren ML, Byers RH, Thomas P, et al. Trends in perinatal transmission of HIV/AIDS in the United States. JAMA. 1999;282:531–8.

33. Institute of Medicine, Committee on Perinatal Transmission of HIV. Reducing the odds: preventing perinatal transmission of HIV in the United States. Washington, DC: National Academy Press; 1999.

34. Centers for Disease Control and Prevention. Achievements in public health: reduction in perinatal transmission of HIV infection—United States, 1985—2005. MMWR Morb Mortal Wkly Rep. 2006;55(21):592–7.

35. Centers for Disease Control and Prevention. Update: trends in AIDS incidence, deaths, and prevalence—United States, 1996. MMWR Morb Mortal Wkly Rep. 1997;46(8):165–73.

36. Palella FJ, Delaney KM, Moorman AC, et al. Declining morbidity and mortality among patients with advanced human immunodeficiency virus infection. N Engl J Med. 1998;338(13):853–60.

37. Antiretroviral Therapy Cohort Collaboration. Life expectancy of individuals on combination antiretroviral therapy in high-income countries: a collaborative analysis of 14 cohort studies. Lancet. 2008;372:293–9.

38. Lee LM, Karon JM, Selik R, Neal JJ, Fleming PL. Survival after AIDS diagnosis in adolescents and adults during the treatment era, United States, 1984–1997. JAMA. 2001;285(10):1308–15.

39. Janssen RS, Valdiserri RO. HIV prevention in the United States: increasing emphasis on working with those living with HIV. J Acquir Immune Defic Syndr. 2004;37(2):S119–21.

40. Centers for Disease Control and Prevention. Subpopulation estimates from the HIV incidence surveillance system—United States, 2006. MMWR Morb Mortal Wkly Rep. 2008;57(36):985–9.

41. Valdiserri RO. Technology transfer: achieving the promise of HIV prevention. In: Peterson JL, DiClemente RJ, editors. Handbook of HIV prevention. New York, NY: Kluwer Academic/Plenum; 2000. p. 267–83.

42. Centers for Disease Control and Prevention. Kaposi's sarcoma and Pneumocystis pneumonia among homosexual men—New York city and California. MMWR Morb Mortal Wkly Rep. 1981;30:305–8.

43. Centers for Disease Control and Prevention. Follow-up on Kapposi's sarcoma and Pneumocystis pneumonia. MMWR Morb Mortal Wkly Rep. 1981;30:409–10.

44. Masur H, Michelis MA, Greene JB, et al. An outbreak of community-acquired Pneumocystis carinii pneumonia: initial manifestation of cellular immune dysfunction. N Engl J Med. 1981;305(24):1431–8.

45. Centers for Disease Control and Prevention. Unexplained immunodeficiency and opportunistic infections in infants—New York, New Jersey, California. MMWR Morb Mortal Wkly Rep. 1982; 31:665–7.

46. Andriote JM. Victory deferred: how AIDS changed Gay life in America. Chicago, IL: University of Chicago Press; 1999.

47. Leo J. The real epidemic: fear and despair: AIDS isolates many of its victims and is changing the gay life-style. Time Magazine. July 4; 1983. pp. 56–8.

48. Kinsella J. Covering the plague. New Brunswick, NJ: Rutgers University Press; 1989.

49. Thomas E. The new untouchables: anxiety over AIDS is verging on hysteria in some parts of the country. Time Magazine, 23 Sep 1985. pp. 24–26.

50. Centers for Disease Control and Prevention. Acquired immune deficiency syndrome (AIDS): precautions for clinical and laboratory staffs. MMWR Morb Mortal Wkly Rep. 1982;31:577–80.

51. Centers for Disease Control and Prevention. Antibodies to a retrovirus etiologically associated with acquired immunodeficiency syndrome (AIDS) in populations with increased incidences of the syndrome. MMWR Morb Mortal Wkly Rep. 1984;33: 377–9.

52. Centers for Disease Control and Prevention. Provisional public health service inter-agency recommendations for screening donated blood and plasma for antibody to the virus causing acquired immunodeficiency syndrome. MMWR Morb Mortal Wkly Rep. 1985;34:1–5.

53. Mason JO. Public health service plan for the prevention and control of acquired immune deficiency syndrome (AIDS). Public Health Rep. 1985; 100(5):453–5.

54. American Public Health Association. Criteria for the development of health promotion and education programs. Am J Public Health. 1987;77:89–92.

55. Research and Decisions Corporation. Designing an effective AIDS prevention campaign strategy for San Francisco: Results from the first probability sample of an Urban Gay Male Community. 3 Dec 1984, San Francisco, CA.

56. McKusick L, Horstman W, Coates TJ. AIDS and sexual behavior reported by Gay men in San Francisco. Am J Public Health. 1985;75:493–6.

57. Wohlfeiler D. Community organizing and community building among Gay and bisexual Men. In: Minkler M, editor. Community organizing and community building for health. New Brunswick, NJ: Rutgers University Press; 1997. p. 230–43.

58. Centers for Disease Control and Prevention. Evolution of HIV/AIDS prevention programs—United States, 1981–2006. MMWR Morb Mortal Wkly Rep. 2006;55:597–603.

59. Bailey ME. Community-based organizations and CDC as partners in HIV education and prevention. Public Health Rep. 1991;106:702–8.

60. Arno PS. The nonprofit sector's response to the AIDS epidemic: community-based services in San Francisco. Am J Public Health. 1986;76:1325–30.

61. Palacios-Jimenez SM. Facilitator's guide to eroticizing safer sex: a psychoeducational workshop approach to safer sex education. New York: Gay Men's Health Crisis; 1986.

62. Booth W. Another muzzle for AIDS education? Science. 1987;238:1036.

63. Kolata G. Erotic films in AIDS study cut risky behavior. New York Times, 3 Nov 1987. p. 18.

64. Johnson JA. AIDS funding for federal government programs: FY1981—FY2009. Congressional Research Service. 23 Apr 2008. http://assets.opencrs.com/rpts/RL30731_20080423.pdf. Accessed 4 Mar 2009.

65. Fineberg HV. Education to prevent AIDS: prospects and obstacles. Science. 1988;239:592–6.

66. Centers for Disease Control and Prevention. Content of AIDS-related materials, pictorials, audiovisuals, questionnaires, survey instruments, and educational sessions in Centers for Disease Control and Prevention (CDC) assistance programs. http://www.cdc.gov/od/pgo/forms/hiv.htm. Accessed 4 Mar 2009.

67. U.S. Public Health Service Executive Task Force on AIDS. Coolfont report: a PHS plan for prevention and control of AIDS and the AIDS virus. Public Health Rep. 1986;101:341–8.

68. Hartgers C, Ameijden EJ, Hoek JA, Coutinho RA. Needle sharing and participation in the Amsterdam Syringe Exchange Program among HIV-seronegative injecting drug users. Public Health Rep. 1992;107:675–81.

69. Strathdee SA, Vlahov D. The effectiveness of needle exchange programs: a review of the science and policy. AIDScience. 2001; 1(16). http://aidscience.org/Articles/aidscience013.12p. Accessed 12 Mar 2009.

70. Gostin LO. The legal environment impeding access to sterile syringes and needles: the conflict between law enforcement and public health. J Acquir Immune Defic Syndr. 1998;18 Suppl 1:S60–70.

71. Lane SD. A brief history. In: Stryker J, Smith M, editors. Dimensions of HIV prevention: needle exchange. Menlo Park, CA: Henry J. Kaiser Family Foundation; 1993. p. 1–9.

72. Thomas SB, Quinn SC. The burdens of race and history on Black Americans' attitudes toward needle exchange policy to prevent HIV disease. J Public Health Policy. 1993;14:320–47.

73. Committee on the Prevention of HIV Infection among Injection Drug Users in High Risk Countries. Preventing HIV infection among injecting drug users in high-risk countries: an assessment of the evidence. Washington, DC: National Academies Press; 2007.

74. Wodak A, Cooney A. Do needle syringe programs reduce HIV infection among injecting drug users: a comprehensive review of the international evidence. Subst Use Misuse. 2006;4(1):777–813.

75. Hurley SF, Jolley DJ, Kaldor JM. Effectiveness of needle-exchange programmes for prevention of HIV infection. Lancet. 1997;349:1797–800.

76. Des Jarlais DC, Hagan H, Friedman SR, et al. Maintaining low HIV seroprevalence in populations of injecting drug users. JAMA. 1995;274:1226–31.

77. Centers for Disease Control and Prevention. Syringe exchange programs—United States, 2005. MMWR Morb Mortal Wkly Rep. 2007;56:1164–7.

78. Schwartzapfel B. Swapping politics for science on drug policy. The Nation. 12/21/2009. http://www.thenation.com/doc/20100104/schwartzapfel/print. Accessed on 3 Mar 2010.

79. Centers for Disease Control and Prevention. Impact of new legislation on needle and syringe purchase and possession—Connecticut, 1992. MMWR Morb Mortal Wkly Rep. 1993;42:145–8.

80. Valleroy LA, Weinstein B, Jones TS, Groseclose SL, Rolfs RT, Kassler WJ. Impact of increased legal access to needles and syringes on community pharmacies' needle and syringe sales—Connecticut, 1992–1993. J Acquir Immune Defic Syndr. 1995; 10:73–81.

81. Groseclose SL, Weinstein B, Jones TS, Valleroy LA, Fehrs LJ, Kassler WJ. Impact of increased legal access to needles and syringes on practices of injecting-drug users and police officers—Connecticut, 1992–1993. J Acquir Immune Defic Syndr. 1995;10: 82–9.

82. Compton WM, Horton JC, Cottler LB, et al. A multistate trial of pharmacy syringe purchase. J Urban Health. 2004;81:661–70.

83. Deibert RJ, Goldbaum G, Parker TR, et al. Increased access to unrestricted pharmacy sales of syringes in Seattle-king county, Washington: structural and individual-level changes, 1996 versus 2003. Am J Public Health. 2006;96:1347–53.

84. Fuller CM, Galea S, Caceres W, Blaney S, Sisco S, Vlahov D. Multilevel community-based intervention to increase access to sterile syringes among injection drug users through pharmacy sales in New York city. Am J Public Health. 2007;97:117–24.

85. Gibson DR, Flynn NM, McCarthy JJ. Effectiveness of methadone treatment in reducing HIV risk behavior and HIV seroconversion among injecting drug users. AIDS. 1999;13:1807–18.

86. Williams AB, McNelly EA, Williams AE, D'Aquila RT. Methadone maintenance treatment and HIV type 1 seroconversion among injecting drug users. AIDS Care. 1992;4:35–41.

87. Metzger DS, Woody GE, McLellan T. Human immunodeficiency virus seroconversion among intravenous drug users in- and out-of-treatment: an 18 month prospective follow-up. J Acquir Immune Defic Syndr. 1993;6:1049–56.

88. Metzger DS, Navaline H, Woody GE. Drug abuse treatment as AIDS prevention. Public Health Rep. 1998;113 Suppl 1:97–106.

89. Kleber HD. Methadone maintenance 4 decades later: thousands of lives saved but still controversial. JAMA. 2008;300:2303–5.

90. Des Jarlais DC, Paone D, Friedman SR, Peyser N, Newman RG. Regulating controversial programs for unpopular people: methadone maintenance and syringe exchange programs. Am J Public Health. 1995;85:1577–84.

91. Centers for Disease Control and Prevention. HIV diagnoses among injection-drug users in states with HIV surveillance—25 States, 1994–2000. MMWR Morb Mortal Wkly Rep. 2003;52:634–6.

92. Centers for Disease Control and Prevention. Trends in HIV/AIDS diagnoses—33 states, 2001–2004. MMWR Morb Mortal Wkly Rep. 2005;54: 1149–53.

93. Des Jarlais DC, Marmor M, Friedmann P, et al. HIV incidence among injection drug users in New York city, 1992–1997: evidence for a declining epidemic. Am J Public Health. 2000;90:352–9.

94. Des Jarlais DC, Arasteh K, Perlis T, et al. Converging of HIV seroprevalence among injecting and non-injecting drug users in New York city. AIDS. 2007;21:231–5.

95. Brandt A. AIDS in historical perspective: four lessons from the history of sexually transmitted diseases. Am J Public Health. 1988;78:367–71.

96. Brandt A. No magic bullet: a social history of venereal disease in the United States since 1880. New York, NY: Oxford University Press; 1985.

97. Institute of Medicine, Committee on a National Strategy for AIDS. Confronting AIDS: directions for public health, health care and research. Washington, DC: National Academy Press; 1986.

98. Valdiserri RO. Epidemics in perspective. J Med Humanit Bioeth. 1987;8:95–100.

99. Kosterlitz J. Educating about AIDS. Natl J Aug 30, 1986; 35:2044–9.

100. Woods D, David D, Westover FJ. "America Responds to AIDS:" its content, process and outcome. Public Health Rep. 1991;106:616–22.

101. Keiser NH. Strategies of media marketing for "American Responds to AIDS" and applying lessons learned. Public Health Rep. 1991;106:623–7.

102. Centers for Disease Control and Prevention. Understanding AIDS: an information brochure being mailed to all U.S. households. MMWR Morb Mortal Wkly Rep. 1988;37:261–9.

103. Mason JO, Noble GR, Lindsey BK, et al. Current CDC efforts to prevent and control human immunodeficiency virus infection and AIDS in the United States through information and education. Public Health Rep. 1988;103:255–60.

104. Centers for Disease Control and Prevention. Guidelines for effective school health education to prevent the spread of AIDS. MMWR Morb Mortal Wkly Rep. 1988;37(S-2):1–14.

105. Office of Technology Assessment, U.S. Congress. Review of the public health service's response to AIDS. Washington, DC: U.S. Congress Office of Technology Assessment, OTA-TM-H-24; February 1985.

106. Panem S. The AIDS bureaucracy. Cambridge, MA: Harvard University Press; 1988.

107. Institute of Medicine. The AIDS Research Program of the National Institutes of Health. Washington, DC: National Academies Press; 1991.

108. U.S. General Accounting Office. AIDS Education: Reaching Populations at Higher Risk; Report to the Chairman, Committee on Governmental Affairs, U.S. Senate. Washington, DC: U.S. General Accounting Office; September 1988 (PEMD-88-35).

109. Lorig K, Laurin J. Some notions about assumptions underlying health education. Health Educ Q. 1985;12:231–43.

110. McGinnis JM. Recent history of federal initiatives in prevention policy. Am Psychol. 1985;40:205–12.

111. Minkler M. Health education, health promotion and the open society: an historical perspective. Health Educ Q. 1989;16:17–30.

112. Leviton LC. Theoretical foundations of AIDS-prevention programs. In: Valdiserri RO, editor. Preventing AIDS: the design of effective programs. New Burnswick, NJ: Rutgers University Press; 1989.

113. Centers for Disease Control and Prevention. Compendium of HIV prevention interventions with evidence of effectiveness, March 1999:1–57. http://www.cdc.gov/resources/reports/hiv_compendium/index.htm. Accessed 24 Mar 2009.

114. Kelly JA, Lawrence JS, Hood HV, Brasfield TL. Behavioral intervention to reduce AIDS risk activities. J Consult Clin Psychol. 1989;57:60–7.

115. Valdiserri RO, Lyter DW, Leviton LC, Callahan CM, Kingsley LA, Rinaldo CR. AIDS prevention in homosexual and bisexual men: results of a randomized trial evaluating two risk reduction interventions. AIDS. 1989;3:21–6.

116. Institute of Medicine. Confronting AIDS: update 1988. Washington, DC: National Academy Press; 1988.

117. Turner CF, Miller HG, Moses LE, editors. AIDS: sexual behavior and intravenous drug Use. Washington, DC: National Academy Press; 1989.

118. Miller HG, Turner CF, Moses LE, editors. AIDS: the second decade. Washington, DC: National Academy Press; 1990.

119. Coyle SL, Boruch RF, Turner CF, editors. Evaluating AIDS Prevention Programs: expanded edition. Washington, DC: National Academy Press; 1991.

120. Kelly JA, Murphy DA, Sikkema KJ, Kalichman SC. Psychological interventions to prevent HIV infection are urgently needed: new priorities for behavioral research in the second decade of AIDS. Am Psychol. 1993;48:1023–34.

121. Auerbach JD, Wypijewska C, Brodie HK, editors. AIDS and behavior: an integrated approach. Washington, DC: National Academy Press; 1994.

122. Higgins DL, Galavotti C, O'Reilly K, Sheridan J. Evolution and development of the aids community demonstration projects. In: Corby NH, Wolitski RJ, editors. Community HIV prevention: the Long Beach AIDS Community Demonstration Projects. Long Beach, CA: California State University Press; 1997. p. 5–20.

123. O'Reilly KR, Higgins DL. AIDS Community Demonstration Projects for HIV prevention among hard-to-reach groups. Public Health Rep. 1991; 106:714–20.

124. Centers for Disease Control and Prevention. Community-level prevention of human immunodeficiency virus infection among high-risk populations: The AIDS Community Demonstration Projects. MMWR Morb Mortal Wkly Rep. 1996;45(RR-6):1–24.

125. CDC AIDS Community Demonstration Projects Research Group. Community-level HIV intervention in 5 cities: final outcome data from the CDC AIDS Community Demonstration Projects. Am J Public Health. 1999;89:336–45.

126. Centers for Disease Control and Prevention, National Institutes of Health, Center for Substance Abuse Treatment. Statement on the role of bleach in HIV prevention programs for injecting drug users (IDUs). 5 May 1993. http://www.aegis.com/pubs/Cdc_Fact_Sheets/1993/CDC93150.html. Accessed 4 Feb 2009.

127. Kirby D, Barth RP, Leland N, Fetro JV. Reducing the risk: impact of a new curriculum on sexual risk-taking. Fam Plann Perspect. 1991;23:253–63.

128. Jemmott JB, Jemmott LS, Fong GT. Reductions in HIV risk-associated sexual behaviors among black male adolescents: effects of an AIDS prevention intervention. Am J Public Health. 1992;82:372–7.

129. St. Lawrence JS, Brasfield TL, Jefferson KW, Alleyne E, O'Bannon RE, Shirley A. Cognitive-behavioral intervention to reduce African American adolescents' risk for HIV infection. J Consult Clin Psychol. 1995;63:221–37.

130. Jemmott JB, Jemmott LS, Fong GT. Abstinence and safer sex HIV risk-reduction interventions for African American adolescents. JAMA. 1998;279:1529–36.

131. DesJarlais DC, Casriel C, Friedman SR, Rosenblum A. AIDS and the transition to illicit drug injection—

results of a randomized trial prevention program. Br J Addict. 1992;87:493–8.

132. McCusker J, Stoddard AM, Zapka JG, Morrison CS, Zorn M, Lewis BF. AIDS education for drug abusers: evaluation of short-term effectiveness. Am J Public Health. 1992;82:533–40.

133. El-Bassel N, Schilling RF. 15 month followup of women methadone patients taught skills to reduce heterosexual HIV transmission. Public Health Rep. 1992;107:500–4.

134. Siegal HA, Falck RS, Carlson RG, Wang J. Reducing HIV needle risk behaviors among injection-drug users in the midwest: an evaluation of the efficacy of standard and enhanced interventions. AIDS Educ Prev. 1995;7:308–19.

135. Kelly JA, St. Lawrence JS, Stevenson Y, et al. Community AIDS/HIV risk reduction: the effects of endorsements by popular people in three cities. Am J Public Health. 1992;82:1483–9.

136. Kegeles SM, Hays RB, Coates TJ. The Mpowerment Project: a community-level HIV prevention intervention for young gay men. Am J Public Health. 1996;86:1129–36.

137. Kelly JA, Murphy DA, Washington CD, et al. The effects of HIV/AIDS intervention groups for high-risk women in urban clinics. Am J Public Health. 1994;84:1918–22.

138. DiClemente RJ, Wingood GM. A randomized controlled trial of an HIV sexual risk-reduction intervention for young African-American women. JAMA. 1995;274:1271–6.

139. Lauby JL, Smith PJ, Stark M, Person B, Adams J. A community-level HIV prevention intervention for inner-city women: results of the women and infants demonstration projects. Am J Public Health. 2000;90:216–22.

140. Watkins JD. Report of the presidential commission on the human immunodeficiency virus epidemic. Washington, DC: U.S. Government Printing Office; 1988.

141. Osborn JE. AIDS: an expanding tragedy: the final report of the National Commission on AIDS. Washington, DC: U.S. Government Printing Office; 1993.

142. Bleakley A, Hennessy M, Fishbein M. Public opinion on sex education in US schools. Arch Pediatr Adolesc Med. 2006;160:1151–6.

143. Darroch JE, Landry DJ, Singh S. Changing emphases in sexuality education in U.S. Public Secondary Schools, 1988–1999. Fam Plann Perspect. 2000;32:204–11. & 265.

144. Landry DJ, Darroch JE, Singh S, Higgins J. Factors associated with the contents of sex education in U.S. public secondary schools. Perspect Sex Reprod Health. 2003;35:261–9.

145. Lindau ST, Tetteh AS, Kasza K, Gilliam M. What schools teach our patients about sex: content, quality and influences on sex education. Obstet Gynecol. 2008;111:256–66.

146. O'Donnell L, O'Donnell CR, Stueve A. Early sexual initiation and subsequent sex-related risks among urban minority youth: the reach for health study. Fam Plann Perspect. 2001;33:268–75.

147. Resnick MD, Blum RW. The association of consensual sexual intercourse during childhood with adolescent health risk and behaviors. Pediatrics. 1994;94:907–13.

148. Santelli J, Ott MA, Lyon M, Rogers J, Summers D, Schleifer R. Abstinence and abstinence-only education: a review of U.S. policies and programs. J Adolesc Health. 2006;38:72–81.

149. Society for Adolescent Medicine. Abstinence-only education policies and programs: a position paper of the Society for Adolescent Medicine. J Adolesc Health. 2006;38:83–7.

150. Kirby DB. The impact of abstinence and comprehensive sex and STD/HIV education programs on adolescent sexual behavior. Sex Res Soc Policy. 2008;5:18–27.

151. Robin L, Dittus P, Whitaker D, et al. Behavioral interventions to reduce incidence of HIV, STD, and pregnancy among adolescents: a decade in review. J Adolesc Health. 2004;34:3–26.

152. Kann L, Telljohann SK, Wooley SF. Health education: results from the school health policies and programs study 2006. J School Health. 2007;77:408–34.

153. Centers for Disease Control and Prevention. Trends in HIV- and STD-related risk behaviors among high school students—United States, 1991–2007. MMWR Morb Mortal Wkly Rep. 2008;57:817–22.

154. Centers for Disease Control and Prevention. Acquired immunodeficiency syndrome in correctional facilities: a report of the National Institute of Justice and the American Correctional Association. MMWR Morb Mortal Wkly Rep. 1986;35:195–9.

155. Valdiserri EV, Hartl AJ, Chamblis CA. Practices reported by incarcerated drug abusers to reduce risk of AIDS. Hosp Community Psychiatry. 1988;39:966–72.

156. Schilling R, El-Bassel N, Ivanoff A, Gilbert L, Su KH, Safyer SM. Sexual risk behavior of incarcerated, drug-using women, 1992. Public Health Rep. 1994;109:539–47.

157. Brewer TF, Vlahov D, Taylor E, Hall D, Munoz A, Polk BF. Transmission of HIV-1 within a statewide prison system. AIDS. 1988;2:363–7.

158. Braithwaite RL, Hammett RM, Mayberry RM. Prisons and AIDS: a public health challenge. San Francisco, CA: Jossey-Bass Publishers; 1996.

159. Centers for Disease Control and Prevention. HIV transmission among male inmates in a state prison system—Georgia, 1992–2005. MMWR Morb Mortal Wkly Rep. 2006;55:421–6.

160. National Commission on AIDS. HIV disease in correctional facilities. Washington, DC: National Commission on AIDS; 1991.

161. Brewer TF, Derrickson J. AIDS in prison: a review of epidemiology and preventive policy. AIDS. 1992;6:623–8.

162. Polonsky S, Kerr S, Harris B, Gaiter J, Fichtner RR, Kennedy MG. HIV prevention in prisons and jails:

obstacles and opportunities. Public Health Rep. 1994;109:615–25.

163. May JP, Williams EL. Acceptability of condom availability in a U.S. Jail. AIDS Educ Prev. 2002;14(Suppl B):85–91.

164. Hammett TM, Gaiter JL, Crawford C. Reaching seriously at-risk populations: health interventions in criminal justice settings. Health Educ Behav. 1998;25:99–120.

165. Jurgens R, Ball A, Verster A. Interventions to reduce HIV transmission related to injecting drug use in prison. Lancet Infect Dis. 2009;9:57–66.

166. National Institutes of Health Consensus Development Panel. The impact of routine HTLV-III antibody testing on public health. In: NIH Consensus Develop Conf Statement, 7–9 Jul. Vol 6(5); 1986.

167. Centers for Disease Control and Prevention. Human T-lymphotropic virus type III/ lymphadenopathy-associated virus antibody testing at alternate sites. MMWR Morb Mortal Wkly Rep. 1986;35:284–7.

168. Valdiserri RO. HIV counseling and testing: its evolving role in HIV prevention. AIDS Educ Prev. 1997;9(Suppl B):2–13.

169. Centers for Disease Control and Prevention. Additional recommendations to reduce sexual and drug abuse-related transmission of human T-lymphotropic virus type III/ lymphadenopathy-associated virus. MMWR Morb Mortal Wkly Rep. 1986;35:152–5.

170. Centers for Disease Control and Prevention. Public Health Service guidelines for counseling and antibody testing to prevent HIV infection and AIDS. MMWR Morb Mortal Wkly Rep. 1987;36:509–15.

171. Wasserheit JN, Valdiserri RO, Wood RW. Assessment of STD/HIV prevention programs in the United States: national, local, and community perspectives. In: Holmes KK, Sparling PF, Mardh PA, Lemon SM, Stamm WE, Piot P, Wasserheit JN, editors. Sexually transmitted diseases. New York, NY: McGraw-Hill; 1999. p. 1255–71.

172. Holtgrave DR, Qualls NL, Curran JW, Valdiserri RO, Guinan ME, Parra WC. An overview of the effectiveness and efficiency of HIV prevention programs. Public Health Rep. 1995;110:134–46.

173. U.S. General Accounting Office. AIDS Prevention Programs: high-risk groups still prove hard to reach. Washington, DC: U.S. General Accounting Office; 1991. HRD-91-52.

174. American Public Health Association. Special initiative on AIDS. HIV antibody testing. Washington, DC: American Public Health Association; 1989. p. 1–14.

175. Higgins DL, Galavotti C, O'Reilly KR, et al. Evidence for the effects of HIV antibody counseling and testing on risk behavior. JAMA. 1991;266:2419–29.

176. Weinhardt LS, Carey MP, Johnson BT, Bickham NL. Effects of HIV counseling and testing on sexual behavior: a meta-analytic review of published research, 1985–1997. Am J Public Health. 1999;89:1397–405.

177. Centers for Disease Control and Prevention. Technical guidance on HIV Counseling. MMWR Morb Mortal Wkly Rep. 1993;42(RR-2):8–17.

178. Kamb ML, Fishbein M, Douglas JM, et al. Efficacy of risk-reduction counseling to prevent human immunodeficiency virus and sexually transmitted diseases: a randomized controlled trial. JAMA. 1998;280:1161–7.

179. Valdiserri RO, Aultman TV, Curran JW. Community planning: a national strategy to improve HIV prevention programs. J Community Health. 1995; 20:87–100.

180. Holtgrave DR, Valdiserri RO. Year one of HIV prevention community planning: a national perspective on accomplishments, challenges and future directions. J Public Health Manag Pract. 1996;2:1–9.

181. AIDS Action Foundation. A blueprint for reforming federal AIDS prevention programs. Washington, DC: AIDS Action Foundation; 1993. p. 1–26.

182. Association of State and Territorial Health Officials, Council of State and Territorial Epidemiologists, National Alliance of State and Territorial AIDS Directors. State health agency vision for HIV prevention. Washington, DC: Association of State and Territorial Health Officials; 1993. p. 1–10.

183. Office of Technology Assessment. External review of the federal centers for disease control and prevention's HIV prevention programs: summary and overview. Washington, DC: Office of Technology Assessment; 1994. p. 1–25.

184. Holtgrave DR. Setting priorities and community planning for HIV-prevention programs. AIDS Public Policy. 1994;9:145–51.

185. Kelly J, Effective HIV. Prevention community planning: an assessment of state initiatives. Washington, DC: National Alliance of State and Territorial AIDS Directors; 1994. p. 1–25.

186. Schietinger H, Coburn J, Levi J. Community planning for HIV prevention: findings from the first year. AIDS Public Policy. 1995;10:140–7.

187. Holtgrave DR, Harrison J, Gerber RA, Aultman TV, Scarlett M. Methodological issues in evaluating HIV prevention community planning. Public Health Rep. 1996;111:108–14.

188. Collins C, Franks P. Improving the use of behavioral research in CDC's HIV prevention community planning process. San Francisco, CA: Center for AIDS Prevention Studies, University of California San Francisco; 1996. p. 1–17.

189. Valdiserri RO. Managing system-wide change in HIV prevention programs: a CDC perspective. Public Admin Rev. 1996;56:545–53.

190. Bau I. Asians and Pacific islanders and HIV prevention community planning. AIDS Educ Prev. 1998;10(Suppl A):77–93.

191. Valdiserri RO, Robinson C, Lin LS, West GR, Holtgrave DR. Determining allocations for HIV prevention interventions: assessing a change in Federal Funding Policy. AIDS Public Policy. 1997; 12:138–48.

192. Kreuter MW. PATCH: its origin, basic concepts, and links to contemporary public health policy. J Health Educ. 1992;23:135–9.

193. Jenkins RA, Carey JW. Decision making for HIV prevention planning: organizational considerations and influencing factors. AIDS Behav. 2005;9:S1–8.

194. Jenkins RA, Averbach AR, Robbins A, et al. Improving the use of data for HIV prevention decision making: lessons learned. AIDS Behav. 2005;9:S87–99.

195. Mejia R, Jenkins RA, Carey JW, et al. Longitudinal observation of an HIV prevention community planning group (CPG). Health Promot Pract. 2009; 10:136–43.

196. Freudenberg N, Lee J, Silver D. How Black and Latino community organizations respond to the AIDS epidemic: a case study in One New York city neighborhood. AIDS Educ Prev. 1989;1:12–21.

197. Valdiserri RO, West GR, Moore M, Darrow WW, Hinman AR. Structuring HIV prevention service delivery systems on the basis of social science theory. J Community Health. 1992;17:259–69.

198. Freudenberg N, Trinidad U. The role of community organizations in AIDS prevention in two Latino communities in New York city. Health Educ Q. 1992;19:219–32.

199. Chillag K, Bartholow K, Cordeiro J, et al. Factors affecting the delivery of HIV/AIDS prevention programs by community-based organizations. AIDS Educ Prev. 2002;14(Suppl A):27–37.

200. DiFranceisco W, Kelly JA, Otto-Salaj L, et al. Factors influencing attitudes within aids service organizations toward the use of research-based HIV prevention interventions. AIDS Educ Prev. 1999;11:72–86.

201. Somlai AM, Kelly JA, Otto-Salaj L, et al. Current HIV prevention activities for women and Gay men among 77 ASOs. J Public Health Manag Pract. 1999;5:23–33.

202. Freudenberg N, Eng E, Flay B, Parcel G, Rogers T, Wallerstein N. Strengthening individual and community capacity to prevent disease and promote health: in search of relevant theories and principles. Health Educ Q. 1995;22:290–306.

203. Walsh C, Campbell C, Willingham M. HIV/STD prevention program assessments, U.S. Abstract PO-D36-4382. IX International Conference on AIDS. 6–11 Jun 1993, Berlin; 1992.

204. National Alliance of State and Territorial AIDS Directors. Technical assistance and capacity building assistance for minority communities: a report from the NASTAD STATUS Project. Washington, DC: National Alliance of State and Territorial AIDS Directors; 2001. p. 1–30.

205. American Psychological Association. Behavioral science expertise needed for HIV prevention community planning. Psychology AIDS Exchange. 1996; 20:7.

206. Veniegas RC, Kao UH, Rosales R, Arellanes M. HIV prevention technology transfer: challenges and strategies in the real world. Am J Public Health. 2009;99:S124–30.

207. Taveras S, Duncan T, Gentry D, Gilliam A, Kimbrough I, Minaya J. The evolution of the CDC HIV prevention capacity-building assistance initiative. J Public Health Manag Pract. 2007;13:S8–S15.

208. Miller RL, Bedney BJ, Guenther-Grey C. Assessing organizational capacity to deliver HIV prevention services collaboratively: tales from the field. Health Educ Behav. 2003;30:582–600.

209. Kraft JM, Mezoff JS, Sogolow ED, Neumann MS, Thomas PA. A technology transfer model for effective HIV/AIDS interventions: science and practice. AIDS Educ Prev. 2000;12(Suppl A):7–20.

210. Richter DL, Potts LH, Prince MS, et al. Development of a curriculum to enhance community-based organizations' capacity for effective HIV prevention programming and management. AIDS Educ Prev. 2006;18:362–74.

211. Kelly JA, Somlai AM, DiFranceisco WJ, et al. Bridging the gap between the science and service of HIV prevention: transferring effective research-based HIV prevention interventions to community AIDS service providers. Am J Public Health. 2000;90:1082–8.

212. Copenhaven MM, Fisher JD. Experts outline ways to decrease the decade-long yearly rate of 40,000 new HIV infections in the US. AIDS Behav. 2006;10:105–14.

213. Valdiserri RO. Mapping the roots of HIV/AIDS complacency: implications for program and policy development. AIDS Educ Prev. 2004;16:426–39.

214. Kaiser Family Foundation. 2009 Survey of Americans on HIV/AIDS: summary of findings on the domestic epidemic; 2009. http://www.kff.org/kaiserpolls/upload/7889.pdf. Accessed 5/11/09.

215. U.S. Census Bureau News. An Older and More Diverse Nation by Midcentury. August 14, 2008. Available at: http://www.census.gov/Press-Release/www/releases/archives/population/012496.html. Accessed on 12 May 2009.

216. Adimora AA, Schoenbach VJ, Doherty IA. Concurrent sexual partnerships among Men in the United States. Am J Public Health. 2007;97:2230–7.

217. Adimora AA, Schoenbach VJ, Martinson FE, et al. Heterosexually transmitted HIV infection among African Americans in North Carolina. J Acquir Immune Defic Syndr. 2006;41:616–23.

218. Adimora AA, Schoenbach VJ, Martinson F, Donaldson KH, Stancil TR, Fullilove RE. Concurrent sexual partnerships among African Americans in the rural south. Ann Epidemiol. 2004;14:155–60.

219. Millett GA, Flores SA, Peterson JL, Bakeman R. Explaining disparities in HIV infection among Black and White men: a meta-analysis of HIV risk behaviors. AIDS. 2007;21:2083–91.

220. Centers for Disease Control and Prevention. HIV infection among young Black men who have sex with men—Jackson, Mississippi, 2006–2008. MMWR Morb Mortal Wkly Rep. 2009;58:77–81.

221. Centers for Disease Control and Prevention. HIV prevalence, unrecognized infection, and HIV testing among men who have sex with men—five U.S. cities, June 2004–April 2005. MMWR Morb Mortal Wkly Rep. 2005;54:597–601.

222. Laurencin CT, Christensen DM, Taylor ED. HIV/AIDS and the African American community: a state of emergency. J Natl Med Assoc. 2008;100:35–43.

223. Padian NS, Buve A, Balkus J, Serwadda D, Cates W. Biomedical interventions to prevent HIV infection: evidence, challenges, and the way forward. Lancet. 2008;372:585–99.

224. Nuttal J, Romano J, Douville K, et al. The future of HIV prevention: prospects for an effective anti-HIV microbicide. Infect Dis Clin North Am. 2007;21:219–39.

225. Cutler B, Justman J. Vaginal microbicides and the prevention of HIV transmission. Lancet Infect Dis. 2008;8:685–97.

226. Siegfried N, Muller M, Deeks JJ, Volmink J. Male Circumcision for prevention of heterosexual acquisition of HIV in men. Cochrane Database Syst Rev. 2009; 2:CD003362. Doi: 10.1002/14651858.CD003362.pub2.

227. Warner L, Ghanem KG, Newman DR, Macaluso M, Sullivan PS, Erbelding EJ. Male circumcision and risk of HIV infection among heterosexual African American men attending Baltimore sexually transmitted disease clinics. J Infect Dis. 2009;199:59–65.

228. Leibowitz AA, Desmond K, Belin T. Determinants and policy implications of male circumcision in the United States. Am J Public Health. 2009;99:138–45.

229. Smith DK, Taylor A, Kilmarx PH, et al. Male circumcision in the United States for the prevention of HIV infection and other adverse health outcomes: report from a CDC consultation. Public Health Rep. 2010;125 Suppl 1:72–82.

230. Centers for Disease Control and Prevention. HIV prevention through early detection and treatment of other sexually transmitted diseases—United States. MMWR Morb Mortal Wkly Rep. 1998;47(No. RR-12):1–24.

231. Rotheram-Borus MJ, Swendeman D, Chovnick G. The past, present and future of HIV prevention: integrating behavioral, biomedical, and structural intervention strategies for the next generation of HIV prevention. Annu Rev Clin Psychol. 2009;5:143–67.

232. Watson-Jones D, Weiss HA, Rusizoka M, et al. Effect of herpes simplex suppression on incidence of HIV among women in Tanzania. N Engl J Med. 2008;358:1560–71.

233. Celum C, Wald A, Hughes J, et al. Effect of aciclovir on HIV-1 acquisition in herpes simplex virus 2 seropositive women and men who have sex with men: a randomised, double-blind, placebo controlled trial. Lancet. 1998;371:2109–19.

234. White RG, Orroth KK, Glynn JR, et al. Treating curable sexually transmitted infections to prevent HIV in Africa. J Acquir Immune Defic Syndr. 2008;47:346–53.

235. Centers for Disease Control and Prevention. CDC trials of pre-exposure prophylaxis for HIV prevention; 2009. http://www.cdc.gov/hiv/resources/Factsheets/print/prep.htm Accessed 19 May 2009.

236. Paxton LA, Hope T, Jaffe HW. Pre-exposure prophylaxis for HIV infection: what if it works? Lancet. 2007;370:89–93.

237. Patiel AD, Freedberg KA, Scott CA, et al. HIV pre-exposure prophylaxis in the United States: impact on lifetime infection risk, clinical outcomes, and cost-effectiveness. Clin Infect Dis. 2009;48:806–15.

238. Valdiserri RO. HIV/AIDS stigma: an impediment to public health. Am J Public Health. 2002;92:341–2.

239. Mahajan AP, Sayles JN, Patel VA, et al. Stigma in the HIV/AIDS epidemic: a review of the literature and recommendations for the way forward. AIDS. 2008;22 Suppl 2:S67–79.

240. Kippax S, Holt M. The state of social and political science research related to HIV: a report for the International AIDS Society; 2009. http://www.iasociety.org.

241. Quinn TC, Wawer MJ, Sewankambo N, et al. Viral load and heterosexual transmission of human immunodeficiency virus type 1. N Engl J Med. 2000; 342:921–9.

242. Porco TC, Martin JN, Page-Shafer KA, et al. Decline in HIV infectivity following the introduction of highly active antiretroviral therapy. AIDS. 2004;18:81–8.

243. Fang CT, Hsu HM, Twu SJ, et al. Decreased HIV transmission after a policy of providing free access to highly active antiretroviral therapy in Taiwan. J Infect Dis. 2004;190:879–85.

244. Clements MS, Prestage G, Grulich A, Van de Ven P, Kippax S, Law MG. Modeling trends in HIV incidence among homosexual men in Australia, 1995–2006. J Acquir Immune Defic Syndr. 2004;35:401–6.

245. Castilla J, Romero J, Hernando V, Marincovich B, Garcia S, Rodriguez C. Effectiveness of highly active antiretroviral therapy in reducing heterosexual transmission of HIV. J Acquir Immune Defic Syndr. 2005;40:96–101.

246. Velasco-Hernandez JX, Gershengorn HB, Blower SM. Could widespread use of combination antiretroviral therapy eradicate HIV epidemics? Lancet Infect Dis. 2002;2:487–93.

247. Granich R, Gilks CF, Dye C, De Cock KM, Williams BG. Universal voluntary HIV testing with immediate antiretroviral therapy as a strategy for elimination of HIV transmission: a mathematical model. Lancet. 2009;373:48–57.

248. Vernazza P, Hirschel B, Bernasconi E, Flepp M. Les personnes seropositives ne souffrant d'aucune autre MST et suivant un traitement antirretroviral efficace ne transmettent pas le VIH par voie sexuelle. Bull Med Suisses. 2008;89:165–9.

249. Das-Douglas M, Chu P, Santos GM, et al. Decreases in community viral load are associated with a reduction in new HIV diagnoses in San Francisco. 17th

conference on retroviruses and opportunistic infections; 2010. http://www.retroconference.org/2010/Abstracts/38232.htm. Accessed on 12 Mar 2010.

250. Montaner J, Wood E, Kerr T, et al. Association of expanded HAART coverage with a decrease in new HIV diagnoses, particularly among injection drug users in British Columbia, Canada. 17th conference on retroviruses and opportunistic infections; 2010. http://www.retroconference.org/2010/Abstracts/39866.htm. Accessed 12 Mar 2010.

251. Sheth P, Kovacs C, Kemal K, et al. Persistent HIV RNA shedding in semen despite effective ART. 16th Conference on retroviruses and opportunistic infections; 2009. http://www.retroconference.org/2009/Abstracts/35773.htm. Accessed 18 May 2009.

252. Marcelin AG, Tubiana R, Lambert-Niclot S, et al. Detection of HIV-1 RNA in seminal plasma samples from treated patients with undetectable HIV-1 RNA in blood plasma. 16th conference on retroviruses and opportunistic infections; 2009. http://www.retroconference.org/2009/Abstracts/34040.htm. Accessed 18 May 2009.

253. Katz MH, Schwarcz SK, Kellog TA, et al. Impact of highly active antiretroviral treatment on HIV seroincidence among men who have sex with men: San Francisco. Am J Public Health. 2002;92:388–94.

254. Wilson DP, Law MG, Grulich AE, Cooper DA, Kaldor JM. Relation between HIV viral load and infectiousness. Lancet. 2008;372:314–20.

255. Dieffenbach CW, Fauci A. Universal voluntary testing and treatment for prevention of HIV transmission. JAMA. 2009;301:2380–2.

256. Holtgrave DR. Strategies for preventing HIV transmission. JAMA. 2009;302:1530–1.

257. Rekart ML, Patrick DM, Chakraborty B, et al. Targeted mass treatment for syphilis with oral azithromycin. Lancet. 2003;361:313–4.

258. Pourbohloul B, Rekart M, Brunham RC. Impact of mass treatment on syphilis transmission: a mathematical model. Sex Transm Dis. 2003;30:297–305.

259. Kerani RP, Handsfield HH, Stenger MS, et al. Rising rates of syphilis in the era of syphilis elimination. Sex Transm Dis. 2007;34:154–61.

260. Hogben M, Leichliter JS. Social determinants and sexually transmitted disease disparities. Sex Transm Dis. 2008;35:S13–8.

261. Francis DP, Anderson RE, Gorman ME, et al. Targeting AIDS prevention and treatment toward HIV-1-infected persons. JAMA. 1989;262:2572–6.

262. Valdiserri RO, Holtgrave DR, West GR. Promoting early diagnosis and entry into care. AIDS. 1999;13:2317–30.

263. Panel on Antiretroviral Guidelines for Adults and Adolescent. Guidelines for the use of antiretroviral agents in HIV-1 infected adults and adolescents. Department of Health and Human Services. Dec 1; 2009. p. 1–161. http://www.aidsinfo.nih.gov/ContentFiles/Adultand AdolescentGL.pdf. Accessed 11 Jan 2010.

264. Janssen RS, Holtgrave DR, Valdiserri RO, et al. The serostatus approach to fighting the HIV epidemic: prevention strategies for infected individuals. Am J Public Health. 2001;91:1019–24.

265. Centers for Disease Control and Prevention. Advancing HIV prevention: new strategies for a changing epidemic—United States, 2003. MMWR Morb Mortal Wkly Rep. 2003;52:329–32.

266. Weinhardt LS, Kelly JA, Brondino MJ, et al. HIV transmission risk behavior among men and women living with HIV in 4 cities in the United States. J Acquir Immune Defic Syndr. 2004;36:1057–66.

267. Crepaz N, Lyles CM, Wolitski RJ, et al. Do prevention interventions reduce HIV risk behaviours among people living with HIV? a meta-analytic review of controlled trials. AIDS. 2006;20:143–57.

268. Marks G, Crepaz N, Senterfitt W, Janssen RS. Meta-analysis of high-risk sexual behavior in persons aware and unaware they are infected with HIV in the United States: implications for HIV prevention programs. J Acquir Immune Defic Syndr. 2005;39:446–53.

269. Marks G, Crepaz N, Janssen RS. Estimating sexual transmission of HIV from persons aware and unaware that they are infected with the virus in the USA. AIDS. 2006;20:1447–50.

270. Centers for Disease Control and Prevention. Revised recommendations for HIV testing of adults, adolescents, and pregnant women in health-care settings. MMWR Morb Mortal Wkly Rep. 2006;55(RR-14):1–17.

271. Burke RC, Sepkowitz KA, Bernstein KT, et al. Why don't physicians test for HIV? a review of the US literature. AIDS. 2007;21:1617–24.

272. Centers for Disease Control and Prevention. Persons tested for HIV—United States, 2006. MMWR Morb Mortal Wkly Rep. 2008;57:845–9.

273. Bartlett JG, Branson BM, Fenton K, Hauschild BC, Miller V, Mayer KH. Opt-out testing for human immunodeficiency virus in the United States: progress and challenges. JAMA. 2008;300:945–51.

274. Yarnall KS, Pollak KI, Ostbye T, Krause KM, Michener L. Primary care: is there enough time for prevention? Am J Public Health. 2003;93:635–41.

275. Kitahata MM, Gange SJ, Abraham AG, et al. Effect of early versus deferred antiretroviral therapy for HIV on survival. N Engl J Med. 2009;360:1–12.

276. Centers for Disease Control and Prevention. Incorporating HIV prevention into the medical care of persons living with HIV: Recommendations of CDC, the Health Resources and Services Administration, the National Institutes of Health, and the HIV Medicine Association of the Infectious Diseases Society of America. MMWR Morb Mortal Wkly Rep. 2003;52(No. RR-12):1–24.

277. Thrun M, Cook PF, Bradley-Springer LA, et al. Improved prevention counseling by HIV care providers in a multisite, clinic-based intervention: positive steps. AIDS Educ Prev. 2009;21:55–66.

278. Buffardi AL, Thomas KK, Holmes KK, Manhart LE. Moving upstream: ecosocial and psychosocial correlates of sexually transmitted infections among young adults in the United States. Am J Public Health. 2008;98:1128–36.

279. Valdiserri RO. Sexually transmitted infections among Gay and bisexual men. In: Wolitski R, Stall R, Valdiserri RO, editors. Unequal opportunity: health disparities affecting Gay and bisexual men in the United States. Oxford, England: Oxford University Press; 2008. p. 159–93.

280. Stall R, Mills TC, Williamson J, et al. Association of co-occuring psychosocial health problems and increased vulnerability to HIV/AIDS among urban men who have sex with men. Am J Public Health. 2003;93:939–42.

281. Operario D, Smith CD, Kegeles S. Social and psychological context for HIV risk in non-Gay-identified African American men who have sex with men. AIDS Educ Prev. 2008;20:347–59.

282. Neaigus A, Gyarmathy A, Miller M, Frajzyngier VM, Friedman SR, Des Jarlais DC. Transitions to injecting drug use among non-injecting heroin users: social network influence and individual susceptibility. J Acquir Immune Defic Syndr. 2006;41:493–503.

283. Rich JA, Grey CM. Pathways to recurrent trauma among young Black men: traumatic stress, substance use, and the "Code of the Street". Am J Public Health. 2005;95:816–24.

284. Hooper S, Rosser BR, Horvath KJ, Oakes JM, Danilenko G. An online needs assessment of a virtual community: what men who use the internet to seek sex with men want in internet-based HIV prevention. AIDS Behav. 2008;12:867–75.

285. Hightow L, Leone P, McCoy S, et al. Continued HIV transmission among African American MSM/W on North Carolina College Campuses: expanding sexual networks of internet use and crystal methamphetamine. 16th conference on retroviruses and opportunistic infections; 2009. http://www.retroconference.org/2009/Abstracts/26873.HTM. Accessed 20 May 2009.

286. Ellis RJ, Childers ME, Chemer M, Lazzaretto D, Letendre S, Grant I. Increased human immunodeficiency virus loads in active methamphetamine users are explained by reduced effectiveness of antiretroviral therapy. J Infect Dis. 2003;188:1820–6.

287. Colfax G, Shoptaw S. The methamphetamine epidemic: implications for HIV prevention and treatment. Curr HIV/AIDS Rep. 2005;2:194–9.

288. Mansergh G, Purcell DW, Stall R, et al. CDC consultation on methamphetamine use and sexual risk behavior for HIV/STD infection: summary and suggestions. Public Health Rep. 2006;121:127–32.

289. Collins CV, Hearn KD, Whittier DN, Freeman A, Stallworth JD, Phields M. Implementing packaged HIV-prevention interventions for HIV positive individuals: considerations for clinic-based and community-based interventions. Public Health Rep. 2010;125 Suppl 1:55–63.

290. National Alliance of State and Territorial AIDS Directors and Kaiser Family Foundation. The National HIV Prevention Inventory: The State of HIV Prevention across the U.S.; 2009. http://www.kff.org/hivaids/prevention.cfm. Accessed 26 Feb 2010.

A National Strategic Approach to Improving the Health of Gay and Bisexual Men: Experience in Australia

17

Adrian Mindel and Susan Kippax

Introduction

The key to the Australian response to HIV and AIDS was (and continues to be) partnership: a partnership between government, affected communities, public health, and research institutions (biomedical/clinical, epidemiological, and social).

We begin the chapter with a brief history outlining the early cases and the subsequent epidemiological picture: "know your epidemic". We then describe the partnership—each aspect of it in turn: "know your response". We then illustrate how certain aspects of this partnership worked in practice. We end the chapter with an overall assessment of the success of the response.

Figure 17.1 shows the time-line of the Australian response with special reference to HIV prevention in gay men.

A. Mindel, M.D., FRCP, FRACP, FAChSHM (✉)
University of Sydney, Camperdown, NSW, Australia
e-mail: adrian.mindel@sydney.edu.au

S. Kippax, Ph.D., FASSA
Social Policy Research Centre, University of New South Wales, Sydney, NSW 2052, Australia
e-mail: s.kippax@unsw.edu.au

Brief History: Outlining the Early Cases and the Subsequent Epidemiological Picture of HIV in Australia

The first case of AIDS was diagnosed in Sydney in 1982 [1]. This first case and the first death from AIDS, which occurred in Melbourne in 1983, were in gay men. Between 1983 and 1985, HIV spread rapidly in Australia where some 4,500 men were infected, predominantly in the gay community in Sydney and to a lesser extent in the gay community in Melbourne [2]. Nonetheless, there was considerable concern that HIV was also spreading in injecting drug users (IDU) and that it was only a matter of time until heterosexual spread became more common [3].

Figure 17.2 shows the distribution of HIV infection and AIDS in gay and other homosexually active men (MSM) and in other populations including heterosexual men and women and injecting drug users (non-MSM).

Over the next few years, as the pattern of transmission became more established, it was apparent that spread via injecting drug use had remained at a very low level (about in 5% of the total, but closer to 1% if those who were also MSM were excluded); that transmission from medical procedures (receipt of blood or blood products) had declined from about 14% in 1985–1986 to about 1% in 1991–1992; and that onwards spread into the heterosexual community had not

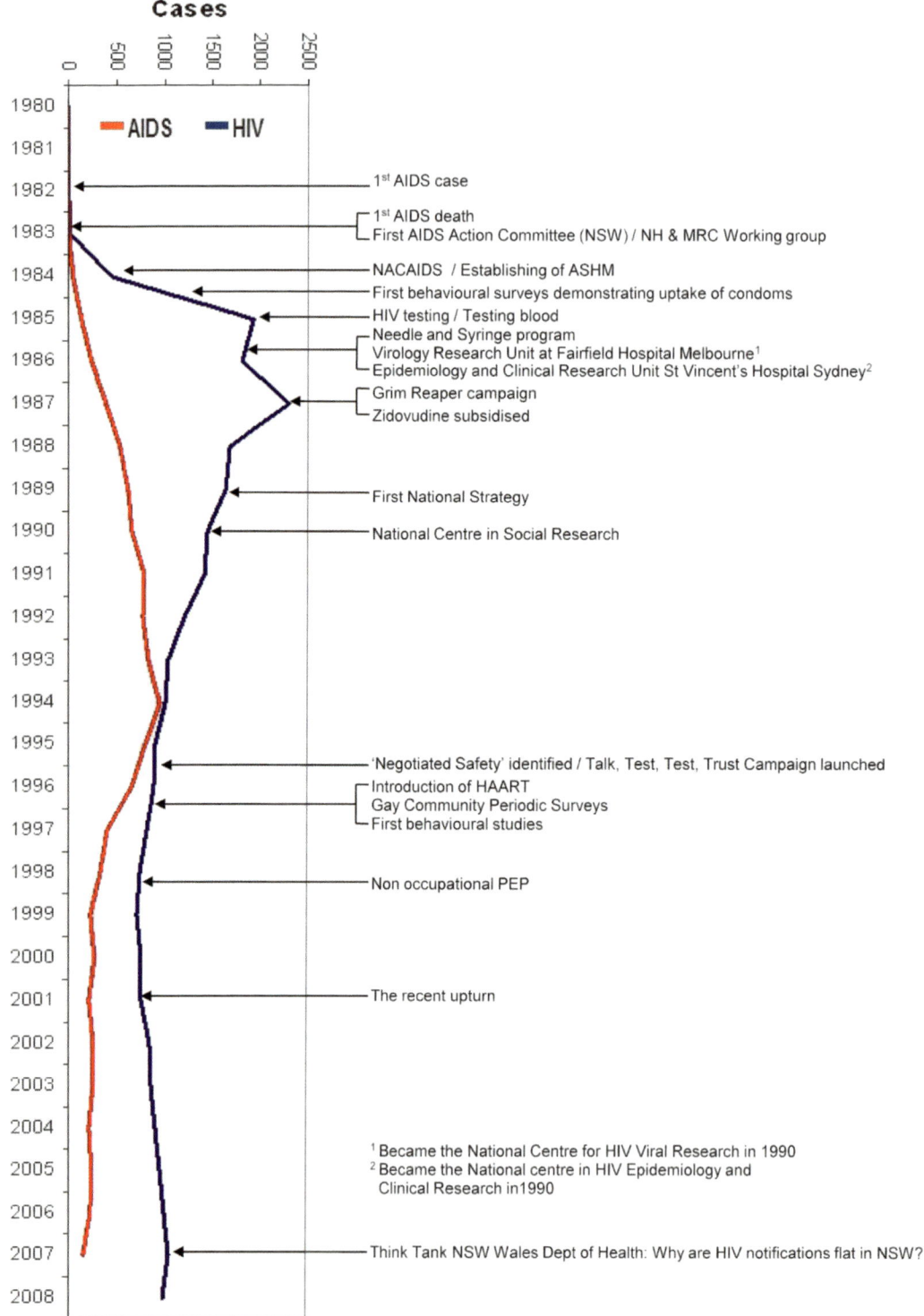

Fig. 17.1 Time-line of the Australian response with special reference to HIV prevention in gay men

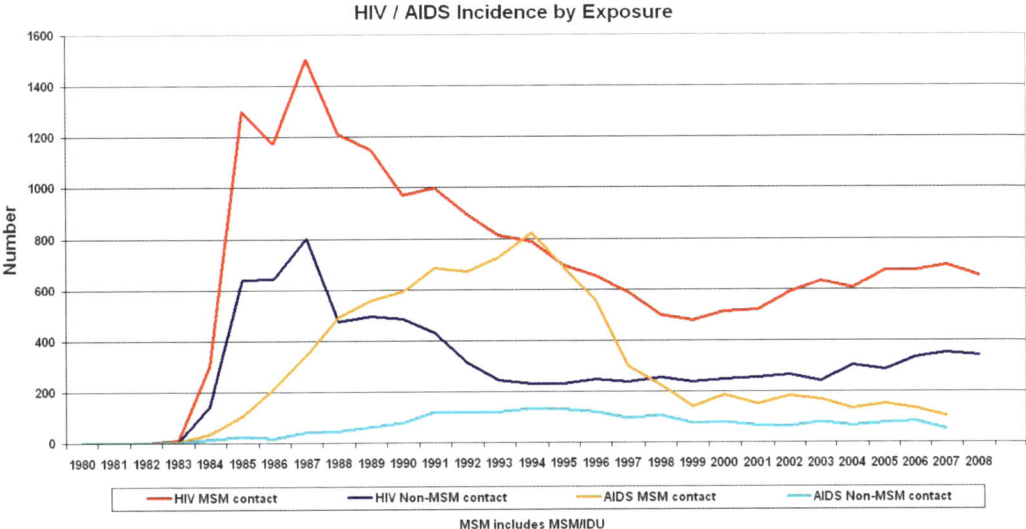

Fig. 17.2 Number of diagnoses of HIV infection and AIDS in Australia by year and exposure category

occurred to any great extent [4, 5]. These successes were attributed mainly to the early and widespread availability of needle and syringe programmes in 1987[1] and rapid expansion of methadone programmes for injecting drug users, the early adoption of condoms by sex workers and testing of the blood supply [6, 7].

Most HIV infections (about 66%) and the highest rates of infection (in 1992 187.5/100,000) were in New South Wales (NSW) with rates in Victoria (66.1/100,00) only about a third of those in NSW [4]. These are the states with the highest overall populations and the highest gay populations in Australia. In fact, most HIV infections continued to occur in gay men in Sydney and Melbourne, the capital cities of NSW and Victoria, respectively.

The peak in HIV incidence occurred in 1987 and incidence declined year on year until 1999. Thereafter, there was a small but steady increase in incidence until 2007 with a slight decline in 2008. Most of the increase between 1999 and 2007 occurred in MSM in Victoria and Queensland and the reasons for this increase is considered in

detail below. The peak in AIDS incidence occurred in 1994 with a dramatic decline from 1994 to 1999. Thereafter the incidence remained steady with a small decease in 2008 [8].

The rate of HIV in the general population in Australia in 2008 (123/100,000) was broadly comparable to the estimated prevalence in New Zealand (100/100,000) and the UK (127/100,000), but considerably lower than the estimated prevalence in France (400/100,000), Italy (400/100,000), Spain (500/100,000), Canada (400/100,000) and the USA (600/100,000). The prevalence in many of the countries in the Asian Pacific area are estimated to be considerably higher ranging from 500/100,000 in Malaysia and Vietnam to 1500/100,000 in Papua New Guinea [8].

Gay and other homosexually active men remain the largest group affected by HIV In Australia [7]. HIV transmission continues to occur mainly through sexual contact between men and in 2004–2008 accounted for 68% of newly diagnosed HIV infections and 86% of newly acquired infection [8].

Community Activism

In their efforts to achieve gay liberation, gay men in both the USA and Australia formed geographically dense social and sexual networks—gay

---

[1]The first needle and syringe programme began in November 1986 in an inner Sydney suburb in contravention of the New South Wales law, but in conformity with harm reduction principles agreed by Australia's political leadership.

communities, and during the late 1970s and early 1980s a close relationship developed between these gay communities. It is these communities that are central to understanding both the early HIV infections rates and the subsequent responses to HIV.

While HIV spread initially among gay men in the USA, the frequent crossing of the Pacific especially between San Francisco and Sydney accounts in part, for the early high infection rates among the population of gay men[2] (compared with other populations) in Australia [9]. The close relationship between the gay communities in both countries also meant that Australian gay men were forewarned, and they responded rapidly to HIV. Gay communities in both countries had been mobilised and active in the gay liberation movement and their members, comprised of highly educated and articulate men who had learnt the arts of advocacy and political lobbying, were quick to respond to the threat of AIDS—particularly, in Sydney, Melbourne and San Francisco and New York.

The first media report of AIDS appeared in the Australian gay press in *The Star* in July 1981: [10] it reported on the disease affecting gay men in the USA, the gay-related immune disease (GRID) or, less kindly, the "gay plague". Along with the announcement of the first case of AIDS and the Sydney blood bank call for the self-exclusion of gay men from the donor pool, came the first official labelling of a "high risk group". Australia experienced its first bout of media panic with headlines such as "US Killer Disease Reaches Australia" and "AIDS—The Killer Disease That's Expected to Sweep Australia" [11]. The reports of AIDS and the hysteria surrounding these reports served as a catalyst to gay activists—first in Sydney and later in other states. Gay men came together to provide voluntary, largely untrained care to people with AIDS in their homes. Individual gay men personally affected, either because they were themselves sick, or because their lovers and friends were sick, later created organisations, such as the Community Support Network (CSN). The Bobby Goldsmith Foundation (BGF) was formed in 1984 to provide financial and material assistance to gay men with AIDS [12]. As well as providing care and support, gay community activists knowing that AIDS threatened to undo all that had been achieved during gay liberation unless men's sexual practice was safe, turned their attention to education programmes and established AIDS Action Committees (AACs)—first in Sydney in May 1983 and then in Melbourne, Canberra and Perth in the same year [2]. One of the very first responses was to advocate and, as early as August 1983, the New South Wales AAC organised a public forum on AIDS, featuring leading health experts in the middle of Sydney's gay community [13].

These AACs later became the AIDS Councils, and by 1985 there was an AIDS Council in each state and territory in Australia [11, 14]. Although there are other AIDS-related non-government organisations, the AIDS Councils and their federal body, the Australian Federation of AIDS Organisations (AFAO) continue as the peak bodies and are the only AIDS-related NGOs funded by governments (state and federal). In New South Wales, for example, the funding has increased from AUD 74,000 (approximately USD 55,000) in 1985 to AUD 5 million (approximately USD 3.75 million) in 1992 with a state-wide staff of 120 employees. Its funding in 2008 was AUD 10.5 million (approximately USD 7.8 million) with a staff of 150 [15, 16]. The purpose of these AACs/AIDS Councils was/is to lobby governments for action and advocate for health and access to drugs and support, and provide education to members of communities and populations, including but not restricted to gay men, injecting drug users, and sex workers, affected by HIV.

Targeting gay community members as early as 1985, the AIDS Council of New South Wales (ACON) produced a pamphlet called "G'day we've got a problem fellas". It suggested that AIDS was transmitted by the exchange of body fluids, but fell short of recommending condoms. A couple of years later a poster produced by ACON and funded by the NSW Health Department

---

[2]Following gay liberation, gay men found sexual freedom in some of the large cities of the USA, Australia and Europe.

called "Rubba Me" was highly sexually explicit and unequivocal in its support of condom use [17]. The AIDS Councils continue to produce HIV-prevention education material, some of it sexually explicit, for distribution in gay bars and sex venues. Some of it has attracted adverse media attention but in the main, the governments (state and federal) have continued to fund this education material. These campaigns targeting gay men have been highly successful in raising awareness of HIV and safe sex, increasing condom use, and producing debate and discussion within gay community [18].

Gay activists were also involved in a long battle to change the laws relating to criminalising "homosexual acts", in particular, the sodomy laws. Their efforts, which began before the advent of AIDS, were successful, and made it easier for a national Australian response. Decriminalisation of homosexuality began in South Australia under a reforming state Labor government in 1972. This was followed by the Federal government legislating for the Australian Capital Territory, and by Victoria in 1980. The first decriminalisation debate in New South Wales occurred in March 1981—the same year that homosexual men in the USA were diagnosed with what was HIV—and in 1984, homosexual acts were decriminalised in New South Wales, and in the same year in the Northern Territory. And although homosexual acts remained illegal in three states—Western Australia, Queensland and Tasmania—until 1990, only in Queensland was the legislation criminalising homosexuality rigorously enforced [11, 19].

Australian Governmental Response

Between the summer of 1984 and the winter of 1985, the Australian Federal government emerged as "the chief owner" of HIV. The critical dates are the national AIDS summits of late 1984 and the Federal budget of August 1985, with for the first time a significant commitment of moneys to AIDS [19]. The Minister of Health at this important moment was Dr. Neal Blewett, a former professor of political science. In between December

1984 and January 1985, Dr Blewett visited the USA, which was "the single most significant influence on my own views about AIDS" [19] (p. 9). He identified a number of aspects of the American situation that shaped the manner in which Australia responded.

The first was the difference he noted between what he called the "Californian cooperative approach" and the "more traditional public health model" adopted in New York. He preferred the former, which was characterised by a partnership between the medical profession and the affected communities, with as great an emphasis placed on education as on medical control, with the integration of gay and other affected communities into both public health campaigns and service delivery [19] (p. 9). So the Australian government built on and incorporated gay activism into its response to the threat of AIDS.

Again, drawing on what he saw in the USA, the anger at Reagan's failure to address AIDS and the bitter political in-fighting, Blewett was convinced that Australia needed a national approach to AIDS, and a national approach that was non-partisan. Blewett did this by cultivating influential figures in the main opposition party, the Liberal Party, and in late 1985 an all-party parliamentary liaison committee on AIDS was established. This committee was (and continued to be) kept informed on all aspects of the epidemic and regularly briefed by national and international AIDS experts. It acted as a sounding board for government policies and programmes and as a conduit for the concerns of other parties. The result at the national level, was "an elite consensus on AIDS policy" [19] (p. 19).

There were important differences between the responses of the two countries: in the USA, AIDS hit the gay community early and hard and, in general, the government response was soft [20, 21]. AIDS organisations were in conflict with the conservative US Federal government, as illustrated by the homophobic Helms Amendment of 1987, which effectively banned harm-reduction-based HIV education on the grounds that it promoted homosexuality [22]. In Australia, the response was primarily a "social" public health response [23]—and remains so. The Minister and those who advised him, including medical and social researchers, believed that it was necessary for public health to address at least two issues: (1) providing treatment, care and support to those infected; and (2) preventing the further spread of infection. Importantly, they were all aware of the central importance of engaging communities at risk of HIV in the Australian response.

Blewett faced little dissent, as the leading AIDS specialists and clinicians in Australia never pushed the traditional public health model, and he also had the support of two important advisory committees he established to pursue an AIDS strategy for Australia. These were the National AIDS Taskforce and the National Advisory Committee on AIDS (NACAIDS). The Taskforce was the more medical of the two and was chaired by Professor David Pennington, Dean of Medicine at Melbourne University, a highly respected haematologist but not an AIDS specialist. The other committee, NACAIDS, which was directly responsible to the Minister, was designed to advise him on educational and social responses to AIDS: "I wanted to use it to signal to the affected communities, the government's commitment to the cooperative approach at the highest level by including their representatives" [19] (p. 14). This committee was chaired by a communications expert, Ita Buttrose, editor of a highly successful women's magazine, who understood the importance of persuasion. It was the job of NACAIDS to produce health promotion material — from *Readers Digest* supplements to erotic and explicit sexual material, designed for use in gay saunas and sex clubs, from condom caricatures on buses to the well-known *Grim Reaper* television campaign. Ita Buttrose was frequently sniped at for her lack of medical knowledge by a media besotted by medical expertise, while the scientific authority of the Taskforce went relatively undisputed — as everyone considered themselves to be experts on education and social questions [6, 24].

Blewett's genius was to have these parallel committees — one essentially medical with a focus on treatment and later, HIV testing, and the other more concerned with prevention and devoted to education and health promotion.

However, as Blewett himself states, relations between the Taskforce and NACAIDS were never smooth. The major focus of tension was HIV testing: in 1985/1986 Pennington and the Taskforce he chaired were advocating testing as the best way to encourage the adoption of safe sexual behaviour and were critical of the current "safe sex" campaign. NACAIDS took an agnostic position on testing leaving the decision to individuals, while some AIDS Councils, notably the AIDS Council of New South Wales (ACON), actively opposed testing. Essentially this was a dispute between strategies based on traditional public health and those based on education. Those who advocated testing argued that knowledge of test status was the best inducement for changing individual sexual behaviour, while those who advocated education argued that promoting safe sexual practices at the community level with the goal of changing social norms would be more likely to prevent HIV transmission. Blewett strove for compromise and was able to keep both strategies alive: "safe sex" campaigns continued, and the number of people coming forward for testing increased as treatments became available. Those AIDS Councils which had opposed HIV testing changed their policy on testing with the proviso it remained voluntary and took place in the context of informed consent and counselling. As Blewett later noted: "I thought it was a fairly satisfactory compromise but received few thanks from either side" [19] (p. 17).

The overall outcome of this and other early tensions was compromise, a compromise that resulted in a partnership between government, affected communities, public health and researchers. Blewett had been persuaded by NACAIDS and the AIDS Councils to invest in peer-led education and community-building programmes and he orchestrated a cost-sharing arrangement with the states stipulating that at least half the AIDS funding was to be spent on education and community programmes [13]. What Blewett understood was that HIV, in particular HIV-prevention, requires that the key players (community activists, clinicians and other public health workers, researchers, educators, policy makers) understand and harness people's ways of actively striving to deal with HIV in their everyday lives. It involves encouraging and enabling people to transform their sexual lives. HIV prevention is essentially about social transformation at the micro- and macro-social levels. He rejected the "contain and control" model of traditional public health with its emphasis on identification of the infected, contact tracing and, if necessary, quarantine. He rejected the model with "the medical men on top, with much less dependence on cooperation and policy input from the affected groups, and with a lesser emphasis on education" [19] (p. 12).

General Population and AIDS

As the evidence for heterosexual transmission became clearer, Australia in line with most income-rich nations began to pay more attention to the "general community", although it never lost sight of the populations most at risk for HIV. The first nationally based television advertisement, the *Grim Reaper* campaign, was launched in April 1987. The television advertisement was intentionally controversial and featured the "Grim Reaper", the archetypal figure of death, playing bowls in a ten-pin bowling alley bowling over men, women and children. The advertisement was supplemented by more detailed written material setting out the ways in which HIV was transmitted and how to prevent it. The campaign aimed to increase awareness and knowledge of HIV and to reposition AIDS as a disease that not only affected gay men but also everyone else.

A report evaluating the *Grim Reaper* campaign [25] concluded that the "assault" phase had exceeded expectations based on changes observed in population responses. The success they argued, should be viewed as a result of the campaign overall and not only the advertising material. The campaign increased awareness of HIV/AIDS and achieved almost universal levels of spontaneous advertising awareness (98%). There was an increase in accurate knowledge of HIV transmission, and fewer Australians associated AIDS with homosexuality (a reduction from 76 to 58%). The campaign helped reduce stigma although the *Grim Reaper* did frighten those who were already

infected and increased the numbers of "worried well". In general, the campaign placed AIDS on everyone's agenda: within a week of launching the campaign, everyone in Australia knew what AIDS was [25]. It also alerted the public to the threat of heterosexual transmission and mobilised school programmes, churches as well as other groups. While the *Grim Reaper* had its detractors, the shift away from "high risk" groups had the outcome of creating the basis for a substantial increase in funding for HIV-prevention programmes.

The Grim Reaper Campaign was followed by a number of other national television, radio and press campaigns. Slowly but surely the early hysteria and responses of panic were replaced by an acceptance by the Australian public that all Australians, including the young, need to be able to access frank and honest information and the means to protect themselves from HIV — condoms, and clean needles and syringes.

From this time on, HIV-prevention had *two* major audiences: the general population targeted by campaigns, which typically were and continue to be funded by the Australian Federal or State governments; and the at-risk groups, including gay men, injecting drug users and sex workers, where campaigns and prevention programmes targeting these populations were and are typically funded by the states, via ear-marked funding from the Federal government.

The five National Strategies that were subsequently developed continued to uphold the Blewett tradition and the decline in HIV transmission speaks to the success of the policies adopted by Blewett and his advisory committees [4, 8].

Five National Strategies

The First National Strategy

The Federal government released its first national HIV/AIDS strategy in 1989 [26], which built on community activism, medical and scientific support, and research that had already been conducted locally and internationally. The strategy had a number of guiding principles, most based on the Ottawa Charter for health promotion [27]. Principles included social justice, equal access, equity and participation, partnership, client focus and freedom from discrimination. The overall goals were to "eliminate transmission of the virus and minimise the personal and social impact of HIV infection". The objectives were set out under six headings: education, prevention, treatment, care and counselling, access and participation, research, and international cooperation. Funding was provided for education and prevention, treatment and service and to train professional caregivers. An evaluation of this policy in 1993 [28] concluded that the education/prevention programmes had resulted in behaviour change in the gay community which had in turn contributed to the stabilisation of the epidemic.

The Second Strategy

The findings from the evaluation of the first strategy informed the approach to the second strategy which maintained the same principles but shifted emphasis from the Federal to the State level in terms of planning and delivery [29]. The second strategy set a national target "to reduce the incidence of new HIV infections in Australia to an annual rate of no more than 2 persons per 100,000 by the year 2000".

A major evaluation of the second strategy was undertaken by Professor Feacham in 1995, 10 years after the start of the epidemic [30]. This evaluation used a variety of methods to determine outcomes including the following: a review of available data and commissioned studies on the incidence and prevalence of HIV/AIDS; the quality and accessibility of services provided to people living with HIV/AIDS; changes in risk practices; how well services and programmes deal with the needs, problems, and challenges created by HIV/AIDS; and the adequacy and appropriateness of organisational and financing arrangements. Overall, the evaluation suggested that although the target of reducing HIV incidence to 2 persons per 100,000 population had not been achieved, the first two strategies were of value.

The Third and Fourth Strategies

As recommended by Professor Feacham, a third national strategy was developed not only to maintain the same principles and goals of the previous strategies but also to strengthen links between STI and hepatitis C services and research [31]. These approaches continued with the fourth strategy [32].

During the life of the fourth strategy, after a period of relative stability in HIV incidence, HIV infections began to rise, particularly in gay men. This was thought to be due to a number of factors including an increase in high risk sexual behaviour in gay men and increasing rates of STIs in these communities. A review of the fourth strategy in 2002 [33], recommended that the national approach be re-energised and that efforts be directed at decreasing the rates of unprotected anal sex in gay men and tackling the increasing incidence of bacterial STIs in the population.

The Fifth Strategy

The fifth strategy was released in 2005 [34]. It built on the successes of the previous strategies and acknowledged the importance of unprotected anal sex and the high rates STIs in relation to HIV in the gay community. Major new recommendations included further enhancing HIV prevention strategies in gay men, in particular reinforcing the importance of condom use and encouraging HIV testing and early diagnosis and treatment of STIs. The strategy was linked to the first ever STI National strategy [35]. The fifth strategy is yet to be evaluated.

Medical/Clinical Response

The clinical response, an essential component of public health response, grew from a number of clusters of medical expertise; in Sydney, at St Vincent's Hospital and the University of New South Wales, and in Melbourne, at the Alfred and Fairfield Hospitals and the University of Melbourne. Over time, clinical research and services were also established in a number of institutions including the Albion Street Clinic and the Burnet Institute and the Australasian Society for HIV Medicine (ASHM).

The Australian Society for HIV Medicine (ASHM)

ASHM was established in the early 1980s by a group of medical practitioners to represent their needs and the organisation was incorporated in 1990 to represent medical practitioners working in the HIV sector [6]. The organisation now has a wide membership including HIV specialists, general practitioners (GPs), researchers and other health professionals. ASHM has provided an important public health role through GP training, promoting research and liaising with governments and NGOs. ASHM receives substantial funding through the Federal Government and trains GPs who wish to work in HIV medicine and prescribe antiretroviral drugs. ASHM is now considered as the leading professional organisation representing HIV health care workers and delivers high quality teaching and training for professionals in Australia and in the Asian Pacific Region. It also has representation of Federal and State Advisory Boards [36].

Availability of Antiretroviral Treatment and the Rapid Drug Approval

The availability of the most appropriate and up to date antiretroviral treatment for all those who need and want it has been and remains an essential aspect of the government response. Discussion about all aspects of current and new treatments is constantly taking place between clinicians, patients, affected communities and the AIDS councils.

The Federal government[3] funds most medical services outside of hospitals including general practice as well as medical research [37]. The national health insurance system aims to provide universal access to health care while allowing personal choice through a substantial private sector. Funding is primarily through Medicare, which derives funds through general taxation. Medicare is Australia's publicly funded universal health care system, operated by the federal government. It provides all citizens and permanent residents affordable treatment by doctors and in public hospitals and supports prescribed medicines and most treatment by doctors [38].

This system has allowed all Australian and New Zealand citizens and permanent residents in Australia with HIV, to be managed under the national health funding scheme. Funding for HIV medications is provided via Medicare through the Pharmaceutical Benefits Scheme, which enables medicines to be dispensed to patients at a subsidised price. HIV medications fall under a programme called the Highly Specialised Drugs Program (S100) and are only able to be dispensed by specialists or medical practitioners associated with a specialist hospital or medical services [39]. The health of many people living with HIV is managed in general practice, as noted above; the training scheme run by ASHM allows GPs to prescribe antiretroviral drugs. In addition, new antiretroviral drugs are rapidly approved following demonstration of efficacy in clinical trials and safety testing.

HIV Testing and Screening

The first HIV tests followed about a year after the discovery of the virus, HIV, in 1983, but it was not until 1985 that testing became widely available through clinical services. Soon after, in April 1985, Australia became the first nation to implement universal screening of blood donations for HIV [2]. The Australian Blood Transfusion Service is a national government organisation where blood is donated for the public good and without payment.

Clinical testing was initially mainly conducted in those hospitals and clinics that had already seen some patients with AIDS. Wide scale testing among men who had sex with men was encouraged

---

[3]Australia has a Westminster style government consisting of a federation of six states and two territories each with its own elected parliament. The Federal government has a leadership role in policy making, particularly in relation to matters of national interest, including public health, research and information management.

and many gay men, particularly those in inner city areas, volunteered for testing, resulting in high testing rates in those communities. In addition testing was also being encouraged for clients of STI clinics, injecting drug users, commercial sex workers and recipients of blood products. Testing is considered to be an important public health strategy in the early diagnosis and treatment of HIV and as a complement to the more general population and community-oriented HIV-prevention education and condom social marketing campaigns. Among gay men in Australia testing rates were and have remained extremely high at around 85% reporting that they have "ever tested" [40]. The AIDS Councils, after some initial hesitation, supported HIV testing, and high rates of testing are a function of engagement in or attachment to the gay community: a study conducted in 1999/2000 showed that while 80–91% of gay men in the major cities in Australia had ever been tested for HIV and 24–50% had been tested in the previous 6 months, testing rates in men who were attached to the gay community were almost twice as high as those who were not attached [41]. Predictors for increased likelihood of being tested include unprotected anal intercourse in the last 6 months, multiple sexual partners, having a sexual partner who is HIV positive, being younger, having friends who are gay and living in Sydney. While high testing rates in those most at risk will increase early detection of HIV, recent mathematical modelling suggests that increased testing will have little impact on the overall number of HIV notifications [42].

Distribution of Condoms

Condoms have been readily available in Australia since before the start of the HIV epidemic and gay men adopted them as a protective measure before public health advocated their use [43]. Free condoms continue to be distributed at STI clinics throughout the country and are always available at gay events, particularly those that attract large crowds. In addition, many gay venues distribute free condoms or have condom vending machines on site. Several studies have evaluated condom use in MSM. MSM continue to use condoms—especially in their casual sexual relations—and behavioural surveillance data indicate that although there has been a steady and significant increase in unprotected anal intercourse with casual partners since 1998, around 65–70% of MSM across Australia who report anal intercourse with casual sexual partners, consistently use condoms with their casual sexual partners [44, 45]. Men in regular relationships are less likely to use condoms when engaging in anal intercourse, but many of them use other harm reduction strategies such as negotiated safety (see below).

The Development and Support of STI Clinical Services

Prior to the HIV epidemic, clinical services specifically for patients with STIs were few and far between and located mainly in larger centres. Many were open just a few hours a week and most had inadequate facilities [46]. However, in the early 1980s, as a consequence of the open access, anonymous nature and free sexual health care offered by these facilities, many gay men were attending STI services and consequently this was a place some chose to attend for HIV testing and care [47]. The importance of STI clinical services (now called sexual health clinics) was recognised by most of the State Governments who used some of their Federal AIDS funding to support existing services and in some cases to develop new services. Sexual health clinics provide advice about safe sex, free condoms, testing for HIV (and other STIs), post exposure prophylaxis and treatment and care for patients with HIV/AIDS. Since 1998, six major clinics have provided useful sentinel surveillance on HIV testing rates and HIV incidence in gay men [7, 48].

Commercial Sex Workers

The commercial sex industry has a long and varied history in Australia and the States and Territories have differed in their legal responses to the industry. Early in the epidemic, Victoria and NSW decriminalised prostitution and several other States and Territories soon followed. This has allowed for extensive health promotion within the industry, the establishment of health and safety regulations for parlours (brothels), wide scale voluntary testing for HIV and STIs and very high levels of condom use. Success, as measured by the virtual absence of HIV in female sex workers [49] has been extraordinary. Whilst it is acknowledged that the majority of commercial sex workers are female, health promotion and condom use in male sex workers has also been successful and resulted in relatively low levels of STIs and HIV in this population group [50]. The inclusion of male sex workers in HIV-prevention is part of the broader approach to risk reduction and health promotion strategies in Australia.

Research and the Importance of the National Centres

The importance of research was recognised by State and Federal governments very early in the epidemic. While early research responses came from clinicians and medical scientists who were dealing with cases of AIDS and from social scientists who were approached by gay men to help them respond to the threat of HIV, in 1986 two units were funded specifically for HIV research. One was the Virology Research unit at Fairfield Hospital in Melbourne and the other the Epidemiology and Clinical Research Unit at St Vincent's Hospital in Sydney. In 1990 these became the National Centre in HIV Virology Research (NCHVR) and the National Centre in HIV Epidemiology and Clinical Research (NCHECR). NCHVR later became the Australian Centre for HIV and Hepatitis Virology Research (ACH [2]), a network or research laboratories around Australia conducting research in HIV and hepatitis virology. One of the major tasks of the NCHECR was HIV (and later STI) surveillance, a key factor in monitoring the epidemic and documenting the possible success and failures of interventions. The third centre The National Centre in HIV Social Research (NCHSR) was established in 1990 [51] and this organisation has been pivotal in conducting behavioural surveillance and a range of social and ethnographic research with gay communities and injecting drug user networks.

All three National Centres seek extra funding via competitive grants and all have been involved in research including basic science, clinical trials, epidemiological surveys and behavioural studies, which has been central to Australia's response. The NCHECR and the NCHSR are the two centres that have worked most closely with communities of MSM, sex workers and injecting drug users in monitoring HIV disease and risk practice. Their surveillance data have informed governments and communities of the current state of and changes in the patterning of the epidemic and of risk.

To illustrate: the NCHSR and the NCHECR together carry out behavioural surveillance monitoring changes in sexual behaviour over time, using cross sectional surveys—the Gay Periodic Community Surveys (GPCS). This long running cross sectional study using a short-form self-complete questionnaire has been used since 1996 and provides twice-yearly, annual or, in smaller states, biennial summary accounts of the sexual practices of gay men, recruited from saunas, sex clubs, bars, gay social venues and clinics and from the various Mardi Gras Fair Days. Over 5000 men are recruited each year and the findings provide both community educators and government with a very clear picture of increases and decreases in risk practice, levels of HIV testing, as well as providing insights into condom use and other harm reduction strategies. The researchers, community, and government have a very good understanding of how HIV and risk and sex are related and what educational and health promotion initiatives are needed as gay men respond to biomedical innovation and to the changing patterning of the epidemic over time. These GPCS findings and those from the longitudinal cohort studies also provide an assessment of the success or otherwise of the ongoing HIV-prevention programmes of the AIDS Councils. Both National Centres publish annual reports: the NCHECR publishes an Annual Surveillance Report that reports on the prevalence and incidence of HIV/AIDS, viral hepatitis and STIs [8], and the NCHSR publishes an annual report on trends in behaviours relating to HIV, viral hepatitis and STIs [52].

The Partnership in Practice

The partnership is nurtured by all players described above: the government (both Federal and State); the public health professionals; specialists and general practitioners; nurses and social workers; the researchers (virologists, clinicians, epidemiologists, and social researchers); and the AIDS Councils and the communities they support and with whom they work. The partnership has taken many forms over the years, which we illustrate in detail below through two *case studies* related to HIV prevention.

The partnership was established in the early days of HIV, as a result of Health Minister Blewett's political insight and also by the advocacy and political skills of members of the gay community and the AIDS Councils they established. For example, the AIDS Council of New South Wales (ACON), knowing it needed research to guide its response, sought advice from social researchers at Macquarie University in Sydney in 1985. Together the social researchers and gay community members designed a study focusing on the social aspects of the prevention of AIDS (the SAPA project), which was funded by the New South Wales Health Department [53]. The partnership between the government health department members, the researchers and the community organisation staff that emerged from this early research project, became a model that has been followed ever since, especially with regard to HIV-prevention. It became the hall-mark of collaboration for AIDS research in Australia.

Social Public Health

A key feature of the SAPA study was that members of ACON did not only suggest that research be done but also remained closely involved with

it through the next 3–4 years. The steering committee—comprising men and women, heterosexual and gay—met about every 6 weeks to develop the questionnaire, the recruitment strategy, and the selection of interviewers, as well as to discuss the results and develop a strategy for the dissemination of results back to the gay community.

Reflexivity was central to the partnership between the researchers and members of ACON. While ACON wanted research to guide and inform their education and HIV-prevention campaigns, researchers wanted input from gay men. The adoption of a reflexive approach to research was a deliberate strategy of the *Macquarie researchers*: the researchers listened to the gay men, read gay porn, and talked about the emotional and sexual relationships between gay men. Together researchers and the gay committee members read and discussed the work of Altman [54, 55], Kinsey, Pomeroy and Martin [56], Freud [57] and Weeks [58–60].

The upshot of this working relationship was the emergence and development of a "social" public health, a public health that recognises the collective nature of epidemics and works with affected communities and social networks to transform social relations [23]. A social public health is underpinned by an acknowledgement of and engagement with the expertise of those at risk. In the case of HIV, such expertise enhanced understanding about what it is to be a sexual being prone to risk-taking behaviours or an injecting drug user. Enquiry is predicated on an involvement sufficient to drive an attempt to understand fully people whom a programme is trying to reach. While objectivity is often raised as a problem in relation to reflexive research, "objectivity" as Deutscher [61] has argued is not a question of emotional distance, but rather it is seeing from the point of view of the other in order to see well [62]. Further, as pointed out by Stephenson and Kippax [63], while reflexive research requires engagement with "others"—in this case gay men—it also requires engagement with science. The *Macquarie researchers'* approach to sexuality research emphasised involvement with research participants and communities, with community organisations and government agencies, and with other researchers and theorists. They tried simultaneously to maintain and traverse the gap between all these interests.

In addition to adopting a policy based on reflexivity, the researchers in this early study made another decision, which stood them in good stead, and that was to focus on the *practice* of groups/networks rather than on the *behaviours* of individuals. These researchers thought it essential to move beyond the naive individualism of the literature on health behaviour change, and to bring collectives and social dynamics into their strategies. This focus on group practices rather than on individual behaviour is also a characteristic of social public health. This approach assumes that personal action or practice is always predicated on social structures and social relations, and at the same time constitutes social structure [64–66]. Sexuality—the focus of the research—is socially constructed, relational and culturally specific [67, 68]. The research had a double object: the *person* as a social actor and the *gay community* as a collective actor. Within a social public health, prevention programmes or interventions are focused on resourcing communities or groups to not only educate and teach skills to their constituent members about changing normative understandings and expectations, but also to act on their own behalf to advocate for change. HIV prevention programmes provide support for social movement.

Social public health is distinguished from medical public health because it includes:

1. A focus on the collective rather than the individual
2. A focus on practice and the structures or "social drivers" that give rise to practice rather than on behaviour
3. A reliance on grass roots expertise as well as medical expertise in the development of health promotion material

So, for example, HIV prevention is not simply understood as the outcome of individuals being counselled by medical or public health experts in the privacy of the clinic, often in the context of HIV testing, to change their behaviour. Within a medical public health approach, it is assumed that

prevention messages are taken up by individuals who are rational and will act to protect themselves and their sexual and drug using partners. In social public health, HIV-prevention is understood as the outcome of communities, which are financed and supported, developing their own HIV prevention programmes on the basis of their own expertise, along with medical and other expertise. In social public health, it is assumed that prevention messages are taken up by members of communities and networks whose practices are regulated by social norms, which are modified in the public sphere via talk and debate.

Adopting such a theoretical approach had and continues to have a strong practical outcome. Effective educational HIV-prevention strategies operate at the intersection of the physical and behavioural actions through which the virus is transmitted and the "meanings" or contexts through which such actions are apprehended and experienced. It is at this intersection where sexual and other risk practices can be reshaped. The theoretical focus on practice is the means by which the practical problems of an educational strategy can be successfully based. In the social transformation model/s, as adopted by social public health, change in practice is understood as social transformation—and the aim of health promotion or prevention education is to facilitate/enable communities/peoples to change normative structures and collective practices, e.g., to make "safe sex" normative among gay men. The changing of social norms is key to sustaining safe sex [53].

Early Response: Condom Use and Negotiated Safety

Condom Use

The empirical findings of studies conducted during the period prior to introduction of successful treatments, support the comparative advantage of "social" over medical/epidemiological public health. During this period, when social public health gained ground, there is no doubt that there was an uptake of condoms and a sustaining of safe sexual practice in Australia [53], in the UK [69],

Europe [70, 71] and in North America [72–76]. The strategies that were in the main most successful were the harm reduction strategies, the strategies based on a mutually acceptable description of safety from the interested positions of official science (both medical and social science) and from affected communities. These were the strategies embraced by social public health.

Gay men largely ignored the call to abstinence. Martin in 1987 [77] and Evans, et al in 1989 [78] documented decreases in the early 1980s in anal intercourse particularly that involving ejaculation, oral-genital sex with ejaculation, and rimming. By 1988 however, there was a return to what appeared to be earlier levels of sexual activity in the USA [79], much of it protected by condoms in an attempt to make sex safe or safer. Similarly, between 1986 and 1996, Australia saw a turn to the use of condoms and an expansion of the sexual repertoire in terms of the adoption of relatively safe sexual practices. [43, 80]

Although early in the epidemic, gay men heeded the medical calls for monogamy this strategy was not adhered to over time. There is some evidence from Martin [77] of a decline in the median number of partners from 5 to 3 in the 12 months prior to interview and a move to one regular or primary partner in the early years of the epidemic. By the time those findings were published, however, findings from a number of studies in Australia [80] and in the USA reviewed by Stall et al. [79] indicate a move back to higher numbers of casual partners and these numbers remained reasonably stable over the next 10 years. Not only did the number of casual partners remain stable during the period between 1987 and 1997 and at higher levels than that reported by Martin [77], but also men in committed primary relationships engaged in casual sex outside their relationship.

In other words, between 1986/7 and 1996/7 in Australia, North America and Western Europe, there was an uptake of certain prevention messages by gay men—increased condom use for anal intercourse and an expansion of the "safe" sexual repertoire, but a turn away from other messages related to abstinence and monogamy. The practice of anal sex was transformed. In Australia, sex positive and often erotic health promotion produced in the main by the AIDS Councils and funded by government was closely associated with a rapid increase in condom use and a concomitant decline in HIV and STI transmission [13]. Although a direct causal relationship between the educational programmes and the decline in HIV is impossible to establish, a study of Sydney gay men documented a significant relationship between attachment to and engagement in gay community and the uptake of condoms and the relative unimportance of knowledge of HIV test status [53].

Negotiated Safety

The medical advance of the HIV antibody test produced in Australia a new harm reduction strategy—negotiated safety—a strategy in which men dispensed with condoms under certain conditions. And nowhere was the partnership between community members and researchers more obvious than in the ways in which gay men understood and incorporated knowledge of their HIV test status into their sexual practice [81].

The notion of "negotiated safety" grew out of researchers' documentation of sexual practice data from the early Social Aspects of the Prevention of AIDS (SAPA) project of 1986/7 [82]. The researchers recognised that the patterning of unprotected anal intercourse that they were documenting differed depending on with whom and under what conditions it was practised. Gay men, especially those who had received a university education and were employed in a professional capacity, were dispensing with condoms with their regular committed sexual partners.

This patterning was not simply understood or positioned by the researchers as 'relapse'. As these researchers and others such as Davies [83] noted, unprotected sexual intercourse in a number of contexts is more or less safe. One such "safe" context is within a primary relationship under "negotiated safety" conditions. The argument advanced then and now is that dispensing with condom use is safe under the following conditions: if the sexual partners are in a primary relationship; are both HIV-antibody negative and aware of each other's negative antibody status; and have reached a clear and unambiguous agreement about the nature of their sexual practice both within and outside their relationship, such that any sexual practice outside their relationship is safe, that is, precludes the possibility of HIV transmission.

Having recognised and documented the practice of dispensing with condoms within certain contexts and under certain conditions, researchers informed the educators within ACON who, in turn, informed their funders in the New South Wales Health Department. Armed with these research data, augmented by qualitative research based on some in-depth interviews with men who were not using condoms with their regular partners, and funded by State Government, ACON developed a campaign called Talk, Test, Test, Trust [84]. From the position of a "gay-informed" health educator, there was recognition that gay men had developed a strategy that might well help them to sustain safe sexual practice.

The aim was to provide realistic and effective HIV/AIDS education material dealing with unprotected anal intercourse within regular relationships for gay men. It was not a decision taken lightly. To advocate the use *and* non-use of condoms presented health promotion professionals with a range of significant education issues. However, given the evidence that gay men, without advice and indeed contrary to current health promotion advice, were employing a range of personal strategies in negotiating sex, the decision was taken to develop a campaign alongside and complementary to condom campaigns. An iterative process was set in motion. An initial evaluation of the campaign and promotion material concluded that the campaign has added to gay men's understanding of how to safely negotiate unprotected sex within relationships [85]. Subsequently social researchers evaluated the strategy and its impact on sexual practice and HIV infections. Evidence from Australia [86, 87] and the Netherlands [88] indicates that negotiated safety campaigns have led to an increase in unprotected anal intercourse between primary partners. However, these same studies have shown that the adoption of such a strategy has not led to an increase in unsafe practice or HIV trans-

missions in either country. Typically men adopting a negotiated safety strategy ensure that both they and their sexual partner are HIV-negative and keep their agreements not to have unsafe sex outside their relationship. More recently the success of "negotiated safety" as a safe sex strategy was illustrated by findings from a study examining the predictors of seroconversion among gay men in Sydney. The results show that "negotiated safety" was a protective strategy for HIV-negative men [89].

The Talk, Test, Test, Trust campaign aroused considerable debate and discussion in the gay press and elsewhere. A study [90] examining the narrative accounts of gay men who had recently seroconverted, showed while men generally adhered to the contracts they negotiated within their primary relationships, negotiated safety posed a threat to men at the beginning of relationships. Findings pointed to difficulties in talking to sexual partners, to misplaced trust, and to poor communication between partners. In response to the debate and results such as these, ACON in early 1998 returned to the issue of negotiated safety. The health promotion professionals re-presented the Talk, Test, Test, Trust campaign and placed more emphasis on talking—particularly early in relationships. The strategy was effective, they argued, but could be made more so. Much later, in the context of recent discussions and research with regard to the practice of "serosorting", [91, 92] ACON returned again to educate young gay men about "negotiated safety".

Negotiated safety is a deliberate strategy on the part of some men in committed/primary relationships to dispense with condoms within their relationships without necessarily giving up sex or anal intercourse outside relationships. It was not a strategy imposed from the outside, but one that was grounded on an already existing practice, that is, the practice of persons in regular committed relationships of dispensing with condoms after informing each other of their negative HIV-status. The safe adoption of such a strategy involves communication, talk, familiarity and ease with one's sexual partner, and trust, but not necessarily fidelity. Not only did gay men choose some strategies and eschew others, they invented their own. The development of this community strategy and its proven effectiveness in Australia add to the already available evidence with reference to the importance of community engagement and involvement in HIV-prevention activities [93].

Medical knowledge was being taken up and socially transformed by those most affected by the epidemic. This occurred with the help of social research and a new social public health that positioned members of affected communities as agents, who had taken up the challenge of HIV and engaged with various pieces of knowledge and understandings—from the medical and social sciences as well as from their own everyday experience—in order to preserve themselves, their partners, and communities [87, 88]. Other strategies based on medical knowledge and advances have also emerged from within gay community: strategies such as "strategic positioning" [94] and "reliance on undetectable viral load" [95]. These strategies have become part of the armoury of gay men in Australia. Some of these are more effective in reducing harm than others, but nonetheless give gay men a number of choices. With the help of educators and on the basis of research, gay men have used and will continue to use medical and other knowledge to fashion prevention strategies that, although they are not 100% risk-free, can be built into the everyday patterning of their lives and be sustained.

Later Response: Upturn in HIV

The second illustration of partnership concerns the upturn in HIV notifications at the beginning of the twenty-first century in Australia. This illustration describes the coming together of all members of the partnership in an attempt to explain and hopefully contain an upturn in HIV.

In general, what became apparent was that although HIV notifications had remained relatively stable and if anything were declining in New South Wales over the period 2001–2006, a different trend was observed in two other states with relatively large populations of gay men and with relatively high prevalence and incident levels of HIV, Victoria and Queensland. In these two states there were substantial increases in HIV notifications recorded over the same period. Increases in HIV notifications were also reported in two less populous states—South Australia and Western Australia.

In response to the above, the Health Promotion Committee of the NSW Ministerial Advisory Committee on HIV/AIDS and Sexually Transmissible Infections organised the NSW Think Tank. The Think Tank was convened in April 2007 to address the differences between the three states and in an attempt to gain some understanding of them [96]. It brought together leaders in HIV epidemiology and social research, clinical sexual health, the HIV community, and officers from the Communicable Diseases and AIDS/Infectious Diseases Branch of the NSW Department of Health and an observer from the Australian Government Department of Health and Ageing.

Over the course of the Think Tank meeting, there were presentations covering HIV surveillance, STI infections in gay men, behavioural surveillance—including time trends in sexual behaviour, HIV testing rates and time trends in community viral load and levels of treatment, and investment in HIV prevention, partnership and capacity. These presentations in modified form were published in a special issue of *Sexual Health* [97] in 2008.

The Think Tank agreed that the observed differences in HIV notifications in Australia reflected differences in HIV incidence and were not primarily an outcome of changes in HIV testing patterns or notification procedures. It was noted that there had been a stabilisation and a subsequent decline in reported rates of unprotected anal intercourse with casual partners (UAI-C) among gay and other homosexually active men in NSW from 2001 to 2006, including among HIV-positive men. This trend was not observed in Victoria or Queensland, where rates of UAI-C have continued to increase to the extent that they now equal or exceed those seen in NSW [44]. As noted in the NSW Think Tank Report [96] (p. 3): "This is the single most important explanation of the differences between the States—but it is not the only one".

A number of other factors have also contributed towards a stabilising of HIV notifications in NSW compared with Victoria and Queensland. These include: a reduction in the proportion of homosexually active men reporting high numbers of casual partners and an increase in the proportion of men reporting no current sexual partners or only having sex with one partner—both since 2003; and a decline in the proportion of serodiscordant relationships, and a concomitant increase in the proportion of seroconcordant relationships [44].

There are other differences between one State and another, but essentially the differences that explain the reduction in HIV notifications in NSW and the increases in HIV notifications in Victoria and Queensland, are associated with changes in risky sexual practices. The "safer" sexual practice observed in New South Wales is in turn highly likely to be related to the comparatively high per capita investment in HIV-prevention in NSW. Compared with the other States, NSW has maintained its investment in HIV overall and in HIV prevention in particular, with reviews and reinvestment implemented as needed [16].

Part of the investment was and continues to be earmarked for comprehensive social marketing initiatives, which targeted both broad and specific audiences of gay men, including HIV-positive men. A comparative analysis of campaign material from NSW and the other two States [96] indicated that the material had engaged with changes in gay community culture and the place of HIV within it and had adopted a wider focus on gay and other homosexually active men's health—in response to evidence that this was an effective way to get HIV prevention messages taken up by men who have sex with men. The analysis also demonstrated that the material was extremely well integrated with other interventions, for example, a comprehensive range of community development and group support programmes, sexual health testing and treatment, mental health and drug harm initiatives.

A heavy emphasis continues to be placed on partnership in NSW by all parties, with a range of mechanisms—including formal and informal committees and meetings, and the sharing of evidence—available and utilised for relationship management, shared problem identification and solving, consensus building, and strategy, policy and programme development. There is a profound sense of engagement and mutual trust and respect between the members of the partnership that is located in the calibre and the commitment of those involved. As Bernard et al [16] (p. 193) note: "An active commitment to and adequate resourcing of HIV prevention by all stakeholders in the HIV partnership—government and non-government departments, researchers and gay community organisations—is crucial if Australia is to respond effectively to HIV among gay men and other men who have sex with men".

While these two examples do not prove conclusively that the NSW approach—the HIV prevention programme funded by NSW Health, informed by epidemiology and social research, and coordinated and managed by the AIDS Council of NSW (ACON)—is effective in reducing HIV transmission, it is a feasible and non-contentious interpretation.

Key Elements of Behaviour Change: Evaluation

Compared with similar high-income countries, Australia has been comparatively successful in responding to HIV. Although there has been some slippage, safe sex has been sustained for 25 years (just under 70% of gay men continue to use condoms 100% of the time with their casual partners). What have we learned?

Two papers recently compared HIV surveillance data from North America, Western Europe and Australia: Sullivan et al. [98] compare annual percentage changes in annual HIV notifications between 1996 and 2000 and 2000–2005 for Australia, Canada, France, Germany, the Netherlands, the UK and the USA. With the exception of Germany, while there was a reduction in annual HIV notifications in all of these countries between 1996 and 2000, Australia had the greatest reduction of 8.1% compared with the 2.9% in the USA, with the other countries falling between these two figures. While all countries experienced an increase in HIV notifications between 2000 and 2005, the USA and Australia experienced the lowest increases of 2.3 and 3.7% respectively. The other countries experienced increases ranging from 12% in Germany to 4.3% in Canada.

Stall et al. [99] report on HIV incidence rates among MSM for the period between 1995 and 2005. With reference to the difference between Australia and the USA in HIV incidence estimates of 0.978 compared with 2.39, Stall et al. [99] (p. 626) conclude as follows: "In short, expected prevalence rates in the Australian case are roughly half those calculated for US MSM by age 40. While such facile comparisons ignore important contextual variables that can drive HIV epidemics at different rates across societies, this difference is so stark that it raises the question of whether it is possible to construct HIV prevention programming and policy to yield far more successful results among gay male communities than have been obtained to date in the United States".

So what is it that works? Our examination of the available data in Australia indicates that there are a number of key elements that give rise to safe sexual practice and a lowering of HIV incidence. Social transformation, which is best achieved via advocacy, public talk and debate, skill building and education, is what is necessary. It is evident that gay men acting together as members of a community rather than individually as unconnected persons, have exercised a collective rationality and the practice of anal sex has been transformed as "safe sex". It is also evident that gay communities will continue to sustain safe sex if informed by research evidence and resourced and supported by government which funds their AIDS Councils to support and educate them. Community norms have been changed in response to both threat of disease and promise of treatment. If *of community* and reinforced by AIDS organisations, effective risk reduction strategies are likely to be sustained by community members.

Australia unlike many other countries in the world, did not adopt an approach in which single interventions were trialled and tested. Indeed it would have been very difficult to do this given the history of the complex HIV-prevention programme established across a range of institutions and organisations. Instead Australian governments,

both Federal and State, have supported and funded community-based HIV prevention programmes alongside more broadly based campaigns targeting the general population. They have also evaluated the programmes that have been put in place. They have done this by relying on the evidence provided by the annual HIV and behavioural surveillance, as well as from a range of research studies, demonstration projects, and process evaluations carried out by the National Centres, independent evaluators, and the AIDS Councils (for example see [18, 97]).

While debate continues about the appropriateness and usefulness of randomised controlled trials (RCTs), there is a growing agreement that such evaluation is of limited use in this context [100, 101]. As Hallett et al. [102] argue, there is tension between indicators for monitoring and evaluation, and variables required for a full and sophisticated understanding of sexual risk. Furthermore, because health promotion builds over time as knowledge increases and social and cultural norms and practices change, health promotion is difficult to evaluate particularly with reference to sexual behaviour change. High quality surveillance data in conjunction with behavioural data and modelling studies are more likely to be of use—especially when evaluating population impact.

It is always difficult to pinpoint what has made for success or failure but unquestionably the Australian success, which has been a sustained success over 25 years, is in part at least a function of the social health model—genuine partnership between government, affected communities, public health and researchers; community-informed health promotion and education alongside evidence-based prevention; and a focus on social relations and social transformation. The Australian government established and continues to fund community-based HIV prevention and support, via the AIDS Councils. These councils are informed by ongoing epidemiological and behavioural surveillance and social research, within a system of health care with a national insurance scheme. Treatment is guaranteed to all those who need and seek it by a highly skilled cadre of health care specialists and general practitioners.

Effective social public health recognises that people are not only individuals but members of groups, networks and collectives. It recognises and indeed relies on the fact that people interact (talk, negotiate, have sex …) *together* and that social relations and their transformation are the bread and butter of change. Safe sex is sustainable because it is *OF* community.

References

1. Penny R, Marks R, Berger J, Marriott D, Bryant D. Acquired immune deficiency syndrome. Med J Aust. 1983;1(12):554–7.
2. Plummer D, Irwin L. Grassroots activities, national initiatives and HIV prevention: clues to explain Australia's dramatic early success in controlling the HIV epidemic. Int J STD AIDS. 2006;17(12): 787–93.
3. Kaldor J. Epidemiological pattern of HIV infection in Australia. J Acquir Immune Defic Syndr. 1993;6 Suppl 1:S1–4.
4. McDonald AM, Crofts N, Blumer CE, et al. The pattern of diagnosed HIV infection in Australia, 1984–1992. AIDS. 1994;8(4):513–9.
5. NCHECR. *HIV/AIDS and related disease: Annual Surveillance Report.* Sydney: National Centre in HIV Epidemiology and Clinical Research, The University of New South Wales, 1997.
6. Bowtell W. *Australia's Response to HIV/AIDS 1982–2005. Report prepared for Research and Dialogue Project on Regional Responses to the spread of HIV/AIDS in East Asia organised by the Japan Center for International Exchange and the Friends of the Global fund to Fight AIDS, Tuberculosis and Malaria (Japan).* Lowy Institute for International Policy, 2005.
7. NCHECR. *HIV/AIDS, Viral Hepatitis and sexually transmissible infections in Australia: Annual Surveillance Report.* National Centre in HIV Epidemiology & Clinical Research, The University of New South Wales, 2008.
8. NCHECR. *HIV/AIDS, Viral hepatitis and sexually transmissible infections in Australia: Annual Surveillance Report.* Sydney: National Centre in HIV Epidemiology & Clinical Research, The University of New South Wales, 2009.
9. Smith GW. *Bugger Me! The Civilising of a Perversion. PhD Thesis.* Sydney, University of New South Wales; 2004.
10. "The first media report of AIDS appeared in the Australian gay press in The Star in July 1981: it reported on the disease affecting gay men in the US, the gay-related immune disease (GRID) or, less kindly, the 'gay plague'" *The Sydney Star.* 1981;2
11. Ballard J. Participation and innovation in a federal system *AIDS in Industrialized Democracies: Passions, Politics and Policies.* New Brunswick: Rutgers University Press; 1992
12. Ariss R. Against death: the practice of living with AIDS. The Netherlands: Gordon and Breach; 1997.
13. Sendziuk P. *Learning to Trust: Australian Responses to AIDS.* Sydney University of New South Wales Press, 2003.
14. Altman D. Power and community: organizational and cultural responses to AIDS. London: Taylor and Francis; 1994.
15. Ariss M. *Against Death: The Practice of Living with AIDS.* Gordon and Breach; 1977.
16. Bernard D, Kippax S, Baxter D. Effective partnership and adequate investment underpin a successful response: key factors in dealing with HIV increases. Sex Health. 2008;5(2):193–201.
17. Donovan R, Chan LK. RUBBA ME: New South Wales HIV/AIDS Campaigns 1984–2004. University of New South Wales; 2007.
18. Wilson A, Fowler D, Spina A, Wise M. Evaluation of NSW HIV/AIDS Health Promotion Plan 2001–2003. Sydney: NSW Health Department; 2004.
19. Blewett N. AIDS in Australia: the primitive years: reflections on Australia's policy response to the AIDS epidemic. Sydney: Australian Health Policy Institute at the University of Sydney; 2003.
20. Kramer L. Reports from the holocaust: the making of an AIDS activist. New York: St. Martin's Press; 1989.
21. Shilts R. And the band played on: politics, people and the AIDS epidemic. New York: St Martin's press; 1987.
22. Patton C. Inventing AIDS. New York; London: Routledge; 1990.
23. Henderson K, Worth H, Aggleton P, Kippax S. Enhancing HIV prevention requires addressing the complex relationship between prevention and treatment. Glob Public Health. 2009;4(2):117–30.
24. Blewett N. *AIDS in Australia: The Primitive Years. Reflections on Australia's policy response to the AIDS Epidemic.* Commissioned Paper Series 2003/07. Sydney: Australian Health Policy Institute, University of Sydney; 2003.
25. Taylor WT, Proudfoot A, Hazell E, Mitchell N. *Australian Market Research. Measurement of Effectiveness of 'Assault' Phase of NAVAIDS AIDS Campaign.* Sydney: 1987.
26. National HIV/AIDS Strategy. A policy information paper. Canberra Australian Government Publishing Service; 1989.
27. WHO. The Ottawa Charter for Health Promotion. Paper presented at: First International Conference on Health Promotion 21 November, 1986; Ottawa.
28. Report of the evaluation of the National HIV/AIDS strategy: report to the Minister for Health, Housing and Community Services and the intergovernmental Committee on AIDS by National Evaluation Steering Committee. Canberra: AGPS; 1992.

29. National HIV/AIDS Strategy 1993–1994 to 1995–1996. Valuing the past … investing in the future. Canberra Australian Government Publishing Service; 1993.
30. Feachem RGA. Valuing the past… investing in the future. Evaluation of the National HIV/AIDS Strategy 1993–1994 to1995–1996: Looking Glass Press for Publications and Design (Public Affairs), Commonwealth Department of Human Services and Health; 1995.
31. National HIV/AIDS Strategy 1996–1997 to1998–1999. A strategy framed in the context of sexual health and related communicable diseases: Looking Glass Press for Publications and Design (Public Affairs), Commonwealth Department of Health and Family Services; 1996.
32. National HIV/AIDS Strategy 1999–2000 to 2003–2004: Changes and Challenges. Canberra: Commonwealth Department of Health and Ages Care; 2000.
33. Moodie R, Edwards A, Payne M. Review of the National HIV/AIDS Strategy 1999–2000 to 2003–2004: Getting back on track… revitalising Australia's response to HIV/AIDS 2002.
34. National HIV/AIDS Strategy 2005–2008. Revitalising Australia's Response: Commonwealth of Australia; 2005.
35. National Sexually Transmissible Infections Strategy 2005–2008: Commonwealth of Australia; 2005.
36. ASHM. Australasian Society for HIV Medicine. Background information and discussion. http://www.ashm.org.au/
37. Leeder S. The Australian health system. Telemed J. 2000;6(2):201–4.
38. The Australian Health Care System: The national healthcare funding system Canberra: Australian Government - Department of Health and Ageing.
39. Highly Specialised Drugs Program. Browse by Section 100 Item List. Canberra: Australian Government - Department of Health and Ageing.
40. Imrie J, Frankland A. Annual Reports of Trends in Behaviour 2008: HIV/AIDS, hepatitis and sexually transmissible infections in Australia. Sydney: National Centre in HIV Social Research, University of New South Wales; 2008.
41. Hull P, Van de Ven P, Prestage G, et al. Gay community periodic survey Sydney 1996–2002. Sydney: National Centre in HIV Social Research, The University of New South Wales; 2003.
42. NCHECR. Mathematical models to investigate recent trends in HIV notifications among men who have sex with men in Australia. Sydney: National Centre in HIV Epidemiology and Clinical Research, The University of New South Wales, 2008.
43. Kippax S, Race K. Sustaining safe practice: twenty years on. Soc Sci Med. 2003;57(1):1–12.
44. Zablotska IB, Prestage G, Grulich AE, Imrie J. Differing trends in sexual risk behaviours in three Australian states: New South Wales, Victoria and Queensland, 1998–2006. Sex Health. 2008;5(2): 125–30.
45. NCHSR. HIV/AIDS, hepatitis and sexually transmissible infections in Australia: Annual reports of Trends in Behaviour 2008. Sydney: National Centre in HIV Social Research, The University of New South Wales, 2008.
46. Lewis M. Sexually Transmitted Diseases Resurgent. Thorns on the rose: the history of sexually transmitted diseases in Australia in international perspective. Canberra: Australian Government Publishing Service; 1998:271–353.
47. Lewis M. A Modern Plague: The Advance of HIV/AIDS. Thorns on the rose: the history of sexually transmitted diseases in Australia in international perspective. Canberra: Australian Government Publishing Service; 1998:407–470.
48. NCHECR. HIV/AIDS, Hepatitis C and sexually transmissible infections in Australia: Annual Surveillance Report. Sydney: National Centre in HIV Epidemiology and Clinical Research, The University of New South Wales, 1999.
49. Egger S, Harcourt C. Prostitution in NSW: the impact of deregulation. In: Easteal P, McKillop S, editors. Women and the law. Canberra: Australian Government: Australian Institute of Criminology; 1993.
50. Estcourt CS, Marks C, Rohrsheim R, Johnson AM, Donovan B, Mindel A. HIV, sexually transmitted infections, and risk behaviours in male commercial sex workers in Sydney. Sex Transm Infect. 2000;76(4):294–8.
51. NCHSR. National Centre in HIV Social Research. http://nchsr.arts.unsw.edu.au/
52. NCHSR. HIV/AIDS, hepatitis and sexually transmissible infections in Australia: Annual Report of Trends in Behaviour 2009. Sydney: National Centre in HIV Social Research, The University of New South Wales, 2009.
53. Kippax S, Connell RW, Dowsett GW, Crawford J. Sustaining Safe Sex: Gay Communities Respond to AIDS (Social Aspects of AIDS). London: The Falmer Press; 1993.
54. Altman D. Coming out in the seventies. Sydney: Wild and Wooley; 1979.
55. Altman D. The Homosexualization of America: the Americanization of the Homosexual. New York: St Martin's Press; 1982.
56. Kinsey A, Pomeroy W, Martin C. Sexual behavior in the human male. Philadelphia: Saunders; 1948.
57. Freud S. Three essays on the theory of sexuality. In: Strachey J, editor. The standard edition of the complete psychological works, vol. 7. London: Hogarth Press; 1964. p. 123–243.
58. Weeks J. Homosexual politics in britain from the nineteenth century to the present. London: Quartet; 1977.
59. Weeks J. Sex, politics and society: the regulation of sexuality since 1800. London: Longman; 1981.
60. Weeks J. Sexuality and its discontents. London: Routedge and Kegan Paul; 1985.
61. Deutscher M. Subjecting and objecting. St Lucia, Queensland: University of Queensland Press; 1983.

62. Haraway DJ. Simians, cyborgs, and women: the reinvention of nature. New York: Routledge; 1991.
63. Stephenson M, Kippax S. Minding the gap: subjectivity and sexuality research. In: Maiers W, Bayer B, Duarte E, Jorna R, Scharaube E, editors. Challenges to theoretical psychology. Ontario: Captus Press Inc; 1999. p. 383–400.
64. Giddens A. The constitution of society: outline of the theory of structuration. Berkeley: University of California Press; 1986.
65. Harre R. Social being: a theory for social psychology. Oxford: Blackwell; 1979.
66. Kippax S. Understanding and integrating the structural and biomedical determinants of HIV infection: a way forward for prevention. Curr Opin HIV AIDS. 2008;3(4):489–94.
67. Gagnon J, Simon W. Sexual Conduct. The sources of human sexuality. London: Hutchinson; 1974.
68. Caplan P. The cultural construction of sexuality. London; New York: Tavistock; 1987.
69. Hickson FC, Reid DS, Davies PM, Weatherburn P, Beardsell S, Keogh PG. No aggregate change in homosexual HIV risk behaviour among gay men attending the Gay Pride festivals, United Kingdom, 1993–1995. AIDS. 1996;10(7):771–4.
70. Moatti JP, Souteyrand Y. HIV/AIDS social and behavioural research: past advances and thoughts about the future. Soc Sci Med. 2000;50(11):1519–32.
71. Moatti JP, Souteyrand Y. AIDS in Europe: new challenges for the social sciences. London and New York: Routledge; 2000.
72. Stall RD, Coates TJ, Hoff C. Behavioral risk reduction for HIV infection among gay and bisexual men. A review of results from the United States. Am Psychol. 1988;43(11):878–85.
73. Schechter MT, Craib KJ, Willoughby B, et al. Patterns of sexual behavior and condom use in a cohort of homosexual men. Am J Public Health. 1988;78(12):1535–8.
74. Moran JS, Janes HR, Peterman TA, Stone KM. Increase in condom sales following AIDS education and publicity, United States. Am J Public Health. 1990;80(5):607–8.
75. Myers T, McLeod DW, Calzavara L. Responses of gay and bisexual men to HIV/AIDS in Toronto, Canada: community-based initiatives, AIDS education and sexual behaviour. Unpublished work. Toronto: HIV Social, Behavioural and Epidemiological Studies Unit, Faculty of Medicine, University of Toronto, Canada, 1991.
76. Remis RS, Major C, Calzavara L, Myers T, Burchell A, Whittingham EP. The HIV Epidemic among Men who have Sex with Other Men: the Situation in Ontario in the Year 2000. Canada: Department of Public Health Services, University of Ontario; 2000.
77. Martin JL. The impact of AIDS on gay male sexual behavior patterns in New York City. Am J Public Health. 1987;77(5):578–81.
78. Evans BA, McLean KA, Dawson SG, et al. Trends in sexual behaviour and risk factors for HIV infection among homosexual men, 1984–1987. BMJ. 1989; 298(6668):215–8.
79. Stall RD, Hays RB, Waldo CR, Ekstrand M, McFarland W. The Gay '90s: a review of research in the 1990s on sexual behavior and HIV risk among men who have sex with men. AIDS. 2000;14 Suppl 3:S101–14.
80. Prestage G, Mao L, Fogarty A, et al. How has the sexual behaviour of gay men changed since the onset of AIDS: 1986–2003. Aust N Z J Public Health. 2005;29(6):530–5.
81. Kippax S, Kinder P. Reflexive practice: the relationship between social research and health promotion in HIV prevention. Sex Education. 2002;2(2): 91–104.
82. Kippax S, Crawford J, Davis M, Rodden P, Dowsett G. Sustaining safe sex: a longitudinal study of a sample of homosexual men. AIDS. 1993;7(2): 257–63.
83. Davies PM. Safer sex maintenance among gay men: are we moving in the right direction? AIDS. 1993;7(2):279–80.
84. Kinder P. A new prevention education strategy for gay men: responding to the impact of AIDS on gay men's lives. Paper presented at: 11th International AIDS Conference 1996; Vancouver.
85. Mackie B. Report and Process Evaluation of the Talk Test Test Trust … Together HIV/AIDS Education Campaign. Sydney: AIDS Council of New South Wales; 1996.
86. Kippax S, Noble J, Prestage G, et al. Sexual negotiation in the AIDS era: negotiated safety revisited. AIDS. 1997;11(2):191–7.
87. Crawford JM, Rodden P, Kippax S, Van de Ven P. Negotiated safety and other agreements between men in relationships: risk practice redefined. Int J STD AIDS. 2001;12(3):164–70.
88. Davidovich U, de Wit JB, Stroebe W. Assessing sexual risk behaviour of young gay men in primary relationships: the incorporation of negotiated safety and negotiated safety compliance. AIDS. 2000;14(6):701–6.
89. Jin F, Crawford J, Prestage GP, et al. Unprotected anal intercourse, risk reduction behaviours, and subsequent HIV infection in a cohort of homosexual men. AIDS. 2009;23(2):243–52.
90. Kippax S, Slavin S, Ellard J, et al. Seroconversion in context. AIDS Care. 2003;15(6):839–52.
91. Mao L, Crawford JM, Hospers HJ, et al. "Serosorting" in casual anal sex of HIV-negative gay men is noteworthy and is increasing in Sydney, Australia. AIDS. 2006;20(8):1204–6.
92. Zablotska IB, Imrie J, Prestage G, et al. Gay men's current practice of HIV seroconcordant unprotected anal intercourse: serosorting or seroguessing? AIDS Care. 2009;21(4):501–10.
93. Anderson R. Successes in HIV control, fact or fiction? Paper presented at: XIII International AIDS Conference; July 9–14, 2000; Durban, South Africa.
94. Van de Ven P, Murphy D, Hull P, Prestage G, Batrouney C, Kippax S. Risk management and harm

reduction among gay men in Sydney. Critical Public Health. 2004;14(4):361–76.

95. Van de Ven P, Mao L, Fogarty A, et al. Undetectable viral load is associated with sexual risk taking in HIV serodiscordant gay couples in Sydney. AIDS. 2005;19(2):179–84.

96. NSW Health: "A Think Tank: Why are HIV notifications Flat in NSW 1998–2006?' Concensus Statement. Sydney: NSW Health Department; 2007.

97. Fairley C, Grulich AE, Imrie JC, Pits M. Investment in HIV prevention works: a natural experiment. Sex Health. 2008;5(2):207–10.

98. Sullivan PS, Hamouda O, Delpech V, et al. Re-emergence of the HIV epidemic among men who have sex with men in North America, Western Europe, and Australia, 1996–2005. Ann Epidemiol. 2009;19(6):423–31.

99. Stall R, Duran L, Wisniewski SR, et al. Running in place: implications of HIV incidence estimates among urban men who have sex with men in the United States and other industrialized countries. AIDS Behav. 2009;13(4):615–29.

100. Nutbeam D. Evaluating health promotion—progress, problems and solutions. Health Promot Int. 1998;13(1):27–44.

101. Kippax S. Sexual health interventions are unsuitable for experimental evaluation. In: Stephenson JM, Imrie J, Bonell C, editors. Effective Sexual Health Intervensions: issues in experimental evaluation. Oxford: Oxford University Press; 2003. p. 17–34.

102. Hallett TB, White PJ, Garnett GP. Appropriate evaluation of HIV prevention interventions: from experiment to full-scale implementation. Sex Transm Infect. 2007;83 Suppl 1:i55–60.

Reducing Disparities in Sexual Health: Lessons Learned from the Campaign to Eliminate Infectious Syphilis from the United States

18

Jo A. Valentine and Susan J. DeLisle

Introduction

All Americans should have equal opportunities to live healthy lives regardless of their income, education, or racial/ethnic background. However, difficult living conditions have made health and wellness elusive for many Americans, creating circumstances that increase poor health outcomes, including disparate rates of sexually transmitted diseases. In particular the persistent high rate of primary and secondary (P&S) syphilis in some of American's most vulnerable populations has been characterized as a sentinel event, signaling a failure in public health capacity to ensure the health of American communities [1, 2]. *The National Campaign to Eliminate Syphilis* (SEP), launched in October 1999, was designed to improve public health capacity, and thereby improve infant health, reduce HIV transmission, reduce health care costs, and eliminate a long-standing glaring health disparity.

In the early 1990s, when primary and secondary (P&S) syphilis was at its peak in the United States, black Americans were accounting for

J.A. Valentine (✉)
Division of STD Prevention, Centers for Disease Control and Prevention, 1600 Clifton Rd., NE, MS E-02, Atlanta, GA 30333, USA
e-mail: jxv2@cdc.gov

S.J. DeLisle
Health Consultant, Atlanta, GA, USA
e-mail: quepasasue@aol.com

more than 80% of the reported cases; [3] and continuing today racial/ethnic minorities and sexual minority populations not only experience higher rates for P&S syphilis but also for all of the reportable bacterial sexually transmitted diseases (STDs). For example between 2005 and 2009, chlamydia rates increased by 26% among blacks, 4% among American Indians/Alaska Natives, and 13% among Hispanics for disparity rates compared to whites of 12:1, 4:1, and 3:1 respectively. In 2009 black Americans accounted for 71% of gonorrhea cases for a rate 20 times higher than the rate for whites and more than 50% of P&S syphilis for a rate that was 8 times higher than the rate for whites (Fig. 18.1). Hispanics Americans accounted for as much as 15% of P&S syphilis, and the disparity in gonorrhea rates for this population was larger in the Northeast (four times higher than whites) [4].

Prior to 1999 there had been multiple focused attempts to eradicate or eliminate infectious syphilis as a public health threat [5, 6]. It is important here to note the difference between *eradication* and *elimination* as was described during the *Dahlem Workshop on the Eradication of Infectious Diseases* (March 1997). At this meeting *eradication* was defined as the permanent reduction to zero of the worldwide incidence of infection caused by a specific agent as a result of deliberate efforts (e.g., smallpox). In contrast, the *elimination* of a disease was defined as the reduction to zero of the incidence of the disease in a defined geographical area as a result of deliberate efforts (e.g., neonatal

S.O. Aral, K.A. Fenton, and J.A. Lipshutz (eds.), *The New Public Health and STD/HIV Prevention: Personal, Public and Health Systems Approaches*, DOI 10.1007/978-1-4614-4526-5_18,
© Springer Science+Business Media New York 2013

Rate (per 100,000 population)

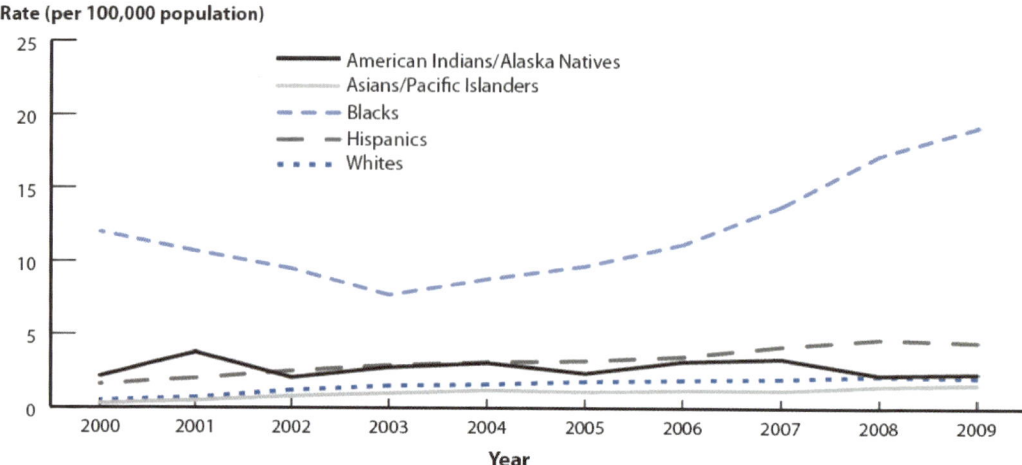

Fig. 18.1 P&S Syphilis by Race/Ethnicity

tetanus). Under elimination conditions intervention measures are required to be ongoing; whereas with a successful eradication interventions are no longer needed [7].

With the advent and widespread availability of penicillin, the *eradication* of syphilis initially seemed simple: identify the case, treat the person and his or her partners, and transmission would be stopped. "Syphilis is something of a natural wonder," wrote William J. Brown in 1962. "Upon examining its characteristics, one is almost amazed that the disease has managed to survive at all in this day and age, let alone increase continually year after year" [8]. Unlike other infectious organisms, syphilis still remains easy to diagnose and treat. As the former Centers for Disease Control and Prevention (CDC) Director, Dr. Jeffery Koplan said at the launch of the 1999 SEP, "Syphilis is not a 21st century disease; it should not even have been a twentieth century disease" [9].

The 1999 SEP sought to better address a variety of individual factors and social determinants that sustain the infectious syphilis epidemic by promoting public health interventions at the: (1) individual, (2) community, and (3) structural levels [2]. Such interventions, it was hoped, would lead to the overall enhancement of public health capacity and improve individual health and community wellness. Designed to be a collaborative effort between the CDC and a wide range of partners working in the public and private sectors at

national, state, and local levels, the mission of the SEP was the promotion of health and quality of life by preventing, controlling, and reducing endemic transmission of syphilis from the United States. More specifically the goal of the plan was to *eliminate* sustained transmission of infectious syphilis, and the national goal set in 1999 was to reduce P&S syphilis cases to <1,000 (rate: 0.4 per 100,000 population) and to increase the number of syphilis-free counties to 90% by 2005 [10]. Therefore, despite previously unsuccessful initiatives to *eradicate* syphilis, it was believed that this new more modest elimination goal was plausible for the United States, given the historically low rates of P&S syphilis in the late 1990s, the geographically limited disease incidence, and the availability of inexpensive and effective diagnostic tests and therapy [11].

When CDC initiated the SEP in 1999, P&S syphilis had reached its lowest point since reporting began in 1941, declining as much as 88% between 1990 and 2000 alone, but, as has been seen repeatedly with infectious syphilis, the P&S rate began increasing again by 2001, and has continued to do so each year since [12]. Significant successes in some American communities notwithstanding, and overall rates that continue to this day to be relatively low compared to other STDs, syphilis remains *something of a natural wonder*, although this wonder may have less to do with the organism itself than it does with personal behavior and community environments. As is true for other STDs, as well as the myriad of health and social challenges facing many of Americans today, individual factors and social determinants that maintain the ongoing transmission of syphilis are complex and interrelated [13–15].

Multidisciplinary Strategies for Syphilis Prevention and Control

Developed in collaboration with partners internal and external to CDC, the 1999 SEP provided national leadership for syphilis research and surveillance, as well as the development and testing of effective biomedical and behavioral interventions to reduce syphilis transmission in the United States. The plan was predicated upon the understanding that eliminating syphilis would require combining intensified traditional approaches [16] to STD control with innovative efforts to generate new synergy to enhance the effectiveness of syphilis elimination activities. The SEP looked specifically to emerging approaches from HIV prevention activities and other forms of community-level formative research [17]. It was believed that by bringing together usual STD prevention strategies (e.g., screening and partner notification) with more contemporary innovations (e.g., community-based participatory research) the effectiveness of syphilis prevention and control could be increased.

Five strategies were laid-out in the 1999 SEP: (1) enhanced surveillance, (2) community involvement and partnerships, (3) rapid outbreak response, (4) expanded clinical and laboratory services, and (5) enhanced health promotion. The five strategies were deemed essential to improving STD prevention and control responses, as well as for shoring up general public health capacity in many communities experiencing persistent and significant disparities in sexual health. In addition to increased fiscal support to state and local programs, CDC also provided direct technical assistance to state and local health departments in the form of *Rapid Response Team* (RRT) deployments [18], *Program Assessments* [19], *Epi-AID* deployments [20], and other research, technical assistance, and evaluation support.

Cross-Cutting and Intervention Strategies

In the 1999 SEP *Enhanced Surveillance* and *Strengthened Community Involvement and Partnerships* were defined as *cross-cutting* in that they were essential to guide, evaluate, and facilitate syphilis prevention and control activities. The strategies of *Rapid Outbreak Response, Expanded Clinical and Laboratory services,* and *Enhanced Health Promotion* were defined as *intervention strategies* and relied upon the *cross-cutting strategies* for more effective application. These five strategies provided a framework for program planning and a focus for program activities. They emphasized the importance of collecting timely and enhanced data, including behavioral and social data in addition to morbidity, and using these data to inform interventions, while continually involving affected communities, and the organizations serving them, in the development and execution of intervention strategies. The three *intervention strategies* themselves focused on strengthening key program actions, expediting response to syphilis increases, increasing case finding through expanded screening, testing and clinical services, and enhancing health promotion messages.

Enhanced Surveillance and Outbreak Response

Surveillance data used to determine the burden of syphilis, as is true for many infectious diseases, are usually outdated due to the processes involved in collecting, reporting, and analyzing data. Epidemics are dynamic events, and they often change quickly. As epidemics progress through relatively predictable stages [21], it is critical to apply social, behavioral, and epidemiological sciences to forecasting and predicting disease trajectories rather than simply describing what has occurred in the past. The SEP called for such forecasting to enhance public health capacity to better address syphilis and other STDs.

Enhanced Surveillance is essential for improving the implementation of the intervention strategy *Outbreak Response.* Interrupting transmission of any communicable disease has at its foundation the development of a sensitive surveillance system with an urgent and robust response to changes in incidence. For syphilis, detecting and determining when an outbreak occurs is complex and quite challenging as there are numerous built-in delays in how information ultimately reaches a surveillance system. A diagnosis of syphilis is generally not based solely on a laboratory test result. A confirmatory test, a clinical examination, a record review, and a patient interview may also be required before a diagnosis is considered complete. The time taken to conduct these processes can result in at least a 3–4 week delay before the case report actually reaches a surveillance system. At best, data analyses often occur 1–2 months after a case, or cluster of cases, has been detected. Therefore, knowledge of outbreaks most often occurs through real time communication between local workers rather than through any formal data system. As there is also no standard definition of a syphilis outbreak that is universally applicable [22], it is incumbent upon local area staff to be familiar with their local epidemiology to detect changes in syphilis case numbers and shifts in risk factors, geography, or demographics. Local jurisdictions with high rates of syphilis can find it challenging to detect focal or new outbreaks against a backdrop of endemic disease while other jurisdictions with low rates need to have a very low threshold for what determines an outbreak.

The SEP called for locally specific outbreak response plans; and although thoughtful and time-consuming work usually went into development of these outbreak response plans, once an outbreak had been declared, many local programs were still challenged with garnering and marshaling the fiscal and human resources necessary to implement and sustain an effective outbreak response [23, 24]. Outbreak response is labor-intensive and can require an ongoing effort of up to several months before any appreciable decrease in cases occurs. In fact, at the onset of an outbreak, it is quite common to see a steep rise in cases because of increased case-finding activities. For many health departments, mounting a

sustained response to a syphilis outbreak means mobilizing staff from other health department programs, forgoing other duties, and even suspending lesser priority public health activities. Relatively rural counties can spend substantial resources for housing and travel of deployed staff, straining local budgets. Given these kinds of conditions the availability of federal Rapid Response Teams was an important asset to state and local programs. However, over time as resources began to shrink at the federal level, this resource also became increasingly limited.

Community Involvement and Organizational Partnerships

By engaging communities and building new organizational partnerships, a number of local STD programs expanded their service capacity for syphilis elimination. Often times these stronger relationships were the result of engagement with community members and stakeholder groups in the course of HIV prevention work. Indeed, as the SEP was being implemented it became evident that when STD and HIV programs are integrated or work well together it can allow for a broader range of social and behavioral data to be shared, informing surveillance analyses and guiding health promotion activities.

Public health programs, including some STD programs, have commonly relied upon community mobilization and partnerships with other organizations, public and private to provide effective services [25, 26]. For the purposes of the 1999 SEP, *community involvement* and *organizational partnerships* was defined as *collaborative relationships with syphilis-affected communities and the health and social service organizations that represented and served them, in both the public and private sectors, and at the local, state, and national levels* [2]. By improving STD program relationships with affected communities and establishing new partnerships, it was reasoned that state and local STD programs would be better able to address a number of individual and social determinants of health such as long-standing community distrust and lack of access to support services [27].

Engaging affected communities and establishing organizational partnerships for syphilis prevention and control can: (1) facilitate effective communication, (2) restore, build, and maintain trust, (3) improve access to and utilization of services, (4) ensure the development of culturally competent [28] interventions, and (5) mobilize community capacity to support syphilis prevention, control, and elimination [29]. To support this commitment to partnership with affected communities and community organizations, as part of the 1999 SEP, CDC stipulated that at least one-third of syphilis elimination awarded funds be used in direct support of community organizations (COs) that represented and served the affected populations. As this was a significant departure for the Division of STD Prevention, there was both internal and external opposition to such a requirement. The objections were numerous: potential for creating a division among COs in the community; lack of COs in rural areas; lack of health department expertise in community development and experience in working with COs; and resistance to the concept of involving community advocates in health department actions and interventions (investigations) that are legally within the purview and responsibility of health departments.

Moreover, as the SEP was being implemented it also became evident that the concepts of community-involvement and organizational partnership were being defined differently based on the persons and institutions involved. Social science and health policy literature argues that such differences frequently have to do with degrees of and rights to power in the relationships [30, 31]. This kind of incongruence of understanding can result in competition, conflict, or apathy. As the editors noted in the book, *Nonprofits and Government: Collaboration and Conflict*, the relationships between government institutions and partners can be both symbiotic and adversarial with events or opportunities continually coloring or governing their interactions [32]. These kinds of outcomes were also seen in the implementation of the SEP [33]. Yet there were also a number of valuable successes as well, including: (1) expanded outreach health education and screening capacity; (2) consumer input into the development of interventions; (3) culturally competent health education messages, materials, and methods; (4) increased community-level STD knowledge and risk reduction skills; (5) private business support for public health events and activities; and (6) increased civic support for STD services [34–36].

Unfortunately the paucity of syphilis elimination funding ultimately led to a situation where the remaining set-aside of funds became insufficient to augment a CO staff position or even pay for the increased administrative burden of contracting and oversight of funding organizations external to the health department. Furthermore both states and cities have competing contracting rules, accounting policies, and other bureaucratic hurdles that mirror or even overshadow those of CDC. This combination of governmental bureaucracies frequently resulted in funding delays of over 1 year and often undermined the effectiveness of this strategy. After repeated requests from state and local health departments to cease this set-aside practice, CDC made the CO support completely optional in FY 2010, and in many cases it now no longer occurs.

Enhanced Health Promotion

Community engagement and partnerships with other agencies has been important to the quality of the strategy *Health Promotion* in the syphilis elimination effort. Tailored interventions, especially those aimed at achieving primary prevention must consider community characteristics such as cultural identity and experiences in the methods, messages, and messengers of these services [37]. Successful community participation in public health efforts is best accomplished when affected community members collaborate in equal partnership with health professionals to determine health goals, implement interventions, and evaluate outcomes [38]. In 2005, CDC released a *Syphilis Elimination Effort (SEE) Community Mobilization Toolkit* [39] to assist state and local health departments in building coalitions and alliances needed to mobilize specific target audiences for syphilis prevention and control. Target-specific materials in the kit provided resources to increase local awareness, visibility, and salience of the syphilis elimination program. The kit also provided guidance and tools for involving, mobilizing, and sustaining community efforts not only for syphilis but also for a variety of public health issues.

Expanded Clinical and Laboratory Services

Improving access to high quality syphilis diagnostic and treatment services remains a core strategy for syphilis elimination. In 1931, Thomas Parran wrote, "The whole health problem in the control of syphilis comprises just two elements: (1) Every infected person must take treatment, and (2) facilities for diagnosis and treatment must be made freely available [25].

As simplistic as we later learned this to be, in many parts of the country, providing this basic public health service to populations at risk continues to be challenging. Disinvestment in local STD programs, loss of experienced program staff, or deployment of clinic staff to support non-STD activities have all had a negative impact on local capacity to treat infected individuals or to contact and notify exposed sex partners.

As syphilis is increasingly diagnosed in the private sector, effective public-private partnerships with jointly agreed upon clinical management protocols are critical. The SEP specifically called for local STD programs to educate private practitioners in high incidence areas in order to make them aware of their public health roles and responsibilities in STD control (e.g., accurate disease staging, appropriate therapy, disease reporting, and patient participation in partner services) [40].

Good clinical services are dependent upon good diagnostic tests and laboratory services. However, the inability to cultivate *Treponema pallidum* on artificial media, problems related to the microscopic diagnosis of the disease and long periods of unapparent infection have resulted in serologic tests being the most frequent means of establishing a diagnosis of syphilis [41]. In addition, these tests are the only means whereby responses to therapy can be monitored. The urgent need to modernize syphilis diagnostic techniques with the development of both rapid treponemal and non-treponemal (point-of-care) tests became increasingly apparent as the SEP was being implemented. With better diagnostic tests, new opportunities for syphilis testing in traditional (e.g., clinical) as well as nontraditional sites (e.g., community centers, outreach, correctional facilities) could be facilitated. Testing for syphilis alongside with HIV has become more common, and studies in Europe have highlighted the potential benefits of utilizing oral fluid assays as an adjunct to outreach screening [42]; however, further research is needed to validate the performance of these new tools for syphilis. Partnerships between CDC, the Food and Drug Administration (FDA), and National Institutes of Health (NIH) are required to determine the most appropriate course of action to facilitate licensing of such tests in the United States.

Partner Services

A hallmark of syphilis prevention and control is, *Partner Services*. This program component is usually carried out by Disease Intervention Specialists (DIS) in local STD programs. The effective provision of *Partner Services* links together *Enhanced Surveillance*, and *Expanded Clinical and Laboratory Services* with *Enhanced Health Promotion*. It further affects the quality of *Community Involvement and Partnerships* because in many instances the program staff responsible for elements from these three strategies are the DIS staff. Although crucial to the delivery of quality syphilis prevention and control services, unfortunately, in many project areas, DIS staff have not been able to keep abreast of the rapidly changing social contexts for syphilis transmission or the demands of dealing with different patient groups and their expectations. For example, DIS staff in some STD programs continue to lack even regular access to computers, any standardized guidance on internet interventions, or the skills to intervene effectively with newly impacted populations such as men-who-have-sex-with-men (MSM).

In 2006 the SEP was updated, expanding the strategies included in the 1999 plan by building upon the lessons learned in the first 5 years of implementation, as well as the changing epidemiological context [33, 43, 44]. The updated SEP was also augmented by a technical monograph of theoretically driven and evidence-based discussion papers examining each of the expanded strategies. The monograph summarized the published literature relevant to each of the SEP's methods and included recommendations for implementation going forward. The monograph chapters also included guidance for how the respective strategies could be evaluated at the local and national levels [34].

A Multidisciplinary Plan with Interdisciplinary Methods

The SEP was clearly intended to support *multidisciplinary* approaches to the prevention and control of infectious syphilis, less explicit, however, was the need for *interdisciplinary* execution [45]. For many staff working in STD prevention and control at the time of the 1999 launch of the SEP, continuing through the implementation of the updated 2006 plan, and including those working at the federal level, the emphasis on the interdependence of the strategies demanded a profound expansion of the more traditional approaches to STD control. This need for multidisciplinary approaches implemented in interdisciplinary fashion proved to be a significant challenge for the syphilis elimination effort.

Dealing with the Diversity of the US Syphilis Epidemic

Diverse Populations

The populations experiencing higher rates of syphilis have become more diverse since the launch of the SEP in 1999. In the fall of 1999 the infectious syphilis epidemic was mainly concentrated in the southeastern United States among disadvantaged African American heterosexual populations [46]. The rate of P&S syphilis reported in African-Americans was at that time 30 times greater than the rate reported in whites. More traditional STD prevention and control methods, that focused on increasing access to and utilization of testing and treatment services, by engaging affected communities and relevant health and social service providers, proved highly effective at reducing the epidemic and thereby the disparities in burden. For 2009, compared with whites, the overall 2009 rate for blacks was only nine times higher.

By the mid-2000s, as STD programs were achieving important successes with the heterosexual epidemic, there began to be a substantial resurgence of P&S syphilis among MSM, and the syphilis rates increased significantly for MSM across all racial and ethnic groups. This diversity in the affected populations continues to demand greater program flexibility to effectively respond. Further complicating efforts, STD programs in a number of communities are forced to address infectious syphilis epidemics that are at different epidemiological phases among different populations [47].

Because the US epidemic of infectious syphilis disproportionately affects disadvantaged ethnic minority communities and men who have sex with men (MSM), the persons who are most at risk for the disease are also often burdened by other negative determinants of health (e.g., poverty, homelessness, substance abuse). These determinants can not only impact access to STD health care but also adversely affect STD health-care-seeking.

Men Who Have Sex with Men

At the inception of the 1999 syphilis elimination campaign, the P&S syphilis rates among MSM were low. Studies suggest that perhaps one third to one half of the decline in P&S syphilis rates between 1990 and 1995 was attributed to AIDS mortality among this population [48]. By the time the SEP was updated in 2006, however, the

United States was experiencing a resurgence of all STDs, particularly syphilis, among MSM [49]. As early as 2004, more than 60% of P&S cases were estimated to have occurred in MSM. In 2009, the rate of reported P&S syphilis among men (7.8 cases per 100,000 males) was 5.6 times higher than the rate among women (1.4 cases per 100,000 females). In 2009, 62% of P&S syphilis cases, in the 44 states and the District of Columbia that provided information about the gender of the sex partners, occurred among MSM. With continuing declines in the heterosexual rates of P&S syphilis, many STD programs across the United States shifted their focus to the reemerging epidemics among MSM. Early on the social marketing and outreach efforts that addressed syphilis outbreaks were often tailored more to predominantly white gay men or MSM in general. Interventions were frequently conducted in such settings as gay bars and bathhouses, and focused significantly on the role of Internet in sexual risk-taking and STD prevention [50].

However, already in 2004 the rate of P&S syphilis among blacks was once again increasing markedly. The increase seen in blacks in 2004 was the first since 1993, and the disparity between black and white rates of P&S syphilis also increased. In 2004, the P&S rate among blacks was 5.6 times higher than that among whites [51] and by 2009, the P&S rate among black men was eight times higher than that among white men [12]. During the time period 2005–2009, among black men 15–19 years old, the P&S rates increased 167%, and rates among black men 20–24 years old increased 212% (Fig. 18.2).

To promote more evidence-based approaches to syphilis elimination, beginning in FY 2008, STD programs were required to develop and submit evidence-based action plans (EBAPs) for each of their syphilis elimination activities. A review of the 2009 syphilis elimination EBAPs showed that only about 10% of the then current activities specifically targeted black MSM. Recognizing the need to better target MSM of color, and black MSM in particular, CDC began conducting formative studies focusing specifically on black MSM to provide more culturally competent sexual health interventions.

Heterosexuals

While still not at the levels seen in the early 1990s, the 52% rate of infectious syphilis among blacks in general has continued to exceed the rates seen for all other ethnic groups. In addition to the rising rates among black men, the P&S syphilis rate among black women now stands at more than 20 times higher than the rate among white women (Fig. 18.3). With this constant threat of reemergence of infectious syphilis among heterosexuals comes the potential risk for a reemergence of congenital syphilis in the United States. Between 2008 and 2009 the rate of congenital syphilis decreased during 2008–2009 (from 10.4 to 10.0 cases per 100,000 live births), but it is important to note that this is still higher than the rate achieved in 2005 when the rate reached a low point of 8.2 cases per 100,000 live births.

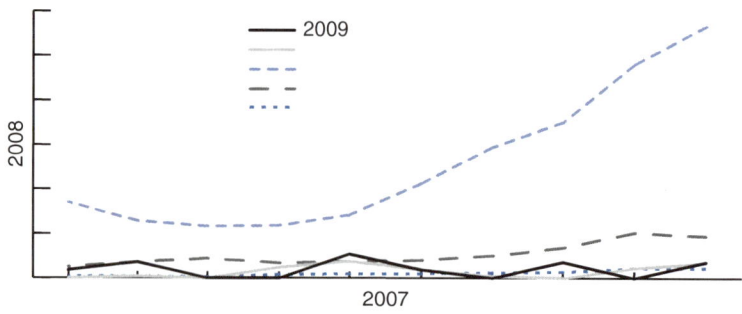

Fig. 18.2 P &S Rates in Males 15–19 by Race/Ethnicity

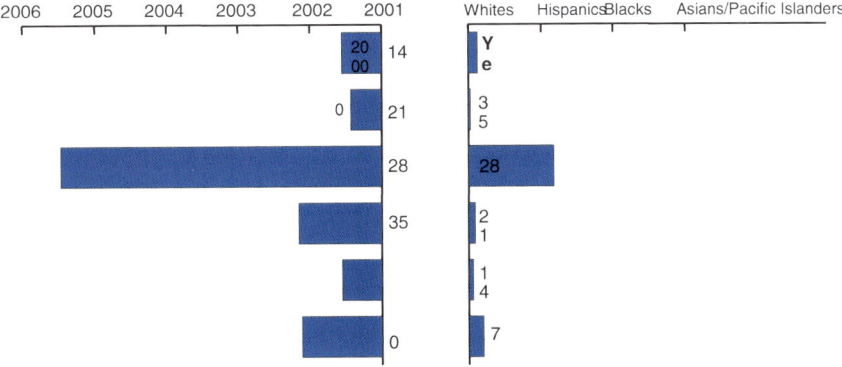

Fig. 18.3   2009 P&S Rates by Race/Ethnicity and Gender

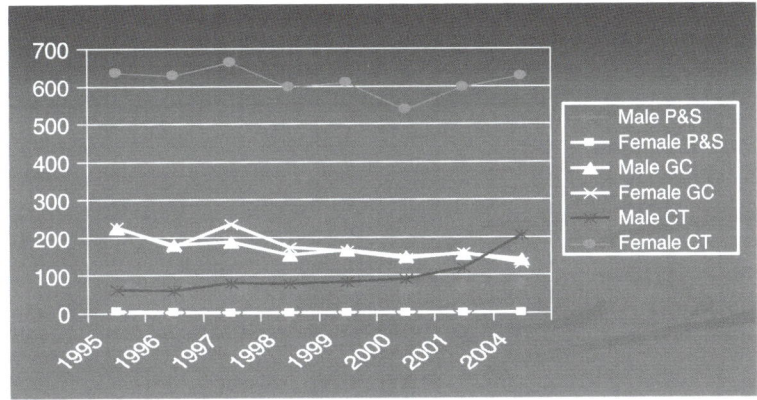

Fig. 18.4   P&S Syphilis, Gonorrhea, Chlamydia Rates by Sex, New York City

Although most cases of congenital syphilis occur among infants whose mothers have had some prenatal care, late or limited prenatal care has been associated with congenital syphilis. Failure of health care providers to adhere to maternal syphilis screening recommendations also continues to contribute to the occurrence of congenital syphilis [52]. STDs programs around the country are expected to diligently monitor heterosexual epidemics, particularly among disadvantaged populations, and respond effectively to outbreaks as they occur.

Epidemic Phases and Interventions

An outbreak response to syphilis looks very different from the sustained initiative often needed to address endemic disease. STD programs involved in the syphilis elimination effort have been challenged to implement multiple population-specific interventions in the context of evolving and changing syphilis epidemics. Phases for sexually transmitted infections can vary substantially. The reported bacterial STDs as an example illustrate the complexity facing STD prevention and control programs. In Fig. 18.4 below depicting STDs in New York City, syphilis is in an endemic phase, gonorrhea is in a declining phase, and Chlamydia in a hyper-endemic phase, with the male Chlamydia epidemic in a growth phase. Different interventions are required for different phases of an epidemic.

A closer examination of the data from New York City in this case shows that for P&S syphilis there was a steep increase among men, which is

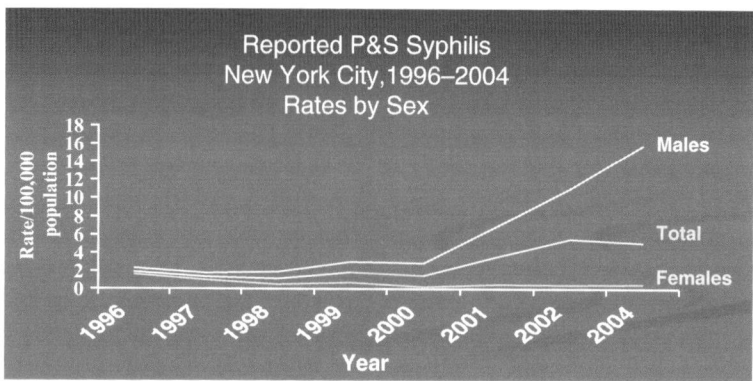

Fig. 18.5 P&S Syphilis Rates by Sex, New York City

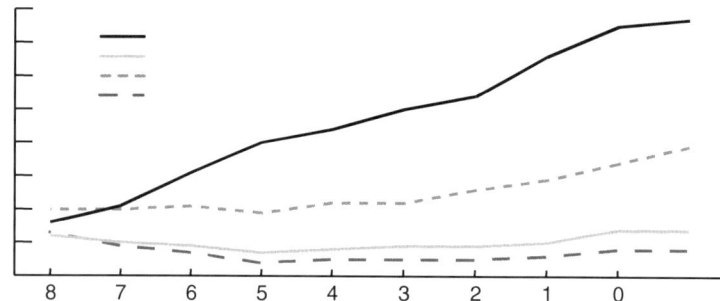

Fig. 18.6 P&S Syphilis STD Clinic vs. Non-STD Clinic Reporting Source

almost imperceptible when looking at rates in the aggregate (Fig. 18.5). In this scenario, P&S syphilis rates among men are in a completely different epidemic phase than that for women, highlighting the need for tailored population-specific interventions. Programmatic nimbleness has heretofore not been the strongest suit of state and local programs or of the CDC when it comes to STD control.

Differing Communities

In 1998 national surveillance data showed that only 28 (0.9%) of 3115 US counties accounted for 50% of P&S syphilis cases, and were disproportionately in the southern part of the country (19 of 28 counties) [53]. By 1999, 80% of US counties reported P&S syphilis rates equal to or less than the Healthy People 2010 objective of 0.2 cases per 100,000 persons [54]. In 2009, the

13 states with the highest rates of P&S syphilis accounted for 75% of all US cases, and once again 10 of these 13 states were in the South. However, different from previous syphilis epidemics, the current US infectious syphilis epidemic occurs mainly in urban settings, whatever the region of the country affected. For example, in 2009, more than 40% of P&S cases were reported from urban areas such as Los Angeles County, California and Harris County (Houston), Texas, Cook County (Chicago), Illinois, and Fulton County (Atlanta), Georgia [55].

The current epidemic of P&S syphilis necessitates a combination of interventions, and increasingly involves both public and private sectors, as more persons seek STD services in facilities other than the conventional local health department STD clinic (Fig. 18.6).

The social context of American communities (e.g., demographics, socioeconomic conditions, sociopolitical structures) can impact both epidemiological factors as well as individual behaviors, affecting the transmission of STDs, including syphilis [56].

"Robbing Peter to Pay Paul"

For both MSM and heterosexual populations, syphilis elimination interventions require approaches that take into account multiple factors at a variety of levels, including: individual, interpersonal, community, and institutional levels. To be most effective prevention and control efforts have to be holistic and operational on many fronts [57, 58]. Although both the 1999 and 2006 plans called for more population-specific tailored approaches, many state and local programs were largely unable to address the evolving and changing epidemics in different populations and communities, particularly as already limited resources continued to dwindle.

Through the cooperative agreement, *Comprehensive STD Prevention Systems* (CSPS), CDC provides fiscal support for STD prevention and control to state and city project areas [59]. Funds for syphilis elimination are awarded through this funding mechanism. Syphilis elimination funds are intended to support infrastructure, interventions, evaluation, research, community outreach, and clinical and laboratory services to project areas with high syphilis morbidity.

Following a series of allocation formulas based on recent morbidity trends, in 2008 CDC, after consultation with state and local health departments, instituted a funding formula based on 2-year averages of P&S morbidity burden. By this formula a high morbidity area (HMA) is defined as a project area that has a minimum of 100 P&S syphilis cases or a P&S case rate greater than 2.2/100,000 population with a minimum of 60 P&S cases. Project areas that have graduate from HMA-status continue to receive supplemental syphilis elimination funding for 2 years after graduating from the HMA-status, because they are considered to be project areas at significant risk for syphilis reemergence [60]. Although the new formula provides a more equitable distribution of fiscal resources based on

disease burden, at least initially it also translated into significant funding losses for some project areas and led in some instances charges of *Brown's Law* [61]. However, the new formula has brought valuable resources to struggling project areas commensurate with their disease burden and better enabled CDC to redirect funds more quickly as P&S cases fluctuate. In an era of relatively flat funding for STD prevention and control, this more consistent distribution is an imperative.

Arguably the concept of the STD program *project area* complicates the equitable disbursement of syphilis elimination funds. While for most of the United States, a *project area* is identified as a state, there are a number of cities that are also designated as independent STD program project areas. Like the state project areas, city project areas not only receive direct funding from CDC for syphilis elimination activities, but they also receive separate general STD funding and direct assistance (federal staff) support. For example, in FY2007, the *state* of Texas and the *city* of Chicago both received approximately $1 million each in syphilis elimination funds. The *state* of Illinois also received syphilis elimination funds in the amount of just under $400,000. As a result, in FY2007, for Texas the syphilis elimination funds investment per case was approximately $1000 per P&S case, while for Chicago the investment was about $2500 per case. For the *state* of Illinois, the investment was closer to the national mean of $3300 per case (Fig. 18.7). The 2008 funding formula leveled the allocation of financial resources for syphilis elimination but did not address the provision of other federal STD resources in general.

Early in the 1990s, state and local STD programs began suffering from an erosion of federal, state and local resources both in funding and staffing. Not only did federal fiscal funding begin to decline, but also federal assignees that once supplied significant staffing resources to local areas were essentially halved between 1990 and 1999. Historically federal staff have significantly bolstered local efforts, and as their numbers have diminished, a critical source of STD program staffing has been lost. During this same time period state, city and county governments also

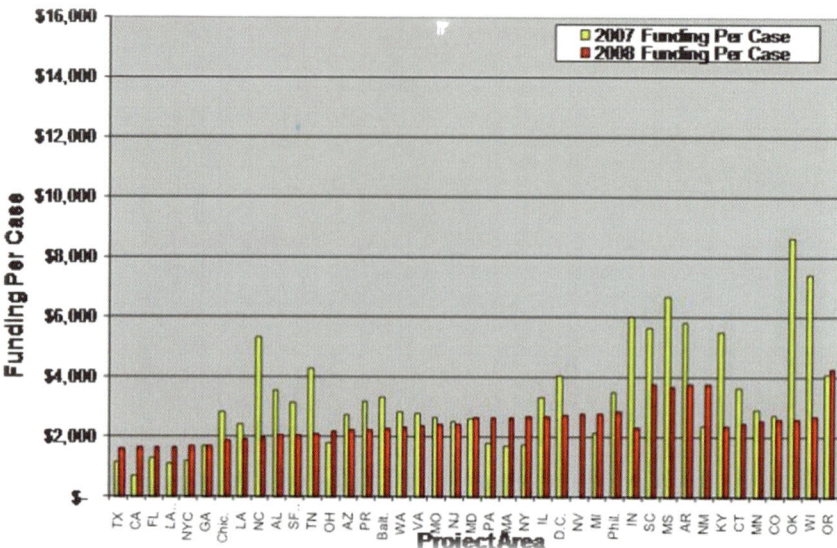

Fig. 18.7   Syphilis Elimination Funding Per Case 2007 & 2008

began to institute various fiscal restraints, including such things as hiring freezes, so that even
when the syphilis elimination funding formula
brought new resources to HMAs, many of the
local programs were still unable to hire critical
staff. With the inability to hire new personnel
many core program infrastructure needs have
gone unaddressed. Such things as the purchasing
and upgrading of computer and other equipment,
facility maintenance, and staff training in evaluation, epidemiology, and new interventions have
been sacrificed. The net effect to state and local
programs has been a diminished capacity to
incorporate new technologies and interventions
and to hire staff with broader skills to effectively
implement the strategies of the SEP.

In area after area, the reduction of both fiscal
and personnel resources has meant that scarce
resources are moved away from one group in
order to respond to higher rates of syphilis rates
in another. Indeed the *National Campaign to
Eliminate Syphilis* was never funded at the level
initially requested in the 1998 *Report to Congress*
[62], a level that might have better supported
innovation and adaptation. CDC continues to
provide technical assistance and support, however, although these committed efforts have usually ensured effective training and epidemiological

analyses, as well as some limited program
staffing, such efforts have proven insufficient for
building vital long-term, sustainable program
infrastructure. Inevitably the federal deployments
have to end.

In the first year of the required evidence-based
action plans, 170 EBAPs addressed the following
interventions: community outreach (~35%), partner notification (~15%), screening (~35%), provider education initiatives (~6%) and other (~6%)
activities, targeting MSM, black, correctional,
and Hispanic populations. Ultimately, however,
faced with complex challenges and diminished
resources, many state and local programs returned
to more traditional interventions, such as partner
services and outreach screening in various community-based settings, even as performance indices for these interventions disappointed, and a
growing body of literature was calling for more
comprehensive approaches.

Although the SEP was written to enable
adaptability for local jurisdictions with high
syphilis morbidity to tailor their programmatic
efforts to meet the unique challenges encountered in their respective communities, the plan
itself was in many cases also adversely affected
by policies, bureaucracies, and individual
behaviors.

Determinants of Health and Syphilis Disparities

A number of factors contribute to a person's current state of health. They may be biological, socioeconomic, psychosocial, behavioral, or social in nature. Many diseases and conditions cluster in socially and economically vulnerable populations, and disparities in diseases may occur by gender, race/ethnicity, education, income, disability, geographic location, and sexual orientation. Social determinants of health such as poverty, inadequate access to health care, lack of education, stigma, and racism and other forms of social discrimination are often associated with disparities in health, and in particular sexual health [63].

At the end of 2010, the highest reported infectious syphilis rates were in MSM. The reasons for the increases are complex. With the availability and widespread use of highly active antiretroviral therapy (HAART) for HIV infection, greater numbers of HIV-positive persons are living healthier lives free from the ravages of AIDS. An entire generation of young MSM also have never experienced their contemporaries dying in large numbers, so sex does not seem so dangerous anymore. The resurgence of syphilis in MSM seen early in the current decade is in part attributable to a resurgence of high-risk sexual behaviors (e.g., high rates of new sex partner acquisition and partner change rates, unprotected penetrative sex) across the United States [64]. However, other determinants (e.g., homophobia and racial discrimination) also impact the spread of syphilis in many MSM networks [65, 66]. Similarly, recurring outbreaks of infectious syphilis among black heterosexual populations can also be attributed to individual risk taking behavior (e.g., prostitution, and high rates of new partner acquisition particularly among heterosexual men), as well as community-level and structural-level factors such as cultural differences, language barriers, impediments to healthcare seeking, and concerns about confidentiality or discrimination.

Individual Level Factors

For the most part STD program services are designed to address the individual-level factors for STD transmission. STD prevention program professionals are trained to emphasize testing, treatment, and partner services. Prevention for STDs, including syphilis prevention, is primarily achieved through disease interruption which relies on testing and treatment (secondary prevention), and risk reduction counseling which seeks to get individuals to reduce their sexual risk behavior (primary prevention) [67]. While these individual-level interventions do work for some, for many others these interventions have fallen short as evidenced by the numbers of persons with repeat sexually transmitted infections [68, 69]. Moreover few STD programs are equipped to provide substance abuse counseling although recreational drug use (e.g., crystal-methamphetamine, crack cocaine), as well as alcohol use, both of which have been linked to risky sexual behavior in both MSM and heterosexual populations [70]. Additionally, mental stress associated with social discrimination (e.g., racism, classism, and homophobia) and social isolation has been found to be associated with increased sexual risktaking. Finally for both MSM and heterosexual populations studies suggest that "safer sex fatigue" [71] is reducing the effectiveness of prevention messages.

Community and Structural Level Factors

In the May 1998 the CDC convened a consultants' meeting to develop the components of action plan for the campaign to eliminate syphilis from the United States. A central theme that emerged from this meeting was the understanding of infectious syphilis in the United States as a *social disease,* as the 1998 meeting report states:

> In otherwise healthy individuals and communities, syphilis is a disease that is easily diagnosed and treated, and its transmission is easily interrupted. Across the work groups, the consultants

recommended that the elimination of syphilis requires an identification and examination of the impact of social factors in the persistence of syphilis. The current US syphilis epidemic largely affects some of the country's most disadvantaged and distressed individuals and communities, persons that are also besieged by a number of other detrimental conditions, such as: poverty, high unemployment, and inadequate educational and health care resources. Many of these same individuals and communities are further negatively impacted by racism and discrimination based on their social and economic status, factors that may indeed influence the availability, accessibility and acceptability of current STD prevention and treatment services [72].

It is important to note that these recommendations were developed during comparatively better economic times than today. For example, a central socio-economic determinant relevant to the prevention and control of syphilis is poverty, which often leads to inadequate income and impoverished living conditions, compelling some individuals to exchange sex for money, food, housing, and drugs [73, 74]. In May 2011, while the overall seasonally adjusted unemployment rate in the United States was at 9%, the rate for black Americans was approximately 16%. For black Americans age 16–19 years the unemployment rate was at 40.7% [75]. Inadequate income also negatively can also affect access to health care resulting in delayed or no health-care-seeking. In a number of instances evidence suggests that even if a disadvantaged person does seek health care, the provider may not be equipped to deliver quality STD health care. In many rural areas, with large geographical distances, transportation for economically disadvantaged persons is a significant barrier to accessing health care, whether they are MSM or heterosexual. Moreover in rural settings where social networks can be small, for many STD patients there are significant concerns about confidentiality.

In urban areas, social venues such as bars, bath-houses, and large social gatherings commonly referred to as "circuit parties" have been linked to increased sexual risk behavior and syphilis transmission, particularly among MSM populations [76]. These links can cross multiple jurisdictions when more affluent members of at-risk populations have the means to travel easily [77].

As a result, infectious syphilis among participants at an urban gathering in the Northeast can also fuel a syphilis outbreak in the Midwest [78]. The explosive use of the internet has promoted both the meeting of sexual partners and broadly advertised social venues, so that electronically arranged private sexual liaisons have become increasingly common for MSM as well as heterosexuals [79]. Sexual encounters can now be arranged anonymously over the internet, thus bringing a new definition and dynamic to social networks.

Yet while the internet was broadening sexual networks for many, for African Americans, data suggests that racial and ethnic discrimination has continued to keep social and sexual networks limited, thereby concentrating opportunities for transmission of infection [80]. For example, as the SEP was underway, it became increasingly clear that in many African American communities the high incarceration rates of African American men, primarily due to drug law enforcement and mandatory sentencing, was disrupting the social ecology of these communities. Increasingly African American women, many of whom have only one sexual partner, knowingly enter into relationships with men who have many more [56, 81]. Over the course of the SEP implementation, it became clear that community and societal characteristics often provide fertile contexts for the reseeding and resurgence of infectious syphilis in affected populations; and traditional individual-level approaches (e.g., partner services, risk reduction counseling) needed to be modified to more effectively respond to these complex environments.

To be successful, a syphilis elimination campaign, like other efforts to reduce health disparities for communities and populations, demands more comprehensive approaches that take into account the balance between individual responsibility (e.g., sexual behavior) and broader social factors (e.g., access to quality STD services). Upstream factors such as employment, housing and quality of living environments, social relationships, and education that are critical to the health of populations. Social determinants have been defined as "the circumstances, in which people are born, grow up, live, work and age, and the systems put in place to deal with illness, circumstances that are in turn shaped by a wider set of forces: economics, social policies, and politics" [82]. As comprehensive as the 1999 and updated 2006 syphilis elimination plans were in recognizing the impact of a variety of determinants of health, state and local health department STD program partners were in many cases not sufficiently prepared for or resourced to effectively address most of these important determinants.

Implications of Infectious Diseases in the Elimination of Health Disparities

Disrupting the cycle of an infectious disease, such as syphilis, requires the incorporation of organism-specific interventions in addition to addressing the individual and social determinants of health. Depending on the life cycle of the organism, transmission of disease can happen rapidly with profound affects to individual and community health. Without a vaccine to offer lifetime immunity, if conditions remain the same an individual may likely experience repeat infections [83]. Chronic disease surveillance and epidemiological analysis generally focus on monitoring trends over a long period of time (6 months- 1 year) but such an approach usually not sufficient for infectious diseases. Interrupting disease transmission requires a more urgent approach with rapid data assessment leading to rapid response. STD program bureaucracies, whether they be at the local, state, or federal level are often severely challenged to move that quickly. Contracts have to be let. Staff have to be trained and deployed. Communities have to be mobilized. And if the epidemic moves to another population that is substantially different then the response process usually has to begin again when the resources are redirected.

Furthermore, the factors surrounding the transmission of an STD such as syphilis are often highly stigmatized (e.g., sex for drugs or survival, prostitution, bath houses,) and many of the groups affected are also often marginalized, significantly complicating reaching at-risk populations with health promotion interventions. The stigma associated with all STDs often makes reluctant participants of those who are affected and infected and can mean little community- or peer-support for healthier lifestyle choices and actions. Sexual partnerships and networks may be established and dissolved unpredictably and in relatively short time periods.

Furthermore, despite efforts on the part of many local STD programs, attempts to mobilize communities and groups around syphilis also proved to be challenging in the context of an ongoing HIV epidemic, and in the midst of other larger STD epidemics like chlamydia, gonorrhea, and even genital herpes. Echoing the words of Dr. Jeffery Koplan, too much of the American public syphilis was and remains a disease of a past century. Key stakeholders did not embrace the more *bug-specific* focus of syphilis elimination when they considered the breadth of threat to the wellness of their respective communities. A combination of these factors often made the kind of sustained enthusiasm needed to implement syphilis elimination community-level interventions difficult [84].

Lessons Learned from the Syphilis Elimination Campaign

Though we have learned much during this latest effort to eliminate syphilis from the United States, five overarching lessons stand out:

Access to Care Is Essential

Access to effective clinical care is paramount for early diagnosis, treatment, and patient counseling for syphilis. In 2002 researchers reported that US physicians were screening for STDs at levels well below recommended guidelines, and that case reporting was also below the level legally mandated [85]. Under-screening contributes to missed opportunities for diagnosis while under reporting, especially by private providers, contributes to a misrepresentation of the burden of disease. This lack of screening and subsequent treatment impeded the effectiveness of the syphilis elimination effort.

Financial, structural, personal, and interpersonal barriers can also limit access to STD health care services. Relevant to syphilis prevention and control are such structural barriers as the lack of health care facilities, the lack of trained and motivated health care providers that provide STD services; and even long wait times. For example, findings from the clinical services reviews done as part of the comprehensive *Syphilis Elimination Program Assessments* revealed that local STD programs experienced challenges with patient scheduling/turn-aways, maintaining adequate staff coverage to provide care, and timely reporting of lab results [86]. Individual level barriers to accessing health care may include perception of risk, personal shame, and substance abuse which can impede healthier decision-making. Although recent reforms to the US health care system promise to increase the availability of services to more persons at risk for syphilis and other STDs, there still remains the question of acceptability for persons who may feel socially threatened in health-care settings, or who may be subject to less than quality health care delivery.

As syphilis is increasingly diagnosed in the private sector, especially among MSM, more effective public-private partnerships with jointly agreed upon clinical management protocols are needed. Private practitioners also have a public health role and responsibility in STD control. However, private practice incentives such as reimbursement structures are lacking, and many private providers also are reluctant to report cases and involve public health departments in the interview of patients and sex partners fearing a negative client reaction to the process.

Expanded Partnerships are Critical

In addition to the lessons learned (and relearned) about working with private providers, was the lesson that partnership-building very often had to begin within the local health department, within the state health department, and even within the CDC. The separation of STD and HIV programs limits routine integration of prevention interventions. Although both programs are dedicated to the promotion of sexual health, their missions sometimes compete and their methods sometimes conflict. For example, interventions to expand HIV testing uptake in order to reduce undiagnosed prevalent HIV infections did not always permit opportunities for concomitant syphilis testing, even though the prevention of syphilis strengthens HIV prevention. There continues to be an urgent need to modernize syphilis diagnostic techniques with the development of both rapid treponemal and non-treponemal (point-of-care) tests, as such a development could increase opportunities to combine syphilis testing with HIV testing especially for population sub-groups at risk for both infections.

To a large extent, STD, HIV, and Hepatitis epidemics overlap in heterosexual and MSM populations. However, prevention messages primarily have remained categorically targeted. This means that individuals and communities are often bombarded with conflicting information given that some diseases are curable, others are treatable but not curable, and others can be prevented with a vaccine. At the core, however, prevention is often similar (e.g., use of condoms, limiting number of sex partners, knowing infection status). Outreach workers who deliver prevention services often receive training or have expertise in only one disease but not in others, yet all are attempting to reach the same at risk populations. Lessons learned from the syphilis elimination effort, particularly in this economically challenging era, instruct that it is more efficient and effective for all prevention workers be able to provide comprehensive information, services, and referrals in the best interest of promoting health and preventing disease.

Furthermore new conceptual frameworks like *health equity* and s*exual health* require the engagement of new partners to better incorporate and improve STD prevention with community wellness. As an example, given the link between drug use and syphilis risk, drug treatment is an important component and most syphilis elimination STD programs did not provide or support access drug treatment services. To support syphilis prevention and control, STD programs, at all levels, will need to reach out to other providers in a manner that respects the commitment and expertise of these different providers. It was learned on multiple occasions that expecting other partners to adopt the syphilis elimination agenda without the same in return from STD programs did not build critical bridges for better health. In too many instances partnering institutions have been asked and expected to take on additional syphilis prevention and control tasks without either authority over these tasks or compensation.

Diverse Epidemics Require Different Approaches

As the trajectory of the infectious syphilis epidemic has changed, state, local, and federal governmental bureaucracies have struggled to move quickly enough to mount the most effective responses. Programs are generally complex and the skill sets of can vary greatly across program activities. Such variation can mean substantial challenges for implementing new approaches quickly. Too many times during the syphilis elimination effort the delay between the detection of a new syphilis outbreak and the execution of control efforts allowed for the outbreak to worsen. Moreover, traditional methods of case finding such as increased screening in correctional settings, or outreach screening in venues such as bathhouses often proved to be of little disease-detection value [87]. Similarly, partner services, touring of venues, and clustering were often equally ineffective [88]. Although syphilis epidemics among MSM have occurred in the past, the context and circumstances surrounding this shift in the epidemic have been very different. As a result, program areas increasingly need individuals skilled in use of the internet and other computer-based interventions, those experienced and skilled in rapid ethnographic assessment and behavioral/social data analysis, and those experienced in working with private-sector HIV care providers and the integration of HIV and STD interventions. However, state, local, or CDC field staff generally do not have these skill sets.

Consequently many state and local program areas have had to scramble to develop or seek such expertise, as they have tried to quickly broaden their program capacity and partnerships.

In 2008, an evaluation of the RRT and general technical assistance support to the project areas was conducted and respondents recommended several changes to how CDC technical assistance is provided going forward [89]. Results of the evaluation favor movement away from the *RRT model*, which in the past provided primarily disease intervention specialist support, and towards a centrally coordinated, multidisciplinary approach. Although the RRT seems to have initially provided much needed person-power and direct service skill early on, the skills increasingly needed by local areas have shifted to include more analysis, planning, and capacity-building. Although the Syphilis Elimination Implementation and Monitoring Group was established in 2005 to facilitate this broader type of assistance, internal Division of STD Prevention differences in perspective and competing priorities impeded access to utilization of this resource.

It Takes more than Money

Although the syphilis elimination effort was never funded at the level originally requested in the 1998 Report to Congress, [62] it became apparent that a multidisciplinary and interdisciplinary approach requires more than financial resources. Financial resources do not change attitudes or efforts to address the multiplicity of factors that drive STD epidemics. Often times more resources actually may inadvertently promote more silos as personnel given the opportunity to work separately readily do so. For example, in the syphilis elimination effort, even in the context of relatively small Program Assessment teams, federal staff worked separately based on disciplines and experience and sometimes competed with each other for the number of program recommendations included in the assessment reports. State and local STD programs would have also benefitted from integrated research agendas that integrating and linked surveillance data with program relevant research questions. Although adequate fiscal resources are certainly necessary to support these kinds of innovations, as the syphilis elimination campaign was implemented it was soon learned that money alone could not ensure an integrated approach. All too often state and local programs simply used the designated funds to support more traditional approaches that did not improve case detection and treatment or prevention.

Effective Program Evaluation Is Challenging but Critical

Indeed the syphilis elimination effort would have benefitted from a more robust and rigorous commitment to program evaluation and program improvement. In an era of limited and shifting resources, which is likely to continue into the future, it has become all the more critical to evaluate the effectiveness of methods and interventions to ensure the best use of ever shrinking dollars. Despite CDC's attempts to assess syphilis elimination program effectiveness by using performance measures [90], structured SE Program Assessments [91], and ultimately the SE Evidence-based Action Plans [92], program evaluation of the syphilis elimination effort has been less than effective. First and foremost program evaluation can be an expensive undertaking, both in dollars and personnel, and many STD programs remain desperate to put what resources they have into direct services, not evaluation. This tension also exists at the federal level. Second, the very diversity of the syphilis HMAs, the affected populations, and the phases of the infectious syphilis epidemic has made a national evaluation impractical, although the 2006 updated plan actually included a comprehensive logic model based on common program elements for syphilis prevention and control. Further, in those instances when state and local programs did undertake their own assessments of program methods and interventions, many remained unwilling to forgo traditional approaches even in the face of unsuccessful outcomes.

Particularly as STD programs are asked to adapt to and even adopt new and unfamiliar frameworks (e.g., sexual health, and social determinants of health) that are arguably grounded in more complex concepts, the need for program evaluation at the structural, community, and individual level only increases. As was learned in the implementation of the SEP, the willingness to conduct program evaluation, accept the outcomes, and adjust program strategies is likely to be challenging for a number of programs, whether they be at the local, state, or federal level.

Conclusions

In 1998 there were just under 7,000 cases of P&S syphilis reported to CDC, and at that time this represented the lowest number of infectious syphilis cases reported since 1958 [93]. This optimistic trend continued in 1999, when 6,657 cases of P&S syphilis were reported to CDC, this new total was now the lowest yearly number of cases reported since 1957 [54]. Based on these syphilis-specific data the elimination of infectious syphilis looked not only plausible but promising. But perhaps these data were not taken in proper context.

Because also in 1998, gonorrhea case reporting data was indicating a reversal in the annual decreases that had been observed in the years preceding. Between 1997 and 1998, the gonorrhea rates for 15- to 19-year-old adolescents had increased from 521.6 per 100,000 to 560.6, and for 20- to 24-year-old young adults increased from 548.4 to 609.6. Except for adults 65 and older, the rates for the other age groups also increased between 1997 and 1998. During 1998, 607,602 chlamydial infections were reported to CDC, exceeding the reported cases of gonorrhea which had reached a total of 355,642 [93]. By 1999, 77% of the now 360,000 reported cases of gonorrhea was among black Americans for a black–white ratio 30:1 [54]. While syphilis elimination might have been plausible, and even promising, arguably the health and wellness of many Americans would have remained significantly deficient.

In retrospect it was perhaps idealistic to launch a campaign to eliminate an infectious disease that (1) has survived with humankind for centuries, (2) is transmitted by intimate interpersonal behavior, and (3) has no vaccine so that repeated infections can occur. As we have seen over time the persistence of infectious syphilis is facilitated by a range of individual, community, and structural determinants over which many of the most affected populations, and even the providers that seek to serve them, may have little to no control.

And yet the campaign to eliminate syphilis from the United States experienced some successes, particularly in the initially targeted populations, heterosexual black Americans. Between 1999 and 2005 there was a 95% reduction in P&S syphilis in women, and a 92% reduction in congenital syphilis. Disparities were reduced. The black–white rate ratio went from 28.6:1 to 5.4:1. Unfortunately these important successes ultimately stalled and have since eroded. In 2009, still more than 50% of all P&S syphilis cases reported to CDC were among black Americans. Compared to white Americans, the overall 2009 rate for black Americans was back up to 9.1 times higher. For some black Americans, particularly black men 15–19 years old, the P&S rates in 2009 increased 167%.

As the national plan to eliminate syphilis from United States was implemented, STD programs were reminded that human sexual behavior is complex and dynamic, involving multiple influences including individual, interpersonal, community, and structural factors. As has been illustrated by Thomas Frieden's *Health Impact Pyramid,* individual level interventions, the kinds most commonly implemented in the syphilis elimination effort, like testing and treatment, and risk reduction counseling, are often expensive and likely to have limited effect at the population level [94].

Addressing a broader array of determinants of sexual health is arguably a more effective strategy for reducing health disparities; however, these concepts are much easier to describe than to implement. If such concepts are not fully operationalized and the determinants of health framework is not generally embraced, and if funding processes are not in place to support the structure this strategy won't work. Plans have to be executed, and as Robert Burns famously wrote, even the best ones can and often do go awry.

In summary, it would seem that epidemics evolve faster than agencies, programs, or research can address them. Bureaucracies are not as adaptable as the organisms they seek to prevent or eliminate. Many of the processes are too cumbersome to mobilize resources or people quickly. Elimination of a non-vaccine preventable disease has never been accomplished, and until such time as a vaccine is available for syphilis, it remains to be seen if elimination of this infection is possible. However, that doesn't mean that it hasn't been important to attempt such a campaign once again, for the effort has taught us how truly complex and interrelated are the human, social, and biological determinants that continue to make STD prevention such a challenge. Perhaps syphilis is not so much a *natural wonder* as it is just a very *opportunistic* infection. As corpas individual behaviors combine with community environments, and are facilitated by social conditions, then this simple organism will not only persist but in too many instances thrive.

References

1. Wasserheit, JN. A barometer of community health. Sex Transm Diseases, 2000.
2. Centers for Disease Control and Prevention. The national plan to eliminate syphilis from the United States. Atlanta, Georgia: U.S. Department of Health and Human Services, CDC, National Center for HIV, STD, and TB Prevention, 1999: 1–84.
3. Nakashima AK, Rolfs R, Flock M, Kilmarx P, Greenspan J. Epidemiology of Syphilis in the United States, 1941–1993. Sex Transm Dis. 1996;23(1): 16–23.
4. Centers for Disease Control and Prevention. Sexually Transmitted Disease Surveillance 2009. Atlanta: U.S. Department of Health and Human Services; 2010. www.cdc.gov/std/stats.
5. Baumgartner L. Syphilis eradication: a plan for action now. In: Venereal Diseases Branch, (ed.), Proceedings of the World Forum on Syphilis and Other Treponematoses. Washington, D.C.: Public Health Service; 1964:26–32.
6. Cates Jr W, Rothenberg RB, Blount JH. Syphilis control. The historic context and epidemiologic basis for interrupting sexual transmission of Treponema pallidum. Sex Transm Dis. 1996;23(1):68–75.

7. Centers for Disease Control and Prevention. Principles of Disease Elimination and Eradication. Morbidity and mortality weekly report, December 31, 1999/48(SU01); 23–7.

8. Brown, WJ. A plan for the eradication of syphilis. Read before the section on preventive medicine. Southern Medical Association, Fifty-Sixth Annual Meeting. Miami Beach, FL. November 1962.

9. Koplan J. Syphilis elimination: history in the making-opening remarks. Sex Transm Dis. 2000;27(2):63–5.

10. Further information available from the Office of Management and Budget. Executive Office of the President website at http://www.whitehouse.gov/omb/mgmt-gpra/gplaw2m.html. Last accessed on October 2005.

11. MMWR. June 26, 1998/47(24);493–497. Primary and Secondary Syphilis—United States, 1997.

12. Centers for Disease Control and Prevention. *Sexually Transmitted Disease Surveillance 2009 Supplement, Syphilis Surveillance Report*. Atlanta, GA: U.S. Department of Health and Human Services, Centers for Disease Control and Prevention, December 2010.

13. Institute of Medicine (IOM). Eng, T.R., and Butler, W.T., (eds.), *The Hidden Epidemic: Confronting Sexually Transmitted Diseases*. Washington, DC: National Academy Press, 1997

14. Aral SO, Holmes KK. Social and behavioral determinants of epidemiology of STDs. Industrialized and developing countries. In: Holmes KK et al., editors. Sexually transmitted diseases. 3rd ed. New York: McGraw Hill; 1999. p. 39–76.

15. Dean, HD, Fenton, KA. Addressing Social Determinants of Health in the Prevention and Control of HIV/AIDS, Viral Hepatitis, Sexually Transmitted Infections, and Tuberculosis. Public Health Reports/2010 Supplement 4/Volume 125.

16. Barrow RY, Berkel C, Brooks LC, Groseclose SL, Johnson DB, Valentine JA. Traditional sexually transmitted disease prevention and control strategies: tailoring for African American communities. Sex Transm Dis. 2008;35(12 Suppl):S30–9.

17. O'Leary A, editor. Beyond condoms: alternative approaches to HIV prevention. New York: Kluwer; 2003.

18. Centers for Disease Control and Prevention. National Syphilis Elimination Rapid Response Team Procedures Guide. Atlanta:CDC; 2003.

19. Centers for Disease Control and Prevention. Lessons Learned and Emerging Best Practices from the National Syphilis Elimination Program Assessment. Atlanta, GA: U.S. Department of Health and Human Services, 2004.

20. Centers for Disease Control and Prevention. Emergency preparedness and response. http://www.bt.cdc.gov/publications/feb08phprep/appendix/appendix5.asp

21. Wasserheit JN, Aral SO. The dynamic topology of sexually transmitted disease epidemics: Implications for prevention strategies. J Infect Dis. 1996;174 Suppl 2:S201–13.

22. Finelli L, Levine W, Valentine J, St. Louis M. Syphilis outbreak assessment. Sex Transm Dis. 2001;28(3):131–5.

23. Centers for Disease Control and Prevention. Division of STD Prevention Rapid Response Team and Technical Assistance Assessment: Lessons Learned, Report to the Director. Atlanta: CDC; 2008.

24. Centers for Disease Control and Prevention. Lessons Learned & Emerging Best Practices from the National Syphilis Elimination Program Assessment. Atlanta: CDC; 2004.

25. Parran T. The eradication of syphilis as a practical public health objective. JAMA. 1931; 97(2)

26. Brown WJ. A plan for the eradication of syphilis. South Med J. 1962;56:840–43.

27. Centers for Disease Control. Principals of Community Engagement. Public Health Practice Program Office, Atlanta, GA: 1997.

28. U.S. Department of Health and Human Services, What is Cultural Competency?, Office of Minority Health (HHS), Available at http://www.omhrc.gov/templates/browse.aspx?lvl=2&lvlID=11.

29. Wallerstein N. Power between evaluator and community: research relationships with New Mexico's health communities. Social Science & Medicine. 1999; 49.

30. Morgan LM. Community participation in health: perpetual allure, persistent challenge. Health Policy Plan. 2001;16(3):221–30.

31. Robertson A, Minkler M. New health promotion movement: a critical examination. Health Educ Q. 1994;21(3):295–312.

32. Boris ET, Steuerle CE. Nonprofits and government: collaboration and conflict. Washington, D.C.: The Urban Institute Press; 2006.

33. Centers for Disease Control and Prevention. Lessons Learned & Emerging Best Practices from the National Syphilis Elimination Program Assessment. Atlanta, GA: US Department of Health and Human Services, September 2004.

34. Centers for Disease Control and Prevention. The Syphilis Elimination Technical Appendix. Atlanta, GA: US Department of Health and Human Services. May 2006.

35. Centers for Disease Control and Prevention. Syphilis Elimination Listening Tour April-June 2005, Summary of Findings. Atlanta, GA: US Department of Health and Human Services, September 2005.

36. Cheney M, John R, Brennan L. A syphilis elimination media campaign in Oklahoma County. Cases Public Health Commun Market. 2008;2:11–38. www.cases-journal.org/volume2.

37. Israel BA, Checkoway B, Schulz A, Zimmerman M. Health education and community empowerment: conceptualizing and measuring perceptions of individual, organizational, and community control. Health Educ Q. 1994;21(3):149170.

38. Office of Minority Health. US Department of Health and Human Services. What is Cultural Competency? URL: www.minorityhealth.hhs.gov/templates/browse.aspx?lvl=2&lvlID=11.

39. Centers for Disease Control and Prevention (CDC). Syphilis Elimination Toolkit webpage. URL: http://www.cdc.gov/std/SEE/description.htm

40. St Lawrence JS, Montaño DE, Kasprzyk D, Phillips WR, Armstrong K, Leichliter JS. STD screening, testing, case reporting, and clinical and partner notification practices: a national survey of US physicians. Am J Public Health. 2002;92(11):1784–8.

41. A manual of tests for syphilis. Larsen SA, Pope V, Johnson RE & Kennedy EJ. (eds.), 9th Ed. 1998. American Public Health Association. Washington, DC.

42. Lambert NL, Fisher M, Imrie J, Watson R, Mercer CH, Parry JV, Phillips A, Iversen A, Perry N, Dean GL. Community based syphilis screening: feasibility, acceptability, and effectiveness in case finding. Sex Transm Infect. 2005;81(3):213–6.

43. Centers for Disease Control and Prevention. Together we can. The National Plan to Eliminate Syphilis from the United States. Atlanta, GA: US Department of Health and Human Services, May 2006: 1–56.

44. Centers for Disease Control and Prevention. Lessons Learned & Emerging Best Practices from the National Syphilis Elimination Program Assessment. Atlanta, GA: US Department of Health and Human Services. Sept 2004.

45. Dyer, JA. Multidisciplinary, interdisciplinary, and transdisciplinary educational models and nursing education. Nursing Education Perspectives/July-August, 2003.

46. Centers for Disease Control and Prevention. *Sexually Transmitted Disease Surveillance 2006 Supplement, Syphilis Surveillance Report*. Atlanta, GA: U.S. Department of Health and Human Services, Centers for Disease Control and Prevention, September 2007.

47. Aral SO Determinants of STD epidemics: implications for phase appropriate intervention strategies. Sex Transmit Infect 2002;78(Suppl I):i3–i13

48. Chesson CW, Dee TS, Aral SO. AIDS mortality may have contributed to the decline in Syphilis rates in the United States in the 1990s. Sex Transm Dis. 2003;30(5):410–24.

49. Fenton KA, Imrie J. Increasing rates of sexually transmitted diseases in homosexual men in Western Europe and the United States: why? Infect Dis Clin North Am. 2005;19(2):311–31.

50. McFarlane M, Kachur R, Klausner JD, Roland E, Cohen M. Internet-based health promotion and disease control in the 8 cities: successes, barriers, and future plans. Sex Transm Dis. 2005;32(10 Suppl):S60–4.

51. MMWR. Primary and Secondary Syphilis —United States, 2003—2004. March 17, 2006/55(10);269–273.

52. Centers for Disease Control and Prevention. Congenital syphilis—United States, 2003–2008. MMWR Morb Mortal Wkly Rep. 2010;59:413–17.

53. MMWR. 1999;48:873–878

54. Centers for Disease Control and Prevention. Sexually Transmitted Disease Surveillance 1999. Atlanta: U.S. Department of Health and Human Services; 2000.

55. Centers for Disease Control and Prevention. Sexually Transmitted Disease Surveillance 2009. Atlanta: U.S. Department of Health and Human Services; 2010.

56. Adimora AA, Schoenbach VJ. Social context, sexual networks, and racial disparities in rates of sexually transmitted infections. J Infect Dis. 2005; 191(Supplement 1):S115–22.

57. Auerbach J. Transforming social structures and environments to help in HIV prevention. Health Aff (Millwood). 2009;28:1655–65.

58. Centers for Disease Control and Prevention (US). Program collaboration and service integration: enhancing the prevention and control of HIV/AIDS, viral hepatitis, sexually transmitted diseases and tuberculosis in the United States. Atlanta: CDC; 2009.

59. Centers for Disease Control. URL: http://www.cdc.gov/od/pgo/funding/grants/glossary.shtm

60. Centers for Disease Control and Prevention. Comprehensive STD Prevention Systems 2009, Program Announcement. Atlanta, GA: U.S. Department of Health and Human Services, 2008.

61. Etheridge EW. Sentinel for health: a history of the centers for disease control. Berkley and Los Angeles, CA: University of California Press; 1992. p. 121.

62. Centers for Disease Control and Prevention. Report to Congress. in The national plan to eliminate syphilis from the United States. Atlanta, Georgia: U.S. Department of Health and Human Services, CDC, National Center for HIV, STD, and TB Prevention, 1999:1–84.

63. Sharpe, TT. McDavid-Harrison, K. Dean, HD. Summary of CDC Consultation to Address Social Determinants of Health for Prevention of Disparities in HIV/AIDS, Viral Hepatitis, Sexually Transmitted Diseases, and Tuberculosis. Public Health Reports/2010 Supplement 4/Volume 125.

64. Douglas JM, Peterman TA, Fenton KA. Syphilis among men who have sex with men: challenges to Syphilis Elimination in the United States. Sex Transm Dis. 2005;32:S80–3.

65. Mayer KH, Mimiaga MJ, Safren SA. Out of the closet and into public health focus: HIV and STDs in Men Who have Sex with Men in middle income and resource-limited countries. Sex Transm Dis. 2010; 37(4):205–7.

66. HIV/STD Risks in Young Men Who Have Sex With Men Who Do Not Disclose Their Sexual Orientation—Six U.S. Cities, 1994–2000. MMWR in *Arch Dermatol*. 2003;139:820–21.

67. Golden MR, Marra CM, Holmes KK. Update on syphilis: resurgence of an old problem. JAMA. 2003,290(11):1510–4.

68. Rietmeijer CA, Van Bemmelen R, Judson FN, Douglas JM Jr. Sex Transm Dis. 2002 Feb;29(2):65–72. Incidence and repeat infection rates of Chlamydia trachomatis among male and female patients in an STD clinic: implications for screening and rescreening.

69. Dunne EF, et al. Rate and Predictors of Repeat Chlamydia trachomatis Infection Among Men. Sex Transm Dis. 2008;35(12):000–0.

70. Bachmann LH, et al. Risk and Prevalence of Treatable Sexually Transmitted Diseases at a Birmingham Substance Abuse Treatment Facility. AJPH. 2000; 90(10):1615–8.

71. Stolte IG, de Wit JB, Kolader M, Fennema H, Coutinho RA, Dukers NH. Association between 'safer sex fatigue' and rectal gonorrhea is mediated by unsafe sex with casual partners among HIV-positive homosexual men. Sex Transm Dis. 2006;33(4): 201–8.

72. Centers for Disease Control. Developing Strategies for Syphilis Elimination in the United States: Consultants' Meeting, May 12–13, 1998. In the National Plan to Eliminate Syphilis from the United States. Atlanta, GA: CDC October 1999.

73. Moran JS, Aral SO, Jenkins WC, et al. The impact of sexually transmitted diseases on minority populations. Public Health Rep. 1989;104:560–5.

74. Thomas JC, Clark M, Robinson J, et al. The social ecology of syphilis. Soc Sci Med. 1999;48:1081–94.

75. United States Department of Labor. Bureau of Labor Statistics. June 3, 2011. http://www.bls.gov/cps/.

76. Mansergh G, et al. CDC Consultation on Methamphetamine Use and Sexual Risk Behavior for HIV/STD Infection: Summary and Suggestions. Public Health Rep. 2006;121(2):127–32.

77. Benotsch EG, Mikytuck JJ, Ragsdale K, Pinkerton SD. Sexual Risk and HIV Acquisition among Men Who Have Sex with Men Travelers to Key West, Florida: A Mathematical Modeling Analysis. AIDS Patient Care STDS. 2006;20(8):549–56. doi:10.1089/apc.2006.20.549.

78. Benotsch EG, Nettles CD, Wong F, Redmann J, Boschini J, Pinkerton SD. Kathleen Ragsdale and John J. Mikytuck sexual risk behavior. Men attending Mardi Gras celebrations in New Orleans, Louisiana. J Community Health. 2007;32(5):343–56. doi:10.1007/s10900-007-9054-8.

79. Berg RC. Barebacking among MSM Internet Users (published online). AIDS Behav. 2007;12(5):822–33. doi:10.1007/s10461-007-9281-0.

80. Hogben M, Leichliter J. Social determinants and sexually transmitted disease disparities. Sex Trans Dis. 2008;35(12):S13–8.

81. Thomas JC, Torrone E. Incarceration as forced migration: effects on selected community health outcomes. Am J Public Health. 2006;96:1762–5.

82. Satcher, D. Include a Social Determinants of Health Approach to Reduce Health Inequities, Public Health Reports/2010 Supplement 4/Volume 125.

83. Phipps W, Kent CK, Kohn R, Klausner JD. Risk factors for repeat syphilis in men who have sex with men. San Francisco Sex Transm Dis. 2009;36(6):331–5.

84. Centers for Disease Control. Principals of Community Engagement. Public Health Practice Program Office, Atlanta, GA: 1997; 6–9.

85. St Lawrence JS, Montano DE, Kasprzyk D, Phillips WR, Armstrong K, Leichliter JS. STD screening, testing, case reporting, and clinical and partner notification practices: a national survey of US physicians. Am J Public Health. 2002;92(11):1784–8.

86. Centers for Disease Control. Lessons Learned and Emerging Best Practices from the National Syphilis Elimination Program Assessment. 2004.

87. Ciesielski C, Kahn R, Taylor M, Gallagher K, Prescot L, Arrowsmith S. Control of syphilis outbreaks in men who have sex with men: the role of screening in nonmedical settings. Sex Transm Dis. 2005; 32(10):S37–42.

88. Oxman GL, Doyle LA. Comparison of the caseÐfinding effectiveness and average costs of screening and partner. Notif Sex Transm Dis. 1996; 23(1):51–7.

89. Centers for Disease Control and Prevention. Rapid response team and technical assistance assessment: Lessons learned. Report to the Director, Division of STD Prevention. Atlanta, GA: CDC August 2008.

90. CDC. 2010 Performance Measures Quick Reference Guide. Atlanta, GA: http://www.cdc.gov/std/program/2010PerformanceMeasuresQuickGuide.pdf

91. Centers for Disease Control and Prevention. Lessons Learned and Emerging Best Practices from the National Syphilis Elimination Programs Assessment. Atlanta, GA: CDC September 2004.

92. CDC. http://www.cdc.gov/stopsyphilis/2009-EBAP-guidance.pdf

93. Centers for Disease Control and Prevention. Sexually Transmitted Disease Surveillance 1998. Atlanta: U.S. Department of Health and Human Services; 1999.

94. Frieden T. A framework for public health action: the health impact pyramid. AJPH. 2010;100:4.

Human Papillomavirus Vaccine and Prevention of Human Papillomavirus-Associated Disease in the USA

19

Lauri E. Markowitz and Susan Hariri

Introduction

The introduction of human papillomavirus (HPV) vaccine has ushered a new era in the prevention of a common sexually transmitted infection that can cause cancer and other benign but serious diseases. Even before it first became available, HPV vaccine was anticipated with enthusiasm for cancer prevention, but there was also concern that the vaccine might detract from secondary prevention of HPV-associated cervical cancers through screening or promote risky sexual behavior. Introduction of HPV vaccine has presented policy, programmatic and communication challenges for public health officials and health-care providers and has required collaboration across disciplines not traditionally involved in immunization, including programs responsible for cancer prevention, sexually transmitted infections, and reproductive health. This chapter focuses on the early years of HPV vaccine introduction in the USA and briefly reviews secondary cervical cancer prevention.

Background

HPV is the most common sexually transmitted infection in the USA. Approximately 6.2 million Americans are newly infected with HPV every year [1]. Of the 100 HPV types currently identified, more than 40 types infect the mucosal surfaces and are sexually transmitted. At least 13 are classified as high-risk or oncogenic HPV types [2]. Most HPV infections are asymptomatic and transient; however, persistent infections with oncogenic HPV types can cause precancerous and cancerous lesions of the cervix, other anogenital cancers (vulvar, vaginal, penile, and anal), and some oropharyngeal cancers [3–5]. Cervical cancer is the most common of the HPV-associated cancers worldwide [6]. However, while cervical cancer remains a leading cause of morbidity and mortality among women in the developing world, widespread implementation of screening with cytologic tests has reduced cervical cancer incidence by over 75% in some developed countries since the 1950s [7]. Currently, an estimated 26,000 HPV-attributable cancers occur in women and men each year in the USA, about half of which (12,000) are cervical cancers (Table 19.1). Among men, oropharyngeal cancers are the most common with about 6,000 new cases diagnosed annually. HPV 16 or 18 are responsible for the majority of all HPV-attributable cancers; approximately 23,000 cancers due to HPV 16 or 18 occur each year. Recent data indicate that the incidence

L.E. Markowitz, M.D. (✉) • S. Hariri, Ph.D.
Division of STD Prevention, Centers for Disease Control and Prevention, 1600 Clifton Rd., NE, MS E-02, Atlanta, GA 30333, USA
e-mail: lem2@cdc.gov

S.O. Aral, K.A. Fenton, and J.A. Lipshutz (eds.), *The New Public Health and STD/HIV Prevention: Personal, Public and Health Systems Approaches*, DOI 10.1007/978-1-4614-4526-5_19, © Springer Science+Business Media New York 2013

Table 19.1 Estimated annual percentage and number of cancers attributable to human papillomavirus (HPV), by sex, USA, 2004–2008

Anatomic area	Average annual number of cases[a]	Estimated percentage of cases attributable to HPV (range)[b]	Estimated percentage of cases attributable to HPV16/18 (range)[b]	Estimated average annual number of cancers attributable to HPV	Estimated average annual number of cancers attributable to HPV16/18
Females					
Cervix	11,967	96 (95–97)	76 (–)	11,500	9,100
Vulva	3,136	51 (37–65)	44 (30–58)	1,600	1,400
Anus[c]	3,089	93 (86–97)	87 (82–91)	2,900	2,700
Oropharynx	2,370	63 (50–75)	60 (46–72)	1,500	1,400
Vagina	729	64 (43–82)	56 (35–76)	500	400
Total (female)	21,291			18,000	15,000
Males					
Oropharynx	9,356	63 (50–75)	60 (46–72)	5,900	5,600
Anus[c]	1,678	93 (86–97)	87 (82–91)	1,600	1,500
Penis	1,046	36 (26–47)	31 (22–42)	400	300
Total (male)	12,080			7,900	7,400
Total	**33,371**			**25,900**	**23,400**

Adapted from: MMWR 2012 [5]

[a]Defined by histology and anatomic site; Watson M. et al. 2008 [3]

[b]Gillison M. et al. 2008 [4]

[c]Some squamous cell rectum cancer also included, assumed to be miscoded anal. Oropharynx includes the palatine and lingual tonsils, the posterior one-third (base) of the tongue, the soft palate, and the posterior pharyngeal wall

of HPV-attributable oropharyngeal cancers has been increasing among men in the USA, [8] leading to speculation that oropharyngeal cancers may become more common than cervical cancers in the USA, where cervical cancer screening and treatment are available. Anal cancer is increasing in both women and men [9].

Some genital HPV types are classified as low-risk because they are not associated with cancer; however, low-risk HPV can cause benign diseases in both men and women. HPV 6 and 11 cause 90% of genital warts, a common sexually transmitted disease with potentially serious psychological and other consequences. HPV 6 and 11 are also causally related to recurrent respiratory papillomatosis [10].

Secondary Prevention: Cervical Cancer Screening

Screening for secondary prevention of HPV-associated cancers is only recommended for cervical cancer. Cervical cytology tests are designed to detect precancerous cervical lesions and, despite having only moderate sensitivity [11], are effective in detecting precancers if applied repeatedly and at recommended intervals. Cytology screening tests include conventional Papanicolaou (Pap) tests and liquid-based cytology. In the USA, cervical cancer screening recommendations were revised in 2012 after the US Preventative Services Task Force (USPSTF) and a multidisciplinary group, including the American Cancer Society/American Society for Colposcopy and Cervical Pathology/American Society for Clinical Pathology (ACS/ASCCP/ASCP), reviewed new evidence [12, 13]. Previously, recommendations varied by organization, although all stated that screening should start at age 21 years or within 3 years of onset of sexual activity. Recommendations for use of molecular tests that detect high risk (HR) HPV were made only by some groups [14]. Since 2012, there is agreement among all organizations on the starting age for screening, and the new recommendations state that screening should begin at age 21 years [12, 13]. While there are slight differences in other aspects of the recommendations, all groups

recommend screening in women aged 21 to 65 years with cytology (Pap test) every 3 years. For women aged 30 to 65 years who want to lengthen the screening interval, screening can be done with a combination of cytology and HPV testing ("co-testing") every 5 years. "Co-testing" in this age group every 5 years is preferred by ACS/ASCCP/ASCP. Screening recommendations will continue to be reviewed and evaluated as vaccination rates increase and new data on molecular tests become available.

It should be noted that despite overall reduction in cervical cancer rates in the past few decades, geographic and racial disparities remain as reflected in lower cervical cancer screening and higher incidence and mortality rates among certain populations [15–17]. Survey results suggest that racial/ethnic minorities such as Hispanics and Asians, women without health insurance, women with less than a high school education, and foreign-born women are screened less frequently than the national average. Moreover, particular groups such as African American women and women living in rural areas such as Appalachia have higher cervical cancer rates than the national average [15].

HPV Vaccines

Two prophylactic HPV vaccines have been licensed in the USA and in many countries worldwide (Table 19.2). These vaccines are virus-like particle (VLP) vaccines made from recombinant L1 capsid protein of the HPV virus and are not infectious. The bivalent vaccine (Cervarix, produced by GlaxoSmithKline) and the quadrivalent vaccine (Gardasil, produced by Merck & Co, Inc.) both target HPV types 16 and 18 [18, 19]. The quadrivalent vaccine also targets HPV types 6 and 11. In addition to targeted HPV types, there are other differences between the two vaccines including the producer cells used to express the L1 protein and the adjuvants. Both vaccines are given intramuscularly in a three-dose series over the course of 6 months.

Large clinical programs were undertaken by both manufacturers to provide data needed for licensure. Pivotal efficacy trials were conducted

Table 19.2 Human papillomavirus (HPV) vaccines licensed in the USA and recommendations for vaccination, 2006–2011

	Quadrivalent HPV vaccine	Bivalent HPV vaccine
Manufacturer	Merck and Co, Inc.	GlaxoSmithKline
HPV types	HPV 6,11,16,18	HPV 16,18
Year of licensure for females	2006	2009
Year of licensure for males	2009	Not licensed for use in males
ACIP recommendation, 2006	Females: Routine vaccination of females aged 11 or 12 years[a] and for females through age 26 years if not previously vaccinated	
ACIP recommendation, 2009	Females: Either vaccine for routine vaccination of females aged 11 or 12 years[a] and for females through age 26 years if not previously vaccinated	
	Males: Males aged 9 through 26 years may be vaccinated, but vaccine for males not included in routine immunization schedule	
ACIP recommendation, 2011	Females: Either vaccine for routine vaccination of females aged 11 or 12 years[a] and for females through age 26 years if not previously vaccinated	
	Males: Routine vaccination of males aged 11 or 12 years and for males through age 21 years if not previously vaccinated[a,b]	

ACIP Advisory Committee on Immunization Practices
Males: Routine vaccination of males aged 11 or 12 years[a] and for males through age 21 years if not previously vaccinated[b]

in over 18,000 women aged 15–25 years (bivalent HPV vaccine) and over 20,000 women aged 16–26 years (quadrivalent HPV vaccine). Cervical precancer lesions (cervical intraepithelial neoplasia grade 2 and 3 or adenocarcinoma in situ) due to HPV vaccine types were used as the primary endpoints for the efficacy trials. Among women naïve to the relevant HPV vaccine types, both vaccines were shown to have high efficacy (>93%) for protection against vaccine type-related cervical precancer lesions [20, 21]. The quadrivalent vaccine also was shown to have high efficacy (99%) against HPV 6, 11-related genital warts [22]. Neither vaccine demonstrated therapeutic efficacy; among women who had infection at the time of vaccination there was no impact on prevention of progression to disease. Immunogenicity studies conducted in persons aged 9–15 or 10–14 years to bridge the antibody titers to those in women in the efficacy studies demonstrated that antibody titers after vaccination are higher in the younger age group [23, 24]. In safety studies, the major adverse events were

injection sites reactions and no major safety concerns were identified prelicensure.

A direct comparison between the two vaccines using data from the clinical trials is difficult because of differences in study populations and assays used to detect HPV antibody and HPV DNA. A comparative immunogenicity trial of the two vaccines was conducted by one of the manufacturers [25]. This study found higher antibody titers after the bivalent HPV vaccine compared with the quadrivalent HPV vaccine. Injection site reactions were more frequent after the bivalent vaccine but both vaccines were well tolerated.

To obtain licensure of quadrivalent HPV vaccine in males, additional efficacy studies were conducted in heterosexual men and men who have sex with men (MSM); endpoints were HPV vaccine type-related genital warts, other external genital lesions and anal intraepithelial neoplasia. High efficacy was found for prevention of vaccine type-related endpoints among men who were naïve to the relevant HPV type at the time of vaccination [26, 27].

Vaccine Licensure and Recommendations for Females

The quadrivalent HPV vaccine was licensed by the Food and Drug Administration (FDA) in June 2006 for use in females aged 9 through 26 years [18]. In October 2009, the bivalent HPV vaccine was licensed for use in females aged 10 through 25 years [19]. Following licensure by FDA, national recommendations for vaccine use are made by the Advisory Committee on Immunization Practices (ACIP). Other professional groups make recommendations as well; these are usually consistent with ACIP recommendations but may differ slightly [28]. When making recommendations, ACIP and other groups take into consideration a variety of factors in addition to efficacy and safety, including epidemiology and burden of infection and disease, acceptability, and cost effectiveness.

In 2006, ACIP recommended routine vaccination of females aged 11 or 12 years with quadrivalent HPV vaccine [18]. The target age group of 11 or 12 years was selected to reach girls prior to sexual initiation [29], since HPV vaccines are not therapeutic and are most efficacious if administered before exposure to HPV through sexual contact. This age also allowed HPV vaccine to be incorporated into the adolescent vaccination schedule. Two other vaccines had been licensed and recommended for children age 11 or 12 years: meningococcal conjugate vaccine and tetanus, diphtheria, and acellular pertussis vaccine. These three vaccines became part of the "adolescent platform" [30].

HPV vaccine was also recommended for females aged 13 through 26 years who had not been previously vaccinated. Females not yet sexually active in this age group are expected to receive the full benefit of vaccination. Although sexually active females in this age group might have been infected with HPV 6, 11, 16, or 18, studies in the USA suggest that only a small percentage of sexually active females have been infected with more than one of these HPV types [31–33]. Therefore, although overall vaccine effectiveness would be lower when administered to a population of females who are sexually active, the majority of females in this age group will have some benefit from vaccination.

When bivalent HPV vaccine was licensed by FDA in 2009, ACIP updated recommendations stating that either HPV vaccine is recommended for routine and catch-up vaccination of females (Table 19.2) [19]. The availability of a second HPV vaccine raised questions about whether a preference should be expressed for one vaccine [34]. While the vaccines both provide high protection against HPV types 16 and 18, only one vaccine provides protection against HPV types 6 and 11, which cause genital warts. Pediatricians and other subspecialty groups also emphasized the potential protection afforded by the quadrivalent HPV vaccine against recurrent respiratory papillomatosis, a rare but serious disease caused by HPV types 6 and 11 [10]. Other differences between the two vaccines include potentially greater cross protection against some oncogenic non-vaccine HPV types phylogenetically related to HPV 16 and 18 [21, 35] and higher titers produced by the bivalent HPV vaccine [25]. In 2009, ACIP did not express a preference for either vaccine but stated differences between them [19].

ACIP recommendations state that the availability of HPV vaccination does not obviate the need for, and should be integrated with, ongoing cervical screening programs. Since the two vaccines target HPV 16 and 18 that cause about 70% of cervical cancer, cervical cancer screening is still recommended for vaccinated women to prevent cancers due to other HPV types [18, 28]. Nevertheless, it has been acknowledged that as vaccine coverage increases, cervical cancer screening recommendations might need to be reconsidered [28].

Vaccine Licensure and Recommendations for Males

At the time of FDA licensure of quadrivalent HPV vaccine in females in 2006, efficacy data required for licensure for males were not yet available. In October 2009, based on data from a clinical trial in males showing 89% efficacy for protection against HPV vaccine type-related genital warts, as well as safety data, quadrivalent HPV vaccine was licensed for use in males aged 9 through 26 years for prevention of genital warts. Soon after, data from a sub-study in MSM demonstrated efficacy for prevention of anal precancer lesions [26]. These data were submitted to FDA and quadrivalent HPV vaccine received an indication for prevention of anal cancer in both males and females in December 2010 [36, 37]. There are no data on efficacy of the vaccine to prevent the most common HPV-associated cancer in males—oropharyngeal cancer.

After licensure of the vaccine for males in October 2009, ACIP provided guidance that the vaccine could be used in males aged 9 through 26 years, but did not include vaccine for males in the routine immunization schedule (Table 19.2) [38]. Reasons included lack of data on prevention of cancers in males at that time, programmatic and fiscal challenges at the state and local level for implementing vaccination of females, the higher burden of HPV-associated cancers in females, and cost-effectiveness studies demonstrating additional costs for adding male HPV vaccination to female vaccination, potentially with relatively minimal benefits if there is high coverage in females.

Arguments have been made for and against routine vaccination of males. Arguments against inclusion of males in the vaccination program center on economic analyses showing that if coverage is high in females, vaccination of males is not a good use of health dollars [39]. Arguments in favor of male vaccination include those related to equity, the direct benefit provided to males by vaccination and the potential for increases in herd immunity resulting in decreased transmission to females. In addition, even with high coverage in females (which might provide indirect protection for males), MSM, who have the highest risk of HPV-associated anal cancers, would not be impacted [40]. Some supported a more targeted recommendation or stronger encouragement of vaccination of MSM, since this group has a high burden of HPV-associated disease [41]. Targeting males based on sexual orientation at an age when they would most benefit from vaccine would be difficult, since disclosure of sexual orientation is infrequent before onset of sexual activity or in early adolescence [42].

In October 2011, after review of additional data including vaccine efficacy for protection against anal precancers in males, the burden of HPV-associated disease in males, and the status of the female vaccination program (see Vaccine Coverage), safety and cost effectiveness, ACIP revised its recommendation and recommended routine vaccination of males at age 11 or 12 years, and vaccination through age 21 years for those not previously vaccinated [43]. For MSM, vaccination was recommended through age 26 years for those not previously vaccinated (Table 19.2).

Cost-Effectiveness of HPV Vaccination

Cost-effectiveness analyses for HPV vaccine are complex due to several factors: the multiple HPV types and multiple outcomes from HPV infection, the long time interval between infection and cancer outcomes, and the secondary prevention measures that exist for cervical cancer [44]. Importantly, there are uncertainties regarding many of the assumptions used in the cost-effectiveness models [45].

A variety of different models have been published examining the cost-effectiveness of vaccination in the USA as well as in other developed countries, estimating the incremental cost per quality-adjusted life year (QALY) gained by adding HPV vaccination of females to existing cervical cancer screening programs [46–51]. Some models considered herd immunity while others did not, and there are differences in the basic structure of the models as well as in the assumptions used. Extensive modeling has been done by the manufacturers [48, 52, 53] as well as by modelers independent of manufacturers [49–51, 54]. In all studies published to date, female vaccination with either bivalent or quadrivalent HPV vaccine was found to be a cost-effective use of public health resources, with the cost per QALY gained by vaccinating girls ranging from about $3,000 to about $45,000. Some studies have also examined cost-effectiveness of catch-up vaccination of females and found that HPV vaccination becomes less cost-effective as the age at vaccination increases beyond the early teenage years [49]. Other models found that catch-up vaccination of females would be cost effective through the mid-twenties [48].

Five published studies have estimated the cost-effectiveness of male HPV vaccination in the USA [39, 48, 51, 55, 56]. In all models, the cost-effectiveness of adding males to a female vaccination program depends on the vaccine coverage of females. As vaccine coverage of females increases, the cost per QALY gained by male vaccination increases, since female vaccination is presumed to protect male partners and little additional benefit would be gained by vaccination of males if most females are vaccinated. Male vaccination at age 12 years, when added to a female-only vaccination program, costs about $20,000–$40,000 per QALY using the more favorable assumptions and about $75,000 to more than $250,000 per QALY using those less favorable [39, 55, 56]. Vaccination of adult males becomes less cost-effective as age at vaccination increases, particularly above age 21 [57]. A cost-effectiveness analysis found that vaccination of MSM would cost <$50,000 per QALY through age 26 years [58].

Vaccine Financing

In the USA there is both public and private financing for vaccines. The Vaccines for Children Program (VFC), started in 1994, supplies private and public health-care providers with federally purchased vaccines as recommended by ACIP for use among eligible children ages 0–18 years [59]. VFC eligible children include those uninsured, Medicaid eligible, or American Indian or Alaska Native. Public sector funding for immunization also supports a program that is authorized by Section 317 of the Public Health Service Act. Through this program, federal funds are available to state and local health departments which can be used for various immunization-related activities and services for both children and adults.

Both the quadrivalent and bivalent HPV vaccines were included in the VFC program at the time recommendations were made for each vaccine [60]. Although quadrivalent HPV vaccine was not recommended for routine use in males in 2009, it was included in the VFC program, meaning that eligible males could obtain the vaccine at no cost. Individual states make decisions regarding use of funds authorized by 317 or state funds to provide HPV vaccine to non-VFC-eligible females or to all females in certain age groups. State-related differences in vaccine financing may contribute to differences observed in vaccine coverage by state [61, 62].

HPV vaccine is one of the most expensive vaccines recommended routinely for children and adolescents in the USA. In 2010, the federal contract price per dose of the quadrivalent HPV vaccine was $108 and of the bivalent HPV vaccine was $96 [63]. Both vaccines are more expensive in the private sector. Most vaccines recommended for routine use by ACIP are covered by insurance; however, there may be some delay in coverage after recommendations are made.

Implementation of HPV Vaccination and Provider Practices

Vaccines are delivered in both the public and private sectors in the USA, primarily in traditional primary care medical settings (e.g., pediatrician, family physician, internist, gynecologist practices, community health centers). A national survey conducted 18 months after vaccine licensure found that 98% of all pediatricians and 87% of family practitioners were administering HPV vaccine in their offices [64]. In five counties in North Carolina, a survey conducted soon after recommendations were issued revealed that the majority of obstetrics-gynecology practices were also administering vaccine and that 74% of family practice, 75% of pediatric, and 64% of obstetrics-gynecology practices had HPV vaccine available in their offices [65].

A variety of barriers to vaccination from the provider perspective have been identified. In a national survey conducted post-licensure, 47% of pediatricians reported failure of some insurance companies to cover HPV vaccination and 24% reported upfront costs of stocking the vaccine as barriers [64]. In Texas, 2 years after licensure, inadequate insurance coverage was reported as a barrier by 76% of physicians responding to a survey [66]. In North Carolina, providers who had concerns about high upfront cost of stocking the vaccine and late reimbursement were less likely to stock the vaccine [65].

Since a provider recommendation has major influence on vaccine acceptance [67], the strength of a provider recommendation is of prime importance for achieving high vaccine coverage. In a national survey conducted 18 months after licensure, over 94% of pediatricians and 93% family physicians reported recommending HPV vaccine to their females patients, but strength of the recommendation varied by age: only 56% of pediatricians and 50% of family physicians were "strongly" recommending vaccine for 11–12 year olds compared with 90% and 85% for 13–15 year olds [64]. Surveys in specific states soon after vaccine introduction reported similar findings; in Texas, 75% of providers always or usually recommended the vaccine for 11–12 year olds compared with 87% for 13–17 year olds [66]. Studies have found that obstetric-gynecologists' intent to recommended vaccine is high [68].

Vaccination of adolescents in primary provider settings (the "medical home") has a variety of challenges including lack of preventive health visits for adolescents and the need for three doses to complete the HPV vaccine series. Since adolescents have less routine preventive visits than do younger children, it is difficult to complete three doses over a 6-month period [69]. Because of this, other venues have been explored for delivery of adolescent vaccinations. While less common than vaccination in the "medical home," vaccines have been delivered in the school setting, either through school-based health clinics (SBHC) or through immunization campaigns located in schools. Only a minority of schools in the USA have an SBHC, comprising an estimated 2000 SBHCs nationwide. Among existing SBHCs, 84% were found to be administering vaccines to adolescents and 80% were offering

HPV vaccine [70]. Schools delivering HPV vaccine reported the main barriers as difficulties in reimbursement (billing) and determination of VFC eligibility, rather than parental refusal. A variety of other barriers to school-based vaccination has been reviewed [71]. School-located vaccination clinics (SLV), established temporarily for purposes of vaccination are being utilized as well. Pilot studies are ongoing to determine feasibility of delivery of HPV vaccine in SLV clinics in the USA.

Immunization Requirements for School Attendance and Other Legislative Issues

Immunization requirements for school attendance have been effective in raising immunization rates among children and adolescents in the USA [72]. All states have requirements for elementary school attendance for routine childhood vaccines and most states have some middle school vaccination requirements. However, efforts to encourage state requirements for HPV vaccine, which occurred less than 6 months after quadrivalent HPV vaccine licensure and were led by industry efforts, raised a variety of philosophical, legal, policy, and political concerns [73–75]. While concern about adolescent sexuality was suggested as a potential major reason for opposition to immunization requirements for school attendance, it was soon clear that many other issues contributed to the resistance. Specific factors identified by interviews with key informants were newness of the vaccine, sexually transmitted nature of HPV, non-transmissibility of HPV in the classroom setting, discomfort with the vaccine manufacturer's involvement, and the price of the vaccine [76]. Opposition to these requirements was not only from those who opposed government interference with parental autonomy and social conservatives, but also public health and policy makers who felt it was too soon to consider these initiatives [73, 77].

In a position paper by the National Vaccine Advisory Committee, it was recommended that a variety of factors be taken into account when considering adolescent mandates, including vaccine cost, funding, supply, safety, effectiveness, community and school district support, and adequate time for planning and implementation [77]. Other groups, such as the Association of Immunization Managers, also issued statements that mandates should only be considered only after an appropriate vaccine implementation period [78]. The manufacturer abandoned lobbying efforts in the face of widespread opposition in early 2007 [79].

Within one year of quadrivalent HPV vaccine licensure, 24 states and the District of Columbia had proposed legislation requiring HPV vaccination before school enrollment [80]. However, by 2008 only two jurisdictions had passed laws requiring HPV vaccination for girls entering sixth grade and both had broad "opt-out" provisions. These were implemented in the 2009–2010 school year; it is not clear whether they led to increased uptake or whether the broad "opt-out" provisions eliminated any impact of these laws. Broader "opt-out" provisions for HPV vaccine have raised concerns in immunization programs that such policies could lead to similar policies for other vaccines. Policies that have permitted personal belief exemptions have been associated with higher incidence of some vaccine preventable diseases [81]. In addition to legislation for school immunization requirements, other laws for HPV vaccine have been introduced and passed. These include laws to require insurance coverage and education about HPV and HPV vaccine [80]. The impact of these measures is being evaluated.

For a brief time in 2009, HPV vaccine was required for female immigrants applying for visas to enter the USA or to adjust their immigration status. This was due to wording in the Immigration and Nationality Act amended in 1996, that vaccines recommended for US residents by ACIP be required for immigrants [82]. While new vaccines recommended by ACIP had been included as a requirement since the act was amended, it was not until 2009 when HPV vaccine was included that controversy arose [83]. ACIP was unaware that its recommendation for HPV vaccine for the US population would be translated as such by this act. In December 2009, CDC revised guidance to state that vaccines required for immigrants must be age-appropriate for the immigrant applicant, protect against a disease that has the potential to cause an outbreak, and protect against a disease that has been eliminated or is in the process of being eliminated in the USA [84]. HPV vaccine and zoster vaccine were removed from the list of required vaccines for immigrant applicants.

Vaccine Coverage

Information on the progress of the immunization programs is mainly obtained from the National Immunization Survey (NIS), which uses provider verified records to determine vaccine coverage. National- and state-specific vaccine coverage has been measured among 13–17 year olds through NIS-Teen since 2006 [61, 62, 85, 86]. HPV vaccine initiation (receipt of at least one dose) among females increased from 25% in 2007 to 49% in 2010. In 2010, coverage with three doses of HPV vaccine was 32% [62].

There has been wide variation in HPV vaccine coverage by state, with three dose coverage ranging from a low of 18% to a high of 55% in 2010 [61]. Reasons for differences by state are not completely understood. Some states provide vaccine for all children regardless of VFC eligibility ("universal states"); variations in financing could account for some of the differences. Other factors likely also contribute. While an increasing number of states have middle school entry vaccination requirements for other vaccines recommended for adolescents, only two jurisdictions have requirements for HPV vaccine and these include broad opt-out provisions [80]. Between 2008 and 2009, 13 states had a greater than 15 percentage point increase in coverage with ≥1 dose of HPV vaccine, including only one of the jurisdictions which had adopted a middle school entry vaccination requirement. While increases in HPV vaccine uptake are expected over time, a statistical model that examined vaccine utilization (incorporating parental attitudes toward HPV vaccine) projected that without school mandates, three dose coverage would not reach 70% until 22 years after vaccine introduction [87].

In 2009 and 2010, NIS-Teen data found some differences for HPV vaccine initiation and completion by poverty status [61, 62]. In 2010, adolescent females 13–17 years living below the federal poverty level initiated the HPV series at a similar rate to those living at or above poverty level but three dose coverage was lower in this group [62]. Vaccine initiation among whites was lower than among Hispanics and American Indian/Alaskan Native but receipt of three HPV doses among those who initiated the vaccine series was lower among blacks and Hispanics compared with whites [62]. Local studies have provided further information on vaccine uptake and potential differences in subgroups. In a managed care organization in California, black race was associated with lower vaccine initiation [88], while a study in North Carolina found no differences between blacks and whites [89]. In one county in New York state, Hispanics were less likely than whites to have initiated the vaccine series [90]. Because there are race/ethnicity differences in cervical cancer morbidity and mortality in the USA [17], lower vaccine uptake or completion rates in some groups could increase existing disparities.

While NIS-Teen data are used to monitor progress of the vaccination program in the target age group, vaccine coverage data are also available from other national surveys, including the National Health and Nutrition Examination Survey [91], Behavioral Risk Factor Surveillance System [92], National Survey of Family Growth [93], and National Health Interview Survey [94]. Coverage data for older age groups are available from some of these surveys as well as, showing coverage among 19–26 year olds was about 11% in the first few years after licensure [91, 94, 95].

Vaccine Safety

Data from prelicensure safety studies are carefully reviewed before licensure of any vaccine. However, because rare events may not be detected, post-licensure studies are also conducted. Monitoring and communication about vaccine safety are critical as events temporally associated with vaccination can be falsely attributed to vaccination and anti-vaccine groups can use safety data to garner opposition to vaccination [96].

Post-licensure safety monitoring in the USA occurs through a variety of systems and HPV vaccine was included in these routine monitoring activities [97]. The Vaccine Adverse Event Reporting System (VAERS), a national passive surveillance system managed jointly by CDC and FDA, receives reports of adverse events after vaccination from multiple sources, including health-care providers, vaccine recipients, parents and guardians of vaccine recipients, and manufacturers. VAERS has many limitations typical of passive surveillance systems and data need to be interpreted with caution; many events may have occurred coincidentally following vaccination and not all reported events can be validated. Other limitations include underreporting, inconsistency in the quality and completeness of reported data, stimulated reporting due to news coverage, and reporting biases [98]. VAERS data are publicly available and have been analyzed by groups not familiar with these limitations or by those opposing vaccination, leading to claims that the vaccine is unsafe [99].

A formal evaluation of HPV vaccine VAERS data by CDC and FDA was conducted after over 23 million doses of quadrivalent HPV vaccine were distributed (June 2006 through December 2008). VAERS received 12,424 reports of adverse events occurring after administration of quadrivalent HPV vaccine with or without other vaccines, 772 (6%) of which met the criteria for a serious adverse event. The pattern of adverse events was similar to that reported for other vaccines given in the same age group except for reports of syncope and venous thromboembolic events (VTE). Of the VTE cases reviewed, 28 (90%) of 31 had a known risk factor for VTE, including 20 who were receiving estrogen containing birth control medications and 10 who had underlying hematologic laboratory abnormalities resulting in a hypercoaguable state. Thirty-two deaths were reported to VAERS and underwent extensive review; no patterns were identified in the types of deaths reported and none were considered related to vaccine [100].

Because VAERS is not designed to provide a definite assessment of risk, the safety of vaccines is also monitored in the Vaccine Safety Datalink (VSD), a collaborative project between CDC and ten large US managed care organizations that collects demographic, medical care, and vaccination data on more than 9.5 million members annually. With more than 600,000 doses of quadrivalent HPV vaccine administered to females in VSD between August 2006 and October 2009, data did not indicate that quadrivalent HPV vaccine was statistically associated with syncope, VTE, Guillan Barré Syndrome, stroke, allergic reactions, anaphylaxis, or seizures [101]. Monitoring of some outcomes will continue until one million doses have been administered in the VSD population. Monitoring will also be done for the bivalent HPV vaccine and for the quadrivalent HPV vaccine in males.

Parental Attitudes and Vaccine Acceptability

Vaccination of Females

Multiple studies have been conducted both before and after licensure to determine HPV vaccine acceptability by parents for their adolescent daughters and most have found high levels of parental acceptability [102, 103]. Studies conducted post-licensure have determined predictors of vaccination and reasons for non-vaccination. These studies found that a sizable minority of parents of unvaccinated daughters reported that they did not intend to have their daughter vaccinated in the next year [89, 90, 104, 105]. In North Carolina, about 30% of parents of unvaccinated daughters reported that they probably or definitely would not get their daughter vaccinated, with no differences by race/ethnicity [89]. Nationally, in 2008–2009, 27% of parents of unvaccinated girls were "not likely at all" to have their daughter vaccinated in the next year and an additional 14% were "not too likely" [104]. In New York State, a study found that 17% of parents had refused vaccine or reported that they would refuse vaccine for their daughter if offered. Hispanic ethnicity and lower

perceptions of vaccine safety were associated with non-vaccination [90].

Studies examining reasons for non-vaccination found common themes among parents, including the need for more information, feeling the vaccine is too new, and feeling their daughter is too young to receive the vaccine [67, 89, 104, 106, 107]. While concern that vaccination would promote early sexual debut was raised prelicensure, most post-licensure studies have not identified this as a major factor for vaccine refusal [89]. However, concern about adverse behavioral consequences has been identified as a concern in some studies post-licensure and has been associated with non-vaccination [103, 108]. One national study reported that 22% of parents strongly or somewhat agreed that vaccination of daughters would send a message that it was "okay to have sex" [108]. In contrast, a study in North Carolina found that less than 1% of parents reported concern that vaccine would lead to the daughter having sex as a main reason for not having initiated vaccination [89]. There are also differences between studies with regard to the impact of religiosity on vaccine acceptance [68, 103, 109, 110].

Consistent with data from providers and coverage surveys, data from studies of parents found a higher likelihood of intent to vaccinate or of vaccination of older girls. A national study of nurses, found that 48% of parents reported being extremely or somewhat likely to vaccinate a daughter age 9–12 years, 69% a daughter 13–15 years, and 86% a daughter 16–18 years [111]. In North Carolina, vaccine initiation soon after vaccine became available was 17.5% among 16–18 year olds, but only 6.4% among 10–12 year olds, and 7.5% 13–15 year olds. Among those for whom a provider recommended vaccine, the most common reason for non-vaccination was that the daughter was too young [89]. Qualitative studies also found that the recommended age in early adolescents was a concern [92, 93]. A related reason for non-vaccination was that the daughter was not sexually active, reported as a major reason by 47% of parents of unvaccinated 13–17 year olds in one study [67]. These data illustrate the need for further education about the benefit of vaccination prior to sexual activity.

As for other vaccines, a provider recommendation has been found to be important for decisions about HPV vaccination [67, 89, 106, 111, 112]. However, studies conducted soon after licensure, found that the majority of parents had not spoken to a health-care provider about HPV vaccine or had not received a provider recommendation that their daughter be vaccinated [67, 89].

Vaccination of Males

Numerous studies have evaluated acceptability of male vaccination for providers, parents and patients [113]. However, most were conducted prelicensure and before studies were available on vaccine efficacy in males. In general, these studies found high acceptability, but lower intent to vaccinate males than females. A survey of providers conducted post-licensure of HPV vaccine for males found that intention to recommend the HPV vaccine for males, if recommended for routine use by ACIP and other professional organizations, was high but lower than for females [114]. Physicians were more likely to strongly recommend HPV vaccine at older ages, with 59% strongly recommending at 13–15 years of age and 69% at 16–18 years of age. Studies also show high acceptability of HPV vaccine among MSM and providers who serve MSM [115].

Education and Communication

Communication and education about HPV and HPV vaccine is challenging and has required coordination across various disciplines [116, 117]. Prelicensure studies found gaps in HPV knowledge among health-care providers and the public [118]. Awareness and knowledge of HPV have improved substantially post-licensure, but knowledge gaps still exist [119]. The early increase in awareness among the general public was likely due, in part, to pharmaceutical marketing efforts. Direct to consumer advertising was conducted with the 2006 introduction of quadrivalent vaccine in the USA. In early studies, the most common source of information and knowledge about HPV vaccine was through an advertisement from a drug company [67, 119].

Both industry and public health efforts have focused on framing HPV vaccine as a cervical cancer vaccine. Studies have found that women who received a message indicating that the vaccine protects only against cervical cancer had significantly higher intentions to vaccinate themselves compared with women who read alternate messages [120]. With the licensure of the bivalent HPV vaccine, protection against genital warts also provided by the quadrivalent HPV vaccine was emphasized as a difference between the two vaccines, but the focus of prevention messages remained on cervical cancer [121]. With licensure of the quadrivalent HPV vaccine for use in males, further broadening of education and communication was needed.

HPV Vaccine and Sexual Health Issues

In the USA, HPV vaccine has been incorporated into the routine adolescent vaccination schedule and the focus has been on the adolescent vaccine platform and on prevention of cervical cancer, as studies indicated preference for these messages [120]. On the other hand, reproductive health and sexual health communities have sought to incorporate HPV vaccine into a larger agenda of sexual health. Since the vaccine is recommended before sexual debut, some have proposed that vaccination or discussion about HPV vaccine can provide an opportunity for providers and parents to talk about sexual health issues with their patients or children. One study found that among college females, mother–daughter communication about sex was strongly associated with vaccination [122]. However, it is unclear if HPV vaccine facilitated this communication. A study of 609 mothers of girls aged 11–20 years found that 81% reported having discussed HPV vaccine with their daughters. Among these, 47% reported that discussion of HPV vaccine led to a conversation about sex, leading the authors to suggest that HPV vaccine conversations may provide opportunities for sexual health promotion [123].

It is unclear whether providers would find HPV vaccine an opportunity for delivering sexual health messages. A national survey found that only 42% of pediatricians and 53% of family physicians felt it necessary to discuss issues of sexuality before recommending HPV vaccine. Furthermore, considering it necessary to discuss sexuality prior to recommending HPV vaccination was associated with not strongly recommending vaccination to 11–12 year olds [64]; there is some concern that linking HPV vaccine to sexual health messages may be an impediment to vaccination in the recommended age group.

Monitoring Impact of Vaccination

The major outcomes to be prevented by HPV vaccine (cancers) occur years after infection. Therefore, it will be decades before an impact of vaccination is observed on these outcomes. The USA has excellent cancer registries that will be able to monitor the incidence of cervical and other HPV-associated cancers [3]. To determine earlier impact of vaccination, several more proximal outcomes are being monitored including HPV prevalence, genital warts, and cervical precancers. In the USA, challenges to establishing a unified monitoring system for any of the outcomes include lack of national Pap registries, incomplete vaccine registries, and lack of unique identifiers to link medical records. A variety of efforts are ongoing to monitor biologic outcomes from HPV prevalence to cancer [97].

Impact of Vaccination on Cervical Cancer Screening

High coverage of HPV vaccine is expected to eliminate, or at least significantly reduce, the incidence of precancerous and cancerous lesions associated with HPV types 16 and 18 [124–127]. While lowering the burden of these lesions is the intended benefit of the vaccines, there may be unintentional consequences to screening efforts. In particular, elimination of HPV 16/18-related lesions in the population will result in lower posi-

tive predictive values (PPV) for both cytology- and HPV-based tests [124, 125, 127]. Moreover, since cytologic tests detect HPV 16/18 as well as other low-grade lesions, it has been argued that a preferential reduction in high-grade cervical lesions will negatively impact the analytic accuracy of cytology-based tests, which would result in only modest increases in the negative predictive value of cytology [127]. Therefore, despite a lower PPV, HPV-based test performance may be superior to cytology tests in vaccinated populations. Vaccination has also been hypothesized to decrease the accuracy of diagnostic procedures currently in place [126, 127]. Specifically, cervical lesions that arise in a vaccinated cohort may be more likely low-grade and associated with non-oncogenic types. These will be more difficult to appreciate on colposcopic exams.

Annual cytology screening is common practice in the USA despite recommendations for longer intervals between testing. This overscreening already leads to overdiagnosis with attendant costs and negative emotional consequences [16] and may be even less efficient in vaccinated cohorts. However, establishing different guidelines for vaccinated individuals in the USA will be challenging given the low coverage in 11 or 12-year-old female cohorts, and incomplete protection in females under 26 years of age who are recommended for catch-up vaccination but who may be vaccinated after exposure to HPV types in the vaccines. Future screening guidelines will have to consider vaccination coverage in the population and the effects on test performance in order to ensure maximum efficiency and avoid an unnecessary financial burden on the health-care system.

Conclusions

The discovery of HPV as the central cause of cervical cancer and subsequent development of highly effective HPV vaccines led to a new approach to preventing cervical cancer and other HPV-associated disease. There have been a variety of challenges to implementation of the HPV vaccination program in the USA including delivery of vaccines in adolescence, an age at which there are fewer preventive health visits; communication about this common sexually transmitted infection, which can lead to cancer but usually clears; and concerns about vaccine safety. Although the high cost of vaccine and challenges to widespread implementation remain as barriers, federal programs that provide funding for recommended vaccines to eligible children through age 18 years have the potential to narrow the disparities in cervical cancer morbidity and mortality across socioeconomic and racial groups.

There will be ongoing policy and program issues to address as the HPV vaccine program matures in the USA. The development of second generation vaccines with protection against additional HPV types is ongoing. Policy implications of data from post-licensure monitoring studies will need to be considered. Furthermore, the impact of vaccination on cervical cancer screening programs will require that secondary prevention programs be reevaluated. HPV vaccine holds great promise as an efficient, cost-effective intervention to reduce the burden of HPV-associated cancers and disease. Efforts to increase uptake are needed to realize the full impact of this effective primary prevention measure.

References

1. Weinstock H, Berman S, Cates Jr W. Sexually transmitted diseases among American youth: incidence and prevalence estimates, 2000. Perspect Sex Reprod Health. 2004;36:6–10.
2. Bouvard V, Baan R, Straif K, et al. A review of human carcinogens–Part B: biological agents. Lancet Oncol. 2009;10:321–2.
3. Watson M, Saraiya M, Ahmed F, et al. Using population-based cancer registry data to assess the burden of human papillomavirus-associated cancers in the United States: overview of methods. Cancer. 2008;113:2841–54.
4. Gillison ML, Chaturvedi AK, Lowy DR. HPV prophylactic vaccines and the potential prevention of noncervical cancers in both men and women. Cancer. 2008;113:3036–46.
5. Saraiya M. Burden of Human Papillomavirus–Associated Cancers—United States, 2004–2008. MMWR. 2012; 61;258–61.
6. Ferlay J, Shin HR, Bray F, Forman D, Mathers C, Parkin DM. Estimates of worldwide burden of

cancer in 2008: GLOBOCAN 2008. Int J Cancer. 2010;127:2893–917.
7. Cuzick J, Arbyn M, Sankaranarayanan R, et al. Overview of human papillomavirus-based and other novel options for cervical cancer screening in developed and developing countries. Vaccine. 2008;26 Suppl 10:K29–41.
8. Chaturvedi AK, Engels EA, Pfeiffer RM, et al. Human papillomavirus and rising oropharyngeal cancer incidence in the United States. J Clin Oncol. 2011;29:4294–301.
9. Joseph DA, Miller JW, Wu X, et al. Understanding the burden of human papillomavirus-associated anal cancers in the US. Cancer. 2008;113:2892–900.
10. Lacey CJN, Lowndes CM, Shah KV. Burden and management of non-cancerous HPV-related conditions: HPV-6/11 disease. Vaccine. 2006;24 Suppl 3:S3/35–41.
11. Arbyn M, Bergeron C, Klinkhamer P, Martin-Hirsch P, Siebers AG, Bulten J. Liquid compared with conventional cervical cytology: a systematic review and meta-analysis. Obstet Gynecol. 2008;111:167–77.
12. Moyer VA on behalf of the U.S. Preventive Services Task Force. Screening for Cervical Cancer: U.S. Preventive Services Task Force Recommendation Statement. Ann Intern Med. 2012;156:880–891.
13. Saslow D, Solomon D, Lawson HW, et al. American Cancer Society, American Society for Colposcopy and Cervical Pathology, and American Society for Clinical Pathology screening guidelines for the prevention and early detection of cervical cancer. Am J Clin Pathol. 2012;137:516–42.
14. Smith RA, Cokkinides V, Brooks D, Saslow D, Brawley OW. Cancer screening in the United States, 2010: a review of current American Cancer Society guidelines and issues in cancer screening. CA Cancer J Clin. 2010;60:99–119.
15. Downs LS, Smith JS, Scarinci I, Flowers L, Parham G. The disparity of cervical cancer in diverse populations. Gynecol Oncol. 2008;109:S22–30.
16. Fernandez ME, Allen JD, Mistry R, Kahn JA. Integrating clinical, community, and policy perspectives on human papillomavirus vaccination. Annu Rev Public Health. 2010;31:235–52.
17. Watson M, Saraiya M, Benard V, et al. Burden of cervical cancer in the United States, 1998–2003. Cancer. 2008;113:2855–64.
18. Markowitz LE, Dunne EF, Saraiya M, Lawson HW, Chesson H, Unger ER. Quadrivalent human papillomavirus vaccine: Recommendations of the Advisory Committee on Immunization Practices (ACIP). MMWR. 2007;56:1–24.
19. CDC. FDA licensure of bivalent human papillomavirus vaccine (HPV2, Cervarix) for use in females and updated HPV vaccination recommendations from the Advisory Committee on Immunization Practices (ACIP). MMWR. 2010;59:626–9.
20. Kjaer SK, Sigurdsson K, Iversen OE, et al. A pooled analysis of continued prophylactic efficacy of

quadrivalent human papillomavirus (Types 6/11/16/18) vaccine against high-grade cervical and external genital lesions. Cancer Prev Res. 2009;2: 868–78.

21. Paavonen J, Naud P, Salmeron J, et al. Efficacy of human papillomavirus (HPV)-16/18 AS04-adjuvanted vaccine against cervical infection and precancer caused by oncogenic HPV types (PATRICIA): final analysis of a double-blind, randomised study in young women. Lancet. 2009;374: 301–14.

22. Dillner J, Kjaer SK, Wheeler CM, et al. Four year efficacy of prophylactic human papillomavirus quadrivalent vaccine against low grade cervical, vulvar, and vaginal intraepithelial neoplasia and anogenital warts: randomised controlled trial. BMJ. 2010; 341:c3493.

23. Pedersen C, Petaja T, Strauss G, et al. Immunization of early adolescent females with human papillomavirus type 16 and 18 L1 virus-like particle vaccine containing AS04 adjuvant. J Adolesc Health. 2007;40:564–71.

24. Block SL, Nolan T, Sattler C, et al. Comparison of the immunogenicity and reactogenicity of a prophylactic quadrivalent human papillomavirus (types 6, 11, 16, and 18) L1 virus-like particle vaccine in male and female adolescents and young adult women. Pediatrics. 2006;118:2135–45.

25. Einstein MH, Baron M, Levin MJ, et al. Comparison of the immunogenicity and safety of Cervarix and Gardasil human papillomavirus (HPV) cervical cancer vaccines in healthy women aged 18–45 years. Hum Vaccin. 2009;5:705–19.

26. Palefsky JM, Giuliano AR, Goldstone S, et al. HPV Vaccine against anal HPV infection and anal intraepithelial neoplasia. N Engl J Med. 2011;365: 1576–85.

27. Giuliano AR, Palefsky JM, Goldstone S, et al. Efficacy of quadrivalent HPV vaccine against HPV Infection and disease in males. N Engl J Med. 2011;364:401–11.

28. Saslow D, Castle PE, Cox JT, et al. American Cancer Society Guideline for human papillomavirus (HPV) vaccine use to prevent cervical cancer and its precursors. CA Cancer J Clin. 2007;57:7–28.

29. Mosher WD, Chandra A. JJ. Sexual behavior and selected health measures: men and women 15–44 years of age, United States, 2002. Adv Data. 2006;362:1–55.

30. Middleman AB. New adolescent vaccination recommendations and how to make them "stick". Curr Opin Pediatr. 2007;19:411–6.

31. Dunne EF, Unger ER, Sternberg M, McQuillan G, Swan D, Patel SS C, Markowitz LE. Prevalence of HPV infection among females in the United States. JAMA. 2007;297:813–9.

32. Markowitz LE, Sternberg M, Dunne EF, McQuillan G, Unger ER. Seroprevalence of human papillomavirus types 6, 11, 16, and 18 in the United States: National Health and Nutrition Examination Survey 2003–2004. J Infect Dis. 2009;200:1059–67.

33. Barr E, Gause CK, Bautista OM, et al. Impact of a prophylactic quadrivalent human papillomavirus (types 6, 11, 16, 18) L1 virus-like particle vaccine in a sexually active population of North American women. Am J Obstet Gynecol. 2008;198:e1–11. 261.

34. Schwartz JL. HPV vaccination's second act: promotion, competition, and compulsion. Am J Public Health. 2010;100:1841–4.

35. Brown DR, Kjaer SK, Sigurdsson K, et al. The impact of quadrivalent human papillomavirus (HPV; types 6, 11, 16, and 18) L1 virus-like particle vaccine on infection and disease due to oncogenic non-vaccine HPV types in generally HPV-naive women aged 16–26 years. J Infect Dis. 2009;199:926–35.

36. FDA: Gardasil approved to prevent anal cancer. 2010. Accessed at http://www.fda.gov/NewsEvents/Newsroom/PressAnnouncements/ucm237941.htm.

37. Food and Drug Administration. Product approval-prescribing information [package insert]. Gardasil [human papillomavirus quadrivalent (types 6, 11, 16, and 18) vaccine, recombinant], Merck & Co, Inc: Food and Drug Administration. Accessed at http://www.fda.gov/downloads/BiologicsBloodVaccines/Vaccines/ApprovedProducts/UCM111263.pdf

38. CDC. FDA licensure of quadrivalent human papillomavirus vaccine (HPV4, Gardasil) for use in males and guidance from the Advisory Committee on Immunization Practices (ACIP). MMWR. 2010;59: 630–2.

39. Kim JJ, Goldie SJ. Cost effectiveness analysis of including boys in a human papillomavirus vaccination programme in the United States. BMJ. 2009;339:b3884.

40. Palefsky JM. Human papillomavirus-related disease in men: not just a women's issue. J Adolesc Health. 2010;46:S12–9.

41. Chin-Hong PV, Vittinghoff E, Cranston RD, et al. Age-related prevalence of anal cancer precursors in homosexual men: the EXPLORE study. J Natl Cancer Inst. 2005;97:896–905.

42. Frankowski BL. Sexual orientation and adolescents. Pediatrics. 2004;113:1827–32.

43. CDC. Recommendations on the Use of Quadrivalent Human Papillomavirus Vaccine in Males—Advisory Committee on Immunization Practices (ACIP), 2011. MMWR. 2011;60:1705–8.

44. Brisson M, Van de Velde N, Boily MC. Economic evaluation of human papillomavirus vaccination in developed countries. Public Health Genomics. 2009;12:343–51.

45. Regan DG, Philp DJ, Waters EK. Unresolved questions concerning human papillomavirus infection and transmission: a modelling perspective. Sex Health. 2010;7:368–75.

46. Chesson HW, Ekwueme DU, Saraiya M, Markowitz LE. Cost-effectiveness of human papillomavirus vaccination in the United States. Emerg Infect Dis. 2008;14:244–51.

47. Goldie SJ, Kohli M, Grima D, et al. Projected clinical benefits and cost-effectiveness of a human

papillomavirus 16/18 vaccine. J Natl Cancer Inst. 2004;96:604–15.

48. Elbasha EH, Dasbach EJ, Insinga RP. Model for assessing human papillomavirus vaccination strategies. Emerg Infect Dis. 2007;13:28–41.

49. Kim JJ, Goldie SJ. Health and economic implications of HPV vaccination in the United States. N Engl J Med. 2008;359:821–32.

50. Sanders GD, Taira AV. Cost-effectiveness of a potential vaccine for human papillomavirus. Emerg Infect Dis. 2003;9:37–48.

51. Taira AV, Neukermans CP, Sanders GD. Evaluating human papillomavirus vaccination programs. Emerg Infect Dis. 2004;10:1915–23.

52. Elbasha EH, Dasbach EJ, Insinga RP, Haupt RM, Barr E. Age-based programs for vaccination against HPV. Value Health. 2009;12:697–707.

53. Elbasha EH, Dasbach EJ, Insinga RP. A multi-type HPV transmission model. Bull Math Biol. 2008;70: 2126–76.

54. Chesson HW, Forhan SE, Gottlieb SL, Markowitz LE. The potential health and economic benefits of preventing recurrent respiratory papillomatosis through quadrivalent human papillomavirus vaccination. Vaccine. 2008;26:4513–8.

55. Elbasha EH, Dasbach EJ. Impact of vaccinating boys and men against HPV in the United States. Vaccine. 2010;28:6858–67.

56. Chesson HW, Ekwueme DU, Saraiya M, Dunne EF, Markowitz LE. The cost-effectiveness of male HPV vaccination in the United States. Vaccine. 2011;29: 8443–50.

57. Chesson HW. HPV vaccine cost effectiveness. Presentation before the Meeting of the Advisory Committee on Immunization Practices (ACIP). Atlanta, GA; June 22, 2011. Accessed at http://www.cdc.gov/vaccines/recs/acip/downloads/mtg-slides-jun11/07-5-hpv-cost-effect.pdf

58. Kim JJ. Targeted human papillomavirus vaccination of men who have sex with men in the USA: a cost-effectiveness modelling analysis. Lancet Infect Dis. 2010;10:845–52.

59. Santoli JM, Rodewald LE, Maes EF, Battaglia MP, Coronado VG. Vaccines for Children program, United States, 1997. Pediatrics. 1999;104:e15.

60. Advisory Committee on Immunization Practices Vaccines for Children Program; vaccines to prevent human papillomaviruses. Accessed at http://www.cdc.gov/vaccines/programs/vfc/downloads/resolutions/1009hpv-508.pdf

61. CDC. National, state, and local area vaccination coverage among adolescents aged 13–17 years—United States, 2009. MMWR. 2010;59:1018–23.

62. CDC. National and state vaccination coverage among adolescents aged 13 through 17 – United States, 2010. MMWR. 2011;60:1117–23.

63. Vaccines & Immunizations. CDC Vaccine Price List. Accessed November 28, 2010, at http://www.cdc.gov/vaccines/programs/vfc/cdc-vac-price-list.htm.

64. Daley MF, Crane LA, Markowitz LE, et al. Human papillomavirus vaccination practices: Survey of US physicians 18 months after licensure. Pediatrics. 2010;126:425–33.

65. Gottlieb SL, Brewer NT, Smith JS, Keating KM, Markowitz LE. Availability of human papillomavirus vaccine at medical practices in an area with elevated rates of cervical cancer. J Adolesc Health. 2009;45:438–44.

66. Kahn JA, Cooper HP, Vadaparampil ST, et al. Human papillomavirus vaccine recommendations and agreement with mandated human papillomavirus vaccination for 11-to-12-year-old girls: a statewide survey of Texas physicians. Cancer Epidemiol Biomarkers Prev. 2009;18:2325–32.

67. Caskey R, Lindau ST, Alexander GC. Knowledge and early adoption of the HPV vaccine among girls and young women: results of a national survey. J Adolesc Health. 2009;45:453–62.

68. Barnack JL, Reddy DM, Swain C. Predictors of parents' willingness to vaccinate for human papillomavirus and physicians' intentions to recommend the vaccine. Womens Health Issues. 2010;20:28–34.

69. Rand CM, Szilagyi PG, Albertin C, Auinger P. Additional health care visits needed among adolescents for human papillomavirus vaccine delivery within medical homes: a national study. Pediatrics. 2007;120:461–6.

70. Daley MF, Curtis CR, Pyrzanowski J, et al. Adolescent immunization delivery in school-based health centers: a national survey. J Adolesc Health. 2009;45:445–52.

71. Lindley MC, Boyer-Chu L, Fishbein DB, et al. The role of schools in strengthening delivery of new adolescent vaccinations. Pediatrics. 2008;121 Suppl 1:S46–54.

72. Horlick G, Shaw FE, Gorji M, Fishbein DB. Delivering new vaccines to adolescents: the role of school-entry laws. Pediatrics. 2008;121 Suppl 1:S79–84.

73. Schwartz JL, Caplan AL, Faden RR, Sugarman J. Lessons from the failure of human papillomavirus vaccine state requirements. Clin Pharmacol Ther. 2007;82:760–3.

74. Javitt G, Berkowitz D, Gostin LO. Assessing mandatory HPV vaccination: who should call the shots? J Law Med Ethics. 2008;36:384–95, 214.

75. Udesky L. Push to mandate HPV vaccine triggers backlash in USA. Lancet. 2007;369:979–80.

76. Colgrove J. The ethics and politics of compulsory HPV vaccination. N Eng J Med. 2006;355: 2389–91.

77. Mandates for adolescent immunizations: recommendations from the National Vaccine Advisory Committee. Am J Prev Med 2008;35:145–51.

78. Association of Immunization Managers. Position statement: school and child care immunization requirements. (Accessed at http://www.immunizationmanagers.org/pdfs/SchoolrequirementsFINAL.pdf.)

79. Political intrigue in Merck's HPV vaccine push. Accessed at http//abcnews.go.com/health/story?id=2890402.
80. National Conference of State Legislatures. HPV vaccine. Accessed at http://www.ncsl.org/default.aspx?tabid=14381.
81. Omer SB, Pan WKY, Halsey NA, et al. Nonmedical exemptions to school immunization requirements: secular trends and association of state policies with pertussis incidence. JAMA. 2006;296:1757–63.
82. Immigration and Nationality Act. Accessed at http://immigration-usa.com/ina_96.html.
83. Hachey KJ, Allen RH, Nothnagle M, Boardman LA. Requiring human papillomavirus vaccine for immigrant women. Obstet Gynecol. 2009;114:1135–9.
84. New Vaccination Criteria for U.S. Immigration. Accessed at http://www.cdc.gov/immigrantrefugeehealth/laws-regs/vaccination-immigration/revised-vaccination-immigration-faq.html.
85. Vaccination coverage among adolescents aged 13–17 years—United States, 2007. MMWR 2008; 57:1100–3.
86. National, state, and local area vaccination coverage among adolescents aged 13–17 years–United States, 2008. MMWR 2009;58:997–1001.
87. Dempsey AF, Mendez D. Examining future adolescent human papillomavirus vaccine uptake, with and without a school mandate. J Adolesc Health. 2010;47:242–8. 8.e1–8.e6.
88. Chao C, Velicer C, Slezak JM, Jacobsen SJ. Correlates for human papillomavirus vaccination of adolescent girls and young women in a managed care organization. Am J Epidemiol. 2010;171: 357–67.
89. Gottlieb SL, Brewer NT, Sternberg MR, et al. Human papillomavirus vaccine initiation in an area with elevated rates of cervical cancer. J Adolesc Health. 2009;45:430–7.
90. Rand CM, Schaffer SJ, Humiston SG, et al. Patient-provider communication and human papillomavirus vaccine acceptance. Clin Pediatr. 2010;50:106–13.
91. Taylor L, Hariri S, Sternberg M, Dunne E, Markowitz L. Human papillomavirus vaccine coverage in the United States, National Health and Nutrition Examination Survey, 2007–2008. Prev Med. 2011; 52:398–400.
92. Pruitt SL, Schootman M. Geographic disparity, area poverty, and human papillomavirus vaccination. Am J Prev Med. 2010;38:525–33.
93. Liddon N, Leichliter J, Markowitz L. Human papillomavirus vaccine and sexual behavior among adolescent and young women. Am J Prev Med. 2012;42:44–52.
94. Anhang Price R, Tiro JA, Saraiya M, Meissner H, Breen N. Use of human papillomavirus vaccines among young adult women in the United States: An analysis of the 2008 National Health Interview Survey. Cancer. 2011;117:5560–8.
95. Jain N, Euler GL, Shefer A, Lu P, Yankey D, Markowitz L. Human papillomavirus (HPV) awareness and vaccination initiation among women in the United States, National Immunization Survey-Adult 2007. Prev Med. 2009;48:426–31.
96. Judicial Watch. Judicial watch uncovers new fda records detailing ten new deaths & 140 serious adverse events related to Gardasil. (Accessed at https://www.judicialwatch.org/press-room/press-releases/judicial-watch-uncovers-new-fda-records-detailing-ten-new-deaths-140-serious-adverse-e/
97. Markowitz LE, Hariri S, Unger ER, Saraiya M, Datta SD, Dunne EF. Post-licensure monitoring of HPV vaccine in the United States. Vaccine. 2010;28:4731–7.
98. Varricchio F, Iskander J, Destefano F, et al. Understanding vaccine safety information from the Vaccine Adverse Event Reporting System. Pediatr Infect Dis J. 2004;23:287–94.
99. National Vaccine Information Center. Gardasil and HPV Infection. Accessed at http://www.nvic.org/Vaccines-and-Diseases/hpv.aspx.
100. Slade BA, Leidel L, Vellozzi C, et al. Postlicensure safety surveillance for quadrivalent human papillomavirus recombinant vaccine. JAMA. 2009;302:750–7.
101. Gee J, Naleway A, Shui I, et al. Monitoring the safety of quadrivalent human papillomavirus vaccine: findings from the Vaccine Safety Datalink. Vaccine. 2011;29:8279–84.
102. Allen JD, Coronado GD, Williams RS, et al. A systematic review of measures used in studies of human papillomavirus (HPV) vaccine acceptability. Vaccine. 2010;28:4027–37.
103. Bernat DH, Harpin SB, Eisenberg ME, Bearinger LH, Resnick MD. Parental support for the human papillomavirus vaccine. J Adolesc Health. 2009; 45:525–7.
104. Dorell CG, Yankey D, Santibanez TA, Markowitz LE. Human papillomavirus vaccination series initiation and completion, National Immunization Survey-Teen, 2008–2009 Pediatrics 2011.
105. Fang CY, Coups EJ, Heckman CJ. Behavioral correlates of HPV vaccine acceptability in the 2007 Health Information National Trends Survey (HINTS). Cancer Epidemiol Biomarkers Prev. 2010;19:319–26.
106. Dempsey AF, Abraham LM, Dalton V, Ruffin M. Understanding the reasons why mothers do or do not have their adolescent daughters vaccinated against human papillomavirus. Ann Epidemiol. 2009;19: 531–8.
107. Katz ML, Reiter PL, Heaner S, Ruffin MT, Post DM, Paskett ED. Acceptance of the HPV vaccine among women, parents, community leaders, and healthcare providers in Ohio Appalachia. Vaccine. 2009;27: 3945–52.
108. Allen JD, Othus MKD, Shelton RC, et al. Parental decision making about the HPV vaccine. Cancer Epidemiol Biomarkers Prev. 2010;19:2187–98.
109. Shelton RC, Snavely AC, De Jesus M, Othus MD, Allen JD. HPV Vaccine Decision-Making and Acceptance: Does Religion Play a Role? J Relig Health 2011.

110. Brewer NT, Gottlieb SL, Reiter PL, et al. Longitudinal predictors of human papillomavirus vaccine initiation among adolescent girls in a high-risk geographic area. Sex Transm Dis. 2011;38:197–204.

111. Kahn JA, Ding L, Huang B, Zimet GD, Rosenthal SL, Frazier AL. Mothers' intention for their daughters and themselves to receive the human papillomavirus vaccine: a national study of nurses. Pediatrics. 2009;123:1439–45.

112. Stokley S, Cohn A, Dorell C, et al. Adolescent vaccination-coverage levels in the United States: 2006–2009. Pediatrics. 2011;128:1078–86.

113. Liddon N, Hood J, Wynn BA, Markowitz LE. Acceptability of human papillomavirus vaccine for males: a review of the literature. J Adolesc Health. 2010;46:113–23.

114. Allison M, Kempe A. HPV vaccine for males: physicians' knowledge attitudes and practices In: ACIP meeting October 2010; 2010

115. Reiter PL, Brewer NT, McRee A-L, Gilbert P, Smith JS. Acceptability of HPV vaccine among a national sample of gay and bisexual men. Sex Transm Dis. 2010;37:197–203.

116. Friedman AL, Shepeard H. Exploring the knowledge, attitudes, beliefs, and communication preferences of the general public regarding HPV: findings from CDC focus group research and implications for practice. Health Educ Behav. 2007;34:471–85.

117. Sherris J, Friedman A, Wittet S, Davies P, Steben M, Saraiya M. Education, training, and communication for HPV vaccines. Vaccine. 2006;24 Suppl 3:S3/210–8.

118. Daley MF, Liddon N, Crane LA, et al. A national survey of pediatrician knowledge and attitudes regarding human papillomavirus vaccination. Pediatrics. 2006;118:2280–9.

119. Hughes J, Cates JR, Liddon N, Smith JS, Gottlieb SL, Brewer NT. Disparities in how parents are learning about the human papillomavirus vaccine. Cancer Epidemiol Biomarkers Prev. 2009;18:363–72.

120. Leader AE, Weiner JL, Kelly BJ, Hornik RC, Cappella JN. Effects of information framing on human papillomavirus vaccination. J Womens Health. 2009;18:225–33.

121. CDC. HPV Vaccines. Accessed at http://www.cdc.gov/hpv/vaccine.html.

122. Roberts ME, Gerrard M, Reimer R, Gibbons FX. Mother-daughter communication and human papillomavirus vaccine uptake by college students. Pediatrics. 2010;125:982–9.

123. McRee AL. RP, Gottlieb SL, Brewer NT. Mother–Daughter Communication About HPV Vaccine. J Adolesc Health. 2011;48:314–7.

124. Massad LS, Einstein M, Myers E, Wheeler CM, Wentzensen N, Solomon D. The impact of human papillomavirus vaccination on cervical cancer prevention efforts. Gynecol Oncol. 2009;114:360–4.

125. Franco EL, Cuzick J. Cervical cancer screening following prophylactic human papillomavirus vaccination. Vaccine. 2008;26 Suppl 1:A16–23.

126. Schiffman M. Integration of human papillomavirus vaccination, cytology, and human papillomavirus testing. Cancer. 2007;111:145–53.

127. Castle PE, Solomon D, Saslow D, Schiffman M. Predicting the effect of successful human papillomavirus vaccination on existing cervical cancer prevention programs in the United States. Cancer. 2008;113:3031–5.

Nicola Low, William M. Geisler, Judith M. Stephenson, and Edward W. Hook III

Introduction

Chlamydia trachomatis infection (chlamydia) is the most common notifiable bacterial sexually transmitted infection (STI) worldwide. In the United States of America (USA) in 2009, 1,244,180 cases of chlamydia were reported to the Centers for Disease Control and Prevention (CDC), the largest number of cases ever reported to CDC for any notifiable disease [1]. It has been estimated, from population prevalence surveys, that approximately 2% of sexually active adults aged 18–44 years old in the UK [2] and 2.2% (CI, 1.8–2.8%) of the US population aged

N. Low, M.D., F.F.P.H. (✉)
Division of Clinical Epidemiology and Biostatistics, Institute of Social and Preventive Medicine, University of Bern, Finkenhubelweg 11, 3012 Bern, Switzerland
e-mail: low@ispm.unibe.ch

W.M. Geisler, M.D., M.P.H.
Division of Infectious Diseases, University of Alabama at Birmingham, 703 19th Street South, ZRB 242, Birmingham, AL 35294, USA

J.M. Stephenson, M.D., F.F.P.H.
Institute for Women's Health, University College London, Medical School Building, 74 Huntley Street, London WC1E 6AU, UK

E.W. Hook III, M.D.
Division of Infectious Diseases, University of Alabama at Birmingham, 703 19th Street South, ZRB 242, Birmingham, AL 35294, USA

Jefferson County Department of Health, 4400 6th Ave South, Birmingham, AL 35233, USA

14–39 years [3] are infected with chlamydia. This level of prevalence in the USA translates into an estimated 2,291,000 (95% confidence interval, CI, 1,857,000–2,838,000) chlamydia infections each year [3]. Globally, the World Health Organization (WHO) estimates that there are about 92 million new cases of chlamydia each year [4].

The public health motivation for controlling chlamydia stems not only from the frequency of infection but because of its potential to cause reproductive tract damage in women [5]. Additional complications of chlamydia occur in men, but less commonly, and neonates may also acquire chlamydia from infected mothers at the time of birth. Research in the late 1970s and early 1980s established the associations between *C. trachomatis* and pelvic inflammatory disease (PID) [6] and between PID and tubal infertility [7, 8]. These studies provided empirical support for the conceptual model that chlamydia control is a surrogate for infertility prevention, thereby providing the primary rationale for a commitment of substantial resources for chlamydia control efforts. Hence, policy was based on the scientific rationale that controlling chlamydia transmission could prevent infertility [5, 9–11]; this would be demonstrated over time, not based initially on evidence that chlamydia control would benefit infertility prevention.

Public health policy and interventions take place within a historical and social context. Of interest, at the beginning of the 1980s, when the importance of *C. trachomatis* and its prevention were being recognized, HIV/AIDS had recently

S.O. Aral, K.A. Fenton, and J.A. Lipshutz (eds.), *The New Public Health and STD/HIV Prevention: Personal, Public and Health Systems Approaches*, DOI 10.1007/978-1-4614-4526-5_20,
© Springer Science+Business Media New York 2013

emerged as a fatal new sexually transmitted infection [12]. Governments and public health authorities in industrialized countries responded to the evolving HIV pandemic with mass media and public education campaigns beginning in the mid to late 1980s [13]. The first studies observing ecological associations between reductions in chlamydia cases and the start of efforts to screen young women for asymptomatic infection in Sweden [14, 15] and the USA [16] occurred contemporaneously with the period during which mass reactions to HIV were at their height. Surveillance data in some countries without chlamydia control efforts recorded reductions in cases of syphilis, gonorrhea, chlamydia, and pelvic inflammatory disease, which were interpreted as being the result of behavior change in response to HIV/AIDS [17, 18]. Thus behavioral change in response to fear of HIV/AIDS might have contributed to the observed decline in chlamydia cases in Sweden and the USA, although it is impossible to say by how much.

As for most sexually transmitted infections, there is no effective chlamydia vaccine available currently. Alternative means of control are therefore needed to prevent new infections and sequelae and break chains of chlamydia transmission by identifying existing infections and curing them before complications arise. Screening to detect asymptomatic chlamydia infections in sexually active young women (and sometimes men) accompanied by treatment of infected cases, has been widely recommended as being effective for reducing *C. trachomatis* transmission and preventing reproductive tract complications [19–22]. There are, however, important limitations to currently available evidence and questions remain about the interpretation of the evidence and about implementation and success of screening programs [23–25]. Screening programs are discussed in detail in the section of this chapter, *Public health tools for chlamydia control.*

The objectives of this chapter are to review the evolution and current state of chlamydia control efforts in the USA and UK by describing (1) the biological rationale and theoretical framework for chlamydia control; (2) the development of chlamydia diagnostics; (3) data sources and epidemiology of chlamydia infection; (4) public health tools for chlamydia control and their application

in the USA and UK; (5) possible interpretations of observed trends in chlamydia infection; and (6) future directions for research and practice.

Biological Rationale and Theoretical Framework for Chlamydia Control

There are key biological characteristics of *C. trachomatis* that make detection through screening the cornerstone of most comprehensive chlamydia control programs. The same characteristics, however, also help explain why infection control through screening and treatment is difficult.

C. trachomatis is an obligate intracellular bacterium, which preferentially infects columnar mucosal surfaces of the urogenital tract and rectum, but also infects oropharyngeal mucosa and conjunctiva. *C. trachomatis* has a propensity to cause asymptomatic infection and the genital examination of those infected is often unremarkable [26]. Chlamydia-infected persons can remain asymptomatically infected for months to years and may transmit the infection to other susceptible persons [27]. Immunity after infection by natural clearance or treatment is limited, so repeated infections are common [28]. The asymptomatic clinical presentation of both lower and upper genital tract infections and the potential for prolonged duration of infection are key factors that fuel continued transmission of chlamydia.

Endocervical chlamydial infection can ascend to the upper genital tract in women and lead to complications. Pelvic inflammatory disease (PID) occurs when chlamydial infection involves the uterus, fallopian tubes, and/or ovaries, and can cause scarring that predisposes to additional complications such as infertility and risk for ectopic pregnancy [29]. The timing, frequency and proportion of lower genital tract infections that spread to the upper genital tract in women and cause clinically important disease are not precisely known, but the frequency of progression is thought now to be lower than the estimates of up to 30% suggested in the 1970s and early 1980s [30, 31]. Some studies have found that 2–3% of asymptomatic chlamydia-infected women developed PID in the interval (median 2 weeks) between receiving a chlamydia screening test and returning for treatment of a positive test [32, 33]. The authors hypothesized that this might represent progression of recently acquired chlamydial infections, whilst acknowledging that the interval between infection and testing was not known [32]. The timing of upper genital tract infections amongst women with preoperative *C. trachomatis* in the month after surgical instrumentation also suggests an early onset [34, 35]. Nevertheless, ongoing ascension, or ongoing inflammation are also likely. Subsequent tubal damage is thought to result from cell-mediated immune processes that lead to scarring, fibrosis, and loss of cilial function [36]. These changes in turn lead to an increased risk for ectopic pregnancy and tubal infertility. In a large cohort of women who underwent diagnostic laparoscopy for suspected PID between 1960 and 1984, Weström and colleagues found a strong association between PID and subsequent risk of infertility: the risks of confirmed tubal factor infertility amongst women reporting one, two, or more episodes of PID were 8.0, 19.5, and 40.0%, respectively [37]. Infertility, chronic pain, and ectopic pregnancy have long been seen as "threats to the fecundity of millions of young women" [38].

The theoretical framework for chlamydia control through screening and treatment as an early component of control efforts is consistent with the conceptualization of phases through which sexually transmitted infection epidemics evolve [39]. Screening is an intervention to detect prevalent, asymptomatic infections of varying durations. Treatment of cases detected through screening results in a reduction in the duration of the infectious period [40]. For chlamydial infection, the rationale is as follows: (1) detecting and treating chlamydia infections in women will prevent lower genital tract infections from ascending and causing PID; (2) prevention of PID will prevent ectopic pregnancy and infertility; (3) the majority of chlamydial infections are asymptomatic in both men and women [41] so most cases will only be detected by screening sexually active persons, even if asymptomatic; (4) an initial approach to control requires widespread screening and treatment of a target population defined only by age and maybe gender, such as sexually active women ≤25 years of age, as well as more targeted strategies [39]. Supplementing this rationale are assumptions that repeat chlamydial infection

occurs frequently following treatment [42], therefore partner treatment, education, and repeated testing are necessary components of chlamydia management; that highly sensitive nucleic acid amplification tests (NAATs) for *C. trachomatis* diagnosis can now be performed on noninvasively collected specimens such as urine, providing opportunities for screening in clinical settings where genital examinations may not be feasible; and that when screening reaches a high enough proportion of the target population over time, chlamydia transmission will be interrupted, prevalence will fall, and the incidence of PID, ectopic pregnancy and infertility will fall further. Logically, as generalized epidemics decline and become endemic in certain sexual networks, targeted strategies will become relatively more important [39]. As discussed later in this chapter, translation of this theoretical framework for chlamydia control into practice has not yet achieved a substantial degree of chlamydia control.

Diagnostic Tools for Chlamydia Control

Accurate diagnostic tools for identification of *C. trachomatis* are essential for assessment of the impact of prevention and control efforts. Most chlamydia-infected persons are asymptomatic or have nonspecific examination findings. As a result, testing is a critical component of chlamydia diagnosis and is often needed to facilitate treatment. Until the mid-1990s, the reference standard for chlamydia diagnosis was isolation of *C. trachomatis* in cell culture. First described in 1965 by Gordon and Quan [43], chlamydia culture became more available in the 1970s, facilitating opportunities for chlamydia screening. However, due to the technical demands and costs of culture, chlamydia screening efforts remained limited. By the early 1980s, *C. trachomatis* was linked as an etiologic agent to clinical syndromes, such as urethritis (non-gonococcal and postgonococcal), cervicitis, etc., which facilitated clinical diagnosis of chlamydia-infected patients and syndromic management. In the mid to late 1980s, nonculture chlamydia tests (e.g., direct fluorescent antibody microscopy, enzyme immunoassays, and nucleic acid hybridization tests), which were less expensive and technically less demanding than culture, became available and facilitated more widespread chlamydia screening. However, they had lower test sensitivities than culture [44] and therefore detected fewer infections.

In the mid to late 1990s, NAATs became commercially available. NAATs have the highest sensitivity of all chlamydia diagnostic tests and therefore detect more infections than earlier tests [44]. NAATs can also be performed on less invasively collected specimens (first-void urine in men or women and self-collected vaginal swabs in women) with accuracy similar to that of genital swabs collected on examination; this provides more screening opportunities in nontraditional venues where genital examination might not be feasible. The availability of NAATs for chlamydia research also led to an improved understanding of chlamydia epidemiology, including an appreciation of the asymptomatic nature of chlamydia in the majority of infected patients and risk factors for chlamydia.

Data Sources and Epidemiology of Chlamydia

In both the USA and UK chlamydia is predominantly an infection of young sexually active women and men. There are typically multiple sources of information available for studying chlamydia infection in a population. These can give different pictures of the level, distribution and time trends of infection, depending on who is included in samples of cases (numerator) and the population (denominator). Ideally, the data source used for monitoring should be chosen according to the information required. In general, levels of chlamydia infection in the general population and levels of diagnosed infection reported through surveillance systems are similar in the USA and UK

Surveillance Reports of Chlamydia Infections

National chlamydial surveillance data record the numbers of diagnosed cases reported to national

public health offices in the USA [1] and UK [45]. The data are presented as raw numbers of cases and as a "rate" per 100,000 population, using the total population as the denominator.

Trends in cases detected through surveillance are the timeliest source of information about levels of recognized chlamydia infections in a population. Surveillance data, however, only partially reflect the underlying epidemiology of chlamydia because reported chlamydia case rates may vary over time with changes in diagnostic, testing and reporting practices obscuring whether or not changes in the actual incidence or prevalence of chlamydia have occurred [1]. For example, most reported cases of diagnosed chlamydia are in women, reflecting chlamydia testing practice. This results in higher rates of diagnosed infection in women, even though the prevalence of infection in women and men is similar [2, 3, 41]. There is a very strong correlation between the numbers of chlamydia cases diagnosed and the numbers of tests; in the USA, about 95% of the variance in the diagnosed case rate is explained by the numbers of tests amongst Medicaid and privately insured women [46]. The number of cases diagnosed depends on the number of people tested; the higher the number of people tested, the higher the number of detected cases, even if the underlying prevalence of infection stays the same [47]. It can therefore be difficult to determine, from surveillance data alone, whether the level of chlamydia transmission in a population is changing. Other factors that affect the number of diagnosed chlamydia cases reported in surveillance data include the sensitivity of diagnostic tests, which has increased following the introduction of NAATs; the age and risk profile of people being tested; and the completeness of reporting.

The surveillance data presented here to represent the UK are from England only, because this was the only country for which consistent data could be compiled from published data sources for all years. England accounts for 84% of the UK population. Direct comparisons between the population rate of diagnosed chlamydia cases in the USA and England can be made from 2008 onwards, after chlamydia surveillance systems in England combined to incorporate diagnoses made in both specialist genitourinary medicine

(GUM) clinics (equivalent to sexually transmitted diseases, STD clinics) and those reported from other settings (Figs. 20.1 and 20.2).

The time trends in overall rates of chlamydia diagnoses in the USA and UK show several similarities, after allowing for the differences in sources of data collection. The numbers of reported chlamydia cases detected in the USA and England have increased steadily over time in both sexes (Figs. 20.1 and 20.2). In the USA, from 1990 through 2009, the rate of reported chlamydial infection increased from 87 to 409 cases per 100,000 population [1]. In the UK, the rate of reported chlamydia diagnoses increased from 64 per 100,000 in 1989 (GUM clinics only) to 344 per 100,000 in 2009 (all settings, 208 per

100,000 in GUM clinics) [45]. When chlamydia diagnoses in all settings are considered, rates in men are slightly higher in the UK (281 per 100,000) than the USA (219 per 100,000). Rates of diagnosed chlamydia in women were, however, higher in the USA (592 per 100,000 in 2009) than in the UK (401 per 100,000).

In 2008, specialist GUM clinics accounted for 61% of all chlamydia diagnoses in England, whereas only 17% of chlamydia diagnoses reported in the USA were made in STD clinics. Chlamydia is diagnosed in a similar number of women and men attending STD clinics in the USA (89,943 cases in women, 95,798 in men in 2008) or GUM clinics in England (53,426 cases in women, 53,697 in men in 2008).

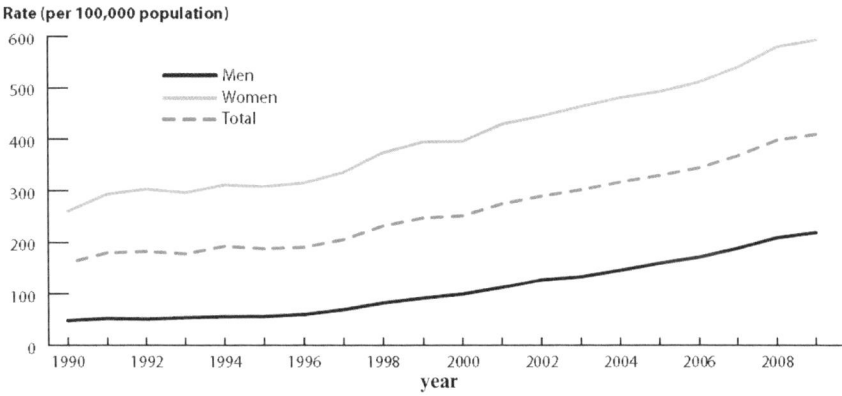

Fig. 20.1 Rates of reported chlamydia infections, US 1990–2009. Data are compiled from reports sent by state STD control programs and health departments. Figure reproduced from CDC STD Surveillance 2009 (Figure 1, p. 10)

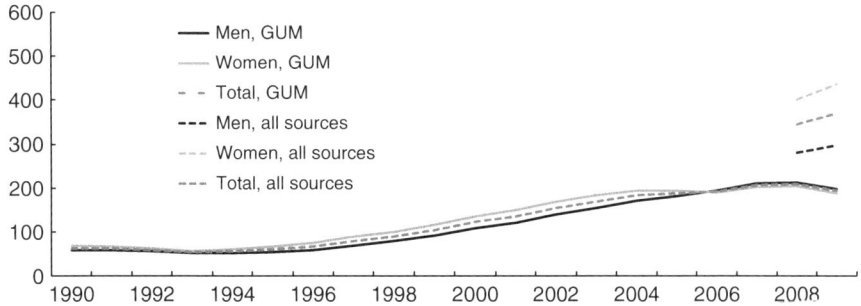

Fig. 20.2 Rates of reported chlamydia infections, England, 1990–2009. Note: Data presented continuously from 1990 onwards are diagnoses made in genitourinary medicine (GUM) clinics only. For 2008–2009, diagnoses made by the National Chlamydia Screening Programme in England, and from laboratories have become available (all sources). Data were compiled from archived reports of case numbers from the Health Protection Agency (formerly Public Health Laboratory Service Communicable Disease Surveillance Centre). Denominator data are mid-year population estimates for women and men of all ages in England from the Office for National Statistics (http://www.statistics.gov.uk/statbase/Product.asp?vlnk=15106)

Surveillance systems in the USA also monitor levels of chlamydia infection in a number of populations, such as women attending federally funded family planning clinics, National Job Training Program entrants and juvenile corrections facilities [48]. These data, which record the positivity rate (number of positive chlamydia tests/number of chlamydia tests done) are used as estimates of prevalence in the populations specified. Trends over time can be monitored but interpretation is complicated if there are changes in test coverage or the risk profile of those tested [46]. In 15- to 24-year-old women tested in federally funded family planning clinics from 1999 to 2006, the trend over time was stable or slightly increasing in most US regions.

Cross-Sectional Prevalence Surveys

Cross-sectional surveys are used to estimate the prevalence of chlamydia in a given population at a given point in time; the number of people who have a disease at a particular time divided by the population at risk [49]. Whilst often referred to as a rate, prevalence is expressed as a percentage. Representative population-based samples provide the least biased estimates of the prevalence of chlamydia in the general population as a whole because individuals from a defined population are sampled at random, irrespective of behavior, symptoms, or healthcare attendance.

There are relatively few large studies providing population-based data about chlamydial prevalence, especially over time, because they are organizationally complex and expensive. Nationally representative surveys were conducted during a similar time period in the USA (the National Health and Nutrition Examination Survey, NHANES) [3] and the UK (the second National Survey of Sexual Attitudes and Lifestyles, Natsal 2) [2] (Table 20.1). Direct comparisons are difficult owing to differences in the types of study populations and their age ranges in published papers. The overall estimated prevalence was around 2% in NHANES (14–39 year olds) and Natsal 2 (18–44 year olds). Importantly, however, the denominator for the Natsal survey included only participants who had ever had sexual intercourse, whilst the NHANES denominator includes nonsexually active persons.

The overall prevalence in both countries is modest, but this hides marked variations according to demographic characteristics. In both countries, the highest prevalence rates were seen in the youngest studied age group in women (14–19 year olds in the USA, 18–24 year olds in the UK) and in slightly older men (20–29 years in the USA, 25–34 years in the UK). Prevalence rates in women and men overall were similar. In the

Table 20.1 Prevalence of chlamydia in general population samples in the USA and UK

Country, survey, year	Response rate	Total tested[a]	Overall % (95% CI)	Women (95% CI)	Men % (95% CI)
US NHANES, 1999–2002					
14–39 years	76%[b]	6,632	2.2 (1.8–2.8)	2.5 (1.8, 3.4)	2.0 (1.6, 2.5)
14–19	–	3,333	3.4 (2.7–4.2)	4.6 (3.7–5.8)	2.3 (1.5–3.5)
20–29	–	1,712	2.5 (1.9–3.4)	1.9 (1.0–3.4)	3.2 (2.4–4.3)
30–39	–	1,587	1.3 (0.7–2.4)	1.9 (1.0–3.5)	0.7 (0.3–1.5)
UK Natsal, 2000					
18–44 years	46%[b]	3,529	–	1.5 (1.1, 2.1)	2.2 (1.5, 3.2)
18–24	–	680	–	3.0 (1.7–5.0)	2.7 (1.2–5.8)
25–34	–	1,456	–	1.7 (1.0–2.8)	3.0 (1.7–5.1)
35–44	–	1,393	–	0.6 (0.3–1.4)	1·0 (0.4–2.5)

[a]Numbers tested, as reported in publications. Prevalence rates estimated from data weighted to represent the general population. Ligase chain reaction (LCx, Abbott Laboratories, Abbott Park, IL) used in both surveys
[b]NHANES response rate calculated from 83% response to household survey and 91.7% of all respondents aged 14–39 years with both chlamydia and gonorrhea test result; Natsal response rate calculated from 65·4% response to household survey for all respondents aged 16–44 years and chlamydia test result from 71% of adults aged 18–44 years invited (random sample of all who reported at least one partner with whom they had sexual intercourse). Analyses were done with weighted data to match the overall age and sex population profile [2]

USA, higher prevalence was associated with both lower levels of income and educational attainment [3]. Chlamydia prevalence was about four times higher in African Americans than whites; after controlling for demographic, economic, and behavioral factors, the odds of infection in African Americans were three times higher [3]. In another nationally representative survey in the USA (the National Longitudinal Study of Adolescent Health, Add Health) [41], the overall prevalence of chlamydia in 18–26 year olds was 4.7% (95% CI 3.9–5.7%) in women and 3.7% (95% CI 2.9–4.6%) in men. In the Add Health survey chlamydia prevalence did not vary markedly by age but was 6.5 times higher in African American than white participants [41].

The distribution of chlamydia in the UK population as a whole was not strongly associated with socioeconomic status, measured as social class, or location and prevalence was not stratified by ethnic group [2]. Nationally representative estimates of chlamydia prevalence amongst different ethnic groups in the UK are not available. There are, however, ethnic group differences in levels of chlamydia positivity amongst people tested in GUM clinics [50] and in non-GUM settings [51] with women and men of black Caribbean ethnicity being more likely than whites to have chlamydia. In both surveys, higher chlamydia prevalence rates were found in those with higher numbers of sexual partners, before and after adjusting for confounding factors. In both countries, however, age remains the only factor that can be reliably used to define a target population for screening.

Changes in chlamydia prevalence over time in the general population have only been measured by the NHANES in the USA, with results from five survey rounds [52]. The data show no statistical evidence of a change in prevalence amongst women aged 14–25 years, who are the target group for annual screening (Fig. 20.3) [52]. There was, however, a fall in chlamydia prevalence amongst the whole NHANES study population, women and men aged 14–39 years of age. The UK Natsal survey is being repeated in 2010–2012, after which population level data from two surveys will be available. The decade separating the surveys includes the time period when widespread chlamydia screening was being introduced in England [53]. Changes over time in the distribution of chlamydia in different age and ethnic groups should be monitored because these could indicate changes in the epidemic phase.

Surveillance for Complications of Chlamydia

While repeated, high quality determinations of chlamydial prevalence using similar methods may be sufficient to track national chlamydial

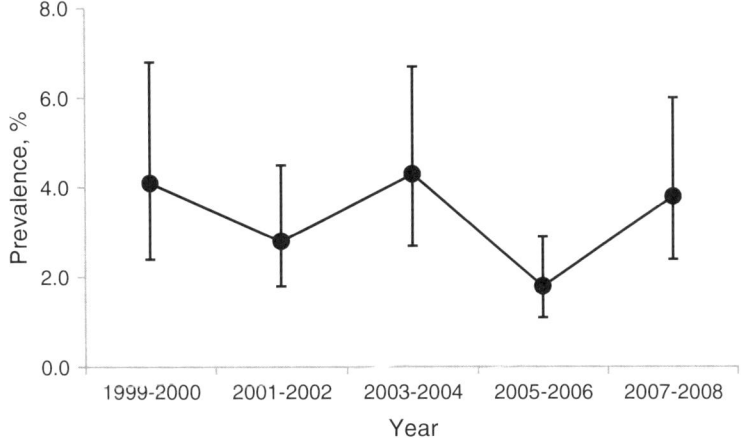

Fig. 20.3 Chlamydia prevalence, 14–25-year-old women, US 1999–2008. Note: Figure produced from data published in Datta et al. [52]. The diagnostic test used in 1999–2000 (Abbott LCx, Abbott Laboratories) was replaced by a different assay (BD ProbeTec ET, Becton Dickinson, Franklin Lakes, NJ) after the first two survey rounds

rates over time, there is more imprecision in measurement of the chlamydial complications, the prevention of which is the main justification for chlamydial screening programs. The reproductive tract complications associated with chlamydia can also be monitored using routine data captured from hospital discharge or from primary care databases. Hospital-based diagnoses in the USA and UK are based on codes published in the International Classification of Diseases (ICD) [54]. Case definitions for diagnoses of conditions such as PID in physicians' offices in the USA [1] and in UK primary care databases [55] might not be comparable. Chlamydia is only one of the possible causes of PID, ectopic pregnancy and infertility. The reported numbers of cases of each condition in surveillance reports usually include all causes because of differences between countries in the use of different ICD subcodes; chlamydia-specific codes exist for PID but appear only to be used in some countries. PID is typically diagnosed by clinical findings, which have poor sensitivity and specificity compared with evaluation for tubal pathology by laparoscopy [56]. Trends in reported rates of these conditions can be influenced by changes in the distribution of infectious and noninfectious causes, as well as in diagnostic practice, case management, health seeking behavior, and the effects of other changes in reproductive health practice and treatment.

Rates of PID reported to surveillance systems have fallen steadily over the past 10–30 years in some countries, including the USA [1], England [55], Australia [57, 58], and Sweden [59, 60]. Several factors might contribute to these trends. PID is now more likely to be managed in outpatient or primary care settings than in hospitals, and the proportion of PID cases requiring hospitalization might have fallen. PID diagnoses in primary care have, however, also fallen in the USA [61], England [55], and Australia [58], so the reduction in these countries has occurred across all settings. In addition, PID can also be a polymicrobial condition [62] and the relative contribution of different organisms might have changed over time. A fall in the contribution of *Neisseria gonorrhoeae* to PID is responsible for part of the decline [29], particularly from the mid-1970s to 1980s [59, 60]. *C. trachomatis* was found in about 30% of PID cases in studies

conducted up to the mid-1990s [29] but more recent data are lacking. Improved antibiotic treatment, more widespread general use of antibiotics active against some of the etiologic agents, or other changes in genital hygiene might also have reduced the incidence and/or severity of PID. Finally, chlamydia control efforts might have contributed to the fall, despite a high continued burden of infection, through timelier chlamydia treatment. PID diagnosis rates have not fallen in all countries, however. In New Zealand, for example, where chlamydia testing and diagnosis rates are high, PID diagnosis rates have remained broadly stable and the contribution of *C. trachomatis* to total PID numbers has increased over time [63, 64].

Ectopic pregnancy can also be monitored through hospital episode statistics. Whilst the diagnosis of ectopic pregnancy is more certain than that for PID, ectopic pregnancy is also multifactorial and chlamydia is only one possible cause. As with PID, there have been changes in diagnostic tools (increasingly sensitive hormone assays and imaging studies) and medical management of ectopic pregnancy is increasing over time; both factors affect the interpretation of time trends. For instance, use of methotrexate for outpatient ectopic pregnancy treatment might have not only simplified management but also reduced reporting. Ectopic pregnancy rates have fallen recently in some countries where chlamydia screening is common, including Denmark and Sweden, but not others, such as New Zealand [64]. In the USA, hospitalizations for ectopic pregnancy from 1997 to 2006 remained at levels from 25,000 to 40,000 per year [61].

Infertility diagnoses are also recorded in hospital episode statistics. Whilst infertility prevention is the final endpoint of chlamydia control, the interpretation of absolute rates and trends is known to be difficult [64]. As for ectopic pregnancy, tubal factor infertility tends to be diagnosed long after the likely age at which chlamydia infection occurred. Diagnosing infertility depends on personal decisions to present for treatment, and access to healthcare providers for infertility evaluation and management. Diagnostic and treatment modalities for infertility have also changed over time and diagnoses made in private clinics might not be included in surveillance efforts.

Public Health Tools for Chlamydia Control

Principles of Infection Control

Thomas Parran, who was tackling syphilis in the USA in the 1930s [65, 66], stated two requirements for effective control, based on his observations of control programs in several European countries (1) that every infected person must be treated and (2) that diagnosis and treatment must be freely available. He operationalized these into five key features for clinical and public health services: (1) a surveillance system for case notification; (2) effective diagnostic methods; (3) easy access to effective treatment; (4) epidemiological investigation to identify and treat the source of infection and contacts, i.e., partner notification; and (5) education for health care workers, the public and patients to promote greater knowledge, interest and early recognition of disease [66]. Parran thus defined the fundamental features of sexually transmitted infection control programs that are adapted and implemented worldwide. The control plan fits into a conceptual framework as a series of three linked levels of intervention, which apply to chlamydia as well as all other sexually transmitted infections [67]. First, effective case management of the individual with chlamydia clearly requires ready access to accurate diagnostic tests and effective treatment, irrespective of clinical presentation. The next level links the individual with chlamydia to management of their recent sexual partner(s), which is needed both to prevent reinfection of the index case and the secondary spread of infection to others. The third level, population-level intervention, requires additional infrastructure to coordinate the control efforts of the first two levels.

Screening Programs

The population level component of a chlamydia control program is screening of asymptomatic individuals. "Screening is a program not a test" is an aphorism coined by Prof. J.A. Muir Gray, former director of the UK National Screening Committee (NSC) [68]. In the case of chlamydia, it emphasizes the fact that, whilst chlamydia screening is delivered by individual health professionals to individuals, reductions in chlamydia incidence in the population can only be achieved if Parran's prescription for easily available good diagnostic tools and treatment are widely implemented in a coordinated, consistent, and continuous manner. Sustained reductions in the transmission of an infectious disease that does not induce lasting immunity can only be expected if infections, reinfections from untreated sex partners, and new infections from future partners are detected and managed in a timely way to reduce the duration of infection [40].

Screening is a public health service in which members of a defined population, who do not necessarily perceive they are at risk of a disease or its complications, are asked a question or offered a test in order to identify those individuals who are more likely to be helped than harmed by further tests or treatment [69]. An ideal chlamydia screening program would be a continuing public health service that ensures that screening is delivered at sufficiently regular intervals to a large enough proportion of the target population to identify and treat asymptomatic chlamydia infections in order to interrupt transmission and prevent reproductive tract complications at a reasonable cost, whilst minimizing harm [12].

National public health agencies in some countries use specific criteria to determine whether a screening program is likely to be an appropriate intervention for a specific disease [70, 71]. In the UK the National Screening Committee (NSC), an independent expert group, is responsible for assessing adherence to criteria listing key aspects about the condition, the test, the treatment, and the program [70]. The criteria have been applied to chlamydia, but conclusions have differed, depending on the interpretation of the evidence available [72–74]. The US Preventive Services Task Force (USPSTF), a panel of non-Federal experts, has similar responsibilities for screening programs and requires that "evidence for the entire preventive service must include studies of sufficient design and quality to provide an unbroken chain of evidence-supported linkages, generalizable to the

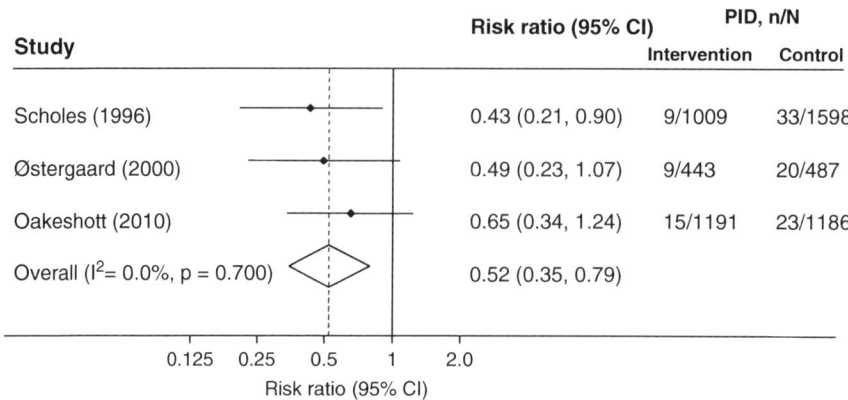

Fig. 20.4 Results of randomized controlled trials of chlamydia screening; incidence of PID in women offered screening compared with control groups. Note: Results of each individual trial shown as *solid black diamond*, with 95% CI shown by lines either side. Overall estimate shown as *open diamond* with point estimate at the vertical points and 95% CI as the horizontal extremes. The *dotted line* runs through the point estimate. Pooled estimate obtained from fixed effects meta-analysis. The I^2 value of zero shows that there is no statistical evidence of heterogeneity between studies, other than that expected by chance

general primary care population, that connect the preventive service with health outcomes" [75].

Evidence Base for the Effectiveness of Chlamydia Screening

There are two stated aims of programs to control genital chlamydial infection: reduction of prevalence and prevention of more costly and often irreversible sequelae [76, 77]. The prevention of PID and its associated sequelae is viewed mainly as an individual level objective; screening of women in routine health care aims to detect and treat chlamydial infection at an early enough stage to reduce PID risk. Partner notification is an integral part of the management to prevent reinfection from current sex partners [76]. The population-level objective of screening (including treatment and partner notification) is to reduce chlamydia prevalence, which requires levels of regular coverage sufficient to interrupt transmission in sexual networks [76]. Reductions in chlamydia prevalence also have an indirect effect on PID in individual women because of reduced risk of exposure to *C. trachomatis*. In fact, several economic evaluations of the cost-effectiveness of chlamydia screening are based on mathemati-

cal modeling studies that present the indirect component of PID prevention resulting from reduced exposure and not the direct effect of interrupting ascending infection [23].

Evidence for the effectiveness of a screening program needs to show that observed reductions in morbidity or mortality were the result of the intervention and not the result of other factors. The study design most likely to minimize the possibility of biases when screening is the intervention is a randomized controlled trial (RCT) with high internal validity [70]. The statements from official bodies have cited the results of both RCTs and ecological time trend studies as evidence supporting the effectiveness of chlamydia screening [19, 22, 78].

While three RCTs have examined the effect of a one-time offer of chlamydia screening for women on the incidence of clinically diagnosed PID of any cause [79–81], the most influential in shaping policy was the first trial, by Scholes et al., published in 1996 [79]. Each study showed a reduction in PID incidence in the intervention group after 1 year (Fig. 20.4). Overall, this suggests that chlamydia screening reduced PID incidence by 48% (95% CI 21, 65%). Whilst all trials are consistent with a reduction in PID incidence, the estimated strength of the effect of screening has become smaller over time, despite the fact that the intensity of the intervention is higher in the more recent trials. With 99% uptake of screening in the most recent trial in the UK [79], the relative risk of PID was 0.65 (95% CI 0.34–1.22) compared with a relative risk of 0.44 (95% CI 0.20–0.90) associated with 64% uptake of screening in the US trial [79]. This probably reflects a lower risk of bias in the conduct of the most recent compared with the earlier trials, for which methodological limitations contributing to an overestimation of the effect of screening have been discussed in detail [12, 23, 24].

The consistency of the effects from the trials is interesting, given the differences between the study populations, which included women selected for being at high risk of chlamydia in the USA [79], unselected high school students in Denmark [80], and students enrolled from further education colleges in the UK [81]. The UK trial is the only one to have examined numbers of PID cases according to their chlamydia infection status at baseline [81]. When all women were screened at baseline, the risk of PID due to any cause in the following year was lower in the screened group (1/63 women with chlamydia) than the control group (7/74, risk ratio 0.17, 95% CI 0.03, 1.01, $p=0.07$).

Evidence from RCTs about the effects of screening on chlamydia prevalence is emerging. The Chlamydia Screening Implementation project in the Netherlands sent annual postal invitations for up to three screening rounds, using a cluster design. Women and men aged 16–29 years old were invited to request a self-sampling kit from an internet website and to mail specimens for chlamydia testing [82]. The uptake of the intervention was lower than expected; of 261,025 people invited in the first round from April 2008 to February 2009, 52,741 (20.2%) requested a chlamydia test package online and 41,638 (16.0%) returned a specimen [82]. Preliminary Results that participation fell in subsequent rounds. Chlamydia positivity in the intervention blocks at the first invitation was the same as in the control block (4.3%) an 0.2% lower at the third invitation (oddas ratio 0.96, CI 0.83, 1.10) [83]. The Australian Chlamydia Control

Evaluation Pilot (ACCEPt) project is a cluster randomized trial evaluating opportunistic chlamydia screening of women and men aged 16–29 years attending general practices, for up to four screening rounds, and results are expected in 2014–2015 [84].

Many studies examining the association between chlamydia screening and changes in prevalence are ecological time trend studies [14–16, 85], which were conducted during the period of HIV prevention campaigns. There are two main reasons why the findings of these studies are difficult to interpret. First, it is not possible to determine the contribution of chlamydia screening relative to the general trend of decreased rates of reported sexually transmitted infections. The usual way of minimizing confounding by other events in time trend studies is to include a period of observation before the introduction of the intervention or to have a control population. In the studies of chlamydia screening, monitoring only began at the start of the intervention (screening of asymptomatic women) and there was no control population.

Second, when an intervention is introduced, the volume of testing increases over the first few years and the population drawn into screening changes. Initially, people at higher risk tend to be preferentially selected. As the number of people tested increases, people at lower risk are included. This means that the percentage of positive tests would be expected to go down over time until both testing and positivity rates reach equilibrium, even if there is no effect on chlamydia transmission in the population at large [12, 46, 73]. This pattern was seen in Sweden, where widespread chlamydia testing began in 1985 [15, 86] and is becoming apparent in participants in chlamydia screening in England (Fig. 20.5) [53, 88]. The largest change in chlamydia positivity rates occurs during the period when the number of tests increases most rapidly. This makes chlamydia positivity unsuitable for monitoring the impact of screening, although this has been suggested as a proxy for changes in population prevalence [87].

Mathematical models that describe the transmission dynamics of C. trachomatis in populations provide a different source of information about the potential effects of chlamydia screening.

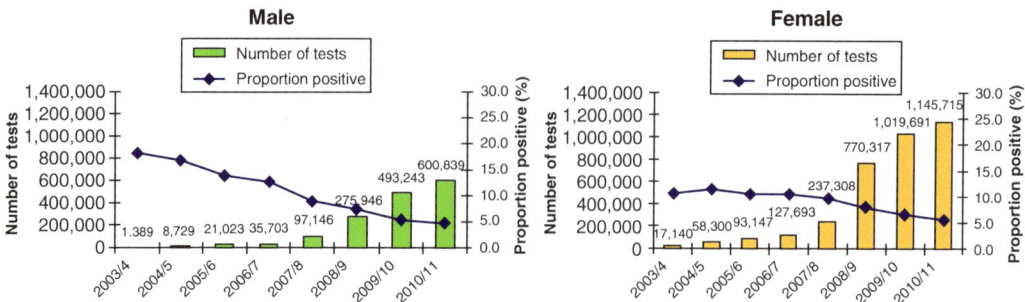

Fig. 20.5 Chlamydia screening test volumes and proportion of positive cases by sex: April 2003–March 2011, England. Note: Slide 10 from NCSP data presentation [88]

While models cannot replace empirical studies of preventive interventions, they may help understand their potential effects under differing circumstances. In a variety of different models, implementing chlamydia screening and treatment of positives at random at a rate of around 0.3 or more per year for 10 years results in a substantial reduction in prevalence [89–92]. This means that individuals receive, on average, a chlamydia test every 3 years. In practice, variations in uptake by sex, geography, risk behavior, or adherence to treatment, partner notification or regular screening could reduce the impact.

Chlamydia Control Strategies in the USA and UK

In this section we summarize chronologically the evolution of chlamydia control activities in the USA (Box 20.1) and the (Box 20.2) UK. In both countries, chlamydia control strategies have been shaped by many factors, including new knowledge about chlamydia epidemiology and clinical manifestations, more sensitive chlamydia diagnostic tests, surveillance trends, resources for testing and treatment, and public policy.

Box 20.1: Chronology of Chlamydia Control in the USA

Chlamydia control strategies in the USA have evolved over the last 25 years from sporadic chlamydia testing and case reporting to specific recommendations about testing, treatment, and partner management from the CDC and other national public health organizations. Chlamydia control efforts in the USA currently are composed of three complementary recommendations: (1) regularly screen persons from population groups with the highest chlamydia prevalence and/or morbidity and provide treatment if their test is positive; (2) test persons with chlamydia-associated syndromes and treat empirically; and (3) provide treatment to sexual partners of chlamydia-infected persons. Key milestones are as follows.

1984   Chlamydia cases were reported by some US states, which represented one of the earliest systematic chlamydia surveillance efforts.

1985   CDC published the first guidelines for chlamydia screening in the USA: "*Chlamydia trachomatis* Infections Policy Guidelines for Prevention and Control" [93]. A risk-based approach emphasizing high-risk women was recommended for chlamydia screening in asymptomatic persons.

1988   Chlamydia screening and prevalence monitoring in women was initiated in the US Department of Health & Human Services (HHS) Region X (Washington, Oregon, Idaho, and Alaska) as a Federal Government (CDC-supported) demonstration project [94]. The primary goal was to demonstrate a reduction in reproductive tract morbidity.

1989   The US Preventive Services Task Force (USPSTF) recommended routine chlamydia screening of sexually active young women [95], supporting CDC recommendations.

(continued)

Box 20.1 (continued)

1993 Chlamydia screening services in federally funded clinics for women were expanded to three more HHS regions (III, VII, and VIII). CDC also published: (1) the "1993 Sexually Transmitted Diseases Treatment Guidelines" [96], which included a recommendation to screen sexually active adolescent females for chlamydia during routine gynecologic examinations and suggested routine screening in females 20–24 years of age and rescreening several months after chlamydia treatment; and (2) "Recommendations for the Prevention and Management of *Chlamydia trachomatis* Infections, 1993" [97] updating the 1985 document.

1994 Chlamydia became a nationally reportable condition through the efforts of the Council of State and Territorial Epidemiologists (CSTE).

1995 Federally supported chlamydia screening services were extended to the remaining HHS regions (I, II, IV, V, VI, and IX), ensuring national chlamydia screening efforts in the public health sector.

1996 Scholes et al. reported results of a randomized controlled trial of chlamydia screening and treatment versus usual care in a Health Management Organization (HMO) population of asymptomatic females [79]. The study demonstrated a reduction in PID incidence in the group that was offered chlamydia screening and treatment.

1997 MMWR reported a 65% decline from 1988 to 1995 in the annual rate of chlamydia test positivity amongst women tested for chlamydia in family planning clinics taking part in the Region X chlamydia demonstration project [98]. Declining trends in chlamydia positivity were also noted in women entering a National Job Training Program from 1990 to 1997 [99] and from chlamydia surveillance data 1994–2000 from the Mid-Atlantic States (Delaware, Washington, DC, Maryland, Pennsylvania, Virginia, and West Virginia) [100].

1998 CDC "1998 Sexually Transmitted Diseases Treatment Guidelines" emphasized annual chlamydia screening in adolescents and continued to suggest screening in 20- to 24-year-old females [101]. From the mid to late 1990s, *C. trachomatis* NAATs were being increasingly used for chlamydia testing. Their increased sensitivity over prior chlamydia diagnostic tests led to an increased number of chlamydia cases detected. Because NAATs could be performed on less-invasively collected specimens (e.g., urine and vaginal swabs), there was now the opportunity to expand chlamydia screening to nontraditional clinical settings where genital examinations were less feasible (e.g., schools, correctional facilities, etc.).

1999 All US states had regulations requiring reporting of chlamydia cases. Commercial and Medicaid plans began voluntary annual reporting of chlamydia screening data in females aged 16–25 years and recorded as being sexually active to the National Committee for Quality Assurance (NCQA) as a Health Plan Employer Data and Information Set (HEDIS) measure [102], which is widely used for comparing quality of health care provision. DHHS published the "Healthy People 2010" objectives for improving health, which included objectives in the STD focus to (1) reduce the proportion of female adolescents and young adults with chlamydia and (2) reduce the proportion of females who have ever required PID treatment. A Healthy People 2010 Mid Course Review showed a fall in PID consultations [103].

2002 The USPSTF Guidelines in 2001 [104] and the CDC "Sexually Transmitted Diseases Treatment Guidelines 2002" [105] both recommended annual chlamydia screening in sexually active females up to age 25 years.

2005 A "Dear Colleague" letter from CDC provided conclusions from a CDC expert consultant meeting on Expedited Partner Therapy (EPT) as a strategy for treatment of partners of patients with chlamydia and/or gonorrhea [106]. CDC concluded that EPT was a useful option to facilitate partner management, especially for male partners of female patients with these infections.

2006 CDC "Sexually Transmitted Diseases Treatment Guidelines, 2006" included EPT as an option for partner management and also included vaginal swabs in women and urine in men as acceptable specimens for *C. trachomatis* NAAT testing [78].

2007 USPSTF updated their chlamydia screening recommendations [19]. A notable difference from the 2001 recommendation was that the upper age limit for annual chlamydia screening in sexually active women decreased from 25 to 24 years. In the same year CDC released a "Dear Colleague" letter about chlamydia screening in men [107]. Recommendations focused on targeted chlamydia screening of males in populations with high chlamydia prevalence.

2009 CDC summarized findings and recommendations from an expert consultation meeting on "Laboratory Diagnostic Testing for *Chlamydia trachomatis* and *Neisseria gonorrhoeae*" [108]. The report recommended urine in men and vaginal swabs in women as the optimal genital specimens for screening by NAAT based on both their ease of collection and the test performance characteristics.

2009 MMWR reported 2007 HEDIS data. CDC-recommended chlamydia screening in women increased from 2000 to 2006, from 25% up to 45% based on the denominator used by HEDIS to define sexual activity [109]. Coverage was 42% in 2007.

Box 20.2: Chronology of Chlamydia Control in the UK

The introduction of recommendations about routine diagnostic testing for chlamydia in the UK has been slow in comparison with countries such as Sweden and the US. Recommendations for routine testing were introduced first in GUM clinics. Key milestones are as follows.

1988   Chlamydia infections diagnosed in GUM clinics became reportable as a category separate from other nonspecific genital infections [110].

1994   A call for "a well designed and evaluated program of screening treatment and contact tracing" for chlamydia was published [111], based on observations from a county in Sweden where screening of asymptomatic women in family planning and abortion clinics had been introduced and the rate of diagnosed cases had fallen between 1984 and 1988 [14].

1996   UK National Screening Committee (NSC) established to advise the government on "the case for implementing new screening programmes… [and] for continuing, modifying or withdrawing existing population screening programmes: in particular programmes inadequately evaluated or of doubtful effectiveness, quality, or value" [112].

1996   The UK Chief Medical Officer (CMO) convened an expert group in response to growing pressure to introduce screening, "because there was no clear professional consensus about who should be "screened" for *Chlamydia* and in which settings… [72]" The purpose of the expert group was "to advise the CMO and Ministers on the issues associated with screening programs for chlamydia for population groups (both male and female) and in different settings." The question of whether to screen for chlamydia was not part of the terms of reference. The findings of Scholes et al.'s randomized trial [79] and ecological data [15, 16] were accepted as "sufficient evidence" of benefit [72]. The report concluded that "the evidence supports opportunistic screening of sexually active women aged under 25." Register based screening was considered "inappropriate" and not recommended. A randomized controlled trial was recommended to find out how cost-effectiveness of screening in non-GUM clinic settings could be maximized [72]. No trial has, however, ever been conducted in the UK

1997   The UK National Centre for the Coordination of Health Technology Assessment Programme commissioned research to address research needs identified by the CMO's expert advisory group. The resulting Chlamydia Screening Studies (ClaSS) project involved a cross-sectional evaluation of chlamydia prevalence of feasibility of postal invitations to mail home-collected specimens for chlamydia testing. Fieldwork began in February 2001 [74].

1998   The UK National Screening Committee (NSC) considered chlamydia as a condition to be appraised for screening [112]. The Chair of the NSC concluded, in an atmosphere of strong pressure to introduce screening, that pilot projects could be set up to examine the feasibility of an opportunistic screening program.

1999   The Department of Health funded 1-year pilot projects of opportunistic screening for chlamydia in women in two areas in England [113]. Half or more of all tests and positives were from general practice with payment to general practitioners for doing tests [114, 115]. 30–50% of women aged 16–24 years in the two areas were screened. The conclusion was that an opportunistic model of urine screening for chlamydial infection was practical and acceptable.

2001   The UK Government launched the first National Strategy for Sexual Health and HIV. This included a commitment to implement national screening for chlamydia, based on the results of the pilot studies [116].

2002   The NSC reported early indications are that chlamydia screening was acceptable to the public and professionals and its plan to begin rolling out national screening [117].

2003   National Chlamydia Screening Programme (NCSP) was launched in England by the Department of Health to "control genital chlamydial infection through the early detection and treatment of asymptomatic infections and prevention of sequelae and onward transmission" [77]. Implementation was phased in to cover all primary care trusts from 2003 to 2008. Annual screening was recommended for all sexually active women and men under 25 years attending a variety of health care settings.

2004   The NSC reported that the NCSP was "a communicable disease control programme rather than a screening programme" [118]. The NSC did not include the NCSP within its national screening programs and did not oversee its implementation.

2005   The Department of Health appointed the Health Protection Agency to oversee the NCSP. A scheme for offering free chlamydia screening tests in some outlets of a major pharmacy chain also began.

(continued)

Box 20.2 (continued)

2006	NSC policy stated that it did not recommend systematic population-based chlamydia screening or chlamydia screening in pregnancy [119]. This policy had not changed by 2011.
2007	The ClaSS project reported that postal, register-based screening was feasible, but unlikely to be cost-effective with uptake of 35% per year [74]. In the same year, an economic analysis based on data collected during the DH pilot studies found that opportunistic screening with 50% coverage per year would only be cost-effective if the progression rate to PID was 10% or more [120].
2008	NCSP was delivered in all 152 primary care trusts in England. In the fiscal year April 2007 to March 2008, an estimated 4.9% of all 15- to 24-year-old women and men had been screened in NCSP settings [53]. In 2008/2009, estimated coverage of chlamydia screening was 16% of all 15 to 24-year-old women and men, combining chlamydia tests from all settings (both NCSP and non-NCSP) outside GUM clinics [121].
2009	Estimated coverage of the NCSP in 2009/2010 was 22% in England including chlamydia tests taken in all non-GUM settings (range 16–26% in different regions).
2009	The National Audit Office reviewed the NCSP [122]. It found that, since the launch of the NCSP, "an estimated £100 million has been spent but the Department [of Health] does not yet know what effect, if any, this has had on reducing the prevalence of the infection." It went on to conclude that the Department of Health does not have a mechanism in place to measure the impact of the NCSP and that it should develop a plan with a clear timeframe for measuring the NCSP's impact on chlamydia and health-related problems.
2010	Estimated coverage of the NCSP in 2010/2011 was 25% in England including chlamydia tests taken in all non-GUM settings (range 19–30% in different regions). The target was 35%.

Differences Between USA and UK Chlamydia Control Policies

Many of the differences in evolution, implementation, evaluation, and monitoring of these chlamydia control activities reflect national differences in traditions of health care provision and public health systems for disease control. Chlamydia control efforts began earlier in the USA than in the UK. The first CDC national recommendations in 1985 [93] and 1993 [97] were based on observed associations between chlamydia and female reproductive tract damage, which resulted in the biological rationale that chlamydia screening would prevent infertility. Subsequent recommendations were strengthened by the publication of the trial by Scholes et al. showing a reduction in the cumulative 1-year incidence of PID in women offered a chlamydia screening test [79]. Chlamydia screening in the USA is now recommended by two national bodies, the CDC [20] and USPSTF [19], although there are differences in policies about the target population age group and recommended

screening frequency. Individual health professionals have the responsibility for implementing the recommendations when they see their patients. Most opportunities for offering chlamydia screening occur in settings other than public STD clinics. There are some initiatives, such as the Infertility Prevention Project, that increase access to free testing for low-income women in selected settings and support training, laboratory performance, and surveillance activities [94] at a regional level.

In the UK National Health Service, public health policy is determined and delivered from a more centralized perspective. Consideration of screening for chlamydia control chlamydia evolved over a period when ideas about screening as a health service were changing in the UK. In the mid to late 1980s in the UK, failures in opportunistic screening for cervical cancer resulted in changes requiring national oversight of quality standards for screening [123]. By the time that the advisory committee on *C. trachomatis* reported its findings [72], the UK National Screening Committee (NSC) had been established

[112]. The NSC appraises evidence about the appropriateness of screening and recommends conditions for which a national "systematic population-based screening programme" should be implemented [124]. In the UK this means a coordinated system of activities to reduce morbidity or mortality, including systematic identification and invitation of the target population at appropriate intervals. Whilst pilot studies and the initial roll out of chlamydia screening were approved [117], the NSC decided in 2004 that chlamydia screening was a disease control program, not a screening program and, since 2006 has not recommended population-based screening for chlamydia or screening for chlamydia in pregnancy. The terminology is confusing because the name has not changed. The National Chlamydia Screening Programme was rolled out in England to offer opportunistic chlamydia screening to sexually active women and men under 25 years and is overseen by the Health Protection Agency not the NSC. Local delivery of chlamydia screening is devolved to individual primary care trusts that employ or contract health care professionals to offer screening. Most screening takes place in community gynecology (family planning) clinics.

Interpretation of Observed Chlamydia Trends in the USA and UK

There is an impression that chlamydia is becoming more prevalent and that this is incompatible with the intensity of chlamydia control efforts, such as those described above [46, 125]. Much of the uncertainty results from the publicity surrounding year on year increases in diagnosed case rates and the subsequent widespread use of surveillance reports of diagnosed cases as a reflection of chlamydia transmission in the population [47], despite published caveats about their interpretation [61].

The trends from the US NHANES population-based data do not show an increase in chlamydia prevalence over time [52]. Rather, the data suggest that chlamydia prevalence might have fallen since 1999 amongst 14- to 39-year-olds overall. A decline amongst the 15- to

25-year-old female age group targeted by the screening recommendations would provide stronger evidence that chlamydia control efforts have played a role in these trends. There are no comparable repeated prevalence data for any other country, but a second survey in the UK is being conducted in 2010–2011 as part of Natsal-3.

Have Chlamydia Control Efforts Achieved Their Aims?

In the past 20 years, many millions of cases of genital chlamydia infection in the USA and the UK have been diagnosed and treated. It remains difficult, however, to determine how many cases of PID, ectopic pregnancy, infertility, and other sequelae could have been, or have been, prevented or whether there has been a reduction in chlamydia transmission at the population level. To show that the aims of chlamydia control efforts have been achieved would require evidence that the introduction of chlamydia screening recommendations was temporally associated with a reduction in chlamydia prevalence and in chlamydial PID, ectopic pregnancy and infertility. This is challenging, in part, because of the temporal dissociation between chlamydia PID (an early complication) and its sequelae (infertility and ectopic pregnancy) that may manifest years later. Other interventions or factors could explain the trends, and consistency across settings and a dose–response relationship between the intensity of the intervention and reduction in the outcome would strengthen claims for a causal effect [126]. As we have shown above, many sources of routinely available information about chlamydia and associated morbidity are indirect and nonspecific, and it is not possible to disentangle the effects of other factors. Thus, even though a national Infertility Prevention Program in the USA provides funding for chlamydia and gonorrhea screening and treatment services for low-income women attending selected healthcare settings [127], it is not currently possible to show at present a direct link between the introduction of chlamydia screening recommendations and prevention of chlamydia-related infertility.

Prevention of PID

RCT evidence links detection and treatment of chlamydia with a reduction in PID (Fig. 20.4) [79–81]. This is an intermediate outcome for infertility. Though it is highly plausible that preventing PID also prevents infertility, the strength of association between chlamydial PID and tubal factor infertility is not known. Taking the results of the three RCTs together, between 64 and 100% of the target population would have to be screened once to achieve a reduction of 50% in the incidence of PID from all causes in the following year (Fig. 20.4). The data from trials cannot be easily extrapolated to determine the expected impact on PID of lower coverage rates on an ongoing opportunistic basis [128].

In the USA there have been reductions in the rates of PID diagnoses since the 1980s, with a steady decline in the late 1980s to mid-1990s and relatively stable rates since 2000 [1]. There were two targets relating to PID in Healthy People 2010. The proportion of females 15–44 years of age who had ever been treated for PID decreased from 8% in 1995 to 5% in 2002, meeting the target. The new target for 2020 is a further reduction to 3.6% [129]. The proportion of childless females 15–44 years of age with fertility problems who had a sexually transmitted disease or required treatment for PID fell from 27 to 22% (42% of the target); there is no further target for 2020. Whilst the targets are not specifically associated with chlamydia control activities, the Infertility Prevention Program is cited as contributing to these declines [103]. It is, however, difficult to know how much of the decline in PID trends can be attributed to chlamydia screening recommendations, since the greatest part of the decline preceded the recommendations, which were first introduced in 1993 [130]. There have been changes in both surveillance and management of PID over time that could affect observed trends. The surveillance definition for PID in the USA has become less specific over time [1]. One would expect this change to increase numbers of reported PID cases in the USA. However, the rates of PID diagnosed in both inpatient and outpatient settings have fallen. The trend for PID management to move more towards the outpatient setting has not been reflected in statistics in the USA [1] or England [55].

In England, where the NCSP has been introduced, there are no targets for reducing PID, although this is a primary objective of the program. Trends in PID diagnoses in primary care, based on a "definite" or "probable" clinical diagnosis show a fall of 10% per year between 2000 (455 per 100,000) and 2008 (189 per 100,000) [55]. The NCSP began its roll out in 2003 and had been introduced in all areas by the end of March 2009, when coverage was 16%. It is unlikely that a 41% reduction in PID diagnoses could be attributed to chlamydia screening at such an early stage in the program.

There might be limitations to the potential impact of chlamydia screening on PID. It is biologically plausible that screening asymptomatic women for chlamydia might only prevent a fraction of PID. If a newly acquired endocervical *C. trachomatis* infection ascends to the upper genital tract and causes asymptomatic PID before screening takes place, then antibiotic treatment might not completely prevent tubal damage, but still may prevent ongoing persisting damage that will lead to infertility. The median duration of untreated chlamydia is estimated to be just over a year [27, 90]. If CDC screening recommendations were fully adhered to and all women had a test every year, chlamydia infections could have been present for an average of 6 months before detection [131], by which time tubal damage might have already occurred. It is still possible that antibiotics could limit the damage caused, but if pathogenesis is the result of host immune responses then antibiotics might not help. There is, however, very little known about the process and timing of ascending infection in relation to the acquisition of *C. trachomatis* or other pathogens [24].

Reducing Chlamydia Transmission

The level and frequency of chlamydia screening needed to achieve a reduction in chlamydia prevalence at the population level are not known.

The lack of baseline data on chlamydia prevalence before the introduction of screening recommendations makes it difficult to have targets that relate directly to reductions in chlamydia transmission [122].

In the USA there are Healthy People 2020 targets for reducing chlamydia test positivity [129] in selected healthcare settings, using it as a proxy for prevalence. If all those eligible in the specified settings are tested and the source populations and diagnostic methods are stable then this is probably a reasonable assumption. The proportion of women 15–24 years of age with chlamydia who attended family planning clinics has been reported for several years. From 1997 to 2003, the percentage of positive tests increased from 5.0 to 6.4%. Part of this increase as been attributed to the increasing use of NAATs for diagnosis [103] so these data do not show whether there might have been a fall in positivity. The Healthy People target for 2010 was 3.0% and this has been revised to 6.7% for 2020. It is not yet clear whether chlamydia control measures have had an impact on population level chlamydia prevalence. The NHANES data show a downward trend for the whole study population, 14–39-year-old women and men between 1999/2000 and 2007/2008 [52]. This is difficult to explain because chlamydia prevalence in the only group to whom screening recommendations are targeted 14–25-year-old women (Fig. 20.3). The data, however, show considerable variability from year to year and wide confidence intervals around the point estimates. Whether or not population prevalence had been higher before the first NHANES survey round is not known.

In England, the NCSP has been introduced more recently but again without establishing the prevalence of chlamydia in the population before the start of the program [122]. The effects of introducing chlamydia screening in England, and increasing screening coverage rapidly, will therefore be difficult to determine. Furthermore, the NCSP does not link tests with individuals so it is not possible to know the numbers of people tested or the number of people being screened regularly. Figure 20.5 shows the issues involved in interpreting chlamydia positivity rates when the coverage of testing is still increasing and the characteristics of the population being tested are changing [46]. In men, a rapid increase in the numbers tested has been accompanied by a decrease in the proportion of positive tests. This is consistent with testing in the earliest years of selected groups of men such as those with symptoms or partners of women with chlamydia. The positivity rate goes down because the number of men with negative tests increases as increasing numbers of asymptomatic men and those with lower levels of behavioral risk are included. In women, the numbers of tests have been much higher and have also increased over time. The positivity rate remained stable until 2007/2008, but has now started to fall.

The most recent data from 2010/2011 show still higher numbers of tests and lower positivity rates in both men and women (overall 5.2% of 1,746,554 tests; 5.6% positive in women; 4.6% positive in men) [88]. It is not possible to determine whether this represents an increase in screening amongst women at lower risk of infection, or a reduction in chlamydia prevalence.

Factors Affecting the Potential Impact of Chlamydia Control

Coverage and Frequency of Chlamydia Screening

It is assumed that higher levels of regular screening coverage will have a greater impact on reducing chlamydia prevalence even if the precise levels required for a clinically meaningful reduction are not known. It is therefore important to know what levels of screening coverage and frequency are attained in routine practice.

In the USA, a routinely available source of chlamydia test coverage is the HEDIS indicator, which records the percentage of the eligible sexually active female population aged 15–25 years receiving a chlamydia test in managed care settings (commercial and Medicaid). The data about tests performed do not distinguish between tests done for screening purposes and those done to investigate symptoms or reported contact with infected partners. From 2000 to 2007, the percentage of eligible women tested increased from 25 to 42% [109]. It is important to note that the percentage tested depends on the denominator, which is the number of women defined as being sexually active [109, 132]. The HEDIS denominator includes only women with an insurance claim for specific reproductive health-related reasons. This underestimates the number of sexually active women because it excludes those who did not make a claim for the specified reasons in a particular year [109, 132]. The HEDIS definition estimates that about 27% of female enrollees aged 15–25 years are sexually active. Population-based data from the National Survey of Family Growth (NSFG) in 1995 show that about 60% of this age group had sexual intercourse in the last 12 months and 62% had used sexual health services [132]. The impact of the size of the denominator on estimated chlamydia test coverage has been examined. Using the HEDIS definition,

41% of sexually active women had a chlamydia test in 2006, compared with 10% using the NSFG estimate, based on women reporting having had sexual intercourse in the last 12 months (Fig. 20.6) [133]. Of note, both methods show that testing coverage in teenage women is lower than for in women in their 20s. The frequency of chlamydia screening is also important for the control of ongoing transmission. Although the CDC recommendation is for annual chlamydia screening, actual screening rates appear substantially lower. When repeat tests in individual women were tracked over time, annual testing levels appeared to be low; only 2% of women enrolled for 2 years had a test in both years and 0.1% of women enrolled for 5 years had a test in every year; on average, a woman received a chlamydia test every 10 years [133].

In England, substantial investment and efforts have been made to increase levels of chlamydia screening amongst asymptomatic young adults in the NCSP (Figs. 20.5 and 20.7). The targets for

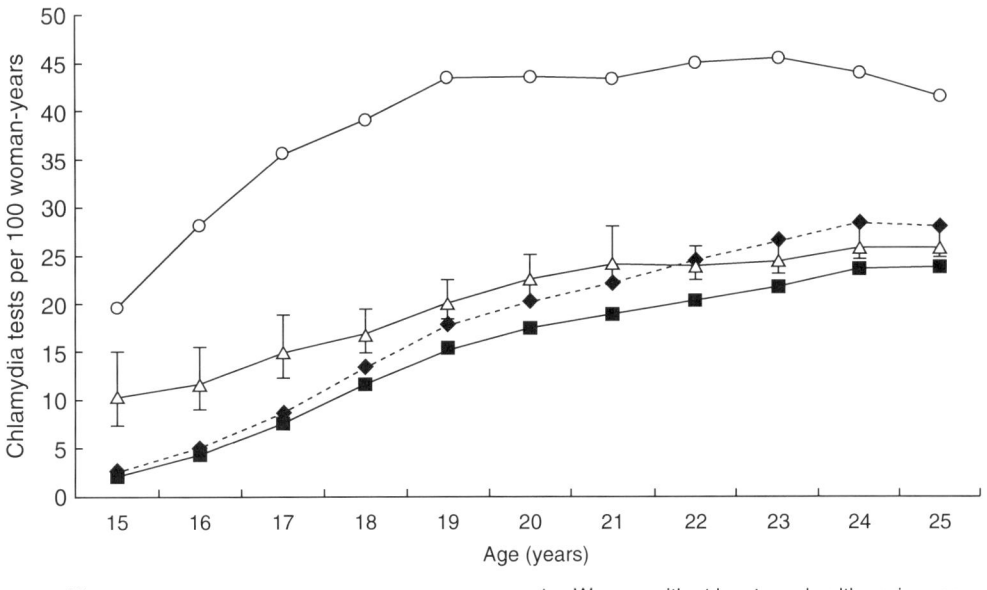

Fig. 20.6 Rates of chlamydia testing per 100 woman years amongst US women aged 15–25 years with health insurance 2006, estimated using different denominators.

Note: *HEDIS* Healthcare Effectiveness Data and Information Set, *NSFG* National Survey of Family Growth. Adapted from Heijne JC et al. [133]

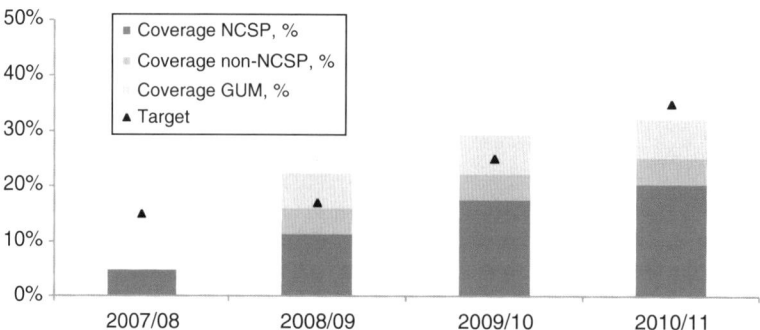

Fig. 20.7 Coverage of chlamydia testing in England, NCSP 2007/2008–2010/2011. Note: NCSP—chlamydia tests reported to the National Chlamydia Screening Programme (NCSP); non-NCSP—chlamydia tests in all settings other than GUM, included in reports from laboratories but not reported to NCSP; GUM—chlamydia tests done in GUM clinics, available from 2008/2009 only. Data include tests done for screening, diagnosis, and partner investigation and are numbers of tests not individuals. Denominator is the mid-year estimate of the population of women and men aged 15–24 years in England. The data collection period is from April 1 to March 31, e.g., April 1 2007 to March 31 2008 is abbreviated as 2007/2008

each year aim to reach coverage levels that predict a reduction in prevalence, based on a mathematical model [92, 122]. Chlamydia tests are done in a variety of settings, not all of which are part of the NCSP, and for a variety of reasons other than screening. The total numbers of chlamydia tests have increased markedly over time and are now at levels that would be expected to have an impact on chlamydia prevalence. In 2010/2011, the number of tests was 32.2% of the number of 15–24 year olds in England (20.3% reported by the NCSP, 7.0% from GUM clinics, and 4.9% from other settings) [88, 134]. Of note, the figures are numbers of tests, not number of individuals; the degree of overestimation is not known and unique individual identifiers are not used so the rate of regular annual testing cannot be calculated. A national audit of the NCSP has recommended that the program should define criteria for success based on reductions in prevalence and a more complete picture of population coverage, including tests done in GUM clinics but excluding multiple tests from the same individuals [122].

Some researchers have suggested that intensive chlamydial screening may have a deleterious effect on control efforts. Brunham hypothesized that intensive chlamydia control activities might have paradoxical effects on chlamydia incidence if widespread early detection and antibiotic treatment prevent immunity from developing after infection and, in that way, make reinfection more likely [135]. This "arrested immunity" hypothesis was based on chlamydia surveillance reports from British Columbia, Canada, which were interpreted as representing population prevalence [125]. A mathematical model could reproduce the observed reported cases over time when 80% of the population was screened each year [135]. The published case rates suggest a screening rate of around 10–20% [47]. This level of coverage may not have a major impact on susceptibility and infection rates at the population level, as observed from the US data on chlamydia test coverage [133] and trends in population prevalence, as measured in repeated cross-sectional surveys [52]. Empirical support for this hypothesis remains weak.

Demographic, Provider, and Health System Factors

The sexual nature of chlamydia infection, stigma and taboos about talking about sex and sexuality, and lack of investment in services for people with sexually transmitted infections are all relevant factors limiting the uptake of chlamydia screening. When screening is delivered as an opportunistic service, adolescents and young adults must feel able to access preventive services regularly and health professionals must feel comfortable taking a sexual history and using all opportunities to offer chlamydia testing. Figure 20.6 shows that the lowest rates of screening are in adolescents who have the highest prevalence of infection. It is known that many chlamydia screening opportunities for adolescents and young women attending health services are missed [136]. In addition, about 25% of 15- to 25-year-old women do not use any health service (from their healthcare plan) [133] and about a third of 11- to 18-year-olds do not have any preventive healthcare visits [137].

Chlamydia screening efforts appear to reach some, but not all, groups of young people at high risk of infection. Chlamydia infections are more uniformly distributed in the population than gonorrhea but there are still demographic and geographic disparities suggesting that the provision and impact of control efforts might differ. National level data mask these differences [1]. In the USA, the Add Health study has been used to examine demographic, geographic, and socioeconomic differences in chlamydia test coverage [138, 139]. Young adults with no health insurance have higher chlamydia prevalence [139] and are less likely than those with any insurance to be tested [138]. Chlamydia test coverage is, however, higher amongst those with public (Medicaid) compared with private health insurance coverage [109, 138] and amongst individuals with inadequate financial income [138]. In the UK, chlamydia test coverage has been found to be higher in areas with higher levels of material deprivation [140]. These findings contrast with reported uptake rates of cervical and breast cancer screening services, which are lower amongst women from deprived and minority ethnic backgrounds.

Partner Notification

Partner notification is sometimes forgotten when referring to "chlamydia screening," but is an integral part of chlamydia case management and control efforts. Mathematical models show that partner notification increases the impact of a strategy that only includes screening with treatment of test positive cases [89]. High levels of repeated infections in the year after treatment for chlamydia, however, suggest that successful partner notification is challenging; detailed information from genotyping of *C. trachomatis* strains in partnerships shows that, whilst new infections are often acquired from new sex partners, reinfection within partnerships is also common [141]. Ensuring the implementation of enhanced methods of partner notification, such as through expedited partner therapy (facilitating treatment of sexual partners without requiring them to undergo counseling or medical assessment) or provision of additional information for partners [142] could help to decrease recurrent chlamydia infections and reach the male partners of women with chlamydia. In the USA, expedited partner therapy is regarded as an option for partner notification [20]. In the UK "accelerated partner therapy" is the term that has been used to allow a medical assessment to be done by telephone or by an accredited pharmacist [143].

Screening Men for Chlamydia

In the USA, chlamydia screening for heterosexual men is not recommended because reviews by CDC and the USPSTF [19] did not provide sufficient evidence of benefit in terms of decreasing chlamydia and its complications in women. CDC recommends that men who have sex with men should have urogenital and/or rectal specimens for chlamydia screening, depending on their sexual practice in the last year [20]. USPSTF guidelines do not cover men who have sex with men [19]. The evidence reviews consider using available resources for screening women to be a higher priority than for men because of the greater morbidity in women. Interestingly, neither review included the Danish RCT that found chlamydia screening is associated with a reduction in the incidence of PID [80]. The screening intervention in that trial included both male and female school students [144] but the outcome was only measured in women. Whilst not a closed community, it is possible that the screening, treatment, and partner notification of men contributed to the effect on PID in women through linked sexual networks. In the NCSP in England, men are included in the target group, even though the Chief Medical Officer's report stated that men would be accessed through partner notification [72] and the pilot studies only included women [114]. The decision to include men might have been based on evidence of similar prevalence in men as in women [2, 145]. The NCSP recommendations do not distinguish between heterosexual men and men who have sex with men.

Partner notification does not identify all infected male sex partners and, even when partners are notified, women often have another episode of infection in the year after being treated for chlamydia [146]. Mathematical modeling studies suggest that screening men in addition to women contributes to decreasing prevalence but does not improve cost-effectiveness because the number of complications averted in men is small.

Moving Forward with Chlamydia Control Efforts

The paradigm of testing and treating as many individuals as possible worked to a great extent for gonorrhea control in the 1970s [131]. The biological differences between *N. gonorrhoeae* and *C. trachomatis*, together with demographic, political, and cultural changes over time, have shown that different approaches to the two infections may be needed. Important scientific advances over the past 30 years in diagnostic, therapeutic, and communications technologies now provide improved tools for use in chlamydial control efforts. NAATs are accurate and acceptable diagnostic tests that have facilitated an expansion of chlamydia testing both inside and outside of traditional health care settings. Azithromycin as single dose treatment has made it easier for antibiotic treatment to be prescribed. The internet has made it possible for people to order specimen collection kits for tests using NAATs. There is limited evidence, however, that these advances have significantly contributed to chlamydia control in either the USA or UK so far, possibly because these advances are still underutilized [147]. It remains to be seen whether the UK Departments of Health will continue to fund an NCSP that has proved unable to demonstrate the impact and cost-effectiveness of its activity. This is not to say that there have not been any benefits to the many millions of individuals who have had a sexually transmitted infection diagnosed and treated in themselves and maybe their sex partner(s). Instead, it demonstrates that there are (still) no magic bullets [148].

Programmatic Research Agenda

RCTs evaluating several rounds of systematic and opportunistic chlamydia screening [82–84] should improve our understanding of the levels of regular screening uptake that can be achieved. Both trials involve men, so they will provide insights into the effectiveness of screening interventions that are more relevant to the NCSP than to current US activities. They will also provide direct evidence of target levels of uptake required to reduce chlamydia prevalence or, if no reduction is observed, the screening levels that need to be exceeded. Additional research questions about the effects of different intervention options or interventions targeted in high prevalence populations would, ideally, be addressed in future RCTs, but it is important to have outcomes that measure the primary endpoints of reduced morbidity [149].

Accurate information about trends in chlamydia prevalence and testing is essential for monitoring the process and outcomes of chlamydia control efforts. Monitoring the uptake of testing requires information that not only spans the different providers of chlamydia testing, but that can also be linked to individuals so that the coverage and frequency of testing can be tracked. Prevalence measured in representative population samples is still the least biased method for examining changes in the level of chlamydia in the population as a whole. The sample size requirements will, however, become more challenging as prevalence falls. Studies that provide more precise data about the prevalence of chlamydia in different populations in different areas of the USA and UK are also needed, particularly if there are geographic areas where chlamydia infection in the general population is high, such as the Southern USA [41, 138]. More intensive targeted control efforts might be required and, in time, such interventions might have greater impact than interventions directed at all young sexually active adults.

Programmatic research involving cohorts of young adults being screened in ongoing control efforts is needed. This would allow the coverage of screening and repeated annual screening, and the uptake of repeated testing following treatment for a positive test to be estimated. These data can then be compared with the outcomes of RCTs of screening interventions and interventions to increase screening rates, and with the predictions from mathematical models about the levels of screening that would be expected to have an impact on chlamydia prevalence or the incidence of PID. At present, such data are not available in England or in the USA. The NCSP provides the environment for such research with around 1.5 million tests and around 90,000 women diagnosed with chlamydia each year outside GUM settings. With modest investment, an integrated research arm could tackle agreed research priorities in an efficient and responsive mode by enrolling even a small proportion of screened individuals into follow-up studies in sentinel sites. Ongoing data from a cohort that can be followed using a unique identifier (i.e., the National Health Service (NHS) number) would then be able to address questions about response to treatment, persistence of infection, risk of reinfection, and hospitalization or outpatient treatment for PID, ectopic pregnancy, infertility, and male complications. There is also the potential for sizeable populations amongst whom the impact of introducing new point-of-care tests [150] into current screening strategies can be evaluated in RCTs.

Making chlamydia testing more easily accessible through home-sampling kits ordered over the internet [151] or provided in pharmacies [53] has been suggested as an innovative way of increasing the coverage of testing and contributing to chlamydia control. In the NCSP, for example, testing in pharmacies accounts for 2–3% of all tests, so this is unlikely to contribute substantially to reducing chlamydia prevalence. The positivity rate amongst those using these methods is, however, generally high (>10%) so they appear to detect infection in a selected group of young people at high risk of having, and transmitting chlamydia. On the other hand, the NCSP has encouraged testing in nonclinical venues such as schools, colleges, and sporting venues, which have had a lower than average yield and have increased apparent screening uptake, but might not be an efficient method of case detection [51]. Future studies of offering tests in non-healthcare settings should collect information about whether or not the individuals taking up these offers have accessed other health services where a chlamydia test should have been offered. If so, then strengthening testing in existing services might be a more efficient use of resources.

Research that identifies and helps to address barriers to chlamydia screening, from the patient and provider standpoints, is needed. At the patient level, lack of health insurance, lack of resources to access preventive health services, lack of awareness of the importance of chlamydia, and possible fears of receiving a positive test result might be relevant. For health care providers, education and beliefs about the benefits and harms of screening should be explored.

Basic Science and Clinical Research Agenda

A large-scale appraisal and reassessment of our understanding of the immunopathogenesis of *C. trachomatis* and the relevance to chlamydia control was undertaken in 2008 [152]. A major research priority is to improve understanding of the way in which tubal damage occurs because the two current hypotheses have different implications for the focus of control efforts. Under the cellular paradigm, inflammatory responses following initial infection occur as soon as the fallopian tube is infected and continue throughout the course of infection. This would mean that the focus of control programs would be on preventing acquisition of infection and detecting and treating existing infections as soon as possible [153]. Under the immunological paradigm, cell-mediated immune responses that are stimulated by repeated infection would be more important in driving tissue damage, so preventing repeat infection would be a greater priority in control programs. Such research would also address the lack of understanding about the timing of PID development, and the relative contributions of direct effects of screening through PID prevention and the indirect effects achieved through reduced transmission and exposure to *C. trachomatis*.

The research agenda also needs to move forward our understanding of the rate of chlamydial PID following lower genital tract chlamydia and of the risk of chlamydial tubal factor infertility following chlamydial PID. Advances that have been made in being able to quantify *C. trachomatis* organism load could be used to obtain more precise estimates of the transmissibility of chlamydia and possibility of ascending infection at different stages or different levels of chlamydia load. This is essential information, not only for evaluation of screening programs, but also for providing information for women about their fertility prospects following a treated chlamydia infection. Improving understanding of transmissibility, protective immunity, and persistent infection will also help with vaccine development, which might eventually provide better prospects for chlamydia control.

Conclusion

Chlamydia control efforts in the USA and UK have raised awareness of genital chlamydia, how it is transmitted, what the potential long-term risks of infection are and how the spread of infection can be prevented. Downward trends in levels of PID from all causes and in chlamydia prevalence in the USA might be partially attributable to ongoing chlamydia control efforts but the evidence to date does not allow a firm conclusion on this. Whilst more remains to be done on reducing stigma, the USA and NCSP efforts

are committed to raising awareness of chlamydia as a sexually transmitted infection and improving knowledge of how it is transmitted and the risks and consequences of acquiring infection. The consensus amongst the public health community is that chlamydia has become a less taboo issue for discussion and action in the UK but STDs, including chlamydia, generally remain highly stigmatized in the USA. There are many innovative advances still to be made in the field of chlamydia control. The biological rationale for chlamydia control through screening of asymptomatic individuals has not been disproven. This chapter shows that there are, however, real questions to be answered about whether or not the current model of chlamydia control can be adapted to achieve measurable and clinically relevant reductions in chlamydia prevalence, PID, and infertility. A program of basic science, clinical, and programmatic research is proposed to address these questions. The commitment to finding innovative ways of controlling chlamydia and its consequences will, however, require a willingness to challenge the paradigm that chlamydia control is simply a matter of doing more testing and treatment.

References

1. Centers for Disease Control and Prevention. Sexually transmitted disease surveillance 2009. Atlanta: U.S. Department of Health and Human Services; 2010.
2. Fenton KA, Korovessis C, Johnson AM, et al. Sexual behaviour in Britain: reported sexually transmitted infections and prevalent genital *Chlamydia trachomatis* infection. Lancet. 2001;358:1851–4.
3. Datta SD, Sternberg M, Johnson RE, et al. Gonorrhea and chlamydia in the United States among persons 14 to 39 years of age, 1999 to 2002. Ann Intern Med. 2007;147(2):89–96.
4. World Health Organization. Global prevalence and incidence of selected curable sexually transmitted infections. Overview and estimates. Geneva: World Health Organisation; 2001.
5. Cates Jr W, Rolfs Jr RT, Aral SO. Sexually transmitted diseases, pelvic inflammatory disease, and infertility: an epidemiologic update. Epidemiol Rev. 1990;12:199–220.
6. Mardh PA, Ripa T, Svensson L, Westrom L. *Chlamydia trachomatis* infection in patients with acute salpingitis. N Engl J Med. 1977;296(24):1377–9.

7. Westrom L. Effect of acute pelvic inflammatory disease on fertility. Am J Obstet Gynecol. 1975; 121(5):707–13.

8. Svensson L, Mardh PA, Westrom L. Infertility after acute salpingitis with special reference to *Chlamydia trachomatis*. Fertil Steril. 1983;40(3):322–9.

9. Washington AE, Katz P. Ectopic pregnancy in the United States: economic consequences and payment source trends. Obstet Gynecol. 1993;81(2):287–92.

10. Washington AE, Arno PS, Brooks MA. The economic cost of pelvic inflammatory disease. JAMA. 1986;255(13):1735–8.

11. Washington AE, Cates WJ, Wasserheit JN. Preventing pelvic inflammatory disease. JAMA. 1991;266(18):2574–80.

12. Low N. Screening programmes for chlamydial infection: when will we ever learn? BMJ. 2007;334(7596):725–8.

13. Berridge V. AIDS in the UK: the making of Policy, 1981–1994. Oxford: Oxford University Press; 1996.

14. Ripa T. Epidemiologic control of genital *Chlamydia trachomatis* infections. Scand J Infect Dis Suppl. 1990;69:157–67.

15. Herrmann BF, Johansson AB, Mardh PA. A retrospective study of efforts to diagnose infections by *Chlamydia trachomatis* in a Swedish county. Sex Transm Dis. 1991;18(4):233–7.

16. Addiss D, Vaughin ML, Ludka D, Pfister J, Davis JP. Decreased prevalence of *Chlamydia trachomatis* infection associated with a selective screening program in family planning clinics in Wisconsin. Sex Transm Dis. 1993;20:28–34.

17. Nicoll A, Hughes G, Donnelly M, et al. Assessing the impact of national anti-HIV sexual health campaigns: trends in the transmission of HIV and other sexually transmitted infections in England. Sex Transm Infect. 2001;77(4):242–7.

18. Coutinho RA, Rijsdijk AJ, van den Hoek JA, Leentvaar-Kuijpers A. Decreasing incidence of PID in Amsterdam. Genitourin Med. 1992;68(6): 353–5.

19. U.S. Preventive Services Task Force. Screening for chlamydial infection: U.S. Preventive Services Task Force recommendation statement. Ann Intern Med. 2007;147:128–34.

20. Centers for Disease Control and Prevention. Sexually transmitted diseases treatment guidelines, 2010. MMWR Recomm Rep. 2010; 59(RR-12); 44–5.

21. Royal Australian College of General Practitioners. Guidelines for preventive activities in general practice. Melbourne: RACGP; 2007.

22. Department of Health. National Chlamydia Screening Programme (NCSP) in England: programme overview; core requirements; data collection. 2nd ed. London: Department of Health; 2004. http://www.dh.gov.uk/assetRoot/04/09/26/48/04092648.pdf. Accessed 6 Sep 2012.

23. Low N, Bender N, Nartey L, Shang A, Stephenson JM. Effectiveness of chlamydia screening: systematic review. Int J Epidemiol. 2009;38(2):435–48.

24. Gottlieb SL, Berman SM, Low N. Screening and treatment to prevent sequelae in women with *Chlamydia trachomatis* genital infection: how much do we know? J Infect Dis. 2010;201 Suppl 2:S156–67.

25. Hay PE, Pittrof RU. Has the effectiveness of a single chlamydia test in preventing pelvic inflammatory disease over 12 months been overestimated? Womens Health (Lond Engl). 2010;6(5):627–30.

26. Stamm WE. *Chlamydia trachomatis* infections of the adult. In: Holmes KK, Sparling PF, Stamm WE, Piot P, Wasserheit JN, Corey L, et al., editors. Sexually transmitted diseases. 4th ed. New York: McGraw Hill Medical; 2008. p. 575–93.

27. Geisler WM. Duration of untreated, uncomplicated *Chlamydia trachomatis* genital infection and factors associated with chlamydia resolution: a review of human studies. J Infect Dis. 2010;201(S2):104–13.

28. Batteiger BE, Xu F, Johnson RE, Rekart ML. Protective immunity to *Chlamydia trachomatis* genital infection: evidence from human studies. J Infect Dis. 2010;201 Suppl 2:S178–89.

29. Paavonen J, Westrom L, Eschenbach D. Chapter 56. Pelvic inflammatory disease. In: Holmes KK, Sparling PF, Stamm WE, Piot P, Wasserheit JN, Corey L, et al., editors. Sexually transmitted diseases. 4th ed. New York: McGraw Hill Medical; 2008. p. 1017–50.

30. Haggerty CL, Gottlieb SL, Taylor BD, Low N, Xu F, Ness RB. Risk of sequelae after *Chlamydia trachomatis* genital infection in women. J Infect Dis. 2010;201 Suppl 2:S134–55.

31. van Valkengoed IG, Morre SA, van den Brule AJ, Meijer CJ, Bouter LM, Boeke AJ. Overestimation of complication rates in evaluations of *Chlamydia trachomatis* screening programmes—implications for cost-effectiveness analyses. Int J Epidemiol. 2004;33(2):416–25.

32. Geisler WM, Wang C, Morrison SG, Black CM, Bandea CI, Hook III EW. The natural history of untreated *Chlamydia trachomatis* infection in the interval between screening and returning for treatment. Sex Transm Dis. 2008;35(2):119–23.

33. Hook III EW, Spitters C, Reichart CA, Neumann TM, Quinn TC. Use of cell culture and a rapid diagnostic assay for *Chlamydia trachomatis* screening. JAMA. 1994;272(11):867–70.

34. Wein P, Kloss M, Garland SM. Postabortal pelvic sepsis in association with *Chlamydia trachomatis*. Aust N Z J Obstet Gynaecol. 1990;30(4):347–50.

35. Qvigstad E, Skaug K, Jerve F. Pelvic inflammatory disease associated with *Chlamydia trachomatis* infection after therapeutic abortion. A prospective study. Br J Vener Dis. 1983;59(3):189–92.

36. Rice PA, Schachter J. Pathogenesis of pelvic inflammatory disease. What are the questions? JAMA. 1991;266(18):2587–93.

37. Westrom L, Joesoef R, Reynolds G, Hagdu A, Thompson SE. Pelvic inflammatory disease and fertility. A cohort study of 1, 844 women with laparoscopically verified disease and 657 control women

with normal laparoscopic results. Sex Transm Dis. 1992;19(4):185–92.

38. Westrom L. Pelvic inflammatory disease. JAMA. 1991;266(18):2612.

39. Wasserheit JN, Aral SO. The dynamic topology of sexually transmitted disease epidemics: implications for prevention strategies. J Infect Dis. 1996;174 Suppl 2:S201–13.

40. Garnett GP. The geographical and temporal evolution of sexually transmitted disease epidemics. Sex Transm Infect. 2002;78 Suppl 1:i14–9.

41. Miller WC, Ford CA, Morris M, et al. Prevalence of chlamydial and gonococcal infections among young adults in the United States. JAMA. 2004;291(18): 2229–36.

42. Hosenfeld CB, Workowski KA, Berman S, et al. Repeat infection with Chlamydia and gonorrhea among females: a systematic review of the literature. Sex Transm Dis. 2009;36(8):478–89.

43. Gordon FB, Quan AL. Isolation of the trachoma agent in cell culture. Proc Soc Exp Biol Med. 1965;118:354–9.

44. Johnson RE, Newhall WJ, Papp JR, et al. Screening tests to detect Chlamydia trachomatis and Neisseria gonorrhoeae infections—2002. MMWR Recomm Rep. 2002;51(RR-15):1–38.

45. Health Protection Agency. STI annual data tables (Topics, Sexually transmitted infections, disease statistics and surveillance). http://www.hpa.org.uk/web/HPAweb&HPAwebStandard/HPAweb_C/1203348026613. Accessed 6 Sep 2012.

46. Miller WC. Epidemiology of chlamydial infection: are we losing ground? Sex Transm Infect. 2008;84(2): 82–6.

47. Low N. Caution: chlamydia surveillance data ahead. Sex Transm Infect. 2008;84(2):80–1.

48. Centers for Disease Control and Prevention. Sexually transmitted disease surveillance 2007 supplement, Chlamydia Prevalence Monitoring Project. Atlanta, GA: U.S. Department of Health and Human Services, Centers for Disease Control and Prevention; 2009.

49. Last JM. A dictionary of epidemiology. Oxford: Oxford University Press; 2001.

50. Low N, Sterne JA, Barlow D. Inequalities in rates of gonorrhoea and chlamydia between Black ethnic groups in South East London: cross-sectional study. Sex Transm Infect. 2001;77:15–20.

51. Simms I, Talebi A, Riha J, et al. The English National Chlamydia Screening Programme: variations in positivity in 2007/2008. Sex Transm Dis. 2009; 36(8):522–7.

52. Datta SD, Torrone E, Kruszon-Moran D, et al. Chlamydia trachomatis trends in the United States among persons 14 to 39 years of age, 1999–2008. Sex Transm Dis. 2011;39(2):92–6.

53. Health Protection Agency. National Chlamydia Screening Programme. NCSP: five years. The fifth annual report of the National Chlamydia Screening Programme 2007/8. London: Health Protection Agency; 2008.

54. World Health Organization. ICD-10. International statistical classification of diseases and related health problems. Tenth Revisionth ed. Geneva: World Health Organization; 1992.

55. French CE, Hughes G, Nicholson A, et al. Estimation of the rate of pelvic inflammatory disease diagnoses: trends in England, 2000–2008. Sex Transm Dis. 2011;38(3):158–62.

56. Simms I, Warburton F, Westrom L. Diagnosis of pelvic inflammatory disease: time for a rethink. Sex Transm Infect. 2003;79(6):491–4.

57. Chen MY, Fairley CK, Donovan B. Discordance between trends in chlamydia notifications and hospital admission rates for chlamydia related diseases in New South Wales, Australia. Sex Transm Infect. 2005;81(4):318–22.

58. Chen MY, Pan Y, Britt H, Donovan B. Trends in clinical encounters for pelvic inflammatory disease and epididymitis in a national sample of Australian general practices. Int J STD AIDS. 2006;17(6):384–6.

59. Westrom L. Decrease in incidence of women treated in hospital for acute salpingitis in Sweden. Genitourin Med. 1988;64(1):59–63.

60. Bjartling C. Osser S, Persson K. The frequency of salping it is and ectopic pregnancy as epidermiological markers of Chlamydia trachomatis Acta Obstct Gynew/Scand 2000;79(2):123–8.

61. Centers for Disease Control and Prevention. Sexually transmitted disease surveillance 2008. Atlanta: U.S. Department of Health and Human Services, Centers for Disease Control and Prevention; 2009.

62. Eschenbach DA, Buchanan TM, Pollock HM, et al. Polymicrobial etiology of acute pelvic inflammatory disease. N Engl J Med. 1975;293(4):166–71.

63. Morgan J, Colonne C, Bell A. Trends of chlamydia infection and related complications in New Zealand, 1998–2008. Sex Health. 2011;8:412–8.

64. Bender N, Herrmann B, Andersen B, et al. Chlamydia infection, pelvic inflammatory disease, ectopic pregnancy and infertility: cross-national study. Sex Transm Infect. 2011;87(7):601–8.

65. Parran T. Shadow on the land—syphilis. New York: Reynal & Hitchcock; 1937.

66. Parran T. The eradication of syphilis as a practical public health objective. JAMA. 1931;97(2):73–7.

67. Low N, Broutet N, Adu-Sarkodie Y, Barton P, Hossain M, Hawkes S. Global control of sexually transmitted infections. Lancet. 2006;368(9551):2001–16.

68. Gray JA. New concepts in screening. Br J Gen Pract. 2004;54(501):292–8.

69. Raffle A, Gray M. Screening: evidence and practice. Oxford: Oxford University Press; 2007.

70. Department of Health. UK Screening Portal. UK National Screening Committee. Programme appraisal criteria. http://www.screening.nhs.uk/criteria. Accessed 6 Sept 2012.

71. National Health Committee. Screening to improve health in New Zealand. Criteria to assess screening programmes. http://www.nhc.govt.nz/publications/PDFs/ScreeningCriteria.pdf. Accessed 20 Oct 2011.

72. Department of Health. CMO's Expert Advisory Group on *Chlamydia trachomatis*. London: Department of Health; 1998.

73. Stephenson JM. Screening for genital chlamydial infection. Br Med Bull. 1998;54(4):891–902.

74. Low N, McCarthy A, Macleod J, et al. Epidemiological, social, diagnostic and economic evaluation of population screening for genital chlamydial infection. Health Technol Assess. 2007; 11(8):1–184.

75. Harris RP, Helfand M, Woolf SH, et al. Current methods of the US Preventive Services Task Force: a review of the process. Am J Prev Med. 2001;20(3 Suppl):21–35.

76. Miller WC. Screening for chlamydial infection: are we doing enough? Lancet. 2005;365(9458):456–8.

77. LaMontagne DS, Fenton KA, Randall S, Anderson S, Carter P, on behalf of the National Chlamydia Screening Steering Group. Establishing the National Chlamydia Screening Programme in England: results from the first full year of screening. Sex Transm Infect 2004;80(5):335–41.

78. Centers for Disease Control and Prevention. Sexually transmitted diseases treatment guidelines, 2006. MMWR Recomm Rep. 2006;55(R-11):1–94.

79. Scholes D, Stergachis A, Heidrich FE, Andrilla H, Holmes KK, Stamm WE. Prevention of pelvic inflammatory disease by screening for cervical chlamydial infection. N Engl J Med. 1996;334(21): 1362–6.

80. Ostergaard L, Andersen B, Moller JK, Olesen F. Home sampling versus conventional swab sampling for screening of *chlamydia trachomatis* in women: a cluster-randomized 1-year follow-up study. Clin Infect Dis. 2000;31(4):951–7.

81. Oakeshott P, Kerry S, Aghaizu A, et al. Randomised controlled trial of screening for *Chlamydia trachomatis* to prevent pelvic inflammatory disease: the POPI (prevention of pelvic infection) trial. BMJ. 2010;340:c1642.

82. van den Broek IVF, Hoebe CJPA, van Bergen JEAM, et al. Evaluation design of a systematic, selective, internet-based, Chlamydia Screening Implementation in the Netherlands, 2008–2010: implications of first results for the analysis. BMC Infect Dis. 2010;10:89.

83. van den Broek IVF, van Bergen JEAM, Brouwers EEHG, et al. Effectiveness of yearly, register based screening for chlamydia in the Netherlands: controlled trial with randomised stepped wedge implementation. BJM 2012;345:e4316.

84. Hocking JS, Spark S, Guy R, et al. The australian chlamydia control effectiveness pilot (ACCEPT): first result from a randomised controlled trail of annuals chlamydia screening in general practice. Abstracts of the 4th joint BASHH-ASTDA meeting in Brighton, UK. 27-29 June 2012. Sex translmfert 2012;88(suppl):A35.

85. Herrmann B, Egger M. Genital *Chlamydia trachomatis* infections in Uppsala County, Sweden,

86. Kamwendo F, Forslin L, Bodin L, Danielsson D. Decreasing incidences of gonorrhea- and chlamydia-associated pelvic inflammatory disease: a 25-year study from an urban area of central Sweden. Sex Transm Dis. 1996;23(5):384–91.

87. LaMontagne DS, Fenton KA, Pimenta JM, et al. Using chlamydia positivity to estimate prevalence: evidence from the Chlamydia Screening Pilot in England. Int J STD AIDS. 2005;16(4):323–7.

88. National Chlamydia Screening Programme. England Quarters 1–4 April 2010–March 2011. National Chlamydia Screening Programme. http://www.chlamydiascreening.nhs.uk/ps/assets/pdfs/data/sha_presentations11/Q1-4%202010-11%20ENGLAND.pdf. Accessed 20 Oct 2011.

89. Kretzschmar M, Welte R, van Den HA, Postma MJ. Comparative model-based analysis of screening programs for *Chlamydia trachomatis* infections. Am J Epidemiol. 2001;153(1):90–101.

90. Althaus CL, Heijne JCM, Roellin A, Low N. Transmission dynamics of *Chlamydia trachomatis* affect the impact of screening programmes. Epidemics. 2010;2(3):123–31.

91. Regan DG, Wilson DP, Hocking JS. Coverage is the key for effective screening of *Chlamydia trachomatis* in Australia. J Infect Dis. 2008;198(3):349–58.

92. Turner KME, Adams EJ, LaMontagne DS, Emmett L, Baster K, Edmunds WJ. Modelling the effectiveness of chlamydia screening in England. Sex Transm Infect. 2006;82(6):496–502.

93. Centers for Disease Control and Prevention. *Chlamydia trachomatis* infections. Policy guidelines for prevention and control. MMWR Recomm Rep. 1985;34(3):53S–74.

94. Centers for Disease Control and Prevention. Infertility Prevention Project. http://www.cdc.gov/std/infertility/ipp.htm. Accessed 6 Sept 2012.

95. U.S. Preventive Services Task Force. Guide to clinical preventive services: an assessment of the effectiveness of 169 preventive interventions. Baltimore: Williams & Wilkins; 1989.

96. Centers for Disease Control and Prevention. Sexually transmitted diseases treatment guidelines. MMWR Recomm Rep. 1993;42(RR-14):1–102.

97. Centers for Disease Control and Prevention. Recommendations for the prevention and management of *Chlamydia trachomatis* infections, 1993. MMWR Recomm Rep. 1993;42(RR-12):1–45.

98. Centers for Disease Control and Prevention. *Chlamydia trachomatis* genital infections—United States, 1995. MMWR Recomm Rep. 1997;46(9): 193–8.

99. Mertz KJ, Ransom RL, St Louis ME. Prevalence of genital chlamydial infection in young women entering a national job training program, 1990–1997. Am J Public Health. 2001;91(8):1287–90.

100. Centers for Disease Control and Prevention. Division of STD prevention. Tracking the hidden epidemics:

1985–1993: declining rates for how much longer? Sex Transm Dis. 1995;22(4):253–60.

trends in STDs in the United States, 2000. http://www.cdc.gov/std/Trends2000/trends2000.pdf. Accessed 6 Sept 2012.

101. Centers for Disease Control and Prevention. Guidelines for treatment of sexually transmitted diseases. MMWR Recomm Rep. 1998;47(RR-1):1–118.

102. Centers for Disease Control and Prevention. Chlamydia screening, HEDIS and managed care. http://www.cdc.gov/std/chlamydia/hedis.htm. Accessed 6 Sept 2012.

103. U.S. Department of Health and Human Services. Midcourse review. Healthy people 2010. Sexually transmitted diseases, 25. http://www.healthypeople. gov/2010/Data/midcourse/html/focusareas/ FA25TOC.htm. Archive accessed 6 Sept 2012.

104. Nelson HD, Helfand M. Screening for chlamydial infection. Am J Prev Med. 2001;20 Suppl 1:95–107.

105. Centers for Disease Control and Prevention. Sexually transmitted diseases treatment guidelines 2002. MMWR Recomm Rep. 2002;51(6):1–78.

106. Centers for Disease Control and Prevention. Expedited partner therapy. Dear Colleague Letter. http://www.cdc.gov/std/DearColleagueEPT5-10-05. pdf. Accessed 6 Sept 2012.

107. Centers for Disease Control and Prevention. Male Chlamydia screening. Dear Colleague Letter. http:// www.cdc.gov/std/chlamydia/Dear-Colleague-Male-CT-Screening-2007.pdf. Accessed 6 Sept 2012.

108. Association of Public Health Laboratories, Centers for Disease Control and Prevention. Laboratory diagnostic testing for *Chlamydia trachomatis* and *Neisseria gonorrhoeae*: expert consultation meeting summary report. 13–15 Jan 2009. Atlanta, GA. http://www.aphl.org/aphlprograms/infectious/std/ documents/ctgclabguidelinesmeetingreport.pdf. Accessed 6 Sept 2012.

109. Centers for Disease Control and Prevention. Chlamydia screening among sexually active young female enrollees of health plans—United States, 2000–2007. JAMA. 2009;302(6):620–1.

110. Communicable Disease Surveillance Centre. Sexually transmitted diseases quarterly report: genital infection with *Chlamydia trachomatis* in England and Wales. Commun Dis Rep CDR Wkly. 1995;5(26):122–3.

111. Taylor-Robinson D. *Chlamydia trachomatis* and sexually transmitted disease. BMJ. 1994;308(6922):150–1.

112. Department of Health. First report of the UK National Screening Committee. London: The Stationery Office; 1998.

113. Department of Health. Second report of the National Screening Committee. London: The Stationery Office; 2000.

114. Pimenta JM, Catchpole M, Rogers PA, et al. Opportunistic screening for genital chlamydial infection. I: acceptability of urine testing in primary and secondary healthcare settings. Sex Transm Infect. 2003;79(1):16–21.

115. Pimenta JM, Catchpole M, Rogers PA, et al. Opportunistic screening for genital chlamydial infection. II: prevalence among healthcare attenders, outcome, and evaluation of positive cases. Sex Transm Infect. 2003;79(1):22–7.

116. Department of Health. National strategy for sexual health and HIV. London: Department of Health; 2001.

117. UK National Screening Committee. Programme director's report. Period: Autumn 2000–Spring 2002; 2002. Report No.: nsc/annualreport2002/1.7.02.

118. UK National Screening Committee. Note of the meeting held on 8 Dec 2004; 2004.

119. UK National Screening Committee. UK Screening Portal. UK NSC policy database. Policies: Chlamydia (adult), Chlamydia (pregnancy). http://www.screening.nhs.uk/policydb.php. Accessed 6 Sept 2012.

120. Adams EJ, Turner KM, Edmunds WJ. The cost effectiveness of opportunistic chlamydia screening in England. Sex Transm Infect. 2007;83(4):267–74.

121. Health Protection Agency. National Chlamydia Screening Programme. The bigger picture. The National Chlamydia Screening Programme. 2008/09 annual report. London: Health Protection Agency; 2009.

122. National Audit Office. Department of Health. Young people's sexual health: the National Chlamydia Screening Programme. Report by the Comptroller and Auditor General. HC 963 Session 2008–2009. London: The Stationery Office; 2009.

123. Cancer of the cervix: death by incompetence. Lancet. 1985;2(8451):363–4.

124. UK National Screening Committee. http://www. screening.nhs.uk/uknsc. Accessed 6 Sept 2012.

125. Rekart ML, Brunham RC. Epidemiology of chlamydial infection: are we losing ground? Sex Transm Infect. 2008;84(2):87–91.

126. Hennekens CH, DeMets D. Statistical association and causation. JAMA. 2011;305(11):1134–5.

127. Centers for Disease Control and Prevention. Infertility and prevention of sexually transmitted diseases 2000–2003. Report to Congress. http://www.cdc. gov/std/infertility/ipp.htm. Accessed 6 Sept 2012.

128. Soldan K, Berman SM. Danish health register study: a randomised trial with findings about the implementation of chlamydia screening, but not about its benefits. Sex Transm Infect. 2011;87(2):86–7.

129. U.S. Department of Health and Human Services. Healthy people 2020. 2011 September. http://www. healthypeople.gov/2020/default.aspx. Accessed 6 Sept 2012.

130. Centers for Disease Control and Prevention. Special focus: surveillance for sexually transmitted diseases. MMWR Recomm Rep. 1993;42(SS-3):1–39.

131. Peterman TA, Gottlieb SL, Berman SM. Commentary: *Chlamydia trachomatis* screening: what are we trying to do? Int J Epidemiol. 2009;38(2):449–51.

132. Tao G, Walsh CM, Anderson LA, Irwin KL. Understanding sexual activity defined in the HEDIS measure of screening young women for *Chlamydia trachomatis*. Jt Comm J Qual Improv. 2002;28(8): 435–40.

133. Heijne JCM, Tao G, Kent CK, Low N. Uptake of regular chlamydia testing by U.S. women: a longitudinal study. Am J Prev Med. 2010;39(3):243–50.

134. National Chlamydia Screening Programme. NHS Vital Signs 2010/11. Primary Care Trust (PCT) and Strategic Health Authority (SHA) specific tables. 1st April 2010 to 31st March 2011. http://www.chlamydiascreening.nhs.uk/ps/assets/pdfs/data/VSI_PCT/VSI_by_PCT_Q1-4_April_2010-March_2011.pdf. Accessed 6 Sept 2012.

135. Brunham RC, Pourbohloul B, Mak S, White R, Rekart ML. The unexpected impact of a *Chlamydia trachomatis* infection control program on susceptibility to reinfection. J Infect Dis. 2005;192(10): 1836–44.

136. Hoover K, Tao G. Missed opportunities for chlamydia screening of young women in the United States. Obstet Gynecol. 2008;111(5):1097–102.

137. Nordin JD, Solberg LI, Parker ED. Adolescent primary care visit patterns. Ann Fam Med. 2010; 8(6):511–6.

138. Nguyen TQ, Ford CA, Kaufman JS, Leone PA, Suchindran C, Miller WC. Infrequent chlamydial testing among young adults: financial and regional differences. Sex Transm Dis. 2008;35(8):725–30.

139. Geisler WM, Chyu L, Kusunoki Y, Upchurch DM, Hook III EW. Health insurance coverage, health care-seeking behaviors, and genital chlamydial infection prevalence in sexually active young adults. Sex Transm Dis. 2006;33(6):389–96.

140. Sheringham J, Sowden S, Stafford M, Simms I, Raine R. Monitoring inequalities in the National Chlamydia Screening Programme in England: added value of ACORN, a commercial geodemographic classification tool. Sex Health. 2009;6(1):57–62.

141. Batteiger BE, Tu W, Ofner S, et al. Repeated *Chlamydia trachomatis* genital infections in adolescent women. J Infect Dis. 2010;201(1):42–51.

142. Trelle S, Shang A, Nartey L, Cassell JA, Low N. Improved effectiveness of partner notification for patients with sexually transmitted infections: systematic review. BMJ. 2007;334(7589):354–7.

143. Estcourt C, Sutcliffe L. Moving partner notification into the mainstream of routine sexual health care. Sex Transm Infect. 2007;83(2):169–72.

144. Ostergaard L, Andersen B, Olesen F, Moller JK. Efficacy of home sampling for screening of *Chlamydia trachomatis*: randomised study. BMJ. 1998;317(7150):26–7.

145. Macleod J, Salisbury C, Low N, et al. Coverage and uptake of systematic postal screening for genital *Chlamydia trachomatis* and prevalence of infection in the United Kingdom general population: cross sectional study. BMJ. 2005;330(7497):940–2.

146. Scott LaMontagne D, Baster K, Emmett L, et al. Incidence and reinfection rates of genital chlamydial infection among women aged 16–24 years attending general practice, family planning and genitourinary medicine clinics in England: a prospective cohort study by the Chlamydia Recall Study Advisory Group. Sex Transm Infect. 2007;83(4):292–303.

147. Maciosek MV, Coffield AB, Edwards NM, Flottemesch TJ, Goodman MJ, Solberg LI. Priorities among effective clinical preventive services: results of a systematic review and analysis. Am J Prev Med. 2006;31(1):52–61.

148. Brandt AM. No magic bullet: a social history of venereal disease in the United States since 1880. 2nd ed. New York: Oxford University Press, Inc.; 1985.

149. Cowan FM, Plummer M. Biological, behavioural and psychological outcome measures. In: Stephenson JM, Imrie J, Bonell C, editors. Effective sexual health interventions. Issues in experimental evaluation. Oxford: Oxford University Press; 2003. p. 111–35.

150. Nadala EC, Goh BT, Magbanua JP, et al. Performance evaluation of a new rapid urine test for chlamydia in men: prospective cohort study. BMJ. 2009;339: b2655.

151. Gaydos CA, Dwyer K, Barnes M, et al. Internet-based screening for *Chlamydia trachomatis* to reach non-clinic populations with mailed self-administered vaginal swabs. Sex Transm Dis. 2006;33(7):451–7.

152. Gottlieb SL, Martin D, Xu F, et al. Summary: the natural history and immunobiology of *Chlamydia trachomatis* genital infection and implications for chlamydia control. J Infect Dis. 2010;201(S2):190–204.

153. Darville T, Hiltke TJ. Pathogenesis of genital tract disease due to *Chlamydia trachomatis*. J Infect Dis. 2010;201(S2):114–25.

Index

Printed by Printforce, the Netherlands